Addressing Food and Nutrition Security in Developed Countries

Addressing Food and Nutrition Security in Developed Countries

Special Issue Editors

Christina M. Pollard
Sue Booth

MDPI • Basel • Beijing • Wuhan • Barcelona • Belgrade

MDPI

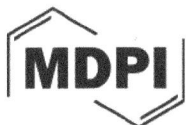

Special Issue Editors

Christina M. Pollard
Curtin University
Australia

Sue Booth
Flinders University of South Australia
Australia

Editorial Office
MDPI
St. Alban-Anlage 66
4052 Basel, Switzerland

This is a reprint of articles from the Special Issue published online in the open access journal *International Journal of Environmental Research and Public Health* (ISSN 1660-4601) from 2018 to 2019 (available at: https://www.mdpi.com/journal/ijerph/special_issues/food_nutrition_security).

For citation purposes, cite each article independently as indicated on the article page online and as indicated below:

LastName, A.A.; LastName, B.B.; LastName, C.C. Article Title. *Journal Name* **Year**, *Article Number, Page Range.*

ISBN 978-3-03921-281-1 (Pbk)
ISBN 978-3-03921-282-8 (PDF)

Cover image courtesy of/copyright of Heather Petty.

Contents

About the Special Issue Editors ix

Christina Mary Pollard and Sue Booth
Addressing Food and Nutrition Security in Developed Countries
Reprinted from: *IJERPH* **2019**, *16*, 2370, doi:10.3390/ijerph16132370 . . . . **1**

Christina M Pollard and Sue Booth
Food Insecurity and Hunger in Rich Countries—It Is Time for Action against Inequality
Reprinted from: *IJERPH* **2019**, *16*, 1804, doi:10.3390/ijerph16101804 . . . . **6**

Merryn Maynard, Lesley Andrade, Sara Packull-McCormick, Christopher M. Perlman,
Cesar Leos-Toro and Sharon I. Kirkpatrick
Food Insecurity and Mental Health among Females in High-Income Countries
Reprinted from: *IJERPH* **2018**, *15*, 1424, doi:10.3390/ijerph15071424 . . . . **19**

Geneviève Jessiman-Perreault and Lynn McIntyre
Household Food Insecurity Narrows the Sex Gap in Five Adverse Mental Health Outcomes
among Canadian Adults
Reprinted from: *IJERPH* **2019**, *16*, 319, doi:10.3390/ijerph16030319 . . . . **55**

Monideepa B. Becerra, Salome Kapella Mshigeni and Benjamin J. Becerra
The Overlooked Burden of Food Insecurity among Asian Americans: Results from the
California Health Interview Survey
Reprinted from: *IJERPH* **2018**, *15*, 1684, doi:10.3390/ijerph15081684 . . . . **70**

Jeromey B. Temple
The Association between Stressful Events and Food Insecurity: Cross-Sectional Evidence from
Australia
Reprinted from: *IJERPH* **2018**, *15*, 2333, doi:10.3390/ijerph15112333 . . . . **81**

Jeromey B. Temple, Sue Booth and Christina M. Pollard
Social Assistance Payments and Food Insecurity in Australia: Evidence from the Household
Expenditure Survey
Reprinted from: *IJERPH* **2019**, *16*, 455, doi:10.3390/ijerph16030455 . . . . **96**

Sue Kleve, Sue Booth, Zoe E. Davidson and Claire Palermo
Walking the Food Security Tightrope—Exploring the Experiences of Low-to-Middle Income
Melbourne Households
Reprinted from: *IJERPH* **2018**, *15*, 2206, doi:10.3390/ijerph15102206 . . . . **111**

Alison Daly, Christina M. Pollard, Deborah A. Kerr, Colin W. Binns, Martin Caraher and
Michael Phillips
Using Cross-Sectional Data to Identify and Quantify the Relative Importance of Factors
Associated with and Leading to Food Insecurity
Reprinted from: *IJERPH* **2018**, *15*, 2620, doi:10.3390/ijerph15122620 . . . . **130**

Jeromey B. Temple and Joanna Russell
Food Insecurity among Older Aboriginal and Torres Strait Islanders
Reprinted from: *IJERPH* **2018**, *15*, 1766, doi:10.3390/ijerph15081766 . . . . **143**

Lauren A. Clay, Mia A. Papas, Kimberly B. Gill and David M. Abramson
Factors Associated with Continued Food Insecurity among Households Recovering from
Hurricane Katrina
Reprinted from: *IJERPH* **2018**, *15*, 1647, doi:10.3390/ijerph15081647 157

Anja Simmet, Peter Tinnemann and Nanette Stroebele-Benschop
The German Food Bank System and Its Users—A Cross-Sectional Study
Reprinted from: *IJERPH* **2018**, *15*, 1485, doi:10.3390/ijerph15071485 167

Leisa McCarthy, Anne B. Chang and Julie Brimblecombe
Food Security Experiences of Aboriginal and Torres Strait Islander Families with Young
Children in An Urban Setting: Influencing Factors and Coping Strategies
Reprinted from: *IJERPH* **2018**, *15*, 2649, doi:10.3390/ijerph15122649 185

**Flora Douglas, Fiona MacKenzie, Ourega-Zoé Ejebu, Stephen Whybrow, Ada L. Garcia,
Lynda McKenzie, Anne Ludbrook and Elizabeth Dowler**
*"A Lot of People Are Struggling Privately. They Don't Know Where to Go or They're Not Sure of What
to Do"*: Frontline Service Provider Perspectives of the Nature of Household Food Insecurity in
Scotland
Reprinted from: *IJERPH* **2018**, *15*, 2738, doi:10.3390/ijerph15122738 207

**Ourega-Zoé Ejebu, Stephen Whybrow, Lynda Mckenzie, Elizabeth Dowler, Ada L Garcia,
Anne Ludbrook, Karen Louise Barton, Wendy Louise Wrieden and Flora Douglas**
What can Secondary Data Tell Us about Household Food Insecurity in a High-Income Country
Context?
Reprinted from: *IJERPH* **2019**, *16*, 82, doi:10.3390/ijerph16010082 230

Elena Carrillo-Álvarez, Tess Penne, Hilde Boeckx, Bérénice Storms and Tim Goedemé
Food Reference Budgets as a Potential Policy Tool to Address Food Insecurity: Lessons Learned
from a Pilot Study in 26 European Countries
Reprinted from: *IJERPH* **2019**, *16*, 32, doi:10.3390/ijerph16010032 247

Timothy J. Landrigan, Deborah A. Kerr, Satvinder S. Dhaliwal and Christina M. Pollard
Protocol for the Development of a Food Stress Index to Identify Households Most at Risk of
Food Insecurity in Western Australia
Reprinted from: *IJERPH* **2019**, *16*, 79, doi:10.3390/ijerph16010079 259

Amanda Lee and Meron Lewis
Testing the Price of Healthy and Current Diets in Remote Aboriginal Communities to Improve
Food Security: Development of the Aboriginal and Torres Strait Islander Healthy Diets ASAP
(Australian Standardised Affordability and Pricing) Methods
Reprinted from: *IJERPH* **2018**, *15*, 2912, doi:10.3390/ijerph15122912 268

**Penelope Love, Jillian Whelan, Colin Bell, Felicity Grainger, Cherie Russell, Meron Lewis
and Amanda Lee**
Healthy Diets in Rural Victoria—Cheaper than Unhealthy Alternatives, Yet Unaffordable
Reprinted from: *IJERPH* **2018**, *15*, 2469, doi:10.3390/ijerph15112469 283

**Sally Mackay, Tina Buch, Stefanie Vandevijvere, Rawinia Goodwin, Erina Korohina,
Mafi Funaki-Tahifote, Amanda Lee and Boyd Swinburn**
Cost and Affordability of Diets Modelled on Current Eating Patterns and on Dietary Guidelines,
for New Zealand Total Population, Māori and Pacific Households
Reprinted from: *IJERPH* **2018**, *15*, 1255, doi:10.3390/ijerph15061255 299

Jill Whelan, Lynne Millar, Colin Bell, Cherie Russell, Felicity Grainger, Steven Allender and Penelope Love
You Can't Find Healthy Food in the Bush: Poor Accessibility, Availability and Adequacy of Food in Rural Australia
Reprinted from: *IJERPH* **2018**, *15*, 2316, doi:10.3390/ijerph15102316 . . . . **311**

Anna Sofia Salonen, Maria Ohisalo and Tuomo Laihiala
Undeserving, Disadvantaged, Disregarded: Three Viewpoints of Charity Food Aid Recipients in Finland
Reprinted from: *IJERPH* **2018**, *15*, 2896, doi:10.3390/ijerph15122896 . . . . **326**

Christina M. Pollard, Bruce Mackintosh, Cathy Campbell, Deborah Kerr, Andrea Begley, Jonine Jancey, Martin Caraher, Joel Berg and Sue Booth
Charitable Food Systems' Capacity to Address Food Insecurity: An Australian Capital City Audit
Reprinted from: *IJERPH* **2018**, *15*, 1249, doi:10.3390/ijerph15061249 . . . . **341**

Sue Booth, Christina Pollard, John Coveney and Ian Goodwin-Smith
'Sustainable' Rather Than 'Subsistence' Food Assistance Solutions to Food Insecurity: South Australian Recipients' Perspectives on Traditional and Social Enterprise Models
Reprinted from: *IJERPH* **2018**, *15*, 2086, doi:10.3390/ijerph15102086 . . . . **358**

Clare Brown, Cara Laws, Dympna Leonard, Sandy Campbell, Lea Merone, Melinda Hammond, Kani Thompson, Karla Canuto and Julie Brimblecombe
Healthy Choice Rewards: A Feasibility Trial of Incentives to Influence Consumer Food Choices in a Remote Australian Aboriginal Community
Reprinted from: *IJERPH* **2019**, *16*, 112, doi:10.3390/ijerph16010112 . . . . **376**

Megan Ferguson, Kerin O'Dea, Jon Altman, Marjory Moodie and Julie Brimblecombe
Health-Promoting Food Pricing Policies and Decision-Making in Very Remote Aboriginal and Torres Strait Islander Community Stores in Australia
Reprinted from: *IJERPH* **2018**, *15*, 2908, doi:10.3390/ijerph15122908 . . . . **387**

Danielle Gallegos and Mariana M. Chilton
Re-Evaluating Expertise: Principles for Food and Nutrition Security Research, Advocacy and Solutions in High-Income Countries
Reprinted from: *IJERPH* **2019**, *16*, 561, doi:10.3390/ijerph16040561 . . . . **401**

About the Special Issue Editors

Christina Mary Pollard (Ph.D.) calls herself a 'pracademic', an experienced public health nutrition practitioner and researcher who has developed, implemented, and evaluated public health nutrition interventions for the government at national, state, and local levels. Her role includes advising on food regulation and development of numerous food and nutrition policies and programs. Policy-driven research is a fundamental component, for example, understanding consumer knowledge, attitudes and beliefs; nutrition profiling; and evaluating mass media campaigns, nutrition interventions, and policies. Dr Pollard has a strong commitment to policy and advocacy to protect and promote public health, particularly for those rendered vulnerable to poor nutrition due to circumstances outside of their control.

Sue Booth (Ph.D.) is a dietitian with over 20 years of experience who has worked in a range of settings—community health, private practice, and in government. Dr Booth has a particular interest in addressing food insecurity. She has a PhD in public health nutrition, and her thesis examined food insecurity amongst homeless young people in Adelaide, South Australia. Her teaching and research interests include food insecurity and the impact of poverty on health, food policy, food democracy, and qualitative research methods. She has written and co-authored a range of materials, including policy papers, books, book chapters, articles, reports, and peer-reviewed papers. Sue teaches in the College of Medicine and Public Health at Flinders University.

International Journal of
*Environmental Research
and Public Health*

MDPI

Editorial

Addressing Food and Nutrition Security in Developed Countries

Christina Mary Pollard [1,*] and Sue Booth [2]

[1] Faculty of Health Science, School of Public Health, Curtin University, GPO Box U1987, Perth 6845, Australia
[2] College of Medicine & Public Health, Flinders University, GPO Box 2100, Adelaide 5000, Australia
* Correspondence: Christina.Pollard@health.wa.gov.au; Tel.: +61-8-9224-1016

Received: 29 June 2019; Accepted: 1 July 2019; Published: 4 July 2019

Abstract: The guest editors of the special issue on *Addressing Food and Nutrition Security in Developed Countries* reflect on the 26 papers that were published as part of this issue and the scope of research contained therein. There is an extensive body of work, which focuses on topics ranging from the prevalence of food insecurity in developed countries, associations and determinants, measurement and monitoring, to reports of the lived experience and coping strategies of people who are living with food insecurity or and those who are a part of the charitable food sector. Very few solutions to address the problem of food insecurity in developed countries were offered, and many challenges highlighted. Further research is required to find the solutions to address the problem of food insecurity in developed countries, and important principles and values are proposed for those undertaking this work to embrace.

Keywords: food security; food insecurity; social assistance; poverty; homeless; nutrition environment; food stress; food affordability; policy; intervention; determinants; food banks; developed countries

---

Improving food and nutrition insecurity has become a public health priority in developed and economically rich countries, such as Australia, Europe, the United Kingdom, Canada, and the U.S. [1]. Food insecurity is costly and has wide-reaching consequences, with its effects extending beyond vulnerable populations. For example, for women residing in high-income countries, food insecurity is associated with an increased risk of depression while conversely, depression is also a predictor of food insecurity [2]. Pregnant women and mothers; women at risk of or are experiencing homelessness; refugees; and those exposed to violence and substance abuse were at the highest risk [2]. In Canada, any experience of food insecurity in both males and females was associated with adverse mental health outcomes [3]. The prevalence of food insecurity among Asian Americans was highest among Vietnamese and lowest among Japanese subgroups and varied by acculturation [4].

Understanding the factors associated with food insecurity can assist in identifying effective responses. Analysis of the 2014 General Social Survey of the Australian population quantified the association between 18 discreet stressful life events and food insecurity. Stressors related to employment and health doubled the likelihood of experiencing food insecurity [5]. Household food insecurity was also associated with receipt of specific social assistance payments in Australia, suggesting that these families were enduring significant financial stress [6]. It is not just welfare-dependent households who are experiencing food insecurity in Australia, the prevalence is increasing in low to middle income groups [7,8]. The complex and interactive nature of the factors associated with food insecurity has also been quantified in one Australian study [8]. Researchers highlighted the need for comprehensive policies and programs that recognize the complex links with other social and public health challenges [1,2,5,9] and recommended the adoption of both nutrition-sensitive and nutrition specific interventions [1].

Long-term food insecurity after disasters is another concern for sociodemographically challenged populations in developed countries. Examination of the impact of Hurricane Katrina on families five years after the event found that higher income, race, and having a partner were protective factors against food insecurity whereas low social support, poor physical and mental health, and being female were risk factors [10].

As governments retreat from the issue, private charitable and not-for-profit sector organizations step in to deliver food and other services to people in need. This is particularly evident in the rapid expansion and proliferation of food banks and charitable food services. In 2017, the population access to Tafel food banks in Germany was such that nearly all residents, including welfare recipients, have access to at least one food bank located in their local district [11]. Public and political debate is continuing about the appropriateness of food banks as the main response to food insecurity in developed countries [1,11].

1. The Experiences of Food Insecurity in Developed Countries and Coping Strategies

Australian Aboriginal and Torres Strait Islander people are significantly more likely to experience food insecurity than their non-indigenous counterparts, particularly those residing in rural or remote areas. There is limited evidence regarding the prevalence of food insecurity among families with young children residing in urban areas. For these families, food insecurity usually occurred intermittently and due to the unaffordability of food relative to income and living expenses, resulting in limited food choice and poorer meal quality. Family support, the main coping strategy, should be considered as an essential safety net in public policy to address food insecurity [12].

The perceptions of frontline service providers on the nature of food insecurity also provide insights on effective interventions. In Scotland, a country-wide study of informants from twenty-five health, social care, and third sector organizations was undertaken. Food insecurity was described as having multiple faces and related factors with concerns being raised regarding those at risk of food insecurity, including working families, young people and women. The difficulty in accepting external help was aptly described as 'stoicism and struggle'. The pessimistic view of the participating community regarding the needs of food insecure groups is of great concern [13]. Australian low- to middle-income families describe similar tensions as they struggle to balance a range of financial, social, physical and personal assets to avoid or alleviate the experience of food insecurity [7].

2. Measurement and Monitoring

Measuring and monitoring of food insecurity and its determinants is a salient concern in some economically developed nations. The absence of robust food insecurity monitoring and surveillance systems in the households of Australia, Scotland and Europe has led researchers to undertake a secondary analysis of related surveys, such as Scotland's Living Costs and Food Survey [14] and Australia's Household Expenditure Survey [6], in order to determine the nature and prevalence of household food insecurity [15]. Food affordability, a key component of food security, has been determined using comparisons of the weekly food expenditure and its ratio to equalized income for households with varying income levels in Scotland [14] and Australia [16,17]. Analysis trends in the relationship between food affordability at the household level and diet quality in Scotland found that poorer households were less likely to achieve recommended dietary intakes over time [14]. However, the authors concluded that robust and comprehensive systems are needed to provide the full picture. Across Europe, a Food Reference Budget has been developed to contribute to the prevention of food insecurity in low income contexts [15].

The same questions are being asked in Australia and New Zealand in the absence of robust and comprehensive food insecurity monitoring systems. Similar to the concept of rental stress, the innovative geographically based Food Stress Index was developed using the Western Australian Government's Food Access and Cost Surveys and relevant sociodemographic census data to determine place-based risk of food stress [16]. Emergency relief service providers and government policy makers are very interested in applying the FSI to identify areas of particular need for food security action.

The Healthy Diets ASAP (Australian Standardized Affordability and Pricing) method assesses the affordability of healthy (recommended) and contemporary (unhealthy) diets. In rural Australia, the price of the contemporary (unhealthy) diet was shown to be more expensive than the recommended healthy diet [18]. Furthermore, a tailored Aboriginal and Torres Strait Islander version tested in five remote communities found similar results, with food alarmingly found to not be affordable in either of these areas [17]. A version was also developed for the contemporary New Zealand diet and assessed with consideration of their dietary recommendations. Expert panels assisted in tailoring the instrument for different population subgroups, including Māori and Pacific households, with the healthy diet again found to be more affordable [19]. The nutritional environment can influence the availability and accessibility of food, which are both components of food insecurity. Nutrition environment measurement tools were applied and they found that in rural and socially disadvantaged communities in Australia, it is harder to access nutritious food at affordable prices [20].

3. Perspectives of Charitable Food Sector and Food Banking Staff and Recipients

The lived experiences of Finnish food aid recipients debunks public perceptions that people are somehow responsible for their own poverty and highlighted the worsening income insufficiency, deepening poverty and the inability of aid agencies to cope [21]. The same phenomena is occurring in Australia where charitable food services persevere with limited resources [22]. There is emerging evidence that traditional food assistance models further stigmatize people and are inadequate. Australian research sought the perspective of users on existing services and ideas for improved models. Empowering and dignified food assistance models that enable choice and reciprocity provide opportunities for social interaction and connection, with links to broader supports being strongly recommended [23].

4. Solutions to Address the Problem of Food Insecurity in Developed Countries

There are limited examples of interventions that are effective in reducing food insecurity in developed countries. Monetary incentives to encourage fruit and vegetable purchases in remote Aboriginal communities show limited success due to the multiple challenges related to the operational running of the community stores, but were highly valued by women with children and accepted by the community [24]. Examination of the decision-making processes of remote community store owners, retailers, and health promotion professionals highlighted the importance of involving store owners and policy makers in the design of interventions [25].

Clearly, further research is required to develop effective interventions to address food insecurity in developed countries. Discrimination, academic expectations, siloed thinking, and cultural differences are some of the challenges to sharing research expertise that must be overcome [26]. Principles and values that can help to drive potential solutions to address these research challenges have been proposed, along with a call for the international research community to adopt them [26].

Author Contributions: C.M.P. and S.B. conceived the topic for the Special Issue and were the guest editors.

Funding: This research received no external funding.

Acknowledgments: We are very grateful to the IJERPH editorial team for their support in assisting us to undertake the Special issue on *Addressing Food and Nutrition Security in Developed Countries.* We thank those who prepared papers for consideration for publication. We congratulate those who published their papers and encourage those with more work to do to continue to publication. We particularly thank the generous people who gave their time to share their experience and expertise in providing thoughtful reviews. The Special Issue would not have been possible without you.

Conflicts of Interest: C.M.P. is a Board Member of Foodbank WA. All views are her own.

References

1. Pollard, C.M.; Booth, S. Food Insecurity and Hunger in Rich Countries—It Is Time for Action against Inequality. *Int. J. Environ. Res. Public Health* **2019**, *16*, 1804. [CrossRef] [PubMed]
2. Maynard, M.; Andrade, L.; Packull-McCormick, S.; Perlman, C.M.; Leos-Toro, C.; Kirkpatrick, S.I. Food Insecurity and Mental Health among Females in High-Income Countries. *Int. J. Environ. Res. Public Health* **2018**, *15*, 1424. [CrossRef] [PubMed]
3. Jessiman-Perreault, G.; McIntyre, L. Household Food Insecurity Narrows the Sex Gap in Five Adverse Mental Health Outcomes among Canadian Adults. *Int. J. Environ. Res. Public Health* **2019**, *16*, 319. [CrossRef] [PubMed]
4. Becerra, M.B.; Mshigeni, S.K.; Becerra, B.J. The Overlooked Burden of Food Insecurity among Asian Americans: Results from the California Health Interview Survey. *Int. J. Environ. Res. Public Health* **2018**, *15*, 1684. [CrossRef] [PubMed]
5. Temple, J.B. The Association between Stressful Events and Food Insecurity: Cross-Sectional Evidence from Australia. *Int. J. Environ. Res. Public Health* **2018**, *15*, 2333. [CrossRef] [PubMed]
6. Temple, J.B.; Booth, S.; Pollard, C.M. Social Assistance Payments and Food Insecurity in Australia: Evidence from the Household Expenditure Survey. *Int. J. Environ. Res. Public Health* **2019**, *16*, 455. [CrossRef] [PubMed]
7. Kleve, S.; Booth, S.; Davidson, Z.E.; Palermo, C. Walking the Food Security Tightrope—Exploring the Experiences of Low-To-Middle Income Melbourne Households. *Int. J. Environ. Res. Public Health* **2018**, *15*, 2206. [CrossRef] [PubMed]
8. Daly, A.; Pollard, C.M.; Kerr, D.A.; Binns, C.W.; Caraher, M.; Phillips, M. Using Cross-Sectional Data to Identify and Quantify the Relative Importance of Factors Associated with and Leading to Food Insecurity. *Int. J. Environ. Res. Public Health* **2018**, *15*, 2620. [CrossRef] [PubMed]
9. Temple, J.B.; Russell, J. Food Insecurity among Older Aboriginal and Torres Strait Islanders. *Int. J. Environ. Res. Public Health* **2018**, *15*, 1766. [CrossRef]
10. Clay, L.A.; Papas, M.A.; Gill, K.B.; Abramson, D.M. Factors Associated with Continued Food Insecurity among Households Recovering from Hurricane Katrina. *Int. J. Environ. Res. Public Health* **2018**, *15*, 1647. [CrossRef]
11. Simmet, A.; Tinnemann, P.; Stroebele-Benschop, N. The German Food Bank System and Its Users—A Cross-Sectional Study. *Int. J. Environ. Res. Public Health* **2018**, *15*, 1485. [CrossRef] [PubMed]
12. McCarthy, L.; Chang, A.B.; Brimblecombe, J. Food Security Experiences of Aboriginal and Torres Strait Islander Families with Young Children in an Urban Setting: Influencing Factors and Coping Strategies. *Int. J. Environ. Res. Public Health* **2018**, *15*, 2649. [CrossRef] [PubMed]
13. Douglas, F.; MacKenzie, F.; Ejebu, O.-Z.; Whybrow, S.; Garcia, A.L.; McKenzie, L.; Ludbrook, A.; Dowler, E. "A Lot of People Are Struggling Privately. They Don't Know Where to Go or They're Not Sure of What to Do": Frontline Service Provider Perspectives of the Nature of Household Food Insecurity in Scotland. *Int. J. Environ. Res. Public Health* **2018**, *15*, 2738. [CrossRef] [PubMed]
14. Ejebu, O.-Z.; Whybrow, S.; Mckenzie, L.; Dowler, E.; Garcia, A.L.; Ludbrook, A.; Barton, K.L.; Wrieden, W.L.; Douglas, F. What Can Secondary Data Tell us about Household Food Insecurity in a High-Income Country Context? *Int. J. Environ. Res. Public Health* **2018**, *16*, 82. [CrossRef] [PubMed]
15. Carrillo-Álvarez, E.; Penne, T.; Boeckx, H.; Storms, B.; Goedemé, T. Food Reference Budgets as a Potential Policy Tool to Address Food Insecurity: Lessons Learned from a Pilot Study in 26 European Countries. *Int. J. Environ. Res. Public Health* **2018**, *16*, 32. [CrossRef] [PubMed]
16. Landrigan, T.J.; Kerr, D.A.; Dhaliwal, S.S.; Pollard, C.M. Protocol for the Development of a Food Stress Index to Identify Households Most at Risk of Food Insecurity in Western Australia. *Int. J. Environ. Res. Public Health* **2018**, *16*, 79. [CrossRef] [PubMed]
17. Lee, A.; Lewis, M. Testing the Price of Healthy and Current Diets in Remote Aboriginal Communities to Improve Food Security: Development of the Aboriginal and Torres Strait Islander Healthy Diets Asap (Australian Standardised Affordability and Pricing) Methods. *Int. J. Environ. Res. Public Health* **2018**, *15*, 2912. [CrossRef]

18. Love, P.; Whelan, J.; Bell, C.; Grainger, F.; Russell, C.; Lewis, M.; Lee, A. Healthy Diets in Rural Victoria—Cheaper than Unhealthy Alternatives, yet Unaffordable. *Int. J. Environ. Res. Public Health* **2018**, *15*, 2469. [CrossRef]
19. Mackay, S.; Buch, T.; Vandevijvere, S.; Goodwin, R.; Korohina, E.; Funaki-Tahifote, M.; Lee, A.; Swinburn, B. Cost and Affordability of Diets Modelled on Current Eating Patterns and on Dietary Guidelines, for New Zealand Total Population, Māori and Pacific Households. *Int. J. Environ. Res. Public Health* **2018**, *15*, 1255. [CrossRef]
20. Whelan, J.; Millar, L.; Bell, C.; Russell, C.; Grainger, F.; Allender, S.; Love, P. You Can't Find Healthy Food in the Bush: Poor Accessibility, Availability and Adequacy of Food in Rural Australia. *Int. J. Environ. Res. Public Health* **2018**, *15*, 2316. [CrossRef]
21. Salonen, A.S.; Ohisalo, M.; Laihiala, T. Undeserving, Disadvantaged, Disregarded: Three Viewpoints of Charity Food Aid Recipients in Finland. *Int. J. Environ. Res. Public Health* **2018**, *15*, 2896. [CrossRef] [PubMed]
22. Pollard, C.M.; Mackintosh, B.; Campbell, C.; Kerr, D.; Begley, A.; Jancey, J.; Caraher, M.; Berg, J.; Booth, S. Charitable Food Systems' Capacity to Address Food Insecurity: An Australian Capital City Audit. *Int. J. Environ. Res. Public Health* **2018**, *15*, 1249. [CrossRef] [PubMed]
23. Booth, S.; Pollard, C.M.; Coveney, J.; Goodwin-Smith, I. 'Sustainable' Rather Than 'Subsistence' Food Assistance Solutions to Food Insecurity: South Australian Recipients' Perspectives on Traditional and Social Enterprise Models. *Int. J. Environ. Res. Public Health* **2018**, *21*, 2086. [CrossRef] [PubMed]
24. Brown, C.; Laws, C.; Leonard, D.; Campbell, S.; Merone, L.; Hammond, M.; Thompson, K.; Canuto, K.; Brimblecombe, J. Healthy Choice Rewards: A Feasibility Trial of Incentives to Influence Consumer Food Choices in a Remote Australian Aboriginal Community. *Int. J. Environ. Res. Public Health* **2019**, *16*, 112. [CrossRef] [PubMed]
25. Ferguson, M.; O'Dea, K.; Altman, J.; Moodie, M.; Brimblecombe, J. Health-Promoting Food Pricing Policies and Decision-Making in very Remote Aboriginal and Torres Strait Islander Community Stores in Australia. *Int. J. Environ. Res. Public Health* **2018**, *15*, 2908. [CrossRef] [PubMed]
26. Gallegos, D.; Chilton, M.M. Re-Evaluating Expertise: Principles for Food and Nutrition Security Research, Advocacy and Solutions in High-Income Countries. *Int. J. Environ. Res. Public Health* **2019**, *16*, 561. [CrossRef] [PubMed]

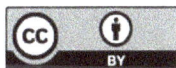

International Journal of
Environmental Research and Public Health

MDPI

Commentary

Food Insecurity and Hunger in Rich Countries—It Is Time for Action against Inequality

Christina M Pollard [1,*] and Sue Booth [2]

[1]   Faculty of Health Science, School of Public Health, Curtin University, Perth 6845, Australia
[2]   College of Medicine & Public Health, Flinders University, Adelaide 5000, Australia;
      sue.booth@flinders.edu.au
*   Correspondence: C.Pollard@curtin.edu.au; Tel.: +61-08-9224-1016

Received: 12 April 2019; Accepted: 18 May 2019; Published: 21 May 2019

Abstract: Household food insecurity is a serious public health concern in rich countries with developed economies closely associated with inequality. The prevalence of household food insecurity is relatively high in some developed countries, ranging from 8 to 20% of the population. Human rights approaches have the potential to address the structural causes, not just the symptoms of food insecurity. Despite most developed countries ratifying the Covenant on Economic, Social and Cultural Rights over 40 years ago, food insecurity rates suggest current social protections are inadequate. The contemporary framing of the solution to food insecurity in developed countries is that of diverting food waste to the hungry to meet the United Nations Sustainable Development Goals agenda (Goals 2 and 12.3). An estimated 60 million people or 7.2% of the population in high income countries used food banks in 2013. Although providing food assistance to those who are hungry is an important strategy, the current focus distracts attention away from the ineffectiveness of government policies in addressing the social determinants of food insecurity. Much of the action needed to improve household food security falls to actors outside the health sector. There is evidence of promising actions to address the social determinants of food insecurity in some developed countries. Learning from these, there is a strong case for government leadership, for action within and across government, and effective engagement with other sectors to deliver a coordinated, collaborative, and cooperative response to finding pathways out of food insecurity.

Keywords: food insecurity; hunger; developed countries; Sustainable Development Goals; social determinants; inequality; food banks

---

1. Introduction

Household food insecurity is a serious public health concern in rich countries with developed economies [1]. For example, in Australia, Canada, Europe, New Zealand, the United Kingdom, and the United States of America (US), improving household food and nutrition security is a public health priority. Food insecurity is costly, has wide-reaching consequences, and its effects extend beyond vulnerable populations. The two main ways of addressing food security in developed countries continue to be measures to respond to poverty including welfare entitlements and food relief [2]. As governments retreat from the issue, third sector organizations step in to deliver services to people in need, evidenced by the rapid proliferation of food banks and charitable food services. As expected, food assistance does little to address the underlying causes of food poverty and insecurity [3]. Clearly the response in developed countries is not working. There are tangible solutions to the problem, what is missing in many countries is the political will to fully acknowledge the problem and take the effective action.

Human rights-focused approaches have the potential to address the impact of government action or inaction, including the structural causes, not just the symptoms, of social inequities. The right to food is bound under international law in Article 25.1, "*Everyone has the right to a standard of living adequate for the health and well-being of himself and of his family, including food, clothing, housing and medical care and necessary social services, and the right to security in the event of unemployment, sickness, disability, widowhood, old age or other lack of livelihood in circumstances beyond his control.*" p. 76 [4]. Enshrined in the International Covenant on Economic, Social and Cultural Rights (ICESCR) Article 11 [5] consenting nation states are obligated to respect, protect and fulfil their commitments, see General Commitment number 12 [5]. Adopted in 1966 [6] with entry into force in 1976, many developed countries have ratified ICESCR including: Australia (1975); Canada, United Kingdom, Great Britain, Northern Island (1976); Japan (1979); and Belgium (1983). The US is a notable exception, signing in 1977 but not yet ratified, and continues to express resistance towards economic and social rights [7].

Countries who are ratified are subject to investigations on their current situation by the Special Rapporteur on the Right to Food. Progress on the realisation of the right to food can be very slow, even in rich countries. Nearly 40 year after ratification, the 2012 Canadian review by the Special Rapporteur, found 57% of people living on social assistance were food insecure and concluded that Canadian cash transfers were insufficient for an adequate standard of living [8]. Although Canada's promotion of labour market participation as a strategy to overcome poverty was commended, it was recommended that their minimum wage legislation should be a 'living wage' [8]. Housing costs were noted as a key reason people were compelled to use food banks.

A sense of urgency to address food insecurity is implicit in the Global Sustainable Development Goals (SDG) which seek actions to realise human rights by 2030, and are determined to end poverty and hunger, in all their forms and dimensions . . . .. Goal 2 (2.1) has a target "*to end hunger and ensure access by all people, in particular the poor and people in vulnerable situations, including infants, to safe, nutritious and sufficient food all year round.*" [9].

2. How You Define Food Insecurity Shapes the Response

How you define and measure a problem influences how you respond to it. Before effective action to address food insecurity can be taken, there is a need to agree on a definition of food security and understand its determinants. A clear definition provides the context for action and assists with identifying the desired outcomes. Since the early 1990s there have been numerous definitions of food insecurity with meanings and actions differing when applied at global, domestic, household, or individual levels. This paper refers to food and nutrition security at the household and individual level in rich countries.

The Committee on World Food Security in 2012, recognising that the response to food insecurity involved multidisciplinary actors who need to speak the same language, sought a standard definition. Food and nutrition security, existing "*when all people at all times have physical, social and economic access to food, which is safe and consumed in sufficient quantity and quality to meet their dietary needs and food preferences, and is supported by an environment of adequate sanitation, health services and care, allowing for a healthy and active life*" p. 8 [10] was adopted. Definitions change and reflect what is socially acceptable at the time. The 2012 definition encompassed some broader aspects of food insecurity, such as sanitation, health services, and care, but moved away from tenets which emphasise non-emergency provision [11], avoiding unorthodox procurement practices (scavenging, stealing, or other coping strategies), social justice, democratic decision making, community self-reliance [12], or providing diets rather than just food [11]. The determinants as well as the extent of the problem are important. Food insecurity is the therefore the limited or uncertain availability of nutritionally adequate or safe foods or limited or uncertain ability to acquire foods in socially acceptable ways [13].

The determinants of food and nutrition insecurity as well as the extent of the problem are important considerations when defining action. Between and within country differences are important considerations, including, but not limited to: geographical differences (e.g., urban versus rural); chronicity and severity levels; political, economic and social drivers; historical government positions; climate impact; and how these factors have changed over time.

3. The Framing of the Issue Determines the Response

The way a problem is framed, or publically portrayed, also shapes the way society responds. Framing food security issues in ways that resonate with the beliefs, priorities and needs of different audiences can mobilize support for action. Within country social inequalities, particularly poverty, lead to food insecurity [2], therefore it would make sense that the problem framing should be in terms of how to address social and economic inequity. Two main frames dominate the way developed countries define the problem of food insecurity and the way government and other key stakeholders' respond—societal benefit and food waste mitigation.

Societal benefit frames household food security in terms of how both individuals and society benefit when all members of society are food secure. Countries with high levels of food security benefit socially, economically, environmentally, and politically. The economic cost of food insecurity is not routinely reported in developed nations however estimates to date suggest they are substantial. Costs related to food insecurity in 2011 in the US were ~A$167.5 billion related to lost productivity, public education expenses, avoidable healthcare costs, and the cost of charity to keep families fed [14]. Food insecurity is associated with a range of physical and mental health issues which contribute significantly to healthcare costs, for example cardiovascular disease [15] and obesity [16]. There is a clear relationship between housing instability, food insecurity and access to health care amongst low income families [17]. Reducing food insecurity would see improvements in health, employment, productivity, and economic viability, and reductions in health care costs. This framing should inform arguments about the need for an urgent response to food insecurity in developed countries, as the cost of inaction is likely to be far more deleterious [14]. The complexity of social disadvantage contributing to poverty, through exposure to adversity throughout the life course and often across generations, should inform the responses to food insecurity [18,19].

Food waste mitigation, *"Waste not want not. Toward zero hunger. Food bank as a green solution to hunger"*, is the contemporary framing used by the 2019 Global Foodbanking Network which frames foodbanks as the solution to hunger (SDG 2) and the environmental impact of food waste (SDG 12.3) [20]. Governments, the commercial sector, the voluntary sector, and social entrepreneurs are increasingly framing food waste diversion to the hungry as a social, economic, and environmental win:win:win [21]. There are significant economic, environmental, and social impacts of food surplus and waste, and countries need to ensure sustainable food systems to remain food secure [21]. The strongest solution to the problem is prevention that is, reducing food surplus at its source through holistic changes in the food system. The framing of the issue of food surplus and waste is currently focussed on recovery as the primary solution that is, reusing waste food for human consumption, an insufficient remedy for long term food insecurity and for food waste [21]. For example, in Australia and the UK, the voluntary sector partners with food businesses to divert food [2,22,23], and in France, food waste redistribution to charities is legislated [24]. Although these approaches may provide some food for relief agencies, unfortunately, the conflating of the two issues does not solve the fundamental and complex problems of either of them [23]. The problem of food surplus/waste distribution is the nature of the food distributed and the manner in which it is provided.

Framing food and nutrition security action within broad policy discourses (for example achieving the SDGs or economic and social policy reform) can generate commitment to act. The United Nation's World Health Organization and Food and Agriculture Organization Driving commitment for nutrition within the UN Decade of Action on Nutrition policy brief frames the argument that taking action on improving nutrition is a win-win option for many sectors and works to achieve at least 12 of the 17 SDGs. Designing frames to resonate with the people who can influence action is important [25].

Framing can be further enhanced to resonate with the people who influence action. For example, financial policy makers would likely be interested in societal benefits in terms of economic rationale (e.g., cost to health systems), civil society groups would be interested in 'the human right to adequate food and to freedom from hunger', and the vulnerability of children to malnutrition may resound with all audiences [25].

Reframing and focusing food insecurity to address the broader sustainable development issues of supporting human rights and sustainable development to create an equitable and prosperous society, will have much broader impacts than the current focus on redistributing food waste. For example, societal benefits in terms of economic rationale (e.g., cost to health systems, workforce productivity) would likely be of interest to financial policy makers; 'the human right to adequate food and to freedom from hunger' may inspire civil society groups; and the focus on vulnerability of children to malnutrition may resound with all audiences [25].

4. The Scale of the Problem of Food Insecurity

A double burden of malnutrition (high rates of undernutrition (including wasting, stunting, and micronutrient deficiencies) co-existing alongside overweight, obesity, and diet-related non-communicable diseases) is commonplace in many countries. In 2017, the absolute number of people affected by undernourishment or chronic food deprivation was estimated to be 821 million and 9 billion adults were overweight or obese. At the same time, 151 million children aged under 5 years were stunted and 38 million were either overweight or obese. Undernutrition contributes to 3.1 million (45% of total) deaths in children under five every year. The UN Decade of Action on Nutrition 2016–2025 (http://www.un.org/nutrition) aims to trigger intensified action to end hunger and eradicate all forms of malnutrition worldwide. Undernourishment, severe food insecurity, and malnutrition is more prevalent in developing economies, 90% of the worlds stunted children live in 36 countries with the highest level of chronic undernutrition. Taking action in these countries is clearly the highest priority to achieve the SDG [26].

5. How Big Is the Problem of Food Insecurity in Developed Countries?

"No Data, No Problem, No Action.", the title of a paper by Friel et al. (2009), captures the crux of the matter in terms of defining the problem of food insecurity in developed countries [27]. Relatively hidden in most developed countries, the population prevalence of food insecurity is largely unreported due to a lack of routine measurement and use of non-comparable measures. Food insecurity is closely associated with poverty and as some countries have no official government statistics, household food insecurity estimations are made using proxy measures such as national poverty lines (50 to 60% of median income) [28]. Estimated food insecurity prevalence is unexpectedly high in some rich countries, for example: Australia and Japan (21.7% of households, ~4.6 million people and 15.7%, ~19.8 million, respectively in 2012—based on 50–60% of the national poverty line); Canada (7.7%, ~1.9 million in 2007/8); the European Union (8.7% or 43.6 million when 27 countries are included); and the US (15% of the population, ~50 million) [28].

Canada and the US regularly monitor household food insecurity, while in other countries, such as the UK, it has been the rapid rise of food banks that has drawn attention to the issue [1]. Food insecurity monitoring using comparable measures should be a mandatory requirement across all countries as without the compulsory requirement national comparable estimates are at risk. Canada, who has monitored food insecurity since 2005, had some jurisdictions opt out of voluntary monitoring, undermining their ability to produce national estimates [29]. The Food and Agriculture Organization (FAO) of the United Nations supports the use of comparable measures of food insecurity to capture its magnitude, severity and causes [30]. The FAO supports an enabling environment for a rapid response to hunger through better data to: shape policies and programs; increase political commitment; support effective co-ordination and evidenced-based decision making. There is an urgent need for most developed countries to commit to using comparable measures and for most, significant effort is needed to meet this recommendation. This surveillance of within- and across-country food insecurity is crucial intelligence for the government and other sector's decision making regarding actions to address food insecurity, and a fundamental requirement for reporting against the SDGs.

6. The Responses to Food Insecurity

Most developed countries respond to food insecurity through the provision of food assistance delivered by the voluntary sector, with very limited government support [31]. Addressing the social determinants of food insecurity is the exception, for example, Norway's political agenda focuses on agricultural support, food pricing regulation, and universal social security [2]. Food assistance is usually in the form of food banks, pantries, parcels, and soup kitchens delivered by the voluntary or charitable sector. The US has embedded government funded food assistance programs: the Supplemental Nutrition Assistance Program (SNAP) of the Food Stamp Act of 1964, provided ~14% of Americans support for household food purchases at a cost of an estimated A$70 billion annually in 2018 [32]; the Special Supplemental Nutrition Program for Women, Infants and Children (WIC) serves 7 million participants a month at a cost of A$5.95 billion in 2016 [33].

Low cost food has been made available through food banks in the US since the late 1960s [34], which began opening in Europe 20 years later, and are now present in all Organisation for Economic Co-operation and Development (OECD) member states [31]. About 60 million people or 7.2% of high income country populations used them in 2013 [28]. The Global Foodbanking Network comprises over 800 food banks in 31 countries [19]. The proportion of the population accessing food banks is relatively high in some developed countries, for example, 12% of the US population (37 million people) in 2009 and 6% (19 million) of those living in the EU used foodbanks in 2011 [28]. It appears that food banks are now a permanent fixture in the response to food insecurity in developed countries, but at what cost?

Countries with relatively low public social spending have greater numbers of foodbank users. For example, the US has 12% of the population using foodbanks and spends 19.7% of Gross Domestic Product (GDP) on social expenditure whereas Belgium has ~1.9% total population using food banks and spent 29.6% of GDP on social expenditure in 2011 [28]. The rapid growth in food banks and public appeals for food donations or money for food suggest a normalisation of food aid in the UK [35] and other developed countries [36]. Despite food banks, food charity, and government programs, food insecurity is a growing problem in rich countries, so what is going wrong?

Each developed country has its own social protection systems or social welfare safety net which, due to reconstructions and cut backs to basic entitlements has meant that food banks have "*become secondary extensions of weakened social safety net*" p. 648 [37]. The inadequacy of developed countries' social protection systems is rendering people vulnerable to food insecurity, as demonstrated by increased food insecurity rates in these countries. In fact, "*Social protections systems, not the least unemployment and child benefits must be recalibrated to take into account the real cost of living and ensure adequate food for all, without compromising on other essentials*" p. X, the Special Rapporteur on the Right to Food [38]. Clearly, food banks can provide emergency food assistance but do not, in and of themselves, offer pathways out of food insecurity in developed nations [31].

The experience of being food insecure and seeking food assistance in rich countries can have negative impacts on the individual as it is traumatic, stressful, and detrimental to one's health and wellbeing [39,40]. In all societies, "*to be mentally healthy you must value and respect yourself*" p. 65 [41]. People who use food assistance in rich countries say they experience stigma, shame, and hopelessness [35,42–45]. Shame is a powerful emotion related to feeling foolish, stupid, ridiculous, inadequate, defective, incompetent, awkward, exposed, vulnerable, and insecure, based on seeing oneself negatively in the eyes of the other [46]. It is the inequality within rich countries that fosters feelings of inferiority, even before needing to seek food assistance. Independence is a core value in Western culture, people who need help to meet a basic need, such as food, are viewed as dependent and dependency is humiliating [47]. This is understandable as needing food assistance and the ways it is currently delivered is not considered socially acceptable, nor should it be in a wealthy country [48]. Another concern is that food banks and pantries strongly influence user's diets, yet are unable to support an adequate dietary intake [49,50]. Trying to address household food insecurity with community-based food interventions is not effective when solutions likely lie upstream in social protection policies [1].

7. What Should or Could Be Done and by Whom

A decade ago, the notion that 'equality is better for everyone' was eloquently expressed by Wilkinson and Pickett (2009) who asserted that to improve the quality of life in rich countries the focus must shift from building material standards and economic growth to finding ways to improve the psychological and social wellbeing of whole societies, essentially by reducing within country inequality [41].

When looking for what could or should be done to address food and nutrition security in developed countries, the discussion paper on addressing the social determinants of non-communicable diseases (NCD) provides a useful framework for multi-sectoral action outside the health sector [51]. Influenced by Friel et al.'s (2015) suggestions to address inequities in healthy eating [52], we adapted the framework for NCD action to one addressing food and nutrition security in developed countries, see Figure 1. Importantly, we have re-ordered the action focus based on potential to reduce food insecurity.

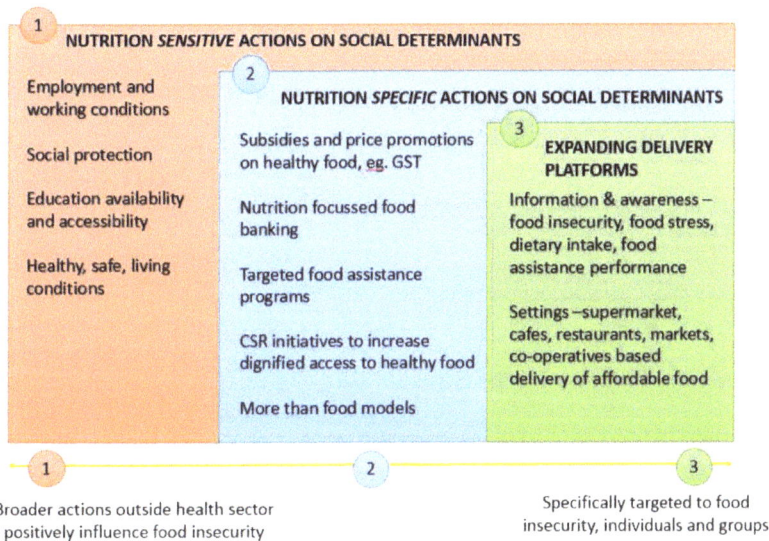

Figure 1. Typology of multi-sectoral actions on food and nutrition security (Adapted from Figure 8 p. 45 Discussion Paper Addressing the Social Determinants of Non-communicable Diseases [52]).

There is evidence to suggest some key actions to take to achieve the SDGs related to address food insecurity in developed countries. The prerequisites for action on the social determinants of food and nutrition security are high-level political commitment, governance mechanisms to facilitate and coordinate multi-sectoral responses, and robust structures for monitoring, evaluation, and accountability. As much of the required action needed to improve food and nutrition security is to be taken by actors outside the health sector, strong advocacy is needed to create cross-sector, cross-government engagement to build a shared understanding of the problem of food insecurity, outline potential actions, and delegations of responsibility. The initial advocacy focus to support the argument for cross-sector action for societal benefit, would include continuing to measure the problem and its impact and using this information to engage various sectors. There is likely to be benefit in high level government leadership bringing together key stakeholders for human development benefit, second to commercial interests. Fine-grained measurement, multilevel monitoring systems, action on the social and environmental determinants of health, and inclusive systems of governance are required to address food insecurity [27].

Political commitment to address nutrition can be created and strengthened over time through strategic action. Baker et al.'s (2018) review of factors that generated political commitment for nutrition action identified the following important drivers, irrespective of country: effective nutrition actor networks; strong leadership; civil society mobilisation; supportive political administrations; societal change and focusing events; cohesive and resonant framing; and robust data systems and available evidence [53]. Private sector interference was found to frequently undermine commitment in high-income countries.

Key actions to build food and nutrition security are in order of potential influence starting with food and nutrition sensitive, followed by food and nutrition specific actions, and lastly expanding delivery platforms. Some examples of promising actions are include:

(1) *Food and nutrition sensitive actions* include core business of non-health actors to address social determinants, including regulating employment and labour conditions, increasing access to education, challenging harmful gender norms, promoting a rights-enhancing legal environment, setting urban development policy or developing social protection programmes. Macro level changes to laws, policies and social structures can redistribute power and resources. All of the actions listed above address the determinants of food insecurity. As a matter of urgency, across government and across sector action is needed to reduce social and economic inequality. Valuable lessons can be learnt from some Scandinavian countries where the social protections systems promote equality [2] and studies from Canada and the UK focussing on reducing financial hardship [54,55]. Government policy to support access to affordable housing without compromising basic needs such as food is recommended [56].

(2) *Food and nutrition specific actions* change conditions of daily life to be those that provide food and nutrition security via interventions including laws, policies, and programmes whose primary purpose is action on the social determinants. Promising actions include: subsidies and price promotions on healthy food to ensure its affordability, for example, the Australian exemption of healthy basic foods from the Goods and Services Tax [57] and in-store price promotions; procurement policies promoting nutrition focussed food banking [58,59]; building support for the nutrition focus in targeted food assistance programs (e.g., SNAP and WIC); Corporate Social Responsibility initiatives to increase dignified access to healthy food and affordable food for all, for example, Lidl's 'Too Good to Waste' boxes selling 5 kilograms of slightly damaged but edible fruit and vegetables for just £1.50 [60]; 'More than food' models of food assistance that provide emergency relief with integrated support services to help people find pathways out of food insecurity [61,62]. Three key principles for the food service aspect of these models are: (1) a client-centred focus; (2) empowering individuals by fostering autonomy and enabling food choice in socially acceptable ways; and (3) providing opportunities for active involvement, social connection, and broader support [63].

(3) *Expanding delivery platforms* use settings to extend the reach of the health sector and extend the reach and impact of health-related information. This includes a focus on non-charitable food-service settings for example, supermarkets, cafes, restaurants, farmers markets, co-operatives, and social enterprise models to ensure affordable food is available to people at high risk of food insecurity in non-stigmatising ways. Government monitoring and surveillance systems, independent of the food industry and the charitable food sector should be developed to contribute country level information to inform appropriate actions. At a minimum these should include using standardised and robust measures of: household food and nutrition security that captures severity and prevalence and includes children (e.g., the United States Department of Agriculture (USDA)'s 18 item U.S. Household Food Security Survey Module where appropriate or part of the suite [64]); food related measures of financial stress (e.g., food stress [65]); routine measure of dietary intake, measured height and weight, and socioeconomic status; and food assistance services performance

indicators. Collectively these build information and intelligence systems to inform the delivery of targeted food insecurity interventions.

The impact of food insecurity is ultimately felt by the individual, the health system and all of society. Although not directly responsible for service delivery of the actions described above, the health sector is well placed to work with other sectors to support them to ensure effective responses to food insecurity. The three main priority actions of the health sector in developed countries to address food and nutrition insecurity are: (1) to provide the technical expertise (nutrition science, public health, food safety, and health promotion) to assist the development of food and nutrition policies to ensure interventions are nutritionally adequate and do not exacerbate health issues; (2) To contribute to the systematic monitoring and surveillance of the performance and outcomes of the comprehensive range of actions described above in terms of food security and other health outcomes; (3) Advocate on behalf of those who are rendered food insecure due to hardship and disadvantage for effective responses to food insecurity across government at all levels and stages of country development across the globe.

There is a key role for academia to provide the evidence base and independent voice to inform and evaluate policy and programs and to challenge existing paradigms and assumptions. The *International Journal of Environmental Research and Public Health* Special Issue on Addressing Food Insecurity in Developed Countries is a good example of how the research community can come together to provide evidence to guide policy and practice [66–86]. There are many opportunities for academics to partner with government, industry, and the third sector to translate research to practice to improve the lives of people rendered food insecure in rich nations.

The problem of food insecurity in developed countries is a growing problem with far reaching public health, social, and economic impacts. There will always be a need for food assistance to address emergency situations. But, this should not distract from the need to address the issue at its cause, in the words of Nelson Mandela, former President of South Africa, *"Overcoming poverty is not a gesture of charity. It is the protection of a fundamental human right, the right to dignity and a decent life."* We call for governments to initiate actions to address the social determinants of food insecurity and to lead a coordinated, collaborative, and cooperative response to finding pathways out of food insecurity guided by the expertise, enthusiasm, and commitment of the third sector and the voices of those who have had the experience.

Author Contributions: Conceptualization, C.M.P. and S.B; Writing—Original Draft Preparation, C.M.P. and S.B.; Writing—Review & Editing, C.M.P. and S.B.

Funding: This research received no external funding.

Conflicts of Interest: Sue Booth declares no conflict of interest. Christina M Pollard is a Board Member of Foodbank Western Australia, her views are her own and do not represent those of Foodbank Western Australia.

References

1. Loopstra, R. Interventions to Address Household Food Insecurity in High-Income Countries. *Proc. Nutr. Soc.* **2018**, *77*, 270–281. [CrossRef]
2. Richards, C.; Kjærnes, U.; Vik, J. Food Security in Welfare Capitalism: Comparing Social Entitlements to Food in Australia and Norway. *J. Rural Stud.* **2016**, *43*, 61–70. [CrossRef]
3. Caraher, M.; Furey, S. *The Economics of Emergency Food Aid Provision. A Financial, Social and Cultural Perspective*, 1st ed.; Palgrave Pivot: London, UK, 2018.
4. General Assembly of the United Nations. Universal Declaration of Human Rights. In *Article 251 (United Nations) Resolution 217A*; General Assembly of the United Nations: Geneva, Switzerland, 1948.
5. Committee on Economic Social and Cultural Rights (CESCR). *General Comment No. 12: The Right to Adequate Food (Article 11)*; Committee on Economic Social and Cultural Rights (CESCR): Geneva, Switzerland, 1999.

6.	United Nations. *Resolution Adopted by the General Assembly. 2200 (XXI). International Covenant on Economic, Social and Cultural Rights, International Covenant on Civil and Political Rights and Optional Protocolo the International Covenant on Civil and Political Rights. In A/RES/21/2200;* United Nations: Geneva, Switzerland, 1966.

7.	Piccard, A.M. The United States' Failure to Ratify the International Covenant on Economic, Social and Cultural Rights: Must the Poor be Always with Us? *Scholar* **2010**, *13*, 231.

8.	De Schutter, O. Report of the Special Rapporteur on the Right to Food, Addendum Mission to Canada*. In *A/HRC/22/50/Add1;* United Nations Human Rights Council: Geneva, Switzerland, 2012.

9.	Global Indicator Framework for the Sustainable Development Goals A/RES/71/313 E/CN.3/2018/2. Available online: unstats.un.org/sdgs/indicators/Global%20Indicator%20Framework%20after%20refinement_Eng.pdf (accessed on 10 April 2019).

10.	Committee on World Food Security. *Coming to Terms with Terminology;* Food and Agriculture Organization: Rome, Italy, 2012; pp. 1–26.

11.	Gottlieb, R.; Fisher, A. Community Food Security and Environmental Justice: Searching for a Common Discourse. *Agric. Hum. Values* **1996**, *13*, 23–32. [CrossRef]

12.	Bellows, A.C.; Hamm, M.W. US-Based Community Food Security: Influences, Practice, Debate. *Food Cult. Soc.* **2002**, *6*, 31–44.

13.	Olson, C.M.; Holben, D.H. Position of the American Dietetic Association: Domestic Food and Nutrition Security. *J. Am. Diet. Assoc.* **2002**, *102*, 1840–1847. [CrossRef]

14.	Shepard, D.S.; Setren, E.; Cooper, D. Hunger in America: Suffering We All Pay for. Center for American Progress. 2011, pp. 1–24. Available online: www.americanprogress.org/wp-content/uploads/issues/2011/10/pdf/hunger_paper.pdf (accessed on 10 April 2019).

15.	Seligman, H.K.; Laraia, B.A.; Kushel, M.B. Food Insecurity is Associated with Chronic Disease Among Low-Income NHANES Participants. *J. Nutr.* **2010**, *140*, 304–310. [CrossRef]

16.	Dinour, L.M.; Bergen, D.; Yeh, M.-C. The Food Insecurity–Obesity Paradox: A Review of the Literature and the Role Food Stamps may Play. *J. Am. Diet. Assoc.* **2007**, *107*, 1952–1961. [CrossRef] [PubMed]

17.	Miewald, C.; Ostry, A. A Warm Meal and a Bed: Intersections of Housing and Food Security in Vancouver's Downtown Eastside. *Hous. Stud.* **2014**, *29*, 709–729. [CrossRef]

18.	Chilton, M.; Knowles, M.; Bloom, S.L. The Intergenerational Circumstances of Household Food Insecurity and Adversity. *J. Hunger Environ. Nutr.* **2017**, *12*, 269–297. [CrossRef]

19.	Chilton, M.M.; Rabinowich, J.R.; Woolf, N.H. Very Low Food Security in the USA is Linked with Exposure to Violence. *Public Health Nutr.* **2014**, *17*, 73–82. [CrossRef] [PubMed]

20.	The Global FoodBanking Network. Waste Not Want Not.Toward Zero Hunger. Food Bank as a Green Solution to Hunger. 2019. Available online: www.foodbanking.org/wp-content/uploads/2019/03/GFN_WasteNot.pdf (accessed on 10 April 2019).

21.	Mourad, M. Recycling, Recovering and Preventing "Food Waste": Competing Solutions for Food Systems Sustainability in the United States and France. *J. Clean. Prod.* **2016**, *126*, 461–477. [CrossRef]

22.	Ruah Community Service. Registry Week 2016 Less Homeless Report. Perth: Ruah. 2016. Available online: https://view.publitas.com/ruah-community-services-1/registry-week-final-report-2016/page/1 (accessed on 10 April 2019).

23.	Caplan, P. Win-Win? Food Poverty, Food Aid and Food Surplus in the UK today. *Anthr. Today* **2017**, *33*, 17–22. [CrossRef]

24.	Angelique Chrisafis. French Law Forbids Food Waste by Supermarkets. Food Banks and Other Charities Welcome Law Making Large Shops Donate Unsold Food and Stop Spoiling Items to Deter Foragers. In The Guardian. Available online: www.theguardian.com/world/2016/feb/04/french-law-forbids-food-waste-by-supermarkets (accessed on 10 April 2019).

25.	World Health Organization and Food and Agriculture Organization of the United Nations. *Driving commitment for nutrition within the UN Decade of Action on Nutrition;* World Health Organization and Food and Agriculture Organization of the United Nations: Geneva, Switzerland, 2018; Available online: https://apps.who.int/iris/bitstream/handle/10665/274375/WHO-NMH-NHD-17.11-eng.pdf?ua=1 (accessed on 6 May 2019).

26. FAO, IFAD, UNICEF, WFP, WHO. *The State of Food Security and Nutrition in the World 2018. Building Climate Resilience for Food Security and Nutrition*; FAO: Rome, Italy, 2018; Available online: https://reliefweb.int/report/ world/state-food-security-and-nutrition-world-2018-building-climate-resilience-food-security (accessed on 6 May 2019).

27. Friel, S.; Vlahov, D.; Buckley, R.M. No Data, No Problem, No Action: Addressing Urban Health Inequity in the 21st Century. *J. Urban Health* **2011**, *88*, 858–859. [CrossRef] [PubMed]

28. Gentilini, U. Banking on Food: The State of Food Banks in High-Income Countries. Institute of Development Studies, IDS Working Papers 2013, 1-18.CSP WORKING PAPER Number 008. Available online: www.ids.ac. uk/publications/banking-on-food-the-state-of-food-banks-in-high-income-countries/ (accessed on 10 April 2019).

29. PROOF Food Insecurity Policy Research. Monitoring Food Insecurity in Canada. Fact sheets. p. 2. Canada: PROOF; 2017:2. Available online: https://proof.utoronto.ca/wp-content/uploads/2016/06/monitoring-factsheet.pdf (accessed on 10 April 2019).

30. Food and Agriculture Organization of the United Nations. Information Systems for Food Insecurity and Nutrition. Available online: www.fao.org (accessed on 10 April 2019).

31. Riches, G. *Food Bank Nations: Poverty, Corporate Charity and the Right to Food*, 1st ed.; Routledge: London, UK, 2018.

32. Mozaffarian, D.; Liu, J.; Sy, S.; Huang, Y.; Rehm, C.; Lee, Y.; Wilde, P.; Abrahams-Gessel, S.; de Souza Veiga Jardim, T.; Gaziano, T. Cost-Effectiveness of Financial Incentives and Disincentives for Improving Food Purchases and Health through the US Supplemental Nutrition Assistance Program (SNAP): A Microsimulation Study. *PLoS Med* **2018**, *15*, e1002661. [CrossRef] [PubMed]

33. Carlson, S.; Neuberger, Z.; Rosenbaum, D. WIC Participation and Costs are Stable. Center on Budget and Policy Priorities 2017. Available online: www.cbpp.org/research/food-assistance/wic-participation-and-costs-are-stable (accessed on 10 April 2019).

34. Ghys, T. Taking Stock of the Ambiguous Role of Foodbanks in the Fight Against Poverty. *J. Poverty Soc. Justice* **2018**, *26*, 173–189. [CrossRef]

35. Purdam, K.; Garratt, E.A.; Esmail, A. Hungry? Food Insecurity, Social Stigma and Embarrassment in the UK. *Sociology* **2016**, *50*, 1072–1088. [CrossRef]

36. Tarasuk, V.; Eakin, J.M. Charitable Food Assistance as Symbolic Gesture: An Ethnographic Study of Food Banks in Ontario. *Soc. Sci. Med.* **2003**, *56*, 1505–1515. [CrossRef]

37. Riches, G. Food Banks and Food Security: Welfare Reform, Human Rights and Social Policy. Lessons from Canada? *Soc. Policy Adm.* **2002**, *36*, 648–663. [CrossRef]

38. Riches, G.; Silvasti, T. *First World Hunger Revisited Food Charity or the Right to Food?* 2nd ed.; Riches, G., Silvasti, T., Eds.; Palgrave Macmillan: Hampshire, UK, 2014.

39. Hecht, A.A.; Biehl, E.; Buzogany, S.; Neff, R. Using a Trauma-Informed Policy Approach to Create a Resilient Urban Food System. *Public Health Nutr.* **2018**, *21*, 1961–1970. [CrossRef]

40. Thompson, C.; Smith, D.; Cummins, S.J.S.S. Medicine: Understanding the Health and Wellbeing Challenges of the Food Banking System: A Qualitative Study of Food Bank Users, Providers and Referrers in London. *Soc. Sci. Med.* **2018**, *211*, 95–101. [CrossRef]

41. Wilkinson, R.; Pickett, K. *The Spirit Level. Why Equality is Better for Everyone*, 2nd ed.; Penguin Books: London, UK, 2010.

42. Middleton, G.; Mehta, K.; McNaughton, D.; Booth, S. The Experiences and Perceptions of Foodbank Amongst Users in High Income Countries: An international Scoping Review. *Appetite* **2018**, *120*, 698–708. [CrossRef]

43. Booth, S.; Begley, A.; Mackintosh, B.; Kerr, D.A.; Jancey, J.; Caraher, M.; Whelan, J.; Pollard, C.M. Gratitude, Resignation and the Desire for Dignity: Lived Experience of Food Charity Recipients and Their Recommendations for Improvement, Perth, Western Australia. *Public Health Nutr.* **2018**, *21*, 831–2841. [CrossRef]

44. Douglas, F.; MacKenzie, F.; Ejebu, O.-Z.; Whybrow, S.; Garcia, A.L.; McKenzie, L.; Ludbrook, A.; Dowler, E. "A Lot of People Are Struggling Privately. They Don't Know Where to Go or They're Not Sure of What to Do": Frontline Service Provider Perspectives of the Nature of Household Food Insecurity in Scotland. *Int. J. Environ. Res. Public Health* **2018**, *15*, 2738. [CrossRef] [PubMed]

45. Garthwaite, K. Stigma, Shame and 'People Like Us': An Ethnographic Study of Foodbank Use in the UK. *J. Poverty Soc. Justice* **2016**, *24*, 277–289. [CrossRef]

46. Scheff, T.J. Shame in Self and Society. *Symb. Interact.* **2003**, *26*, 239–262. [CrossRef]
47. Poppendieck, J. *Sweet Charity? Emergency Food and the End of Entitlement*, 1st ed.; Penguin Group: New York, NY, USA, 1998.
48. Silvasti, T. Participatory Alternatives for Food Charity? Finnish Development in an International Comparison. In *Participation, Marginalisation and Welfare Services—Concepts, Politics and Practice Across European Union Countries*, 1st ed.; Matthies, A.-L., Uggerhoj, L., Eds.; Ashgate: Farnham, UK, 2014; pp. 183–197.
49. Simmet, A.; Depa, J.; Tinnemann, P.; Stroebele-Benschop, N. The Nutritional Quality of Food Provided from Food Pantries: A Systematic Review of Existing Literature. *J. Acad. Nutr. Diet.* **2017**, *117*, 577–588. [CrossRef]
50. Simmet, A.; Depa, J.; Tinnemann, P.; Stroebele-Benschop, N. The Dietary Quality of Food Pantry Users: A Systematic Review of Existing Literature. *J. Acad. Nutr. Diet.* **2017**, *117*, 563–576. [CrossRef]
51. United Nations Development Programme. *Discussion Paper Addressing the Social Determinants of Non-communicable Diseases*; United Nations: New York, NY, USA, 2013; Available online: www.undp.org/content/dam/undp/library/hivaids/English/Discussion_Paper_Addressing_the_Social_Determinants_of_NCDs_UNDP_2013.pdf (accessed on 11 April 2019).
52. Friel, S.; Hattersley, L.; Ford, L.; O'Rourke, K. Addressing Inequities in healthy eating. *Health Promot. Int.* **2015**, *30*, ii77–ii88. [CrossRef] [PubMed]
53. Baker, P.; Hawkes, C.; Wingrove, K.; Demaio, A.R.; Parkhurst, J.; Thow, A.M.; Walls, H. What Drives Political Commitment for Nutrition? A Review and Framework Synthesis to Inform the United Nations Decade of Action on Nutrition. *BMJ Glob. Health* **2018**, *3*, e000485. [CrossRef] [PubMed]
54. Tarasuk, V. Implications of Basic Income Guarantee for Household Food Security. Northern Policy Institute Research Paper No. 24. 2017. Available online: https://proof.utoronto.ca/wp-content/uploads/2017/06/Paper-Tarasuk-BIG-EN-17.06.13-1712.pdf (accessed on 11 April 2019).
55. Loopstra, R.; Laylor, D. Financial Insecurity, Food Insecurity, and Disability: The Profile of People Receiving Emergency Food Assistance from The Trussell Trust Foodbank Network in Britain. June 2017. Available online: https://trusselltrust.org/wp-content/uploads/sites/2/2017/06/OU_Report_final_01_08_online.pdf (accessed on 11 April 2019).
56. Kirkpatrick, S.I.; Tarasuk, V. Housing Circumstances are Associated with Household Food Access among Low-Income Urban Families. *J. Urban Health* **2011**, *88*, 284–296. [CrossRef]
57. Landrigan, T.J.; Kerr, D.A.; Dhaliwal, S.S.; Savage, V.; Pollard, C.M. Removing the Australian Tax Exemption on Healthy Food Adds Food Stress to Families Vulnerable to Poor Nutrition. *Aust. New Zealand J. Public Health* **2017**, *41*, 591–597. [CrossRef] [PubMed]
58. Ross, M.; Campbell, E.C.; Webb, K.L. Recent Trends in the Nutritional Quality of Food Banks' Food and Beverage Inventory: Case Studies of Six California Food Banks. *J. Hunger Environ. Nutr.* **2013**, *8*, 294–309. [CrossRef]
59. Wetherill, M.S.; Williams, M.B.; White, K.C.; Li, J.; Vidrine, J.I.; Vidrine, D.J. Food Pantries as Partners in Population Health: Assessing Organizational and Personnel Readiness for Delivering Nutrition-Focused Charitable Food Assistance. *J. Hunger Environ. Nutr.* **2019**, *14*, 50–69. [CrossRef]
60. Too Good to Waste. Lidl UK. Available online: www.lidl.co.uk/en/Too-Good-To-Waste-15447.htm (accessed on 11 April 2019).
61. Martin, K.S.; Redelfs, A.; Wu, R.; Bogner, O.; Whigham, L. Offering More Than Food: Outcomes and Lessons Learned from a Fresh Start food pantry in Texas. *J. Hunger Environ. Nutr.* **2019**, *14*, 70–81. [CrossRef]
62. Martin, K.S.; Colantonio, A.G.; Picho, K.; Boyle, K.E. Self-Efficacy is Associated with Increased Food Security in Novel Food Pantry Program. *SSM Popul. Health* **2016**, *2*, 62–67. [CrossRef]
63. Booth, S.; Pollard, C.M.; Coveney, J.; Goodwin-Smith, I. 'Sustainable' Rather Than 'Subsistence' Food Assistance Solutions to Food Insecurity: South Australian Recipients' Perspectives on Traditional and Social Enterprise Models. *Int. J. Environ. Res. Public Health* **2018**, *21*, 2086. [CrossRef]
64. Food Security in the U.S Survey Tools. Available online: www.ers.usda.gov/topics/food-nutrition-assistance/food-security-in-the-us/survey-tools.aspx (accessed on 11 April 2019).
65. Landrigan, T.J.; Kerr, D.A.; Dhaliwal, S.S.; Pollard, C.M. Protocol for the Development of a Food Stress Index to Identify Households Most at Risk of Food Insecurity in Western Australia. *Int. J. Environ. Res. Public Health* **2018**, *16*, 79. [CrossRef]
66. Temple, J.B.; Russell, J. Food Insecurity among Older Aboriginal and Torres Strait Islanders. *Int. J. Environ. Res. Public Health* **2018**, *15*, 1766. [CrossRef] [PubMed]

67. Temple, J.B.; Booth, S.; Pollard, C.M. Social Assistance Payments and Food Insecurity in Australia: Evidence from the Household Expenditure Survey. *Int. J. Environ. Res. Public Health* **2019**, *16*, 455. [CrossRef]

68. Temple, J.B. The Association between Stressful Events and Food Insecurity: Cross-Sectional Evidence from Australia. *Int. J. Environ. Res. Public Health* **2018**, *15*, 2333. [CrossRef] [PubMed]

69. Simmet, A.; Tinnemann, P.; Stroebele-Benschop, N. The German Food Bank System and Its Users—A Cross-Sectional Study. *Int. J. Environ. Res. Public Health* **2018**, *15*, 1485. [CrossRef] [PubMed]

70. Salonen, A.S.; Ohisalo, M.; Laihiala, T. Undeserving, Disadvantaged, Disregarded: Three Viewpoints of Charity Food Aid Recipients in Finland. *Int. J. Environ. Res. Public Health* **2018**, *15*, 2896. [CrossRef]

71. Pollard, C.M.; Mackintosh, B.; Campbell, C.; Kerr, D.; Begley, A.; Jancey, J.; Caraher, M.; Berg, J.; Booth, S. Charitable Food Systems' Capacity to Address Food Insecurity: An Australian Capital City Audit. *Int. J. Environ. Res. Public Health* **2018**, *15*, 1249. [CrossRef] [PubMed]

72. McCarthy, L.; Chang, A.B.; Brimblecombe, J. Food Security Experiences of Aboriginal and Torres Strait Islander Families with Young Children in an Urban Setting: Influencing Factors and Coping Strategies. *Int. J. Environ. Res. Public Health* **2018**, *15*, 2649. [CrossRef] [PubMed]

73. Maynard, M.; Andrade, L.; Packull-McCormick, S.; Perlman, C.M.; Leos-Toro, C.; Kirkpatrick, S.I. Food Insecurity and Mental Health Among Females in High-Income Countries. *Int. J. Environ. Res. Public Health* **2018**, *15*, 1424. [CrossRef] [PubMed]

74. Mackay, S.; Buch, T.; Vandevijvere, S.; Goodwin, R.; Korohina, E.; Funaki-Tahifote, M.; Lee, A.; Swinburn, B. Cost and Affordability of Diets Modelled on Current Eating Patterns and on Dietary Guidelines, for New Zealand Total Population, Māori and Pacific Households. *Int. J. Environ. Res. Public Health* **2018**, *15*, 1255. [CrossRef] [PubMed]

75. Love, P.; Whelan, J.; Bell, C.; Grainger, F.; Russell, C.; Lewis, M.; Lee, A. Healthy Diets in Rural Victoria—Cheaper than Unhealthy Alternatives, yet Unaffordable. *Int. J. Environ. Res. Public Health* **2018**, *15*, 2469. [CrossRef]

76. Lee, A.; Lewis, M. Testing the Price of Healthy and Current Diets in Remote Aboriginal Communities to Improve Food Security: Development of the Aboriginal and Torres Strait Islander Healthy Diets Asap (Australian Standardised Affordability and Pricing) Methods. *Int. J. Environ. Res. Public Health* **2018**, *15*, 2912. [CrossRef]

77. Kleve, S.; Booth, S.; Davidson, Z.E.; Palermo, C. Walking the Food Security Tightrope—Exploring the Experiences of Low-To-Middle Income Melbourne Households. *Int. J. Environ. Res. Public Health* **2018**, *15*, 2206. [CrossRef]

78. Jessiman-Perreault, G.; McIntyre, L. Household Food Insecurity Narrows the Sex Gap in Five Adverse Mental Health Outcomes Among Canadian Adults. *Int. J. Environ. Res. Public Health* **2019**, *16*, 319. [CrossRef]

79. Gallegos, D.; Chilton, M.M. Re-Evaluating Expertise: Principles for Food and Nutrition Security Research, Advocacy and Solutions in High-Income Countries. *Int. J. Environ. Res. Public Health* **2019**, *16*, 561. [CrossRef] [PubMed]

80. Ferguson, M.; O'Dea, K.; Altman, J.; Moodie, M.; Brimblecombe, J. Health-Promoting Food Pricing Policies and Decision-Making in very Remote Aboriginal and Torres Strait Islander Community Stores in Australia. *Int. J. Environ. Res. Public Health* **2018**, *15*, 2908. [CrossRef] [PubMed]

81. Ejebu, O.-Z.; Whybrow, S.; Mckenzie, L.; Dowler, E.; Garcia, A.L.; Ludbrook, A.; Barton, K.L.; Wrieden, W.L.; Douglas, F. What Can Secondary Data Tell us about Household Food Insecurity in a High-Income Country Context? *Int. J. Environ. Res. Public Health* **2018**, *16*, 82. [CrossRef] [PubMed]

82. Daly, A.; Pollard, C.M.; Kerr, D.A.; Binns, C.W.; Caraher, M.; Phillips, M. Using Cross-Sectional Data to Identify and Quantify the Relative Importance of Factors Associated with and Leading to Food Insecurity. *Int. J. Environ. Res. Public Health* **2018**, *15*, 2620. [CrossRef] [PubMed]

83. Clay, L.A.; Papas, M.A.; Gill, K.B.; Abramson, D.M. Factors Associated with Continued Food Insecurity among Households Recovering from Hurricane Katrina. *Int. J. Environ. Res. Public Health* **2018**, *15*, 1647. [CrossRef] [PubMed]

84. Carrillo-Álvarez, E.; Penne, T.; Boeckx, H.; Storms, B.; Goedemé, T. Food Reference Budgets as a Potential Policy Tool to Address Food Insecurity: Lessons Learned from a Pilot Study in 26 European Countries. *Int. J. Environ. Res. Public Health* **2018**, *16*, 32. [CrossRef] [PubMed]

85. Brown, C.; Laws, C.; Leonard, D.; Campbell, S.; Merone, L.; Hammond, M.; Thompson, K.; Canuto, K.; Brimblecombe, J. Healthy Choice Rewards: A Feasibility Trial of Incentives to Influence Consumer Food Choices in a Remote Australian Aboriginal Community. *Int. J. Environ. Res. Public Health* **2019**, *16*, 112. [CrossRef]

86. Becerra, M.B.; Mshigeni, S.K.; Becerra, B.J. The Overlooked Burden of Food Insecurity among Asian Americans: Results from the California Health Interview Survey. *Int. J. Environ. Res. Public Health* **2018**, *15*, 1684. [CrossRef]

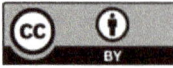

International Journal of
*Environmental Research
and Public Health*

MDPI

Review

Food Insecurity and Mental Health among Females in High-Income Countries

Merryn Maynard [1,*], Lesley Andrade [2], Sara Packull-McCormick [2], Christopher M. Perlman [2], Cesar Leos-Toro [2] and Sharon I. Kirkpatrick [2,*]

[1]   Meal Exchange Canada, Toronto, ON M5V 3A8, Canada
[2]   School of Public Health and Health Systems, University of Waterloo, Waterloo, ON N2L 3G1, Canada;
       landrade@uwaterloo.ca (L.A.); srpackul@uwaterloo.ca (S.P.M.); chris.perlman@uwaterloo.ca (C.M.P.);
       cesar.leos-toro@uwaterloo.ca (C.L.-T.)
*   Correspondence: merryn@mealexchange.com (M.M.); sharon.kirkpatrick@uwaterloo.ca (S.I.K.);
       Tel.: +1-416-657-4489 (M.M.); +1-519-888-4567 (ext. 37054) (S.I.K.)

Received: 5 June 2018; Accepted: 4 July 2018; Published: 6 July 2018

Abstract: Food insecurity is a persistent concern in high-income countries, and has been associated with poor mental health, particularly among females. We conducted a scoping review to characterize the state of the evidence on food insecurity and mental health among women in high-income countries. The research databases PubMed, EMBASE, and psycINFO were searched using keywords capturing food insecurity, mental health, and women. Thirty-nine articles (representing 31 unique studies/surveys) were identified. Three-quarters of the articles drew upon data from a version of the United States Department of Agriculture Household Food Security Survey Module. A range of mental health measures were used, most commonly to measure depression and depressive symptoms, but also anxiety and stress. Most research was cross-sectional and showed associations between depression and food insecurity; longitudinal analyses suggested bidirectional relationships (with food insecurity increasing the risk of depressive symptoms or diagnosis, or depression predicting food insecurity). Several articles focused on vulnerable subgroups, such as pregnant women and mothers, women at risk of homelessness, refugees, and those who had been exposed to violence or substance abuse. Overall, this review supports a link between food insecurity and mental health (and other factors, such as housing circumstances and exposure to violence) among women in high-income countries and underscores the need for comprehensive policies and programs that recognize complex links among public health challenges.

Keywords: food insecurity; mental health; depression; women; scoping review

---

1. Introduction

Food insecurity is a growing and persistent concern in high-income countries [1,2]. In North America, rates of household food insecurity have remained stable or risen in the last several years [3,4]. High rates have also been documented in the UK and Australia [5,6]. According to the Food and Agriculture Organization, "food security exists when all people, at all times, have physical, social, and economic access to sufficient safe and nutritious food that meets their dietary needs and food preferences for an active and healthy life" [7].Conceptualizations of food insecurity in high-income countries primarily focus on the economic aspect; for example, the Household Food Security Survey Module (HFSSM) [8], which is commonly used in the United States and Canada, measures uncertain or inadequate access to food due to financial constraints. This conceptualization aligns with literature linking vulnerability to food insecurity to high rates of poverty, particularly among population subgroups, such as single-parent households, racial/ethnic minorities, and those relying on social assistance [2–4,9–13].

Among population subgroups in high-income countries, food insecurity has been shown to be associated with compromised nutrition [14], poor general health, and a myriad of chronic health conditions [15,16]. Food insecurity has also been shown to be a marker of poor mental health, with studies identifying associations with mood and anxiety disorders and suicidal ideation, particularly among women [16–18]. Indeed, severity of household food insecurity appears to be linked with poor mental health in a dose–response manner, with experiences of severe food insecurity representing extreme chronic stress [19] and possibly acting as an independent determinant of suicidal ideation [20].

The relationship between food insecurity and poor mental health among women is of particular concern given that they are disproportionately impacted by food insecurity [2–4,21]. Women are overrepresented among low-income groups compared to men, with visible minority women and single mothers experiencing high rates of poverty in Canada and the United States [9–11]. Further, the existing literature suggests that women may be particularly vulnerable to poor mental health in conjunction with poverty and food insecurity [12] and for women with children, that the stress associated with these experiences has possible ripple effects, negatively impacting their children's physical and mental health as well [13].

To identify future research needs and inform policy and program responses, we conducted a scoping review to examine the state of the literature on food insecurity and mental health among women living in high-income countries.

2. Materials and Methods

The scoping review was conducted according to steps outlined by Arksey and O'Malley [22]. Scoping reviews, which use systematic search techniques, are appropriate when the aim is to address a broad question, such as querying the state of the evidence on a topic (especially when study designs may vary) and identifying gaps in that evidence [22] to inform future research and practice. As per Arksey and O'Malley [22], steps in the process include identifying the research question, identifying relevant studies, study selection, charting the data, and collating, summarizing, and reporting the results. Reporting follows the PRISMA guidelines [23].

2.1. Identifying Relevant Studies

The systematic search, developed in consultation with a librarian who is an expert in systematic searching, was conducted using the research databases PubMed, EMBASE, and psycINFO to capture records published up to May 2016. Given the range of possible mental health conditions, the search strategy was quite broad. Key words and Medical Subject Headings (MeSH) included "food" OR "nutrition" OR "diet" AND "security" OR "insecurity" OR "insufficiency" OR "scarcity" OR "*adequacy" OR "hunger" OR "poverty" OR "food supply" OR "nutritional requirements/status" AND "anxiety" OR "depression" OR "mental health" OR "mental health disorder" OR "mental health illness" OR "psychosis" OR "emotional disorder" OR "mania" OR "mental disease" OR "phobia" OR "mental disturbance/health/psychology". The key words and MESH headings to capture women included "women" OR "woman" OR "female" OR "pregnancy" OR "sex factors" OR "women's rights" OR "mothers" OR "girl" (note: * indicates a wildcard, which allows searching a range of terms related to a root word). The initial search elicited a total of 13,645 citations (excluding duplicates) (Figure 1).

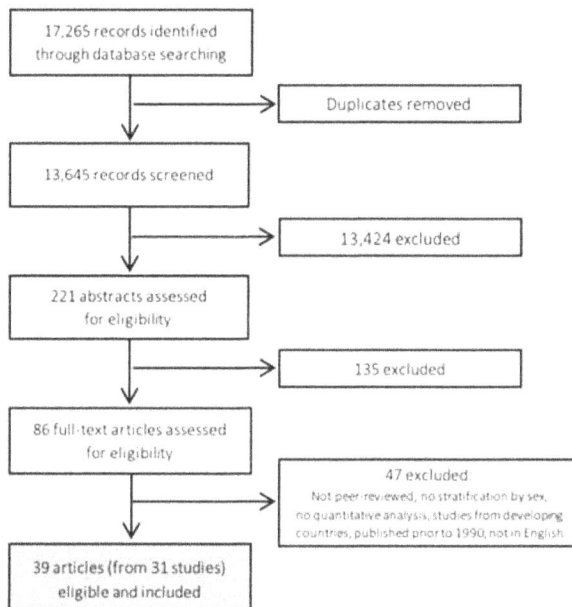

Figure 1. Overview of identification and screening of records for scoping review of literature on food insecurity and mental health among women in high-income countries.

2.2. Study Selection

Articles deemed eligible quantitatively examined associations between food insecurity and indicators of mental health, with a focus on females in high-income countries; studies that included both males and females but reported analyses stratified by sex were also considered. Specific criteria related to age were not applied, allowing consideration of studies reporting on adolescent girls as well as women. Studies published since 1990 (to provide insights into relatively recent research on the topic of food insecurity) were considered.

An initial screening of titles and abstracts was conducted by one author (S.P.-M.) to identify potentially relevant peer-reviewed articles that addressed food insecurity and health, leaving 221 citations for further review (Figure 1). Abstracts for these 221 citations were screened independently by a second author (M.M. or S.I.K.) and discrepancies resolved, leaving 86 citations for full-text review. After full-text screening (conducted independently by two authors), 39 articles remained, representing 31 unique studies/surveys. Separate articles making use of data from the same study or survey were examined and charted to identify salient characteristics related to measurement of food security and mental health and the examination of associations between the two.

2.3. Charting the Data

A data abstraction form guided extraction of the characteristics of interest, including study setting and population, study design, main study objectives, measures used to assess food security and mental health and specific mental health states considered, and analytic approach and findings.

2.4. Collating, Summarizing, and Reporting the Results

The abstracted data were assessed in terms of patterns in measures and tools used and associations between food insecurity and depression (the most frequently examined mental health measure) and other mental health markers. Given that we conducted a scoping rather than a systematic review, formal quality appraisal of studies was not conducted [22]. However, in addition to synthesizing the evidence emerging from this literature, we comment on the characteristics of the available research, in terms of study design for example, to inform future research.

3. Results

3.1. Overview of Included Articles

The characteristics of the 39 articles are outlined in Appendix A. Over half (*n* = 23) were published from 2010 on [15–17,24–43]. The majority (*n* = 34) analyzed data from studies conducted in the United States, three focused on studies conducted in Canada [16,17,32], one was focused on a sample in New Zealand [43], and one was conducted in England [44]. Twenty-eight articles reported on cross-sectional analyses (one also included qualitative data collection [28]) and eleven reported longitudinal analyses (one included qualitative data collection [45]) (Appendix A). Although all studies assessed the association between food insecurity and a mental health condition or state in some manner, the particular research questions and analytic approaches varied. Some studies examined food insecurity and mental health among general samples of the population, whereas others focused on particularly vulnerable population subgroups or sought to assess the feasibility or other properties of tools. Half (*n* = 20) focused on mothers or caregivers, another five studied pregnant women, and several focused on other specific subpopulations, including rural women, those living with disabilities, older women, refugees, women experiencing insecure housing or homelessness, and women at risk for HIV (Appendix A).

3.2. Food Insecurity Measures

Three-quarters (*n* = 30) of the reviewed articles drew upon data collected using a version of the Household Food Security Survey Module (HFSSM), developed by the United States Department of Agriculture [8] (Table 1). The full HFSSM contains 18 items and yields a single score indicating the severity of household food insecurity over the past 12 months or 30 days; ten items refer to adults and eight refer to children in the household [8]. Scores are typically used to categorize households as food secure or food insecure with different levels of severity (since a review of the measure conducted in the early 2000s [46], the categories of food insecurity have been referred to as low and very low food security, replacing earlier labels of food insecure with/without hunger). The HFSSM was compared to household food expenditures and income [8] and associated with compromised dietary intakes [14], supporting its validity in capturing constrained food access due to inadequate finances. Fourteen articles drew upon abbreviated versions of HFSSM, including the six-item subset developed by USDA and the ten adult-referenced items, as well as other adaptations (Table 1).

One article reported on data using a single item drawn from the 12-item Radimer–Cornell scale [47], and another used data collected using the Community Childhood Hunger Identification Project (CCHIP) instrument [48]. Both the Radimer–Cornell and CCHIP tools are used to categorize food security status and were shown to have good specificity and sensitivity compared to evaluations of food security status based on household food inventories, dietary recall data, and other measures among a sample of women living with children in rural New York [49]. These tools were drawn upon in the development of the HFSSM [8].

Three articles drew upon data collected using a single item from the National Health and Nutrition Examination Survey-III (NHANES-III) to assess food insufficiency (defined as "an inadequate amount of food intake due to a lack of money or resources") [50]. As opposed to more comprehensive instruments, measures of food insufficiency are less detailed and may misclassify some households [49,51]. Finally, four articles drew upon data from other single- or multi-measures adapted from prior literature (Table 1).

Table 1. Overview of measures of food security drawn upon in articles ($n = 39$) examining associations between food insecurity and mental health among women in high-income countries.

Measure	Description	Abbreviated and Modified Versions	Articles Using Full Version	Articles Using Modified Versions
Community Childhood Hunger Identification Project	An 8-item scale developed by Wehler et al. [48]. Part of a survey instrument to examine the prevalence of hunger among low-income families. The items address qualitative and quantitative compromises among adults and children. Shown to have good specificity and sensitivity compared to evaluations of food security status based on household food inventories, dietary recall data, and other measures among a sample of women living with children in rural New York [49].	None	None	Wehler et al. 2004 [52]
Household Food Security Survey Module	An 18-item measure developed by the United States Department of Agriculture [8] and used to monitor household food security in the US and Canada. Measures the food security status of a household in the last 12 months. Items ask an adult respondent about anxiety related to the household food supply, running out of food, providing inadequately nutritious food, and substitutions or restrictions in food consumption by adults and/or children in the household due to lack of financial resources. Items are compiled to form a continuous, linear scale that categorizes households into one of four groups; food secure, marginal food secure, low food secure, and very low food secure [8]. Data from the HFSSM have been compared to household food expenditures and income [8] and dietary intakes [14], supporting its validity in capturing constrained food access due to inadequate financial resources.	Six-item short form: uses a subset of the 18-item survey. Does not characterize severe food insecurity and does not contain child-specific items. 10-item adult scale: includes only items referenced to adults in the household. Health Canada modifications: Refers to low food security as "moderate food insecurity" and "severe food insecurity". Less stringent than USDA coding, in that 2+ affirmative responses place an individual into a food insecure category.	Bronte-Tinkew et al. 2007 [53]; Casey et al. 2004 [54]; Chilton et al. 2013 [28]; Corman et al. 2016 [24]; Garg et al. 2015 [25]; Hanson et al. 2012 [15]; Hernandez et al. 2014 [26]; Huddleston-Casas et al. 2009 [55]; Laraia et al. 2006 [56]; Laraia et al. 2015 [27]; Lent et al. 2009 [45]; McCurdy et al. 2015 [29]; Sun et al. 2016 [30]; Trapp et al. 2015 [31]; Health Canada coding; Muldoon et al. 2013 [32]; Tarasuk et al. 2013 [16]	Dressler et al. 2015 [3]; Kaiser et al. 2007 [57]; Laraia et al. 2009 [58]; Martin et al. 2016 [17] (Health Canada coding); Mathews et al. 2010 [54]; Peterman et al. 2013 [58]; Sharpe et al. 2016 [59]; Whitaker et al. 2006 [5]; 15-item adaptation for pregnant Latinas: Hromi-Fielder et al. 2011 [60] Other non-standard adaptations (3-, 4-, or 7-items): Ajrouch et al. 2010 [35]; Davey-Rothwell et al. 2014 [40]; Harrison et al. 2008 [44]; Melchior et al. 2009 [44]; Sidebottom et al. 2014 [33]
National Health and Nutrition Examination Survey-III (NHANES-III) food sufficiency indicators	NHANES-III was a health and nutrition survey conducted by the US Center for Disease Control (CDC). A food sufficiency component was included in the in-home adult questionnaire. Respondents were classified as "food insecure" if they "sometimes" or "often" did not have enough food to eat. Other questions included how many days in the prior month the respondent did not have money for food, reasons for not having enough food, and whether the respondent or child in the household had restricted their food intake due to lack of food [61].	None	Heflin et al. 2005 [62]; Siefert et al. 2007 [63]; Siefert et al. 2001 [64]	None

Table 1. *Cont.*

Measure	Description	Abbreviated and Modified Versions	Articles Using Full Version	Articles Using Modified Versions
New Zealand measure of individual deprivation (NZiDep)	An 8-item scale measuring individual socioeconomic deprivation, specific to New Zealand. The scale has been validated among Maori, Pacific, and White New Zealand citizens [65]; criterion validity relied upon associations with tobacco smoking. Includes three-item composite measure of food security: "In the last 12 months have you personally made use of special food grants or food banks because you did not have enough money for food?" (yes/no), "In the last 12 months have you personally been forced to buy cheaper food so that you could pay for other things you needed?" (yes/no), "In the last 12 months have you personally gone without fresh fruit and vegetables often so that you could pay for other things you needed?" (yes/no).		Carter et al. 2011 [43]	None
Radimer–Cornell scale	A 12-item scale developed by Radimer et al. [47] at Cornell University based on qualitative research with low-income women. Twelve items cover aspects of household, adult, and child food insecurity. The content of the items address food anxiety, monotony of diet, financial constraints, food restriction, insufficient intake, and acquiring food in socially acceptable ways [47,66]. Shown to have good specificity and sensitivity compared to evaluations of food security status based on household food inventories, dietary recall data, and other measures among a sample of women living with children in rural New York [49]. Further information about the evolution of the instrument is available [67].	Single item	None	Sharkey et al. 2011 [41]
Other Multi- or Single-Item Measures			Birmingham et al. 2011 [42]; Klesges et al. 2001 [68]; Sharkey et al. 2003 [69]	None

3.3. Mental Health Measures

Depression and depressive symptoms were the most prevalent mental health states assessed. Associations between food insecurity and depression were examined in 36 articles (Appendix A). Ten articles drew upon measures assessing clinical diagnoses, while the remainder relied upon self-reported symptoms.

Measures are described in Table 2, along with information about their validation. In reviewed articles, authors sometimes noted that measures have been tested for psychometric properties such as internal consistency, in some cases, in the context of the particular study (Appendix A). Data from the short form of the World Health Organization World Mental Health Composite International Diagnostic Interview (CIDI) [70] were drawn upon to establish a clinical diagnosis of depression or anxiety in six articles. To assess depressive symptoms, the Centre for Epidemiologic Studies Depression Scale (CES-D) [71] was used most frequently, drawn upon in 14 articles. For anxiety, one article drew upon data from Spielberger's Trait Anxiety Inventory [72] and another the Hopkins Symptom Checklist Subscale (HSCL) [73]. Some measures targeted specific life stages such as pregnancy and older age; for example, maternal depressive symptoms were assessed with the Kemper three-item screen [74] and the Edinburgh Postpartum Depression Scale [75], while depressive symptoms among older women were assessed using the Geriatric Depression Scale [76].

Various other mental health markers were measured, including perceived control over one's life, perceived stress, quality of life, self-esteem, mastery, general mental health, psychosis, substance abuse, post-traumatic stress disorder, and disordered eating (Appendix A).

Table 2. Overview of measures of mental health drawn upon in articles (*n* = 39) examining associations between food insecurity and mental health among women in high-income countries.

Measure	Description	Abbreviated Versions	Articles Using Full Version	Articles Using Abbreviated Versions
Center for Epidemiologic Studies, Depression Scale (CES-D)	A 20-item self-report scale measuring depressive symptoms in the general population. Components assess depressed mood, feelings of guilt and worthlessness, feelings of helplessness and hopelessness, psychomotor retardation, loss of appetite, and sleep disturbance in the prior week. Validity of the CES-D has been established through correlations with self-reported measures, clinical scores for depression, and other construct validity variables. Reliability and validity has been demonstrated across diverse characteristics of general population samples [71].	10-item short form 12-item short form	Ajrouch et al. 2010 [35]; Davey-Rothwell et al. 2014 [40]; Dressler et al. 2015 [37]; Hanson et al. 2012 [36]; Hromi-Fielder et al. 2011 [36]; Huddleston-Casas et al. 2009 [55]; Laraia et al. 2006 [56]; Laraia et al. 2009 [58]; Lent et al. 2009 [45]; McCurdy et al. 2015 [29]; Siefert et al. 2007 [63]	Bronte-Tinkew et al. 2007 [53]; Garg et al. 2015 [25]; Sharpe et al. 2016 [39]
Cohen's Perceived Stress Scale (PSS)	A 14-item self-report Likert scale that measures the degree of unpredictability of the respondents' life and the degree to which the respondent feels stress regarding these situations. Validated in young adult and post-secondary student population, the PSS correlated with physical and mental health related outcomes [77].	PSS-4 (4-item subset) 10-item short form	Laraia et al. 2006 [56]	Trapp et al. 2015 [31]; Laraia et al. 2015 [27]
Diagnostic Interview Schedule (DIS)	A structured interview designed for non-clinicians to assess and diagnose psychiatric disorders in respondents according to criteria in the Diagnostic and Statistical Manual of Mental Disorders, Fourth Edition (DSM-IV). The DIS has 19 diagnostic modules that cover different types of mental disorders. Within each module, respondents answer whether they have particular symptoms at the present, or have experienced them in the past [78].	None	Melchior et al. 2009 [44]	None
Edinburgh Postpartum Depression Scale (EPDS)	A 10-item self-report scale used to measure risk of postpartum depression in mothers within eight weeks of delivery. Items assess feelings of guilt, sleep deprivation, lack of energy, suicidality, and other general depressive symptoms experienced within the last 7 days. Validity has been examined in a sample of postpartum mothers, 6-weeks post-delivery, and compared with clinician diagnosis of depression [75].	3-item short form	None	Birmingham et al. 2011 [42]
Geriatric Depression Scale (GDS)	A 30-item self-report scale that assesses depression in geriatric populations (≥55 years). Items assess motivation, self-esteem, helplessness, mood, and agitation [76].	15-item short form	Klesges et al. 2001 [68]	Sharkey et al. 2003 [69]
Hopkins Symptom Checklist Subscale (HSCL)	A 58-item self-report scale used primarily with psychiatric outpatients, capturing five symptom dimensions including somatization, obsessive-compulsive, interpersonal sensitivity, depression, and anxiety [73]. Authors discuss a variety of studies in which the validity of the HSCL has been evaluated.	None	Klesges et al. 2001 [68]	None

Table 2. *Cont.*

Measure	Description	Abbreviated Versions	Articles Using Full Version	Articles Using Abbreviated Versions
Kemper 3-Item Screen	A 3-item self-report screening tool designed to assess maternal depressive symptoms. Validity examined with English-speaking mothers with children under 6 years of age, demonstrated 100% sensitivity and 88% specificity [74].	None	Casey et al. 2004 [54]; Chilton et al. 2013 [28]; Sun et al. 2016 [30]	None
Kessler-10 Scale	A 10-item screen developed for the US National Health Interview Survey. Designed to assess symptoms of general psychological distress through items on level of nervousness, hopelessness, lack of energy, depressive feelings, and worthlessness. Validity was examined with adults living in Australia, aged 18 years and older [79].	None	Carter et al. 2011 [43]	None
Patient Health Questionnaire (PHQ-9)	A 9-item questionnaire administered in a primary care setting by clinicians, designed to provide a diagnosis of major depressive disorder according to DSM guidelines. Items assess depressive symptoms and anhedonia experienced within the past 2 weeks. Validity was assessed among patients recruited through primary care offices, with 73% sensitivity and 94% specificity [80].	PHQ-2 (2-item subset)	Harrison et al. 2008 [60]; Sidebottom et al. 2014 [33]	Trapp et al. 2015 [31]
Pearlin's Mastery Scale	A 7-item self-report Likert scale that measures the degree of control respondents feel they have over their lives. Authors note validation with individuals aged 18 to 65 years [81].	None	Heflin et al. 2005 [62]; Laraia et al. 2006 [56]	None
Rosenberg's Self-Esteem Scale	A 10-item self-report Likert scale that assesses level of self-esteem in respondents [82].	None	Laraia et al. 2006 [56]; Laraia et al. 2009 [58]	None
SF-36 Health Survey	A 36-item health survey that consists of 5 physical health scales and 5 mental health scales. The mental component summary score is calculated from scores on 4 subscales; social functioning, role emotional, vitality, and mental health scales [83]. When tested on individuals 16–74 years of age, the SF-36 demonstrated good construct validity in patient population. Authors noted promise in use with the general population [83].	SF-12 (12-item short form)	Lent et al. 2009 [45]	Mathews et al. 2010 [34]
Spielberger's Trait Anxiety Inventory	The Spielberger State–Trait Anxiety Inventory is a 20-item tool commonly used to measure anxiety, with higher scores indicating greater levels of anxiety [72]. The American Psychological Association has noted sensitivity of this inventory to predict distress overtime in caregivers [72].	None	Laraia et al. 2006 [56]	None
World Health Organization World Mental Health Composite International Diagnostic Interview (CIDI)	A comprehensive interview designed to diagnose major depressive disorder, other depressive disorders, anxiety disorders, substance abuse, and impulse control disorders according to the World Health Organization International Classification of Disease (ICD) and DSM criteria [70]. Evaluation studies suggested good test-retest and interrater reliability, and its use in different settings and countries was deemed acceptable [84].	CIDI short form (CIDI-SF), also referred to as screening version	None	Corman et al. 2016 [24]; Heflin et al. 2005 [62]; Hernandez et al. 2014 [26]; Martin et al. 2016 [17]; Siefert et al. 2001 [44]; Whitaker et al. 2006 [59]

3.4. Overview of Findings on Food Insecurity and Mental Health

The majority of cross-sectional analyses examining depression and food insecurity (or food insufficiency) reported some form of association deemed to be significant [16,28,29,32,34–36,38–44,54,56–60,63,64,68,69,85]. Several longitudinal analyses likewise observed relationships between depression and food insecurity, with food insecurity increasing the risk of experiencing depressive symptoms or a depression diagnosis [44,53,62], or changes in food insecurity associated with changes in depression [62]. For example, a longitudinal analysis of data from 8693 parent–child dyads by Bronte-Tinkew et al. [53] found that mothers affected by food insecurity were more likely to report depressive symptoms compared to food-secure mothers. Some authors reported that the relationship functioned in the opposite direction, with depression leading to food insecurity [15,24–26,45], or was bidirectional [55]. For example, Garg et al., who analyzed data from the Early Childhood Longitudinal Study Birth Cohort (*n* = 2917), found that mothers who experienced depression were at greater risk of remaining food insecure over time compared to mothers without depression [25]. Food insecurity and depression were also investigated in relation to other markers of material deprivation; for example, Corman et al. [24] found that women who experienced a major depressive episode at baseline had greater odds of experiencing food insecurity and inadequate housing at follow-up.

Several articles focused on pregnant women and revealed associations between prenatal and postpartum depression and food insecurity [33,36,42,56,60]. Food-insecure pregnant women were at increased risk of experiencing prenatal depressive symptoms compared to their food-secure counterparts [33,36]. Although a comprehensive measure of food insecurity was not used, Birmingham et al. [42] tested depression screening methods in a cross-sectional analysis of 195 mothers of newborns and found that those who had concerns about food were 5.5 times more likely to have a positive postpartum depression screen result.

Anxiety and stress were associated with food insecurity in multiple studies [16,17,32,56,59]. Analyses of cross-sectional data from the 2007–2008 Canadian Community Health Survey (CCHS) by Tarasuk et al. (*n* = 77,053) [16] and Muldoon et al. (*n* = 5588) [32] indicated that severe food insecurity and a self-reported diagnosis of mood or anxiety disorders were associated among women. Siefert et al. [64] found an association between food insecurity and generalized anxiety disorder in a cross-sectional study of 724 US women receiving welfare, but the relationship was not significant when covariates were taken into account. In two studies, one cross-sectional (*n* = 606) [56] and one longitudinal (*n* = 526) [27], Laraia et al. found that food-insecure pregnant women had higher perceived stress compared to food-secure women, and those who had experienced any level of food insecurity during pregnancy or at three months postpartum were more likely to have high perceived stress scores at 12 months postpartum. Martin et al. [17] investigated perceived stress among Canadian adults and found that the prevalence of high levels of stress increased with lower food security status. However, Trapp et al. [31] explored food insecurity among a group of 222 low-income mothers and their children in a cross-sectional analysis and found that levels of perceived stress did not differ between food-insecure and food-secure groups.

Three recent articles explored disordered or emotional eating among women experiencing food insecurity [27,37,39]. Laraia et al. [27] and Sharpe et al. [39] found bivariate associations between food insecurity and disordered or emotional eating; however, in models adjusted for sociodemographic characteristics, Laraia et al. [27] did not observe significant associations between food insecurity and disordered eating behaviors. Dressler et al. [37] examined associations between emotional eating and depression and suggested that emotional eating may mediate associations among food insecurity, mental health, and other food-related outcomes, such as dietary intakes and weight status.

Moreover, some studies examined multiple mental and physical health conditions suggesting comorbid physical and mental health problems increased vulnerability to food insecurity [16,34] and that food insecurity increased vulnerability to poor physical and mental health [41,69]. There was also a focus on implications for others, including children, in the household. For example,

Bronte-Tinkew et al. [53] found that mothers living in food-insecure households reported high rates of depression, which was correlated with fair and poor health in children.

Given that the precise focus of the studies varied, a range of covariates was examined. Several studies examined various forms of social support [15,17,35,52,60,63]. Instrumental social support (e.g., ability to borrow money, help with childcare and transportation) was examined in a study conducted by the Detroit Centre for Oral Health Disparities. Cross-sectional analyses by Siefert et al. [63] (*n* = 824) indicated that the effect of food insufficiency on depression could be reduced with the availability of instrumental social support, while Ajrouch et al. [35] (*n* = 736) found that this protective effect was dampened when respondents experienced high levels of food insecurity-related stress. Using cross-sectional Canadian data, Martin et al. [17] (*n* = 100,401) found associations between food insecurity and feelings of community belonging; for example, the prevalences of living in severely food-insecure households were 18% and 25.6% among women reporting high and low community belonging, respectively. In a cross-sectional analysis, Wehler et al. [52] (*n* = 354) found that financial social support from a sibling reduced the odds of mothers experiencing hunger but did not reduce the odds of children in the same household experiencing hunger. Further, Hanson and Olson [15] (*n* = 225) found that parenting social support (e.g., having someone to talk to and having help in an emergency) did not reduce the odds of a household experiencing persistent vs. discontinuous food insecurity over a period of three years.

The role of childhood and adulthood adverse experiences, including abuse, was also examined. In multivariable models, Wehler et al. [52] found that sexual abuse in childhood increased the odds of adult hunger, and that this appeared to be mediated by experiences of intimate partner violence in adulthood. Sun et al. [30] examined Adverse Childhood Experiences, including abuse, neglect, and household dysfunction, and found that mothers reporting four or more adverse experiences were more likely to report food insecurity, with adjustment for demographic factors. In bivariate analyses, Harrison et al. [60] found that each of food insecurity, intimate partner violence and depressive symptoms were correlated. In multivariable models accounting for demographic factors, Melchior et al. [44] found that intimate partner violence was higher among women who had reported indications of food insecurity two years prior.

4. Discussion

Overall, the evidence reviewed here supports a link between food insecurity and compromised mental health among women in high-income countries. Although longitudinal data were limited, associations between food insecurity and depression appear to operate in both directions. There are multiple plausible potential pathways by which food insecurity and poor mental health may be linked. The experience of food insecurity itself is characterized by worry and anxiety about the household food supply. Toxic stress, which refers to chronic and unyielding stress without adequate social and environmental supports [13], may be one pathway through which food insecurity and mental health are intertwined. Depending on the availability and regularity of finances, periods of household food insecurity can occur repeatedly or chronically; households in the United States that were food insecure in 2016 experienced food insecurity in seven months on average [3]. Therefore, food insecurity may represent a chronic stressor that could contribute to the development of poor mental health. Conversely, a mental health condition could inhibit an individual from maintaining steady employment, thereby increasing vulnerability to food insecurity. Further, Seligman and Schillinger [86] posit that the relationship between food insecurity and poor health is cyclical; food insecurity increases the likelihood of trade-offs in food choices among those who receive low income and challenges the self-management of health conditions. Poor self-management results in higher health care and medication costs for the individual, which further contribute to financial instability and food insecurity [86]. Once an individual enters this cycle, it may be very difficult to exit, particularly in countries where there are disparities in access to health care and social supports, impacting access. Additionally, studies found an association between instances of abuse and depression and food insecurity [26,44,52,60]. The early life stress hypothesis argues that stressors experienced during key developmental periods can enhance vulnerability to mental health outcomes in adult life [87].

The majority of the available literature is cross-sectional, and further longitudinal research could shed light on the nature of the observed relationships and factors that underlie them. For example, research is needed to examine the interconnections among various markers of mental health and experiences of food insecurity across the lifespan, as well as to further examine the influence of potential mediating factors, such as social support or experiences of abuse. Many existing studies have focused on women with children, and pregnant women have also been investigated. A population of growing interest in regards to food insecurity is postsecondary students [88–91]; given that this is a life stage during which vulnerability to poor mental health is also high [89,92,93], research examining the root causes of both issues and how they interact is of public health importance. At the other end of the spectrum, we also identified little research focused on older women.

Food insecurity is a complex and multidimensional phenomenon [51,94] and its measurement is also complex. Many of the reviewed studies relied upon data from the HFSSM, or an adaptation, to assess food security. The HFSSM is considered the standard in household food insecurity measurement in North America and is used widely in research and surveillance [3,4]. While this tool provides an indicator of quantitative deprivation, it focuses on economic access to food and does not capture aspects that are likely to be relevant to mental health, such as the social acceptability of food acquisition strategies [51]. For example, Hamelin et al. have described alienation that accompanies lack of access to adequate food [67], as well as the social implications [95]. Nonetheless, the HFSSM has been widely-used and, within the North American context, provides data that are comparable to those from national surveys [4,8,21]. The Household Food Insecurity Access Scale (HFIAS) [94] is a standardized tool that uses similar questions as the HFSSM and is designed to differentiate food-secure from food-insecure households across cultural contexts; this tool may be appropriate depending on the setting and populations of interest. Whenever feasible, a comprehensive tool is recommended over single or brief measures that may not accurately classify households and cannot provide insights into severity of food insecurity (thus potentially missing the opportunity to shed insights into those who are most vulnerable). Additionally, studies using mixed methods can generate unique information not yielded by a standardized measure such as the HFSSM.

There was greater variety in measures used to assess mental health compared with those used to determine household food security status, the majority involving screening for depressive symptoms, along with diagnostic measures that use more stringent criteria. Many authors noted that these tools had been tested and are widely used, but the range of tools used makes it difficult to compare across studies. As with food insecurity, abbreviated measures, such as those assessing depression and depressive symptoms, may have been limited in sensitivity and specificity compared to full measures, potentially dampening observed relationships or creating spurious effects. While the use of comprehensive measures and greater standardization of tools used to assess depression and other mental health conditions may allow for greater comparability across this body of literature and more robust inferences, it is critical for any study that the measure be well suited to the research question and the population/setting.

Furthermore, much of the existing research has focused on depression; widening this scope could enable policy and program responses that consider the potential range of mental health conditions related to inadequate food access. An emerging area of research is the link between food insecurity and disordered eating; in addition to the studies reviewed here focused on women, recent findings from a study of US adult men and women accessing a food pantry indicated a positive association between food insecurity and indicators of eating disorder pathology, such as binge eating and engaging in compensatory behaviors [96]. Additionally, few studies examined food security in relation to schizophrenia/psychosis or bipolar disorder among females.

The findings of the reviewed articles should be interpreted in light of several considerations. Most of the available research is based on US populations. While several studies were conducted among subpopulations such as women with children and African-American women, more research is needed to assess how food insecurity and mental health interact with other markers of vulnerability (such as single parenthood, insecure housing, drug use, experiences of violence, and immigrant/refugee status) in diverse subgroups. The majority of studies were cross-sectional, and causal inferences were not possible. Additionally, for longitudinal studies, in some cases, it was challenging to ascertain the timing of baseline and follow-up data collections. Adherence to checklists such as STROBE (Strengthening the Reporting of Observational Studies in Epidemiology) [97] could help promote transparency and accurate interpretation. Many authors noted limitations of self-reported data on mental health outcomes and food insecurity [16,17,26,29–32,34,40,44,55,62]. Some also noted temporal incongruence between measures of food insecurity and indicators of mental health [25,39,41] that may have affected their findings. Due to the varied emphases of the studies (including assessing feasibility and other characteristics of measures), a range of covariates and potential confounders were examined; in some cases, they were used to characterize samples whereas in others, they were included in statistical models such that it is difficult to compare estimates from one study to another. Finally, explicit approaches to account for the potential conceptual overlap between food insecurity and mental health indicators, such as feelings of worry or anxiety that are conceptualized as part of the experience of food insecurity and are also markers of psychological distress, were not common.

Considerations related to the review itself also warrant highlighting. We followed methodology for a scoping study [22] and, thus, did not conduct a formal appraisal of the quality of the included evidence, nor weight the evidence. Rather, our objective was to characterize the existing literature as to identify directions for future research. Further, although we employed a systematic search strategy and careful screening, our search was broad and it is possible that some relevant articles were inadvertently excluded. Additionally, we did not consider studies that presented pooled estimates for males and females. Although our interest was in females, this does not preclude the existence of associations between food insecurity and mental health among males, as observed in some reviewed studies that include stratified analyses. Additionally, given that we relied upon published articles, we did not account for publication bias in that research not supporting relationships between food insecurity and mental health may be less likely to have been identified.

5. Conclusions

Overall, this review supports a link between food insecurity and poor mental health among women in high-income countries. Despite gaps, the existing evidence is sufficient to warrant policy and program interventions to address these major public health challenges in a coordinated manner. An underlying theme of the literature is the complex ways in which food insecurity and mental health are connected both to each other and to an array of other issues, such as experiences of violence, housing circumstances, and life transitions such as pregnancy. These links underscore the need for coordinated approaches that consider how policy and program interventions can best address these complex issues and their interactions. Such approaches may be informed by systems methods [98–100] that consider the interplay among factors and how interventions to address one issue may affect another issue, influencing overall health and well-being.

Strategies to address financial inadequacy, such as a guaranteed basic income, have been called for to reduce vulnerability to food insecurity [19,101,102], and could play a role in ameliorating mental health conditions [103]. Additionally, food security screening has been recommended within clinical settings to enable referral to available community resources [13,104–106] (although it is imperative that practitioners have effective resources to which they can make referrals). While addressing the financial circumstances that underlie food insecurity is critical, screening for food access issues among those seeking treatment for mental health conditions could help build momentum in addressing the whole person instead of tackling issues in isolation, for example, helping health practitioners to understand, and potentially address, reasons for non-adherence to recommendations related to diet or other factors. Health and social service settings with integrated care models, in which women have access to a range of services that provide support during periods of food insecurity and poor mental health, may allow complex challenges to be addressed simultaneously [107]. In addition, health care providers are uniquely positioned to support individuals in accessing services such as government income-related benefits, dietary allowance benefits, or legal supports [16,106,108], and alongside individuals with lived experience of vulnerability, to advocate for increased financial supports and access to mental health care.

Author Contributions: S.P.-M., S.I.K., and M.M. developed and conducted the search and screened articles. S.P.-M. and M.M. extracted data and C.L.-T., L.A., and S.I.K. verified data extraction. M.M., L.A. and S.I.K. led the manuscript development and all authors contributed critical revisions.

Funding: This research received no external funding. Open access fees were funded by a Canadian Cancer Society Research Institute Capacity Development Award (grant #702855) held by S.I.K.

Acknowledgments: The authors are grateful to Jackie Stapleton for her guidance on the search strategy and Mona Qutub for her assistance with referencing.

Conflicts of Interest: The authors declare no conflict of interest.

Appendix A

Table A1. Key characteristics of articles (*n* = 39 from 31 studies/surveys) included in scoping review of food insecurity and mental health among women in high-income countries, by measure of food insecurity.

Reference	Sample (Participants (Age), Setting, Race/Ethnicity, Data Source)	Study Design (Sample Size)	Purpose	Food Security Measure	Mental Health Measure	Mental Health States/Conditions	Covariates Considered	Analytic Approach and Key Findings
				Household Food Security Survey Module (HFSSM)				
			Longitudinal analyses					
Bronte-Tinkew et al. 2007 [53]	**Mothers** (mean age, 27.5 years), US, race/ethnicity not specified Early Childhood Longitudinal Study-Birth Cohort (ECLS-B)	Longitudinal (8693)	Examine association between food insecurity and child health, and examine parental depression and behaviors as mediators	USDA HFSSM	CES-D 12-item subset Authors note strong psychometric properties	Symptoms of maternal depression	Parent education, maternal employment, maternal age (at birth), family structure, receipt of food subsidy, child exposure to cigarette smoke, number of well-baby visits, household poverty index ratio	Structural equation modeling; Mothers in food-insecure households reported higher levels of depressive symptoms (β = 0.243, *p* < 0.001), which were associated parent-reported fair or poor health in children at 24 months.
Corman et al. 2016 [54]	**Mothers** (mean age, 25 years) from 75 birth hospitals in 20 US cities; included White, African American, Hispanic, and other races/ethnicities Fragile Families and Child Wellbeing Study	Longitudinal (2965)	Examine association between maternal depression in the postpartum year, housing conditions, and food insecurity	USDA HFSSM	CIDI short form Authors note that the measure has been validated	Clinical diagnosis of a MDE (defined as 3+ symptoms of dysphoria or anhedonia for most of the day for a period of at least 2 weeks) during the postpartum year (assessed at 1 year)	Maternal, paternal, and prenatal housing characteristics (measured at baseline), maternal grandparents' mental illness and child characteristics	Multivariable analysis: Compared to women who did not report depression, mothers who reported depression were more likely to experience inadequate housing at 2–3 years due to lack of heat (aOR 1.57, 95% CI 1.11–2.22) and energy insecurity (aOR 1.69, 95% CI 1.24–2.30). Depression was associated with combinations of hardships, including inadequate housing, housing instability, and food insecurity (aOR 3.85, 95% CI 1.34–11.11).
Garg et al. 2015 [55]	**Low-income mothers** (mean age, 25 years) and their young children in the US, non-Hispanic White, non-Hispanic Black, Hispanic, Asian-Pacific Islander, other races/ethnicities Early Childhood Longitudinal Study, Birth Cohort (ECLS-B)	Longitudinal (2917)	To determine impact of maternal depression on future household food insecurity in low-income households with young children.	USDA HFSSM	CES-D 12 item Authors note that the short form has been previously validated.	Depressive symptoms	Maternal and household characteristics including race/ethnicity, age, marital status, employment, education, mothers' foreign-born status, household income, and maternal self-reported health status.	Multivariable analyses: Maternal depression at baseline (9 months) was associated with food insecurity at follow-up (24 months) (aOR 1.50, 95% CI 1.06–2.12). Mothers who reported depressive symptoms and received WIC at baseline were more likely (aOR 1.59, 95% CI 1.15–2.21) to experience food insecurity at follow-up.

Table A1. *Cont.*

Reference	Sample (Participants (Age), Setting, Race/Ethnicity, Data Source)	Study Design (Sample Size)	Purpose	Food Security Measure	Mental Health Measure	Mental Health States/Conditions	Covariates Considered	Analytic Approach and Key Findings
Hanson et al. 2012 [15]	Low income, rural **mothers** (mean age, 30 years) in US, White and non-White races/ethnicities Rural Low-Income Families: Monitoring Their Well-being and Functioning in the Context of Welfare Reform	Longitudinal (225)	Examine food insecurity and various risk factors, including human capital, social support, and financial situation, among rural low-income families with children.	USDA HFSSM	CES-D 20-item	Depressive symptoms	Education, 3 or more chronic health conditions, food and financial skills, high support for parenting, home ownership at baseline, employment, housing assistance, participation in SNAP assistance, health insurance	Multivariable analyses: Compared to women having no years at risk for depression, women classified as at risk for depression for 2 consecutive years had 4.28 times greater odds of experiencing persistent versus no food insecurity ($p < 0.01$), and 3.65 times greater odds to experience persistent versus discontinuous food insecurity ($p < 0.05$).
Hernandez et al. 2014 [26]	Low-income, urban, unmarried **mothers** (mean age, 28 years) of newborn children recruited from 75 birth hospitals in 20 US cities, White, African American, Hispanic, and other races/ethnicities Fragile Families and Child Well-being Study	Longitudinal (1690)	Examine association between intimate partner violence, depression, and household food insecurity	USDA HFSSM	CIDI short form	Clinical diagnosis of depression; depressive symptoms	Mothers' age, race/ethnicity, education, employment, relationship status, household income, number of children, baseline food security	Multivariable analyses: Mothers reporting depression were twice as likely to be food-insecure two years later compared to mothers who did not report depression (aOR 2.03, 95% CI 1.45–2.84). The relationship between intimate partner violence and food insecurity among women was mediated by depression ($z = 2.89$, $p < 0.01$).
Lent et al. 2009 [45]	Rural, low-income **mothers** (18+ years), recruited through local educators, WIC and Even Start programs in New York, US, majority White. Rural Families Speak: Tracking the Well-Being and Functioning of Rural Families in the Context of Welfare Policies Study	Longitudinal (mixed methods) (29)	Examine the temporal/causal relationship and potential mechanisms between mental health conditions such as depression and household food insecurity	USDA HFSSM	CES-D 20-item, SF-36 Health Survey (mental health scales: Vitality, Social Functioning, Role Emotional, Mental Health)	Depressive symptoms	Not applicable	Unadjusted analyses: High levels of depressive symptoms (according to the CES-D) at wave 2 were correlated with remaining food-insecure at wave 3 ($p = 0.009$); reverse relationship not significant. Unhealthy scores on the mental health scores at wave 2 were also associated with remaining food-insecure at wave 3 ($p = 0.01$). Qualitative analyses suggest that poor mental health contributes to persistence of food insecurity by limiting employment.

Table A1. *Cont.*

Reference	Sample (Participants (Age), Setting, Race/Ethnicity, Data Source)	Study Design (Sample Size)	Purpose	Food Security Measure	Mental Health Measure	Mental Health States/Conditions	Covariates Considered	Analytic Approach and Key Findings
Huddleston-Casasin et al. 2009 [35]	Rural mothers (mean age, 30 years) recruited from programs serving low-income populations 17 US states, included White, African American, Latina, and other races/ethnicities NC-223, Rural Families Speak Study	Longitudinal (413)	Examine direction of the relationship between household food insecurity and depression over three annual waves of data	USDA HFSSM	CES-D 20-item Authors note that reliability in this sample matched that documented for the general population	Depressive symptoms	Age, ethnicity, household income, marital status, education	Structural equation modeling (using data for 413 women, with sensitivity analysis with 184 women who had depression data for three waves): A bidirectional relationship between food insecurity and depression ($X^2/df = 1.835$, RMSEA = 0.068, CFI = 0.989) was observed.
Laraia et al. 2015 [27]	Pregnant women (16+ years), US, included White, Black, other races/ethnicities Pregnancy, Infection, and Nutrition (PIN) Postpartum study, recruited from University of North Carolina Hospitals and private clinics	Longitudinal (526)	To examine relationship between food insecurity and perceived stress, disordered eating, dietary intake, and postpartum weight status	USDA HFSSM, 18 items (between 27 and 30 weeks' gestation) and 6-item short form (12 months postpartum)	Cohen's Perceived Stress Scale (PSS) 10-item, Eating Attitude Test (EAT) 26 item Authors note that Cohen's Perceived Stress has been validated in pregnant women	Perceived stress, disordered eating	Maternal race, age, marital status, education, parity, physical activity, smoking during pregnancy and postpartum, breastfeeding postpartum, poverty level	Multivariable analyses: Women living in food-insecure households during pregnancy had higher levels of perceived stress (β = 3.36, 95% CI 0.79–5.92) and higher scores for disordered eating (β = 1.95, 95% CI 0.25–4.16) at 3 months postpartum and higher levels of perceived stress (β = 3.67, 95% CI 0.94–6.41) at 12 months postpartum compared to those living in food-secure households during pregnancy. Women who experienced any level of household food insecurity during the postpartum period had higher perceived stress (β = 6.12, 95% CI 3.86–8.38), and higher scores for disordered eating (β = 1.79, 95% CI 0.03–3.62) compared to women in food-secure households.

Table A1. *Cont.*

Cross-sectional analyses

Reference	Sample (Participants (Age), Setting, Race/Ethnicity, Data Source)	Study Design (Sample Size)	Purpose	Food Security Measure	Mental Health Measure	Mental Health States/Conditions	Covariates Considered	Analytic Approach and Key Findings
Casey et al. 2004 [54]	Female **caregivers** (age not specified), US, women of African American, White, and Hispanic race/ethnicity Recruited from medical centers in several large US cities	Cross-sectional (5306)	Examine nature of the relationship between depression, food insecurity, and loss of social assistance and its impact on child health	USDA HFSSM	Kemper 3-item screen Authors note sensitivity of 100%, specificity of 88%, and positive predictive value of 66% compared to an 8-item screening instrument	Maternal depressive symptoms	Study site location, race, insurance type, education, and low birth weight	Multivariable analysis: Mothers experiencing food insecurity had greater odds of positive depression screen compared to those from food secure households (aOR 2.69, 95% CI 2.33–3.11). Mothers experiencing a decrease or sanction in food stamp status had increased odds of reporting a positive depression screen, compared to those with no decrease in food stamp status (aOR 1.26, 95% CI 0.97–1.65 and aOR 1.56 95% CI 1.06–2.30, respectively).
Chilton et al. 2013 [28]	**Mothers** (mean age, 26.7 years) in Philadelphia, US, African American, White, Hispanic races/ethnicities Recruited from public assistance programs through the Children's Health Watch study	Cross-sectional (mixed methods) (44)	Explore aspects of exposure to violence related to food insecurity among lone mother households.	USDA HFSSM	Kemper 3-item screen	Maternal depressive symptoms	Not applicable	Descriptive estimates: A higher proportion of mothers living with very low food security reported depressive symptoms (71%) compared to those with low food security (53%) and food-secure (17%) mothers. Women living with very low food security (53%) were more likely to have experienced life-changing violence in childhood compared to those with low food security (33%) and food secure (33%) mothers.
McCurdy et al. 2015 [29]	Low-income **mothers** (mean age, 30.1 years) and children recruited from 7 preschools in low-income urban neighborhoods in the US; included Hispanic and non-Hispanic races/ethnicities	Cross-sectional (166)	To determine correlates of weight, including food security, among low-income, ethnically diverse mothers and examine role of mental health	USDA HFSSM	CES-D 20-item Authors note high internal consistency for the measure and note acceptable internal reliability in this sample	Depressive symptoms	Not applicable	Bivariate analyses: Mothers living in food-insecure households had more depressive symptoms compared to food-secure mothers (t = 2.26, p < 0.02).

Table A1. *Cont.*

Reference	Sample (Participants (Age), Setting, Race/Ethnicity, Data Source)	Study Design (Sample Size)	Purpose	Food Security Measure	Mental Health Measure	Mental Health States/Conditions	Covariates Considered	Analytic Approach and Key Findings
Sun et al. 2016 [30]	**Mothers** (mean age, 24 years) of young children (aged < 4 years), US, non-Hispanic White, non-Hispanic Black, Hispanic, other races/ethnicities, recruited from Philadelphia hospitals.	Cross-sectional (1255)	To examine association between adverse childhood experiences among mothers and household and child food insecurity determine associations with depressive symptoms	USDA HFSSM	Kemper 3-Item Screen, ACEs scale for Adverse Childhood Experiences Authors note that the Kemper 3-item is validated as a proxy for a longer screener with 100% sensitivity, 88% specificity, and 66% positive predictive value, and ACEs scale has been validated and shown to have good test-retest reliability.	Depressive symptoms, adverse childhood experiences, such as abuse, neglect, and household dysfunction	Caregiver's age and self-rated health, caregiver's participation in nutrition programs, race/ethnicity, marital status, employment, education, and child's health insurance,	Depressive symptoms were reported among, 18.4% of women in food-secure households, 48.6% of those in households with low food security, and 54.4% of those in households with very low food security (*p* < 0.01). Multivariable analyses: Mothers who reported depressive symptoms and 4+ adverse childhood experiences were 2.3 times (95% CI 1.0–5.3) as likely to report low food security, 6.6 times (95% CI 2.1–20.5) as likely to report indications of very low food security compared to those reporting depressive symptoms but no adverse childhood experiences. In addition, mothers who reported depressive symptoms and 4+ adverse childhood experiences were 17.6 times (95% CI 7.3–42.6) as likely to report child food insecurity compared to those who reported no depressive symptoms and no adverse childhood experiences.
Trapp et al. 2015 [31]	Low-income children (2–4 years) and **mothers** (18+ years), US, Hispanic, African-American races/ethnicities Steps to Growing Up Health study, primary care-based intervention	Cross-sectional (222)	Examine relationship between food security, diet, and weight status among urban preschool children, and examine whether maternal depression and stress acts as a mediator	USDA HFSSM	PHQ-2, Cohen's Perceived Stress Scale 4-item subset (PSS-4) Authors note that the PHQ-2 has good validity, and identified the sensitivity and specificity of the cutoff used for risk for major depression	Depressive symptoms and perceived stress	Household size, primary home language, marital status, employment, household income	Bivariate analyses: Mothers living in food-insecure households were more likely to report depressive symptoms compared to food-secure mothers (27% vs. 9%; *p* < 0.001), but perceived stress scores were not different between food-insecure and food-secure mothers (*p* = 0.5).

Table A1. *Cont.*

Reference	Sample (Participants (Age), Setting, Race/Ethnicity, Data Source)	Study Design (Sample Size)	Purpose	Food Security Measure	Mental Health Measure	Mental Health States/Conditions	Covariates Considered	Analytic Approach and Key Findings
Laraia et al. 2006 [56]	Low-income **pregnant women** (mean age, 29 years), US, included African American, White, and other races/ethnicities Pregnancy, Infection, and Nutrition (PIN) cohort study, recruited from University of North Carolina Hospitals and private clinics	Cross-sectional (606)	Examine prevalence and determinants of food insecurity among pregnant women from medium- and low-income women	USDA HFSSM	Cohen's Perceived Stress Scale 14-item, Spielberger's Trait Anxiety Inventory 20-item, CES-D 20-item, Rosenberg's Self Esteem Scale 10-item, Pearlin's Mastery Scale 7-item, Levenson's IPC Locus of Control 24-item Authors note stability and internal consistency of measures	Perceived stress, anxiety, depressive symptoms, self-esteem, mastery, locus of control	Mother's age, number of children, household income, education, race, marital status	Multivariable analyses: Perceived stress (aOR 2.24, 95% CI 1.63–3.08), trait anxiety (aOR 2.14, 95% CI 1.55–2.96), depressive symptoms (aOR 1.87, 95% CI 1.40–2.51), and feeling that ones' destiny is up to chance (aOR 1.67, 95% CI 1.20–2.32) were positively associated with household food insecurity. Women living in food-insecure households were less likely to report feelings of mastery over their lives (aOR 0.49, 95% CI 0.35–0.68) and high self-esteem (aOR 0.52, 95% CI 0.38–0.69).
Muldoon et al. 2013 [32]	Adults (18–64 years), Canada 2007–2008 Canadian Community Health Survey	Cross-sectional (sample subset of 5588 reporting indications of food insecurity in the past year)	Examine rates of mental illness among Canadian adults who lived in food-insecure households with and without hunger	USDA HFSSM (Health Canada coding)	Self-reported diagnosis of chronic health conditions diagnosed by a health professional	Clinical diagnoses of mood or anxiety disorders	Education, age, single parent household status, immigrant status	Multivariable analyses: Females experiencing food insecurity with hunger had greater odds (aOR 1.89, 95% CI 1.62–2.20) of reporting a depression diagnosis compared to women who did not report food insecurity with hunger.
Tarasuk et al. 2013 [16]	Adults (18–64 years), Canada 2007–2008 Canadian Community Health Survey	Cross-sectional (77,053)	Examine whether chronic physical and mental conditions health conditions are associated with household food insecurity	USDA HFSSM (Health Canada coding)	Self-reported presence of chronic health conditions diagnosed by a health professional	Clinical diagnoses of mood or anxiety disorders	Age, sex, province, education, household type, median household income, main source of household income, and home ownership	Multivariable analysis: Self-reported diagnoses of 3 or more chronic physical and mental health conditions raised the odds of a woman experiencing severe food insecurity (aOR 2.15, 95% CI 1.50–3.10) compared to fewer or no chronic conditions Among women in food-secure households, 11.6% reported mood or anxiety disorders; among those in marginally food-secure, moderately food-insecure, and severely food-insecure households, the prevalences were 20.3%, 26.8%, and 47.1%, respectively.

Table A1. *Cont.*

Reference	Sample (Participants (Age), Setting, Race/Ethnicity, Data Source)	Study Design (Sample Size)	Purpose	Food Security Measure	Mental Health Measure	Mental Health States/Conditions	Covariates Considered	Analytic Approach and Key Findings
Abbreviated/adapted versions of Household Food Security Survey Module (HFSSM)								
Longitudinal analyses								
Melchior et al. 2009 [44]	**Mothers** of twins (average 35.5 years) from England and Wales, Britain, included White and non-White races/ethnicities. Environmental Risk Study	Longitudinal (1116)	Examine the association between food insecurity and maternal depression, psychosis spectrum disorder, alcohol or drug abuse, and intimate partner violence	USDA HFSSM, 7-item short form	Diagnostic Interview Schedule (DIS)	Depressive symptoms, Psychotic symptoms	Mother's age, income, ethnicity, marital status, household size, mother's employment, mother's reading ability	Multivariable analyses: Food insecurity increased the odds of depression (OR 2.12, 95% CI 1.61–4.93), intimate partner violence (OR 2.36, 95% CI 1.18–4.73), and psychosis (OR 4.01, 95% CI 2.03–7.94) among women two years later. Food insecurity was associated with mental illness comorbidity in mothers—29% of food-insecure mothers had experienced mental health problems or intimate partner violence.
Sidebottom et al. 2014 [63]	**Pregnant women** (mean age, 22 years) recruited from Health Centres in Minneapolis and St. Paul, US, included African American, American Indian, Asian/Pacific Islander, Hispanic (any race), White, and bi/multiracial women Data from the Twin Cities Healthy Start Program	Longitudinal (prenatal and postpartum assessments) (594)	Examine correlates of depression in pregnancy and postpartum period	USDA HFSSM, 4-item subset	PHQ-9 with modification of the item measuring psychomotor issues (split into 2 questions but scored as one) Authors noted sensitivity of 77%, specificity of 94%, and positive predictive value of 59% in primary care populations, with higher values in populations with a high prevalence of depressive disorder	Depressive symptoms	Age, race/ethnicity, foreign-born, lack of social support, abuse of any kind, child protection involvement, living with child's father, drug, alcohol and cigarette use, lack of phone access, and housing instability	Multivariable analyses: Compared to women who had low depressive symptom levels in both the prenatal and postpartum periods, the odds of elevated depressive symptoms prenatally were higher (aOR 2.44, 95% CI 1.43–4.16) among those with low levels of food security. Food security and depressive symptoms in the postpartum period were not related.

Table A1. *Cont.*

Cross-sectional analyses

Reference	Sample (Participants (Age), Setting, Race/Ethnicity, Data Source)	Study Design (Sample Size)	Purpose	Food Security Measure	Mental Health Measure	Mental Health States/Conditions	Covariates Considered	Analytic Approach and Key Findings
Whitaker et al. 2006 [59]	Mothers (18+ years) of 3-year old children, recruited from 75 birth hospitals in 20 US cities. Included White, African American, Hispanic, other races/ethnicities Fragile Families and Child Wellbeing Study	Cross-sectional (2870)	Examine if food security is associated with prevalence of depression and anxiety in mothers and behavior problems in children	USDA HFSSM, 10 adult-referenced items	CIDI short form administered 3 years after child's birth, modified cut-off for a major depressive episode (MDE) based on symptoms of anhedonia	Clinical diagnosis of a MDE or generalized anxiety disorder (GAD) in the prior 12 months	Mother's education, race/ethnicity, relationship status, employment in previous year, binge drinking, illicit drug use, global health, prenatal smoking, prenatal physical domestic violence, household income/poverty ratio, number of children, non-food related material hardship, and whether father was ever in jail	Multivariable analyses: Compared to fully food-secure mothers, experiencing marginal food insecurity increased the odds of experiencing an MDE or GAD (aOR 1.4, 95% CI 1.1–1.8; and aOR 1.7, 95% CI 1.0–2.7, respectively). Compared to fully food-secure mothers, experiencing food insecurity increased the odds of experiencing an MDE or GAD (aOR 2.2, 95% CI 1.6–2.9; and aOR 2.3, 95% CI 1.5–3.6 respectively). Mothers experiencing food insecurity twice as likely to also experience either MDE or GAD compared to food-secure mothers (aOR 2.2, 95% CI 1.6–2.9).
Laraia et al. 2009 [58]	African American, first-time **mothers** (18–35 years) recruited from Special Supplemental Nutrition Program for Women, Infants, and Children (WIC) clinics in North Carolina, US Infant Care, Feeding, and Risk of Obesity observational study	Cross-sectional analysis of longitudinal study, focused on 3-month postpartum baseline data (206)	Identify maternal and household correlates of food insecurity among African-American mothers	USDA HFSSM, 6-item short form	CES-D, Rosenberg Self-Esteem Scale	Depressive symptoms and self-esteem	Maternal age, education, work status, depression score, and self-esteem, as well as household composition (presence of father, grandmother and household size)	Bivariate analyses: Women living in food-insecure households had significantly higher scores on the depressive scale compared to food-secure women (p < 0.05). Multivariable analyses: Depressive symptoms were associated with marginal food security and food insecurity (aRRR * 1.04, 95% CI 1.00–1.08 and aRRR * 1.10, 95% CI 1.04–1.16, respectively). Self-esteem scores were negatively associated with risk for marginal food security and food insecurity (aRRR * 0.91, 95% CI 0.84–0.98, and aRRR * 0.89, 95% CI 0.79–0.99, respectively) * aRRR = adjusted Relative Risk Ratio.

Table A1. *Cont.*

Reference	Sample (Participants (Age), Setting, Race/Ethnicity, Data Source)	Study Design (Sample Size)	Purpose	Food Security Measure	Mental Health Measure	Mental Health States/Conditions	Covariates Considered	Analytic Approach and Key Findings
Mathews et al. 2010 [34]	**Mothers (<25 years)** recruited from the Special Supplemental Nutrition Program for Women, Infants, and Children (WIC) clinics in Butte County, California, US, included White, non-White races/ethnicities	Cross-sectional (155)	Evaluate the prevalence of and associations between food insecurity and health status among women participating in WIC	USDA HFSSM, 6-item short form	SF-12 Health Survey Authors noted that the SF-12 has been validated previously	General mental (and physical) health symptoms	Diet choice score, income, ethnicity, age, education	Bivariate analyses: Women experiencing low or very low food insecurity had significantly lower mental health scores, indicating more mental health symptoms compared to food-secure women ($p < 0.001$). The correlation between food insecurity and mental health scores indicates that as women's food security increased, mental health also increases. Multivariable analyses: The likelihood of having a good mental health score was lower (OR 0.41, 95% CI 0.16–0.73) among those in food-insecure versus those in food-secure households.
Ajrouch et al. 2010 [35]	Female African-American **caregivers (mean age, 30.8 years)** of young children recruited from high-poverty census tracts in Detroit, US Detroit Centre for Research on Oral Health Disparities.	Cross-sectional (multiple waves of data collection, relevant variables were assessed in wave 2) (736)	Explore link between situational stressors, including food insufficiency, psychological distress, and examine social support as a potential mediator	USDA HFSSM, 3-item subset (referred to as food insufficiency) Cronbach's alpha reported as 0.79	CES-D 20-item Authors noted high internal reliability in this sample	Depressive symptoms	Age, self-rated health, and education level	Multivariable analyses: Higher food insufficiency associated with higher depressive symptoms (referred to as psychological distress) ($\beta = 2.88$, $p < 0.001$). At high levels of stress, social support was not a mediator of this relationship.
Hromi-Fiedler et al. 2011 [36]	Low income, **pregnant Latina women** (mean age, 25 years), recruited from local agencies and programs in Hartford, Connecticut, US.	Cross-sectional (135)	Assess relationship between household food insecurity and prenatal depressive symptoms	USDA HFSSM, 15-item subset adapted version for pregnant Latinas Authors note that the adapted version was validated for this population	CES-D 20-item Authors note that the CES-D has been validated with multi-ethnic samples, including Mexican-Americans	Prenatal depressive symptoms	Parity, heartburn during pregnancy, self-reported health during pregnancy, history of depression, Latina subgroup, acculturation	Multivariable analyses: Women experiencing food insecurity were more likely to report high levels of prenatal depressive symptoms compared to those who were food secure (aOR 2.59, 95% CI 1.03–6.52).

Table A1. *Cont.*

Reference	Sample (Participants (Age), Setting, Race/Ethnicity, Data Source)	Study Design (Sample Size)	Purpose	Food Security Measure	Mental Health Measure	Mental Health States/Conditions	Covariates Considered	Analytic Approach and Key Findings
Harrison et al. 2008 [60]	**Pregnant women** in Minneapolis and St. Paul, US; included African American, Asian/Pacific Islander, Hispanic, American Indian, White, bi/multiracial races/ethnicities. recruited from Federally Qualified Health Centres Feasibility study associated with Twin Cities Healthy Start Program	Cross-sectional (1386)	Examine the prevalence, co-occurrence, and inter-correlations of self-reported psychosocial risk factors, including food insecurity.	USDA HFSSM, 4-item subset	PHQ-9, intimate partner violence items, 8 items from the Maternal Social Support Index Authors note high levels of internal reliability, test-retest reliability, sensitivity, and specificity for PHQ-9	Depressive symptoms	Not applicable	Bivariate analyses: Depressive symptoms (r = 0.267), social support (r = 0.194), and intimate partner violence (r = 0.173) were significantly correlated ($p \leq$ 0.0001) with household food insecurity.
Martin et al. 2016 [17]	Adults (18–75 years), Canada Data from the 2009–2010 Canadian Community Health Survey	Cross-sectional (100,401)	To examine the co-occurrence of food insecurity and mental illness across varying levels of stress and community belonging	USDA HFSSM, 10 adult-referenced items (Health Canada coding)	Self-reported diagnosis of a mood or anxiety disorder, subsample (n = 47,942) completed CIDI short form, one item for each of perceived stress and community belonging	Clinical diagnosis of a mood disorder such as depression, bipolar disorder, mania, or dysthymia; or an anxiety disorder such as phobia, obsessive-compulsive disorder, or panic disorder. Past 12 months of major depression from CIDI short form.	Age, marital status, children in house, household income, education, unemployment, and self-perceived physical health, as well as overall stress level and community belonging.	Multivariable analyses: Women living in severely food-insecure households had 18.4% (95% CI 16.7–20.1) greater adjusted prevalence of a mental disorder compared to those living in food-secure households. The prevalence of women reporting high levels of stress increased with worsening food security. Greater proportions of severely food-insecure women reported low community belonging compared to more food-secure women. Interaction between community belonging, food insecurity, and perceived stress not significant.

Table A1. *Cont.*

Reference	Sample (Participants (Age), Setting, Race/Ethnicity, Data Source)	Study Design (Sample Size)	Purpose	Food Security Measure	Mental Health Measure	Mental Health States/Conditions	Covariates Considered	Analytic Approach and Key Findings
Dressler et al. 2015 [7]	Low-income women (18–64 years) recruited from homeless shelters, food pantries, libraries, soup kitchens, and community centers, US, included African American, White, Native American women	Cross-sectional (330)	Examine depression and its relationship with food insecurity, weight status, emotional eating, and dietary intake among low-income women	USDA HFSSM, 6-item short form	CES-D 20-item, emotional eating questions developed using validated questionnaires. Authors note that the CES-D is valid and reliable and note the internal consistency in the sample for both the CES-D and the emotional eating questions	Symptoms of depression and emotional eating	Not applicable	Bivariate analyses: Women categorized as depressed had higher food insecurity scores compared to women who were not depressed (3.2 vs. 1.9, $p < 0.05$). Depression and emotional eating were also associated.
Kaiser et al. 2007 [5]	Women (18+ years) living in California, US, included White, African American, Hispanic/Latino, and other races/ethnicities. 2004 California Women's Health Survey	Cross-sectional (4037)	Identify factors associated with food insecurity	USDA HFSSM, 6-item subset, modified to refer to respondent and not to other adults in household	Indicators of mental or emotional problems	Mental, (physical), or emotional problems that interfere with daily life, feeling depressed or sad, and feeling overwhelmed	Income as a proportion of the federal poverty ratio	Multivariable analyses: Higher food insecurity was associated with feeling depressed or sad for 2+ days in the prior month (aOR 1.61, 95% CI 1.28–2.02), feeling overwhelmed in past 30 days (aOR 3.10, 95% CI 2.49–3.85), and reporting that physical or mental health conditions interfered with normal activities in past 30 days (aOR 1.81, 95% CI 1.45–2.27).
Peterman et al. 2013 [8]	Cambodian women (30–65 years) recruited from clients of the Cambodian Mutual Assurance Association of Lowell, Massachusetts, US Cambodian Community Health Program 2010	Cross-sectional (150)	Examine post-immigration experiences with food, food security status, and correlates among refugee women	USDA HFSSM, 6-item short form	Harvard Program in Refugee Trauma's depression scale; 14 items, previously translated and validated for use in Cambodian refugee populations	Clinical diagnosis of depression	Marital status, receipt of food stamps, income to poverty ratio, acculturation, age	Multivariable analyses: Women experiencing marginal/low/very low food security were more likely (aOR 3.73, 95% CI 1.26–11.05) to be classified as depressed compared to those in food-secure households.

Table A1. *Cont.*

Reference	Sample (Participants (Age), Setting, Race/Ethnicity, Data Source)	Study Design (Sample Size)	Purpose	Food Security Measure	Mental Health Measure	Mental Health States/Conditions	Covariates Considered	Analytic Approach and Key Findings
Sharpe et al. 2016 [39]	Low-income women (25–51 years) recruited from 18 census tracts in which 25% or more of residents had below-poverty income in South Carolina, US, mainly African-American Sisters Taking Action for Real Success (STARS) trial	Cross-sectional (202)	Examine whether on diet quality and psychosocial and behavioral factors are associated with household food security	USDA HFSSM, 6-item short form	CES-D 10 item, emotional eating subscale of the Eating Behavior Patterns Questionnaire Authors noted that the CESD-10 has been validated and that the Eating Behavior Patterns Questionnaire has been shown to have acceptable internal consistency and construct validity in African-American women; authors also identified Cronbach's alphas for both measures in the study sample	Symptoms of depression and emotional eating	Not applicable	Bivariate analyses: Women experiencing food insecurity had significantly higher scores for depressive symptoms (indicating more symptoms) compared to women living in food-secure households (mean score 10.9 (SD 6.1) vs. 8.3 (SD 5.0), t = 3.36, p < 0.001). Women experiencing food insecurity had significantly lower emotional eating scores (indicating higher levels of emotional eating) compared to women living in food-secure households (mean score 10.2 (SD 3.1) vs. 11.4 (SD 3.8), t = 2.45, p < 0.02).
Davey-Rothwell et al. 2014 [40]	Low-income women (18–55 years) at risk for HIV, recruited through street outreach and public advertisements in the US, majority African-American women Data from the CHAT study	Cross-sectional (based on 6-month visit) (443)	Explore food insecurity among drug-using and non-drug-using women and examine the relationship between depression and food insecurity	USDA HFSSM, 4-item subset Authors noted acceptable internal consistency in this sample	CES-D 20-item Authors noted high internal consistency in this sample	Depressive symptoms	Age, race, income, receipt of food stamps	Multivariable analyses: Drug-users were 2.71 times (aOR, 95% CI 1.51–4.88), and non-drug-users were 5.9 times (aOR, 95% CI 2.80–12.45) more likely to experience depression if they were food insecure compared to food secure.

Table A1. *Cont.*

Reference	Sample (Participants (Age), Setting, Race/Ethnicity, Data Source)	Study Design (Sample Size)	Purpose	Food Security Measure	Mental Health Measure	Mental Health States/Conditions	Covariates Considered	Analytic Approach and Key Findings
Radimer–Cornell Scale								
Cross-sectional analyses								
Sharkey et al. 2011 [...]	Urban and rural women (18+ years) living in Brazos Valley, Texas, US, included White and non-White races/ethnicities Brazos Valley Health Status Assessment	Cross-sectional (1367)	Examine health status, mental distress, and household food insecurity among urban and rural women	Radimer–Cornell Scale, first item focused on food deprivation (food we bought did not last and we did not have enough money to buy more) was used to determine presence of household food insecurity Authors noted that the Scale has been shown to be valid for non-white participants	Centre for Disease Control (CDC) and the Behavioral Risk Factor Surveillance Systems (BRFSS) questionnaire to assess health-related quality of life (perceived mental—and general and physical—well-being —thinking about your mental health, which includes stress, depression, and problems with emotions, for how many days during the past 30 days was your mental health not good? Authors noted that the measures have been shown to be valid for non-white populations	Perceived mental health (stress, depression, problems with emotions), referred to as frequent mental distress	Age, race, education, annual household income, employment, rural vs. urban geographic location	Multivariable analyses: Women experiencing food insecurity in the last 30 days were more likely to frequently experience mental distress compared to food-secure women (aOR 2.25, 95% CI 1.59–3.18)

Table A1. *Cont.*

Reference	Sample (Participants (Age), Setting, Race/Ethnicity, Data Source)	Study Design (Sample Size)	Purpose	Food Security Measure	Mental Health Measure	Mental Health States/Conditions	Covariates Considered	Analytic Approach and Key Findings
				Community Childhood Hunger Identification Project (CCHIP) measure				
				Cross-sectional analyses				
Wehler et al. 2004 [52]	Homeless and housed women (mean age, 28 years) recruited from Worcester's homeless shelters and welfare hostels and the Department of Public Welfare office, US, included White, African American, Hispanic, and other races/ethnicities. Worcester Family Research Project	Cross-sectional (354)	Examine factors associated with adult or child hunger among low-income housed and homeless female-headed families	CCHIP: 7 items querying adult and child hunger. Authors noted high level of internal consistency and factor analysis indicated a single-factor solution	Structured Clinical Interview for Diagnostic Statistical Manual (DSM-III-R non-patient edition), Life Experiences Survey	Clinical diagnosis of substance use, depression, posttraumatic stress disorder (PTSD), major life events in adulthood (e.g., violence)	Age, ethnicity, housing status, marital status, acculturation, parenting status, parent substance abuse, foster care status, number and age of children, income, psychological factors (coping and parental hassles), social service utilization, social network size	Exploratory analytic approach identified factors differentiating families with child hunger from those with no hunger; these did not include the mental health factors. Multivariable analyses: The experience of sexual abuse in childhood increased the odds of adult hunger (aOR: 4.23, 95% CI 2.28–7.82); intimate partner violence in adulthood and a PTSD diagnosis appeared to be mediators of the childhood sexual abuse–current hunger association. Financial support from a sibling reduced the odds of experiencing food insecurity.
				NHANES-III food insufficiency indicators				
				Longitudinal analyses				
Heflin et al. 2005 [62]	Mothers (18–54 years) receiving public assistance in urban Michigan, US, included African American, non-Hispanic White races/ethnicities. Women's Employment Study	Longitudinal (753)	Examine effect of food insecurity on the mental health status of welfare recipients over a 3-year period	NHANES-III food insufficiency question. Authors noted that this measure is widely accepted as a valid measure of food insufficiency	CIDI short form, Pearlin Mastery Scale 7 item	Clinical diagnosis of depression, mastery (degree to which individuals perceive themselves to be in control of their own lives)	Household size, marital status, household income, poverty-related stressful life circumstances, neighborhood hazards, domestic violence, experiences of discrimination based on race and gender	Multivariable fixed effects models: Changes in food insecurity significantly predict changes in major depression status after adjusting for changes in household composition and socio-environmental stressors ($\beta = 0.75$, SE 0.24, $p < 0.01$). No association observed between changes in food insufficiency status and changes in mastery.

Table A1. *Cont.*

Reference	Sample (Participants (Age), Setting, Race/Ethnicity, Data Source)	Study Design (Sample Size)	Purpose	Food Security Measure	Mental Health Measure	Mental Health States/Conditions	Covariates Considered	Analytic Approach and Key Findings
				Cross-sectional analyses				
Siefert et al. 2001 [64]	Single women receiving welfare (mean age, 28 years) living in urban Michigan, US; included African-American, White women Women's Employment Study	Cross-sectional (724)	Examine relationship between food insufficiency and physical and mental health among low-income women	NHANES-III food insufficiency question Authors noted that this measure is widely accepted as a valid measure of food insufficiency	CIDI short form Authors noted that acceptable test-retest reliability and clinical validity have been observed	Clinical diagnosis of major depressive disorder and generalized anxiety disorder	Self-rated health, physical limitations, age, number of children in the household, education level, poverty level, employment, poverty-related stressful life events and conditions	Multivariable analyses: Food insufficiency significantly predicted major depressive disorder (aOR 2.21, 95% CI 1.48–3.29). The association between food insufficiency and generalized anxiety disorder, adjusted for covariates, was not significant.
Siefert et al. 2007 [65]	African-American mothers (mean age, 28 years) recruited from 39 high-poverty census areas in Detroit, US Detroit Center for Research on Oral Health Disparities	Cross-sectional (multiple waves of data collection, relevant variables were assessed in wave 1) (824)	Determine correlates of depressive symptoms among low-income mothers	NHANES-III food insufficiency question Authors noted that this measure is widely accepted as a valid measure of food insufficiency	CES-D, 20-item Authors noted that the CES-D is a reliable and well-validated sale, with standard scoring widely used in research, four-factor structure found in the general population has also been found in African-Americans with low socioeconomic status	Depressive symptoms	Living in poorly maintained housing, not being employed, experiences of everyday discrimination, instrumental and emotional social support, age, education, household size, number of children <18 years of age, income	Bivariate analyses: Mothers with depressive symptoms more likely to report household food insufficiency (14.5%) compared to women without depressive symptoms (6%). Multivariable analyses: In models adjusted for income and education, living in a food-insufficient household was associated with 2.5 greater odds (95% CI 1.25–4.98) of maternal depressive symptoms. Instrumental social support was a protective factor.
				Other brief measures				
				Cross-sectional analyses				
Birmingham et al. 2011 [62]	Mothers of newborns (mean age, 25 years), US; included African American, Hispanic, White, Asian, other races/ethnicities, recruited from urban pediatric emergency departments	Cross-sectional (195)	To examine the performance of the Edinburgh Postpartum Depression Scale (EPDS) for screening patients in emergency departments, and examine correlates of postpartum depression	2 items querying worry about the food supply and inability to eat the way you should due to lack of money	EPDS 3-item short form	Postpartum depressive symptoms	Maternal age, ethnicity, education, marital status, employment, maternal health problems, health insurance, household income, household size, father's presence in the home, social support, infant health and health insurance,	Multivariable analyses: Having concerns about food increased odds (aOR 5.5, 95% CI 2.2–13.5) of postpartum depression.

Table A1. *Cont.*

Reference	Sample (Participants (Age), Setting, Race/Ethnicity, Data Source)	Study Design (Sample Size)	Purpose	Food Security Measure	Mental Health Measure	Mental Health States/Conditions	Covariates Considered	Analytic Approach and Key Findings
Carter et al. 2011 [43]	General population (15+ years) in New Zealand, included NZ/European, Maori, Pacific, Asian, and other groups. New Zealand Survey of Families, Income, and Employment, 2002–2010	Cross-sectional (18,090)	Examine association between food insecurity and psychological distress	Food security items from measure of individual deprivation (NZiDep): 3 items querying use of food banks and food compromises due to lack of money for food in last 12 months	Kessler-10 scale	Symptoms of psychological distress	Age, ethnicity, legal marital status, family composition, household income, employment, highest level of education, individual-level deprivation	Multivariable analyses: Women who experienced food insecurity were more likely to report moderate to high levels of psychological distress (OR 2.1, 95% CI 1.8–2.4).
Klesges et al. 2001 [68]	Disabled women (65+ years) living in the community in Baltimore, US, primarily White women. Women's Health and Aging Study	Cross-sectional (1001)	Examine prevalence and correlates of financial difficulty acquiring food	Single item, self-perception of food sufficiency "How often does it happen that you (and your husband) do not have enough money to afford the kind of food you should have?" Authors note that such single-item measures have shown validity in discriminating energy intake differences, but have poor sensitivity and underestimate prevalence	Geriatric Depression Scale (GDS),Hopkins Symptom Checklist subscale for anxiety, 20-item perceived quality of life scale	Symptoms of depression, anxiety, quality of life	Age, marital status, and number of household members	Multivariable analyses: In non-white women, depression was associated with financial difficulty accessing food (aOR 1.13, 95% CI 1.04–1.22). This association not significant among white women after adjusting for covariates.
Sharkey et al. 2003 [69]	Women (60+ years) who are homebound (as a result of disability, illness, or isolation), recruited from meal delivery programs in North Carolina, US, included African-American and White women. Nutrition and Function Study (NAFS)	Cross-sectional (279)	Examine food sufficiency and association with dietary intake and burden of multiple diseases	Four items adapted from a national nutrition evaluation survey, 2 situations related to lack of food, 2 related to making trade-offs between food and other necessities. Authors noted that the items were previously used in a national evaluation of elderly nutrition programs	Geriatric Depression Scale (GDS) 15-item short form	Depressive symptoms	Not applicable	Bivariate analyses: Women experiencing food insufficiency had higher prevalence of 6 or more depressive symptoms (52% vs. 26%, p = 0.03) and disease multi-morbidity (74% vs. 41%, p < 0.001) compared to those who were food sufficient.

References

1. Gregory, C.A.; Coleman-Jensen, A. *Food Insecurity, Chronic Disease, and Health among Working-Age Adults*; Economic Research Report, 235; U.S. Department of Agriculture, Economic Research Service: Washington, DC, USA, 2017. Available online: https://www.ers.usda.gov/webdocs/publications/84467/err-235_summary.pdf?v=42942 (accessed on 27 June 2018).

2. Tarasuk, V.; Mitchell, A.; Dachner, N. Household Food Insecurity in Canada, 2014. 2016. Available online: http://proof.utoronto.ca/resources/proof-annual-reports/annual-report-2014/ (accessed on 27 June 2018).

3. Coleman-Jensen, A.; Rabbitt, M.P.; Gregory, C.; Singh, A. *Household Food Security in the United States in 2016*; Economic Research Report; United States Department of Agriculture: Washington, DC, USA, 2017. Available online: https://www.ers.usda.gov/webdocs/publications/84973/err237_summary.pdf?v=42979 (accessed on 27 June 2018).

4. Tarasuk, V.; Mitchell, A.; Dashner, N. Household Food Insecurity in Canada, 2012. 2014. Available online: http://proof.utoronto.ca/resources/proof-annual-reports/annual-report-2012/ (accessed on 27 June 2018).

5. Bates, B.; Roberts, C.; Lepps, H.; Porter, L. The Food & You Survey: Wave 4. 2017. Available online: https://www.food.gov.uk/sites/default/files/media/document/food-and-you-w4-exec-summary.pdf (accessed on 27 June 2018).

6. Lindberg, R.; Lawrence, M.; Gold, L.; Friel, S.; Pegram, O. Food insecurity in Australia: Implications for general practitioners. *Aust. Fam. Physician* **2015**, *44*, 859–863. [PubMed]

7. FAO. Agriculture and Development Economics Division. *Food Security: Policy Brief.* 2006. Available online: http://www.fao.org/fileadmin/templates/faoitaly/documents/pdf/pdf_Food_Security_Cocept_Note.pdf (accessed on 27 June 2018).

8. Bickel, G.; Nord, M.; Price, C.; Hamilton, W.; Cook, J. *Guide to Measuring Household Food Security*; USDA: Alexandria, VA, USA, 2000. Available online: https://fns-prod.azureedge.net/sites/default/files/FSGuide.pdf (accessed on 27 June 2018).

9. Entmacher, J.; Robbins, K.; Vogtman, J.; Morrison, A. *Insecure and Unequal: Poverty and Income among Women and Families, 2000–2013*; National Women's Law Center: Washington, DC, USA, 2014; Available online: https://nwlc.org/resources/insecure-unequal-poverty-and-income-among-women-and-families-2000-2013/ (accessed on 27 June 2018).

10. Maheux, H.; Chui, T. *Women in Canada: A Gender-Based Statistical Report*; Statistics: Ottawa, ON, Canada, 2011; Available online: https://www150.statcan.gc.ca/n1/pub/89-503-x/89-503-x2010001-eng.htm (accessed on 27 June 2018).

11. Semega, J.L.; Fontenot, K.R.; Kollar, M.A. Income and Poverty in the United States: 2016. Current Population Reports; 2017. Available online: https://www.census.gov/library/publications/2017/demo/p60-259.html (accessed on 27 June 2018).

12. Ivers, L.C.; Cullen, K.A. Food insecurity: Special considerations for women. *Am. J. Clin. Nutr.* **2011**, *94*, 1740S–1744S. [CrossRef] [PubMed]

13. Knowles, M.; Rabinowich, J.; Ettinger de Cuba, S.; Cutts, D.B.; Chilton, M. "Do you wanna breathe or eat?": Parent perspectives on child health consequences of food insecurity, trade-offs, and toxic stress. *Matern. Child Health J.* **2015**, *20*, 25–32. [CrossRef] [PubMed]

14. Kirkpatrick, S.I.; Tarasuk, V. Food insecurity is associated with nutrient inadequacies among Canadian adults and adolescents. *J. Nutr.* **2008**, *138*, 604–612. [CrossRef] [PubMed]

15. Hanson, K.L.; Olson, C.M. Chronic health conditions and depressive symptoms strongly predict persistent food insecurity among rural low-income families. *J. Health Care Poor Underserved.* **2012**, *23*, 1174–1188. [CrossRef] [PubMed]

16. Tarasuk, V.; Mitchell, A.; McLaren, L.; McIntyre, L. Chronic physical and mental health conditions among adults may increase vulnerability to household food insecurity. *J. Nutr.* **2013**, *143*, 1785–1793. [CrossRef] [PubMed]

17. Martin, M.S.; Maddocks, E.; Chen, Y.; Gilman, S.E.; Colman, I. Food insecurity and mental illness: Disproportionate impacts in the context of perceived stress and social isolation. *Public Health* **2016**, *132*, 86–91. [CrossRef] [PubMed]

18. McIntyre, L.; Williams, J.V.A.; Lavorato, D.H.; Patten, S. Depression and suicide ideation in late adolescence and early adulthood are an outcome of child hunger. *J. Affect. Disord.* **2013**, *150*, 123–129. [CrossRef] [PubMed]

19. Jessiman-Perreault, G.; McIntyre, L. The household food insecurity gradient and potential reductions in adverse population mental health outcomes in Canadian adults. *SSM Popul. Health* **2017**, *3*, 464–472. [CrossRef] [PubMed]

20. Davison, K.M.; Marshall-Fabien, G.L.; Tecson, A. Association of moderate and severe food insecurity with suicidal ideation in adults: National survey data from three Canadian provinces. *Soc. Psychiatry Psychiatr. Epidemiol.* **2015**, *50*, 963–972. [CrossRef] [PubMed]

21. Health Canada. *Canadian Community Health Survey, Cycle 2.2, Nutrition (2004): Income-related Household Food Security in Canada*; No. 4696; HC Publisher: Ottawa, ON, Canada, 2007; Available online: https://www.canada.ca/content/dam/hc-sc/migration/hc-sc/fn-an/alt_formats/hpfb-dgpsa/pdf/surveill/income_food_sec-sec_alim-eng.pdf (accessed on 27 June 2018).

22. Arksey, H.; O'Malley, L. Scoping studies: Towards a methodological framework. *Int. J. Soc. Res. Methodol.* **2005**, *8*, 19–32. [CrossRef]

23. Moher, D.; Liberati, A.; Tetzlaff, J.; Altman, D.G.; Grp, P. Preferred reporting items for systematic reviews and meta-analyses: The PRISMA statement (reprinted from annals of internal medicine). *Phys. Ther.* **2009**, *89*, 873–880. [PubMed]

24. Corman, H.; Curtis, M.A.; Noonan, K.; Reichman, N.E. Maternal depression as a risk factor for children's inadequate housing conditions. *Soc. Sci. Med.* **2016**, *149*, 76–83. [CrossRef] [PubMed]

25. Garg, A.; Toy, S.; Tripodis, Y.; Cook, J.; Cordella, N. Influence of maternal depression on household food insecurity for low-income families. *Acad Pediatr.* **2015**, *15*, 305–310. [CrossRef] [PubMed]

26. Hernandez, D.C.; Marshall, A.; Mineo, C. Maternal depression mediates the association between intimate partner violence and food insecurity. *J. Womens Health* **2014**, *23*, 29–37. [CrossRef] [PubMed]

27. Laraia, B.; Vinikoor-Imler, L.C.; Siega-Riz, A.M. Food insecurity during pregnancy leads to stress, disordered eating, and greater postpartum weight among overweight women. *Obesity* **2015**, *23*, 1303–1311. [CrossRef] [PubMed]

28. Chilton, M.M.; Rabinowich, J.R.; Woolf, N.H. Very low food security in the USA is linked with exposure to violence. *Public Health Nutr.* **2013**, *17*, 1–10. [CrossRef] [PubMed]

29. McCurdy, K.; Kisler, T.; Gorman, K.S.; Metallinos-Katsaras, E. Food- and health-related correlates of self-reported body mass index among low-income mothers of young children. *J. Nutr. Educ. Behav.* **2015**, *47*, 225–233. [CrossRef] [PubMed]

30. Sun, J.; Knowles, M.; Patel, F.; Frank, D.A.; Heeren, T.C.; Chilton, M. Childhood adversity and adult reports of food insecurity among households with children. *Am. J. Prev. Med.* **2016**, *50*, 561–572. [CrossRef] [PubMed]

31. Trapp, C.M.; Burke, G.; Gorin, A.A.; Wiley, J.F.; Hernandez, D.; Crowell, R.E.; Grant, A.; Beaulieu, A.; Cloutier, M.M. The relationship between dietary patterns, body mass index percentile, and household food security in young urban children. *Child. Obes.* **2015**, *11*, 148–155. [CrossRef] [PubMed]

32. Muldoon, K.A.; Duff, P.K.; Fielden, S.; Anema, A. Food insufficiency is associated with psychiatric morbidity in a nationally representative study of mental illness among food insecure Canadians. *Soc. Psychiatry Psychiatr. Epidemiol.* **2013**, *48*, 795–803. [CrossRef] [PubMed]

33. Sidebottom, A.C.; Hellerstedt, W.L.; Harrison, P.A.; Hennrikus, D. An examination of prenatal and postpartum depressive symptoms among women served by urban community health centers. *Arch. Womens Ment. Health* **2014**, *17*, 27–40. [CrossRef] [PubMed]

34. Mathews, L.; Morris, M.N.; Schneider, J.; Goto, K. The relationship between food security and poor health among female WIC participants. *J. Hunger Environ. Nutr.* **2010**, *5*, 85–99. [CrossRef]

35. Ajrouch, K.J.; Reisine, S.; Lim, S.; Sohn, W.; Ismail, A. Situational stressors among African-American women living in low-income urban areas: The role of social support. *Women Health* **2010**, *50*, 159–175. [CrossRef] [PubMed]

36. Hromi-Fiedler, A.; Bermúdez-Millán, A.; Segura-Pérez, S.; Pérez-Escamilla, R. Household food insecurity is associated with depressive symptoms among low-income pregnant Latinas. *Matern. Child Nutr.* **2011**, *7*, 421–430. [CrossRef] [PubMed]

37. Dressler, H.; Smith, C. Depression affects emotional eating and dietary intake and is related to food insecurity in a group of multiethnic, low-income women. *J. Hunger Environ. Nutr.* **2015**, *10*, 496–510. [CrossRef]

38. Peterman, J.N.; Wilde, P.E.; Silka, L.; Bermudez, O.I.; Rogers, B.L. Food insecurity among Cambodian refugee women two decades post resettlement. *J. Immigr. Minor. Health* **2013**, *15*, 372–380. [CrossRef] [PubMed]

39. Sharpe, P.A.; Whitaker, K.; Alia, K.A.; Wilcox, S.; Hutto, B. Dietary intake, behaviors and psychosocial factors among women from food-secure and food-insecure households in the United States. *Ethn Dis.* **2016**, *26*, 139–146. [CrossRef] [PubMed]

40. Davey-Rothwell, M.A.; Flamm, L.J.; Kassa, H.T.; Latkin, C.A. Food insecurity and depressive symptoms: Comparison of drug using and nondrug-using women at risk for HIV. *J. Commun. Psychol.* **2014**, *42*, 469–478. [CrossRef] [PubMed]

41. Sharkey, J.R.; Johnson, C.M.; Dean, W.R. Relationship of household food insecurity to health-related quality of life in a large sample of rural and urban women. *Women Health* **2011**, *51*, 442–460. [CrossRef] [PubMed]

42. Birmingham, M.C.; Chou, K.J.; Crain, E.F. Screening for postpartum depression in pediatric emergency department. *Pediatr. Emerg. Care* **2011**, *27*, 795–800. [CrossRef] [PubMed]

43. Carter, K.N.; Kruse, K.; Blakely, T.; Collings, S. The association of food security with psychological distress in New Zealand and any gender differences. *Soc. Sci. Med.* **2011**, *72*, 1463–1471. [CrossRef] [PubMed]

44. Melchior, M.; Caspi, A.; Howard, L.M.; Ambler, A.P.; Bolton, H.; Mountain, N.; Moffitt, T.E. Mental health context of food insecurity: A representative cohort of families with young children. *Pediatrics* **2009**, *124*, e564–e572. [CrossRef] [PubMed]

45. Lent, M.D.; Petrovic, L.E.; Swanson, J.A.; Olson, C.M. Maternal mental health and the persistence of food insecurity in poor rural families. *J. Health Care Poor Underserved.* **2009**, *20*, 645–661. [CrossRef] [PubMed]

46. Wunderlich, G.S.; Norwood, J. *Food Insecurity and Hunger in the United States: An Assessment of the Measure*; National Academies Press: Washington, DC, USA, 2006; Available online: https://www.nap.edu/catalog/11578/food-insecurity-and-hunger-in-the-united-states-an-assessment (accessed on 27 June 2018).

47. Radimer, K.L.; Olson, C.M.; Greene, J.C.; Campbell, C.C.; Habicht, J.P. Understanding hunger and developing indicators to assess it in women and children. *J. Nutr. Educ.* **1992**, *24*, 36S–44S. [CrossRef]

48. Wehler, C.A.; Scott, R.I.; Anderson, J. The community child hunger identification project: A model of domestic hunger—Demonstration project in Seattle, Washington. *J. Nutr. Educ.* **1992**, *24* (Suppl. 1), 29S–35S.

49. Frongillo, E.A., Jr.; Rauschenbach, B.S.; Olson, C.M.; Kendall, A.; Colmenares, A.G. Questionnaire-based measures are valid for the identification of rural households with hunger and food insecurity. *J. Nutr.* **1997**, *127*, 699–705. [CrossRef] [PubMed]

50. Briefel, R.R.; Woteki, C. Development of food sufficiency questions for the third national health and nutrition examination survey. *J. Nutr. Educ.* **1992**, *24* (Suppl. 1), 24S–28S. [CrossRef]

51. Tarasuk, V. Discussion Paper on Household and Individual Food Insecurity. 2001. Available online: https://www.canada.ca/en/health-canada/services/food-nutrition/healthy-eating/nutrition-policy-reports/discussion-paper-household-individual-food-insecurity-2001.html (accessed on 27 June 2018).

52. Wehler, C.; Weinreb, L.F.; Huntington, N.; Scott, R. Risk and protective factors for adult and child hunger among low-income housed and homeless female-headed families. *Am. J. Public Health* **2004**, *94*, 109–115. [CrossRef] [PubMed]

53. Bronte-Tinkew, J.; Zaslow, M.; Capps, R.; Horowitz, A.; McNamara, M. Food insecurity works through depression, parenting, and infant feeding to influence overweight and health in toddlers. *J. Nutr.* **2007**, *137*, 2160–2165. [CrossRef] [PubMed]

54. Casey, P.; Goolsby, S.; Berkowitz, C.; Frank, D.; Cook, J.; Cutts, D.; Black, M.M.; Zaldivar, N.; Levenson, S.; Heeren, T.; et al. Maternal depression, changing public assistance, food security, and child health status. *Pediatrics* **2004**, *113*, 298–304. [CrossRef] [PubMed]

55. Huddleston-Casas, C.; Charnigo, R.; Simmons, L.A. Food insecurity and maternal depression in rural, low-income families: A longitudinal investigation. *Public Health Nutr.* **2009**, *12*, 1133–1140. [CrossRef] [PubMed]

56. Laraia, B.A.; Siega-Riz, A.M.; Gundersen, C.; Dole, N. Psychosocial factors and socioeconomic indicators are associated with household food insecurity among pregnant women. *J. Nutr.* **2006**, *136*, 177–182. [CrossRef] [PubMed]

57. Kaiser, L.; Baumrind, N.; Dumbauld, S. Who is food-insecure in California? Findings from the California Women's Health Survey, 2004. *Public Health Nutr.* **2007**, *10*, 574–581. [CrossRef] [PubMed]

58. Laraia, B.A.; Borja, J.B.; Bentley, M.E. Grandmothers, fathers, and depressive symptoms are associated with food insecurity among low-income first-time African-American mothers in North Carolina. *J. Am. Diet. Assoc.* **2009**, *109*, 1042–1047. [CrossRef] [PubMed]

59. Whitaker, R.C.; Phillips, S.M.; Orzol, S.M. Food insecurity and the risks of depression and anxiety in mothers and behavior problems in their preschool-aged children. *Pediatrics* **2006**, *118*, e859–e868. [CrossRef] [PubMed]

60. Harrison, P.A.; Sidebottom, A.C. Systematic prenatal screening for psychosocial risks. *J. Health Care Poor Underserved.* **2008**, *19*, 258–276. [CrossRef] [PubMed]

61. United States Centers for Disease Control and Prevention. Third National Health and Nutrition Examination Survey (NHANES III), 1988–94: NHANES-III Household Adult Data File Documentation, Ages 17+. Available online: https://wwwn.cdc.gov/nchs/nhanes/nhanes3/DataFiles.aspx (accessed on 27 June 2018).

62. Heflin, C.M.; Siefert, K.; Williams, D.R. Food insufficiency and women's mental health: Findings from a 3-year panel of welfare recipients. *Soc. Sci. Med.* **2005**, *61*, 1971–1982. [CrossRef] [PubMed]

63. Siefert, K.; Finlayson, T.L.; Williams, D.R.; Delva, J.; Ismail, A.I. Modifiable risk and protective factors for depressive symptoms in low-income African American mothers. *Am. J. Orthopsychiatr.* **2007**, *77*, 113–123. [CrossRef] [PubMed]

64. Siefert, K.; Heflin, C.M.; Corcoran, M.E.; Williams, D.R. Food insufficiency and the physical and mental health of low-income women. *Women Health* **2001**, *32*, 159–177. [CrossRef] [PubMed]

65. Salmond, C.; Crampton, P.; King, P.; Waldegrave, C. NZiDep: A New Zealand index of socioeconomic deprivation for individuals. *Soc. Sci. Med.* **2006**, *62*, 1474–1485. [CrossRef] [PubMed]

66. Kendall, A.; Olson, C.; Frongillo, E.A., Jr. Validation of the Radimer/Cornell measures of hunger and food insecurity. *J. Nutr.* **1995**, *125*, 2793–2801. [PubMed]

67. Hamelin, A.M.; Beaudry, M.; Habicht, J.P. Characterization of household food insecurity in Québec: Food and feelings. *Soc. Sci. Med.* **2002**, *54*, 119–132. [CrossRef]

68. Klesges, L.M.; Pahor, M.; Guralnik, J.M.; Shorr, R.I.; Williamson, J.D. Financial difficulty acquiring food among elderly disabled women: Results from the Women's Health and Aging Study (WHAS). *Am. J. Public Health* **2001**, *91*, 68–75. [PubMed]

69. Sharkey, J.R. Risk and presence of food insufficiency are associated with low nutrient intakes and multimorbidity among homebound older women who receive home-delivered meals. *J. Nutr.* **2003**, *133*, 3485–3491. [CrossRef] [PubMed]

70. World Health Organization. WHO WMH-CIDI Instruments. *World Health Organization.* 2018. Available online: https://www.hcp.med.harvard.edu/wmhcidi/about-the-who-wmh-cidi/ (accessed on 27 June 2018).

71. Radloff, L.S. The CES-D scale: A self-report depression scale for research in the general population. *Appl. Psychol. Meas.* **1977**, *1*, 385–401. [CrossRef]

72. American Psychological Association. The State-Trait Anxiety Inventory (STAI). 2018. Available online: http://www.apa.org/pi/about/publications/caregivers/practice-settings/assessment/tools/trait-state.aspx (accessed on 27 June 2018).

73. Derogatis, L.R.; Lipman, R.S.; Rickels, K.; Uhlenhuth, E.H.; Covi, L. The Hopkins Symptom Checklist (HSCL): A self-report symptom inventory. *Behav. Sci.* **1974**, *19*, 1–15. [CrossRef] [PubMed]

74. Kemper, K.J.; Babonis, T.R. Screening for maternal depression in pediatric clinics. *Am. J. Dis. Child.* **1992**, *146*, 876–878. [CrossRef] [PubMed]

75. Cox, J.L.; Holden, J.M.; Sagovsky, R. Detection of postnatal depression: Development of the 10-item Edinburgh Postnatal Depression Scale. *Br. J. Psychiatry* **1987**, *150*, 782–786. [CrossRef] [PubMed]

76. Yesavage, J.A.; Brink, T.L.; Rose, T.L.; Lum, O.; Huang, V.; Adey, M.; Leirer, V.O. Development and validation of a geriatric depression screening scale: A preliminary report. *J. Psychiatr. Res.* **1982**, *17*, 37–49. [CrossRef]

77. Cohen, S.; Kamarck, T.; Mermelstein, R. A global measure of perceived stress. *J. Health Soc. Behav.* **1983**, *24*, 385–396. [CrossRef] [PubMed]

78. Weiner, I.B.; Craighead, W.E. Diagnostic Interview Schedule for DSM-IV (DIS-IV). In *The Corsini Encyclopedia of Psychology*; John Wiley & Sons Inc.: Hoboken, NJ, USA, 2009.

79. Andrews, G.; Slade, T. Interpreting scores on the Kessler Psychological Distress Scale (K10). *Aust. N. Z. J. Public Health* **2010**, *25*, 494–497. [CrossRef]

80. Kroenke, K.; Spitzer, R.L.; Williams, J.B.W. The PHQ-9: Validity of a brief depression severity measure. *J. Gen. Intern. Med.* **2001**, *16*, 606–613. [CrossRef] [PubMed]

81. Pearlin, L.I.; Menaghan, E.G.; Lieberman, M.A.; Mullan, J.T. The stress process. *J. Health Soc. Behav.* **1981**, *22*, 337–356. [CrossRef] [PubMed]

82. Rosenberg, M. *Society and the Adolescent Self-Image*; Princeton University Press: Princeton, NJ, USA, 1965.

83. Brazier, J.E.; Harper, R.; Jones, N.M.B.; O'Cathain, A.; Thomas, K.J.; Usherwood, T.; Westlake, L. Validating the SF-36 health survey questionnaire: New outcome measure for primary care. *Br. Med. J. Gen. Pract.* **1992**, *305*, 160–164. [CrossRef]

84. Wittchen H-UU. Reliability and validity studies of the WHO—Composite International Diagnostic Interview (CIDI): A critical review. *J. Psychiatr. Res.* **1994**, *28*, 57–84.

85. Weinreb, L.; Wehler, C.; Perloff, J.; Scott, R.; Hosmer, D.; Sagor, L.; Gundersen, C. Hunger: Its impact on children's health and mental health. *Pediatrics* **2002**, *110*, e41. [CrossRef] [PubMed]

86. Seligman, H.K.; Schillinger, D. Hunger and socioeconomic disparities in chronic disease. *N. Engl. J. Med.* **2010**, *363*, 6–9. [CrossRef] [PubMed]

87. Garner, A.S.; Shonkoff, J.P.; Siegel, B.S.; Dobbins, M.I.; Earls, M.F.; Garner, A.S.; Shonkoff, J.P. Early childhood adversity, toxic stress, and the role of the pediatrician: Translating developmental science into lifelong health. *Pediatrics* **2012**, *129*, e224–e231. [PubMed]

88. Bruening, M.; van Woerden, I.; Todd, M.; Laska, M.N. Hungry to learn: The prevalence and effects of food insecurity on health behaviors and outcomes over time among a diverse sample of university freshmen. *Int. J. Behav. Nutr. Phys. Act.* **2018**, *15*. [CrossRef] [PubMed]

89. Bruening, M.; Argo, K.; Payne-Sturges, D.; Laska, M.N. The struggle is real: A systematic review of food insecurity on postsecondary education campuses. *J. Acad. Nutr. Diet.* **2017**, *117*, 1767–1791. [CrossRef] [PubMed]

90. Farahbakhsh, J.; Hanbazaza, M.; Ball, G.D.C.; Farmer, A.P.; Maximova, K.; Willows, N.D. Food insecure student clients of a university-based food bank have compromised health, dietary intake and academic quality. *Nutr. Diet.* **2017**, *74*, 67–73. [CrossRef] [PubMed]

91. Bruening, M.; Brennhofer, S.; van Woerden, I.; Todd, M.; Laska, M. Factors related to the high rates of food insecurity among diverse, urban college freshmen. *J. Acad. Nutr. Diet.* **2016**, *116*, 1450–1457. [CrossRef] [PubMed]

92. O'Connell, M.E.; Boat, T.; Warner, K. *Preventing Mental, Emotional, and Behavioral Disorders among Young People: Progress and Possibilities*; National Academies Press: Washington, DC, USA, 2009. Available online: https://www.ncbi.nlm.nih.gov/books/NBK32775/ (accessed on 27 June 2018).

93. Kessler, R.C.; Berglund, P.; Demler, O.; Jin, R.; Merikangas, K.R.W.E. Lifetime prevalence and age-of-onset distributions of DSM-IV disorders in the National Comorbidity Survey replication. *Arch. Gen. Psychiatry* **2005**, *62*, 593–602. [CrossRef] [PubMed]

94. Coates, J.; Swindale, A.; Bilinsky, P. *Household Food Insecurity Access Scale (HFIAS) for Measurement of Food Access: Indicator Guide*; FANTA III; Food and Nutrition Technical Assistance: Washington, DC, USA, 2007; Available online: https://www.fantaproject.org/monitoring-and-evaluation/household-food-insecurity-access-scale-hfias (accessed on 27 June 2018).

95. Hamelin, A.-M.; Habicht, J.-P.; Beaudry, M. Food insecurity: Consequences for the household and broader social implications. *J. Nutr.* **1999**, *129*, 525S–528S. [CrossRef] [PubMed]

96. Becker, C.B.; Middlemass, K.; Taylor, B.; Johnson, C.; Gomez, F. Food insecurity and eating disorder pathology. *Int. J. Eat. Disord.* **2017**, *50*, 1031–1040. [CrossRef] [PubMed]

97. Vandenbroucke, J.P.; Von Elm, E.; Altman, D.G.; Gøtzsche, P.C.; Mulrow, C.D.; Pocock, S.J.; Poole, C.; Schlesselman, J.J.; Egger, M. Strengthening the Reporting of Observational Studies in Epidemiology (STROBE): Explanation and elaboration. *PLoS Med.* **2007**, *4*, 1628–1654. [CrossRef] [PubMed]

98. Sterman, J.D. Learning from evidence in a complex world. *Am. J. Public Health* **2006**, *96*, 505–514. [CrossRef] [PubMed]

99. Mabry, P.L.; Marcus, S.E.; Clark, P.I.; Leischow, S.J.; M'Endez, D. Systems science: A revolution in public health policy research. *Am. J. Public Health* **2010**, *100*, 1161–1163. [CrossRef] [PubMed]

100. Friel, S.; Pescud, M.; Malbon, E.; Lee, A.; Carter, R.; Greenfield, J.; Cobcroft, M.; Potter, J.; Rychetnik, L.; Meertens, B. Using systems science to understand the determinants of inequities in healthy eating. *PLoS ONE* **2017**, *12*, e0188872. [CrossRef] [PubMed]

101. Tarasuk, V. Implications of a basic income guarantee for household food insecurity. In *Basic Income Guarantee Series*; Research Paper No. 24; Northern Policy Institute: Thunder Bay, ON, USA, 2017; Available online: http://proof.utoronto.ca/wp-content/uploads/2017/06/Paper-Tarasuk-BIG-EN-17.06.13-1712.pdf (accessed on 27 June 2018).
102. Public Policy and Food Insecurity Fact Sheet. *PROOF Food Insecurity Policy Research*; Public Policy and Food Insecurity Fact Sheet: Toronto, ON, USA, 2016; Volume 41, Available online: http://proof.utoronto.ca/wp-content/uploads/2016/06/public-policy-factsheet.pdf (accessed on 27 June 2018).
103. Forget, E.L. The town with no poverty: The health effects of a Canadian income guaranteed annual income field experiment. *Can. Public Policy* **2011**, *37*, 283–305. [CrossRef]
104. American Academy of Pediatrics Council on Community Pediatrics, Committee on Nutrition. Promoting food security for all children. *Pediatrics* **2015**, *136*, e1431–e1438.
105. Tarasuk, V.; Cheng, J.; de Oliveira, C.; Dachner, N.; Gundersen, C.; Kurdyak, P. Association between household food insecurity and annual health care costs. *Can. Med. Assoc. J.* **2015**, *187*, E429–E436. [CrossRef] [PubMed]
106. Holben, D.H.; Marshall, M.B. Position of the academy of nutrition and dietetics: Food Insecurity in the United States. *J. Acad. Nutr. Diet.* **2017**, *117*, 1991–2002. [CrossRef] [PubMed]
107. McGorry, P.; Tanti, C.; Stokes, R.E.A. Australia's national youth mental health foundation—Where young minds come first. *MJS* **2007**, *187*, 5–8.
108. Pinto, A.D.; Bloch, G.; Bloch, G. Framework for building primary care capacity to address the social determinants of health. *Can. Fam. Physician* **2017**, *63*, 476–482.

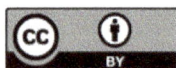

International Journal of
Environmental Research and Public Health

MDPI

Article

Household Food Insecurity Narrows the Sex Gap in Five Adverse Mental Health Outcomes among Canadian Adults

Geneviève Jessiman-Perreault and Lynn McIntyre *

Department of Community Health Sciences, Cumming School of Medicine, University of Calgary,
Calgary, AB T2N 1N4, Canada; gjessima@ucalgary.ca
* Correspondence: lmcintyr@ucalgary.ca; Tel.: +1-403-220-8664

Received: 1 October 2018; Accepted: 22 January 2019; Published: 24 January 2019

Abstract: The sex gap (i.e., the significant difference in an outcome between men and women) in the occurrence of a variety of mental health conditions has been well documented. Household food insecurity has also repeatedly been found to be associated with a variety of poor mental health outcomes. Although both sex and household food insecurity have received attention individually, rarely have they been examined together to explore whether or how these indicators of two social locations interact to impact common mental health outcomes. Using a pooled sample (N = 302,683) of the Canadian Community Health Survey (2005–2012), we test whether sex modifies the relationship between household food insecurity assessed by the Household Food Security Survey Module and five adverse mental health outcomes, controlling for confounding covariates. Although the sex gap was observed among food secure men versus women, males and females reporting any level of food insecurity were equally likely to report adverse mental health outcomes, compared with those reporting food security. Therefore, household food insecurity seems to narrow the sex gap on five adverse mental health outcomes.

Keywords: household food insecurity; mental health; sex; Canadian adults

---

1. Introduction

The sex gap (i.e., the significant difference in the occurrence of a health outcome between males and females) in mental health conditions has been consistently documented and re-examined [1–3]. The sex gap in mental health outcomes (typically cited as a nearly 2:1 ratio for women versus men reporting depression [4]) has also remained stable across decades. While the exact mechanism underlying drivers of the sex gap in mental health outcomes remains elusive, researchers have begun to examine the sex gap in the context of other important social determinants of health such as age [5], marital status [6], and sexual orientation [7]. This study examines the relationship between sex and five common mental health outcomes in the context of household food insecurity.

1.1. Household Food Insecurity in Canada and Adverse Mental Health Outcomes

Household food insecurity is operationally defined as the lack of access to food because of financial constraints [8] and in Canada, it is measured through national survey responses to the Household Food Security Survey Module (HFSSM) [9,10]. Using this metric, recent national estimates indicate that in 2012, 12.5% of Canadian households experienced some form of food insecurity (4.1% marginal food insecurity, 5.7% moderate food insecurity, and 2.7% severe food insecurity) [8]. Certain subsets of the population—groups most often associated with material deprivation—have a disproportionate risk of reporting household food insecurity; this includes Indigenous Canadians, African Canadians, households that rely on social assistance as their main income source, lone-mother led households, and those who rent rather than own their own home [8].

There is a large and robust body of literature establishing the relationship between household food insecurity and a variety of physical health problems. Adults and children living in food insecure households report poorer physical health; increased physical limitations; and higher prevalence of diabetes mellitus, heart disease, and other chronic conditions [11–13]. Furthermore, those living in food insecure households with pre-existing chronic health problems, such as diabetes, experience increased difficulties managing those conditions [14].

In addition to being associated with poorer physical health, there is a growing body of evidence that household food insecurity is associated with poor mental health and an increased risk of reporting certain mental health conditions, including psychological distress [15], mood and anxiety disorders [12,15], suicidal ideation [15], self-reported fair/poor mental health [16,17], depression [13,17–19], and psychiatric morbidity [20]. Recent research has reported that increasing severity of household food insecurity is associated with a graded increase in the risk of reporting six common mental health outcomes among Canadian adults [21].

Household food insecurity is hypothesized to be associated with poor mental health because of the unique social, physical, and psychological stresses associated with being in a food insecure household [22]. Interestingly, there is evidence that the relationship between household food insecurity and mental health could be bidirectional. Managing a food insecure household is extremely difficult and requires substantial planning [23]; therefore, individuals with pre-existing mental health conditions may be at increased risk of becoming food insecure as a result of the impact of the known symptoms of mental health conditions, such as a lack of energy, fatigue, loss of interest, and impairment of decision making, on the ability of the individual to manage a food insecure household [24,25].

1.2. Household Food Insecurity, Gender/Sex, and Mental Health

Much of the research studying the impact of gender (i.e., the sociocultural expression of biological sex) on household food insecurity and mental health has been conducted on lone mothers. Researchers focusing on this topic have observed that a disproportionate number of food insecure households are led by mothers with a history of depression, psychosis spectrum disorder, or domestic violence [24]. Mothers reporting household food insecurity are also at increased risk of either a major depressive episode or a generalized anxiety disorder at every level of household food insecurity severity (21% for moderate, 30.3% for severe) compared with food secure mothers (16.9%) [19]. Food insecure women may occupy a distinct social position that makes them more susceptible to food management stressors. For example, women have been shown to protect other household members against food insecurity by reducing their food intake to allow other household members to have more food [26,27]. Moreover, women predominantly hold the responsibility for providing and preparing food, which, in the context of food insecurity, may increase levels of stress felt by women [27].

Comparatively little research has been conducted on the mental health of males reporting household food insecurity. The results from in-depth interviews indicate that food insecure men report similar precursors to mental illness as women, such as feelings of powerless, guilt, embarrassment, shame, inequity, and frustration [28]. These emotions, in conjunction with heightened levels of stress associated with food insecurity, could plausibly result in higher levels of mental health conditions. In cross-sectional surveys, men experiencing household food insecurity report a higher prevalence of mood or anxiety disorders compared with food secure men, but those figures are lower than the rates of mood and anxiety disorders observed in food insecure women [12]. Past research on the mental health of males has highlighted that simply being male may not provide equal privilege in mental health, particularly for males who occupy different social locations of disadvantage [29]. We suggest that household food insecurity may be one such social location of disadvantage for males.

This study's research questions are specifically as follows:

1. How is household food insecurity related to the reporting of five adverse mental health outcomes (depressive thoughts in the past month, anxiety disorders, mood disorders, suicidal ideation, and self-reported mental health) in Canadian adult men and women?

2. How is the sex gap in the reporting of five adverse mental health outcomes in Canadian adults changed by concurrent consideration of household food insecurity status, controlling for common socio-demographic covariates?

2. Materials and Methods

2.1. Data Source

The study sample (N = 302,683) was generated by pooling four cycles (Cycle 3.1 [2005], 2007–2008, 2009–2010, and 2011–2012) of the Canadian Community Health Survey (CCHS). The CCHS is a nationally representative series of cross-sectional surveys structured to collect information annually on a variety of issues relating to health including health status, health care utilization, and health determinants [30]. The target population, sampling procedure, and sample sizes are all determined by Statistics Canada. The CCHS is divided by health region and reflects estimates according to health region and province/territories, as well as the Canadian population as a whole. The CCHS collects data from a randomly selected person within a household aged 12 or older residing in a dwelling in the ten provinces and three territories. Individuals living on reserves or Crown land, in institutions, in remote regions, or who are members of the Armed Forces are not included in the survey. The CCHS data sample represents approximately 98% of the Canadian population aged 12 years or older [30]. It is important to note that the survey only captures biological sex, and not gender per se.

The CCHS questions are designed for computer-assisted interviewing with pre-programmed questions, content flow, and allowable responses (ranges or answers). Half of the interviews take place by telephone, while the other half take place in person. Participation in the CCHS is voluntary and responses are kept strictly confidential [30].

Given the difference in sample sizes between the four cycles, the existing survey weights (determined by Statistics Canada) were adjusted depending on their contribution to their total pooled sample sized. Once the individual cycles' sample weights were adjusted, the cycles were combined and the pooled dataset was treated as one sample from a single population with a sample size of N = 515,421 prior to exclusions.

2.2. Exclusion Criteria

The population of interest in this study is working-age Canadian adults, aged 18–64 years, living in the ten provinces. Children aged 12–17 years were excluded from the dataset as mental health concerns differ in youth from adulthood, as do experiences of food insecurity in food insecure households [31]. Respondents aged 65 and older were excluded because seniors have the lowest levels of household food insecurity of the adult demographic in Canada, likely related to receiving seniors' pensions [32]. They also report different mental health problems including more cognitive impairment than working-age adults [33]. In addition, because of challenges of food supply related to isolated geographic areas such as Canada's Northern Territories [34], only respondents from the 10 provinces were included.

Provincial participation in the CCHS is dependent on whether modules of the survey were considered core or optional content in each survey cycle; the measurement of household food insecurity via the Household Food Insecurity Survey Module (HFSSM) was optional in the CCHS 3.1; for that cycle, Newfoundland, Labrador, New Brunswick, Manitoba, and Saskatchewan declined participation [35]. In the 2009–2010 cycle, Prince Edward Island and New Brunswick declined participation in the HFSSM [36]. Pooling four cycles and bootstrapping circumvents problems related to generalizability of the results to the ten provinces, given a substantial sample size was still collected in each of the provinces. Given its importance to the research question, only households who provided a response to the HFSSM were included. After applying exclusions, the total sample size was N = 302,683.

2.3. Measures

2.3.1. Household Food Security Survey Module

Household food insecurity in Canada is measured through the HFSSM. This 18-item questionnaire has been internationally validated and translated into many languages [9]. The HFSSM assesses the food security situation of adults as a group and children as a group within the household over the past 12 months. The HFSSM includes 10 questions measuring household food insecurity in adults and 8 questions measuring household food insecurity in children [30]. Typically, Statistics Canada will compile these to create a derived variable measuring three levels of household food security—food secure, moderate food insecurity, and severe food insecurity. For this study, a four-category household food insecurity variable was used, adding marginal food insecurity, which has demonstrated predictive power in increasing risk of chronic conditions in Canadian adults [12,19,20,37,38]. A description of the creation of the four-level household food insecurity variable is available in Appendix A.

2.3.2. Mental Health Outcome Variables

Five common mental health outcomes collected in the CCHS were included in the analysis: depressive thoughts in the past month, anxiety disorders, mood disorders, mental health status, and suicidal thoughts in the past year. All five outcomes were self-reported, because of the nature of the survey, but respondents were asked to only respond affirmatively to the anxiety and mood disorder questions if they had been so diagnosed by a health professional. These mental health conditions were selected based on their high response rates and their relatively high prevalence rates in Canada. The module including some mental health variables was optional content; as a result, two of the outcomes used in this study (suicidal thoughts, depressive thoughts) were not asked in all provinces. A detailed description of the five mental health outcome variables is presented in Appendix B.

2.3.3. Demographic and Socioeconomic Covariates

Six demographic variables (age, sex, household composition, homeownership, and highest education level in household) were included as covariates and were assessed for effect modification or confounding on the relationship between household food insecurity and adverse mental health outcomes. In addition, variables that measure respondents' race (White, Asian, Indigenous, Other), immigration status (immigrated less than 10 years ago, immigrated 10 or more years ago, Canadian-born), main income source (wages, government assistance, other sources), and inflation-adjusted household income (low income, medium-high income) were also included in the analysis. These covariates were included because of their known association with increased levels of household food insecurity [12,16,17,20,39]. Referent groups were selected based on the lowest prevalence of household food insecurity.

Finally, a cycle variable (2005, 2007/2008, 2009/2010, 2011/2012) was included to determine whether macro-level economic events, such as the 2008–2009 recession in Canada, modified or confounded the relationship between household food insecurity and adverse mental health outcomes.

2.4. Statistical Analysis

Data analysis was conducted at the Prairie Research Data Centre (RDC) using STATA statistical software (version 14, StataCorp, College Station, TX, USA). All estimates were generated with sample weights and 500 bootstrap replicates to approximate the Canadian population, that is, 18–64 year old individuals living in the ten provinces.

Univariate descriptive analyses of all study variables were followed by crude binary logistic regression analyses to assess the proportion of each mental health outcome by level of household food security and by sex, separately, in Canadian adults. Sex-adjusted binary logistic regression models were generated to assess the relationship between household food insecurity and the five mental health outcomes. Finally, interaction terms were created for sex and household food insecurity, and those interactions were included in the sex-adjusted binary logistic regression models to assess for effect modification with each mental health outcome. Reduced (by the removal of non-significant covariates) binary logistic regression analyses were conducted on sex-stratified datasets (one dataset for each sex) to visualize the sex gap for each level of household food insecurity on the odds of reporting five adverse mental health outcomes compared with those who are food secure.

3. Results

Table 1 presents the prevalence and 95% confidence intervals (95% CI) of the study variables. The prevalence of adverse mental health outcomes in this population ranged from 5.3% (5.2%–5.4%) reporting fair/poor mental health to 20.0% (19.6%–20.3%) responding that they had had depressive thoughts in the past month. Approximately 11.8% of the population fulfilled the criteria for some level of household food insecurity (3.7% marginal, 6.7% moderate, and 1.4% severe). Females comprised 50.9% (50.8%–50.9%) of the population.

Table 1. Prevalence (%) and 95% confidence intervals (CI) of study variables (N = 302,683). CCHS—Canadian Community Health Survey.

Variable	Categories	Percent	95% CI
	Outcome		
Depressive Thoughts in the Past Month	Yes	20.0	19.6–20.3
Anxiety Disorders	Yes	5.8	5.7–6.0
Mood Disorders	Yes	7.2	7.0–7.3
Suicidal Thoughts in the Past Year	Yes	19.7	18.7–20.7
Mental Health Status	Fair/Poor	5.3	5.2–5.4
	Exposure		
	Food Secure	88.2	88.0–88.4
Household Food Insecurity Level	Marginal Food Insecurity	3.7	3.5–3.8
	Moderate Food Insecurity	6.7	6.5–6.9
	Severe Food Insecurity	1.4	1.3–1.5
Covariate	**Categories**	**Mean**	**Standard Deviation**
Age	Continuous (18–64)	42.8	13.5
Covariate	**Categories**	**Percent**	**95% CI**
Sex	Male	49.1	49.1–49.2
	Female	50.9	50.8–50.9
	Unattached, living alone	12.5	12.3–12.7
	Single living with others	5.1	5.0–5.3
Household Composition	Couple, no kids	25.3	25.0–25.5
	Couple with kids <25	45.0	44.7–45.3
	Lone parent, kids <25	6.1	5.9–6.3
	Other/multi-family	6.0	5.9–6.2
	Common-law or Married	65.2	64.9–65.4
Marital Status	Divorced, Widowed, or Separated	9.2	9.0–9.4
	Single	25.7	25.4–25.9
Inflation-Adjusted Income [a]	Low	5.8	5.6–5.9
	Med-High	94.2	94.1–94.4
	Wages & Salary	88.9	88.7–89.1
Income Source	Social Assistance [b]	9.3	9.2–9.5
	Other [c]	2.7	2.6–2.8
	White	79.2	78.9–79.6
Race	Asian	11.7	11.4–11.9
	Indigenous	2.6	2.5–2.7
	Other [d]	6.5	6.3–6.7

Table 1. *Cont.*

Covariate	Categories	Percent	95% CI
Education	Post-Secondary Degree	80.5	80.2–80.7
	Some Post-Secondary	5.4	5.2–5.5
	High School Grad	9.8	9.7–10.0
	Less than High School	4.4	4.2–4.5
Immigration	Immigrated ≥10 years	15.7	15.5–16.0
	Immigrated <10 years	7.5	7.3–7.7
	Canadian Born	76.7	76.4–77.0
Homeownership	Homeowner	73.5	73.1–73.8
	Renter	26.5	26.2–26.9
Cycle of CCHS	3.1	22.2	22.1–22.3
	2007/2008	25.5	25.4–25.6
	2009/2010	25.6	25.6–25.7
	2011/2012	26.6	26.6–26.7

[a] Derived from respondent's total household income before taxes adjusted by Canadian inflation rates for the year the respondent was surveyed [40]. Inflation adjusted income was ranked (low-lower middle, middle, upper middle, and highest) based on the number of people in household and national income thresholds [41,42]. The four-level variable was dichotomized into low and medium-high income. [b] includes the following: benefits from Canada or Quebec pension plan, old age security and guaranteed income supplement, provincial or municipal social assistance or welfare, and child tax benefit. [c] includes the following: retirement pensions, child support, alimony, employment insurance, worker's compensation board, and other. [d] includes those who identify as Black, Latin American, Arab, and Other (multi-racial).

Table 2 presents results from the crude binary logistic regression analysis. The odds ratios were converted to prevalence, and 95% CI are reported for each mental health outcome by level of household food insecurity and by sex, separately. Table 2 also presents the crude sex gap in the reporting of depressive thoughts in the past month, anxiety disorders, mood disorders, suicidal thoughts in the past year, and fair or poor mental health in this population. Table 2 shows that females have a higher prevalence of reporting four out of five mental health outcomes, prior to adjusting for covariates. Males and females have a statistically significant equal prevalence of reporting having had suicidal thoughts in the past year, prior to adjusting for covariates.

Table 2. Results from crude binary logistic regression of household food insecurity and by sex, separately, on five adverse mental health outcomes, presented as prevalence (%) and 95% confidence intervals.

Variable Category	Depressive Thoughts in the Past Month	Anxiety Disorders	Mood Disorders	Suicidal Thoughts in the Past Year	Fair/Poor Mental Health
Household Food Insecurity Level					
Food Secure	17.5 (17.2, 17.9)	4.8 (4.7, 4.9)	5.8 (5.7, 5.9)	16.8 (15.7, 17.8)	4.0 (3.9, 4.1)
Marginally Food Insecurity	31.1 (28.7, 33.5)	9.9 (9.1, 10.8)	11.4 (10.5, 12.2)	25.6 (21.2, 30.0)	9.2 (8.3, 10.1)
Moderately Food Insecurity	39.8 (37.8,41.7)	13.6 (12.8, 14.3)	17.4 (16.6, 18.3)	24.8 (22.0, 27.7)	15.0 (14.2, 15.8)
Severely Food Insecurity	59.3 (55.2, 63.4)	25.4 (23.5, 27.3)	34.2 (32.0, 36.4)	41.0 (36.1, 45.9)	31.1 (28.9, 33.4)
Sex					
Male	15.1 (14.6, 15.7)	4.1 (4.0, 4.3)	5.0 (4.8, 5.2)	20.9 (19.4, 22.4)	4.8 (4.6, 5.0)
Female	24.7 (24.1, 25.2)	7.5 (7.3, 7.7)	9.3 (9.1, 9.5)	18.8 (17.5, 20.1)	5.8 (5.6, 6.0)

Table 3 presents the sex-adjusted odds of reporting five adverse mental health outcomes for each level of household, compared with those reporting household food security. All five adverse mental health outcomes show increasing odds of reporting adverse mental health outcomes with increasingly severe household food insecurity adjusted for sex, compared with those who are food secure. No interaction, that is, no effect modification, was observed between household food insecurity and sex for any of the five adverse mental health outcomes. Table 3 shows, however, after that the sex gap for four of the five mental health conditions persists when controlling for household food insecurity. In sum, household food insecurity at any level is associated with increased odds of reporting five mental health outcomes, compared with those reporting food security, and the sex gap remains when household food insecurity is held constant for all mental health conditions, except suicidal thoughts in the past year.

Table 3. Sex-adjusted binary logistic regression models of household food insecurity and five adverse mental health outcomes, including food insecurity and sex interactions.

Variable Category	Model 1: Depressive Thoughts in the Past Month	Model 2: Anxiety Disorders	Model 3: Mood Disorders	Model 4: Suicidal Thoughts in the Past Year	Model 5: Fair/Poor Mental Health
	Odds Ratio (95% Confidence Interval)				
	Household Food Insecurity Level (food secure = ref)				
Marginal Food Insecurity	2.3 ** (2.0, 2.8)	2.2 ** (1.9, 2.7)	2.3 ** (1.9, 2.7)	1.8 * (1.3, 2.6)	2.4 ** (2.1, 2.9)
Moderate Food Insecurity	3.2 ** (2.8, 3.7)	2.8 ** (2.5, 3.2)	3.2 ** (2.9, 3.6)	1.8 ** (1.4, 2.4)	4.3 ** (3.8, 4.8)
Severe Food Insecurity	8.2 ** (6.3, 10.6)	6.3 ** (5.4, 7.3)	8.4 ** (7.2, 9.7)	3.0 ** (2.2, 4.1)	11.0 ** (9.2, 13.1)
	Sex (male = ref)				
Female	1.9 ** (1.8, 2.0)	1.8 ** (1.7, 1.9)	1.9 ** (1.8, 2.0)	0.9 * (0.7, 1.0)	1.2 ** (1.1, 1.2)
Marginal * Female	0.8 (0.7, 1.0)	0.9 (0.8, 1.2)	0.9 (0.7, 1.0)	0.9 (0.6, 1.5)	1.0 (0.8, 1.2)
Moderate * Female	0.9 (0.7, 1.1)	1.1 (0.9, 1.3)	1.0 (0.9, 1.2)	0.9 (0.6, 1.2)	1.0 (0.8, 1.1)
Severe * Female	0.7 (0.5, 1.0)	1.2 (0.9, 1.4)	1.0 (0.9, 1.3)	1.3 (0.9, 2.0)	1.0 (0.8, 1.2)

$* p < 0.05, ** p < 0.001.$

Figures 1–5 visualize the results from the reduced binary logistic regression analysis stratified by sex. These figures show, separately for males and females, the adjusted odds ratio of respondents experiencing each level of household food insecurity in turn reporting five mental health outcomes, compared with those reporting that they are food secure. The results, adjusted for significant covariates, show that males and females with any level of household food insecurity have no statistically significant difference in the odds ratio for each mental health outcome, compared to those reporting household food security.

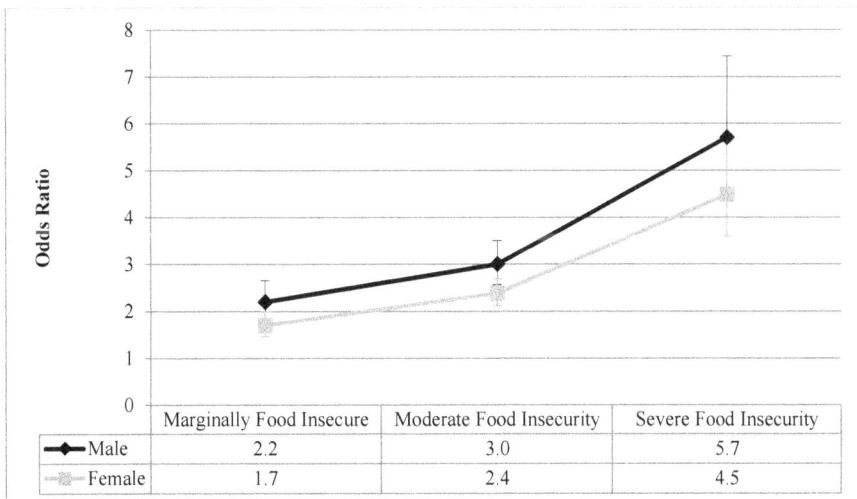

	Marginally Food Insecure	Moderate Food Insecurity	Severe Food Insecurity
Male	2.2	3.0	5.7
Female	1.7	2.4	4.5

Figure 1. Odds ratio of reporting depressive thoughts in the past month for each level of household food insecurity stratified by sex, compared with food secure; results from reduced binary logistic regression.

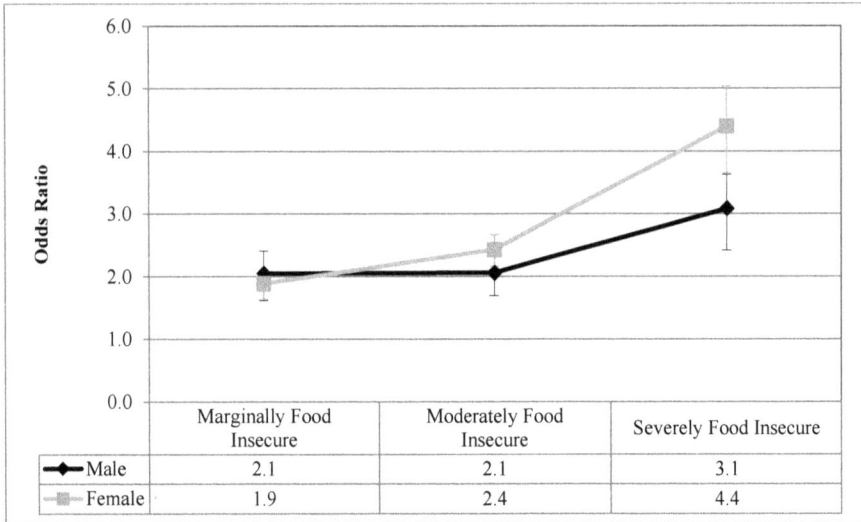

Figure 2. Odds ratio of reporting anxiety disorders for each level of household food insecurity stratified by sex, compared with food secure; results from reduced binary logistic regression.

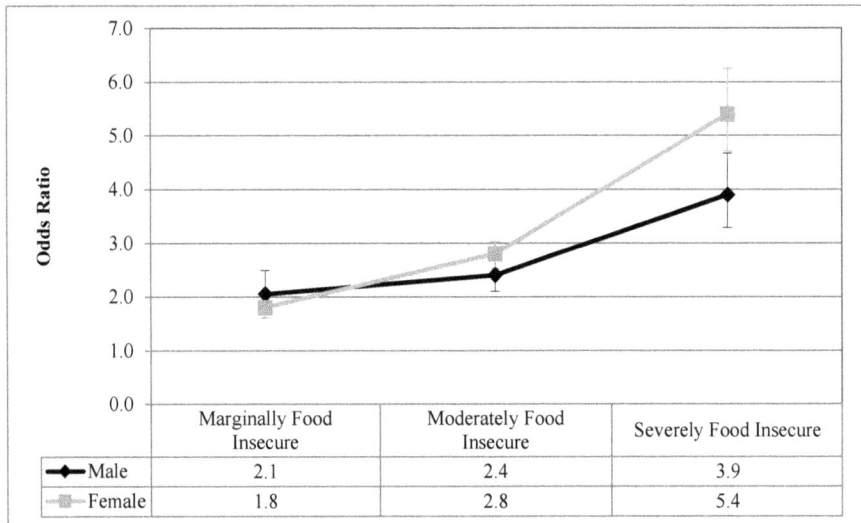

Figure 3. Odds ratio of reporting mood disorders for each level of household food insecurity stratified by sex, compared with food secure; results from reduced binary logistic regression.

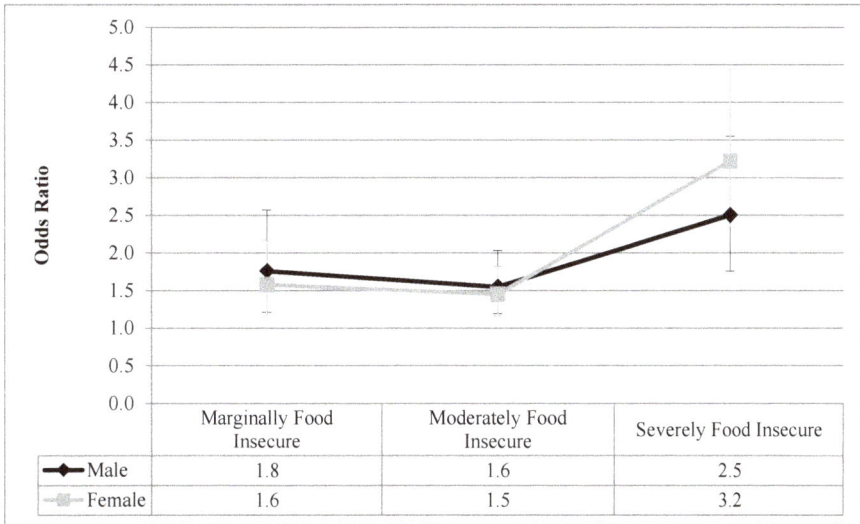

Figure 4. Odds ratio of reporting suicidal thoughts in the past month for each level of household food insecurity stratified by sex, compared with food secure; results from reduced binary logistic regression.

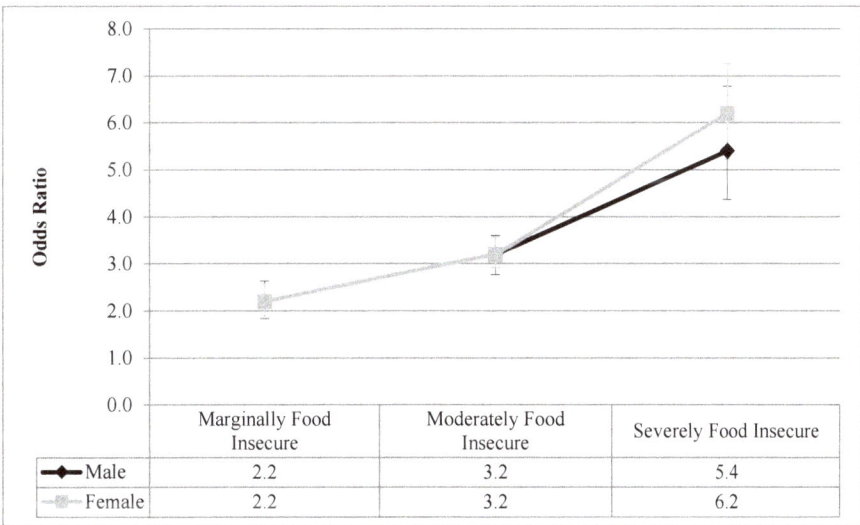

Figure 5. Odds ratio of reporting fair/poor mental health status for each level of household food insecurity stratified by sex, compared with food secure; results from reduced binary logistic regression.

4. Discussion

In recent years, mental health researchers have recognized that separate social locations such as sex and race must be considered together, but in much of the scholarship focusing on mental health conditions, these locations are often treated as independent variables [43]. This type of analysis results in a lack of observability of within-group differences among individuals in different social categories.

From a review of the literature, sex and household food insecurity are two important variables related to the reporting of adverse mental health outcomes. Empirically, this study examined how sex and household food insecurity interact and how that statistical interaction impacts the reporting of mental health outcomes. We first showed that, prior to the inclusion of household food insecurity in the analysis, females reported higher prevalence of depressive thoughts in the past month, anxiety disorders, mood disorders, and fair or poor mental health, compared with males (Table 2), which is aligned with decades of reporting on the sex gap in common mental health outcomes [1–3]. Table 3 shows that even after controlling for sex, household food insecurity was associated with high odds ratios of reporting five common mental health outcomes compared with food secure respondents, and these odds ratios increase with the severity of household food insecurity. Upon analyzing the interaction between household food insecurity and sex (Table 3), sex was found to not be an effect modifier on the relationship between household food insecurity and all five adverse mental health outcomes. Therefore, males and females reporting each level of household food insecurity had statistically equal odds ratios of reporting these adverse mental health outcomes, compared with those who are food secure. In order to confirm this finding, sex-stratified reduced binary logistic regression analyses were conducted for each mental health outcome, and the results are presented graphically in Figures 1–5. The overlapping confidence intervals at each level of household food insecurity indicate that males and females, at each level of household food insecurity, report statistically similar odds of five common mental health outcomes, compared with food secure respondents. Males and females who experience household food insecurity (a chronically stressful experience) may be equally at risk of reporting mental health problems due to their disadvantaged position. It appears that working age adult males' lower rates of reporting or succumbing to mental health outcomes [44,45] are reduced to non-significance once household food insecurity is considered.

This is a novel finding and indicates that the often-reported sex gap in mental health may be true among those who are food secure (who represent most Canadian adults), but among a distinctly disadvantaged population (food insecure), males and females appear to experience a similar mental health burden. Another study focused on the interactions between household food insecurity and sex and its relationship with mental health outcomes, in a high-income country. Carter and associates [46] examined the association between a binary food insecurity measure and psychological distress in New Zealand for males and females separately. The authors found that the sex gap was substantially reduced in the stratified model, but that food insecure females had slightly higher odds of psychological distress than males (using a *p*-value of <0.1), compared with those who are food secure [46]. The present study advances this work by examining this relationship using a more precise four-level household food insecurity measure that was generated using an internationally adopted and validated tool (i.e., HFSSM). In addition, the present study examines five common adverse mental health outcomes.

Much of the research on the impact of gender on household food insecurity and mental health has been conducted with a study population comprised of females only [16,17,19]. Our results indicate that the relationship between household food insecurity and five adverse mental health outcomes is equally strong in males. Therefore, the chronic stresses associated with household food insecurity [22] could be narrowing the commonly observed sex gap in mental health. This study's findings could indicate that the experience of males and females in food insecure households may be similar. Both groups likely experience substantial psychological, physical, and social stresses (e.g., guilt, shame, powerlessness, and inequality) [22,28] as a result of not having enough money to feed themselves or their families.

Our findings suggest that males and females in a food insecure household experience a similar mental health burden as a result of sharing a more similar social location compared with food secure members of their own sex. The sex gap in mental health outcomes that is often reported for the general population is largely comprised of food secure respondents and appears to have masked the food insecure sub-group's experience of mental health problems, if this important variable is not considered.

4.1. Limitations

The CCHS does not survey some groups that are particularly vulnerable to household food insecurity and mental health problems, specifically First Nations people living on-reserve, homeless populations, and those living in remote regions [47,48]. Researchers estimate that there could be as many as 470,000 additional food insecure people living in Canada that are not included in Statistics Canada's estimate [49]. We cannot assume that the social location of household food insecurity for men and women in these circumstances is the same as the CCHS sample.

While it would be preferable to speak only in terms of gender, the CCHS only delineates by sex and, therefore, sex is used as a variable of interest in this study. Given the self-reported nature of the CCHS, there is potential for measurement error in the mental health outcomes, particularly as a result of social desirability bias—this would result in an underestimation of mental health burden.

The CCHS uses two methods of data collection—computer assisted telephone interviewing (CATI) and computer-assisted person interviewing (CAPI). While there is some evidence in the literature of statistically equal prevalence of self-reported mental health status using CATI and CAPI [50], face-to-face interviewing yields slightly higher reporting of household food insecurity than CATI [51]. This may result in an underestimation of household food insecurity for those responding using CATI.

Finally, type 1 error (the probability of rejecting a null hypothesis that is in fact true [52]) is a threat with a large sample size. In order to circumvent this problem, a bootstrapping method was employed, which effectively narrowed the confidence intervals to increase the difficulty of rejecting the null hypothesis.

4.2. Strengths

This study employs a large and robust dataset, with enough power to examine a four-level household food insecurity variable, using the internationally validated HFSSM. This study uses a nationally representative survey that results in generalizable findings to 98% of the Canadian population aged 18–64 living in the ten provinces. The use of a four-level household food insecurity variable is rare in the literature, despite the predictive power of the marginal group [12,19,37,38].

Finally, this study is novel in that it is one of only two studies to examine the interaction between sex, household food insecurity, and mental health outcomes in high-income countries [46], and the first to examine this phenomenon in Canada, with a four-level food insecurity variable.

5. Conclusions

Although the sex gap in mental health outcomes has been observed and re-examined for decades, few studies have considered whether these important social determinants, sex and food insecurity, have a multiplicative effect on the odds of reporting of mental health problems.

This study showed that the well-documented sex gap in mental health outcomes was reduced to non-significance when household food insecurity was reported. Therefore, household food insecurity appears to act as a chronically stressful condition that overwhelms the capacity of males to either withstand reporting mental health conditions or actually succumb to them. This study suggests that household food insecurity is a social location with public health implications. The high odds of reporting adverse mental health outcomes seen among males experiencing household food insecurity, compared with food secure males, suggest that there is a distinct mental health burden among males experiencing household food insecurity, and that this previously overlooked group is deserving of further study.

Finally, household food insecurity is a modifiable stressor within the complex interplay of sex and mental health. Given the lack of a sex gap in mental health among those with household food insecurity, addressing food insecurity with progressive policy change could result in mental health gains for women, as well as men who share this vulnerability.

Author Contributions: Conceptualization, G.J.P. and L.M.; methodology, G.J.P. and L.M.; formal analysis, G.J.P.; investigation, G.J.P. and L.M.; writing—original draft preparation, G.J.P. and L.M.; writing—review and editing, G.J.P. and L.M.; visualization, G.J.P.; supervision, L.M.; funding acquisition, G.J.P. and L.M.

Funding: This study was funded by a Programmatic Grant in Health and Health Equity from the Canadian Institutes of Health Research (CIHR) (grant no. FRN 115208) and a CIHR graduate student award.

Acknowledgments: The authors thank and acknowledge the assistance of the staff at the Prairie Regional Data Centre for their advice and guidance.

Conflicts of Interest: The authors declare no conflict of interest.

Appendix A

Table A1. Description of Household Food Insecurity Variable Derived from Household Food Security Survey Module.

Level of Household Food Insecurity	Description of Level	Number of Affirmative Responses
Food Secure	No financial constraints on the ability to fill household's food need.	0 to adult or child food situation questions
Marginally Food Insecure	Worry about running out of food due to financial constraints.	1 food situation question
Moderately Food Insecure	Reductions in quality and/or quantity of food due to financial constraints.	2–5 adult food situation questions or 2–4 child food situation questions
Severely Food Insecurity	Reductions in food intake, missing meals and at its most extreme going a full day without food.	6+ adult food situation questions or 5+ child food situation questions

* adapted from [8].

Appendix B

Table A2. Description of Outcome Variables Included in Study.

Name of Variable	Level of Measurement	Survey Question	Description
Depressive Thoughts in the Past Month	Binary (Yes, No)	"During the past month, about how often did you feel sad or depressed?"	Those who responded all of the time, most of the time, some of the time were coded into the "yes" group. All other respondents were coded into the "no" group.
Major Depressive Episodes in the Past Year	Binary (Yes, No)	The Composite International Diagnostic Interview Short Form (CIDI-SF) measures Major Depressive Episodes (MDE). This subset of questions assesses the depressive symptoms of respondents who felt depressed or lost interest in things for 2 weeks or more in the last 12 months. Respondents are screened into the CIDI-SF based on affirmative responses to the following 2 screening questions, if a respondent answers affirmatively to the screening questions, their depression level is measured based on 7 additional questions.	The classification of depression is based on an affirmative response to the original screening question and 5 out of 9 of the depression questions. This corresponds to a 90% predictive probability of caseness, which closely aligns with the DSM-5 diagnostic guidelines for MDE in adults [53]. This probability expresses the chance that the respondent would have been diagnosed as having experienced a Major Depressive Episode in the past 12 months had they completed the CIDI Long-Form [30].
Anxiety Disorder	Binary (Yes, No)	"Do you have an anxiety disorder such as phobia, obsessive-compulsive disorder or a panic disorder?"	Respondents are reminded that the question is only referring to those conditions diagnosed by a health professional.
Mood Disorder	Binary (Yes, No)	"Do you have a mood disorder such as depression, bipolar disorder, mania or dysthymia?"	Respondents are reminded that the question only refers to those conditions diagnosed by a health professional.
Suicidal Thoughts in the Past Month	Binary (Yes, No)	"Have you ever seriously considered committing suicide or taking your own life? Has this happened in the past 12 months?"	This variable was recoded into a dichotomous variable. In addition, those who answered "not applicable: were coded into the "no" group, given they answered negatively to this question in an earlier prompt.
Self-Reported Mental Health Status	Binary (Fair/Poor, Good/Very Good/Excellent)	"In general, would you say your mental health is: excellent, very good, good, fair, or poor?"	This variable was recoded into a dichotomous variable. "Fair/poor" or "Good/very good/excellent". This variable has been validated and is a reliable measure of general mental health [54].

References

1. ESEMeD/MHEDEA 2000 Investigators; Alonso, J.; Angermeyer, M.C.; Bernert, S.; Bruffaerts, R.; Brugha, T.S.; Bryson, H.; de Girolamo, G.; de Graaf, R.; Demyttenaere, K.; et al. Prevalence of mental disorders in Europe: Results from the European Study of the Epidemiology of Mental Disorders (ESEMeD) project. *Acta Psychiatr. Scand.* **2004**, *109*, 21–27. [CrossRef] [PubMed]
2. Blazer, D.G.; Kessler, R.C.; McGonagle, K.A. The prevalence and distribution of major depression in a national community sample: The National Comorbidity Survey. *Am. J. Psychiatry* **1994**, *151*, 979–986. [CrossRef] [PubMed]
3. Kessler, R.C.; Berglund, P.; Demler, O.; Jin, R.; Koretz, D.; Merikangas, K.R.; Rush, A.J.; Walters, E.E.; Wang, P.S. The epidemiology of major depressive disorder. *JAMA* **2003**, *289*, 3095. [CrossRef] [PubMed]
4. Kessler, R.C. Epidemiology of women and depression. *J. Affect. Disord.* **2003**, *74*, 5–13. [CrossRef]
5. Patten, S.B.; Williams, J.V.A.; Lavorato, D.H.; Wang, J.L.; Bulloch, A.G.M.; Sajobi, T. The association between major depression prevalence and sex becomes weaker with age. *Soc. Psychiatry Psychiatr. Epidemiol.* **2016**, *51*, 203–210. [CrossRef] [PubMed]
6. Simon, R.W. Revisiting the relationship among gender, marital status, and mental health. *Am. J. Sociol.* **2002**, *107*, 1065–1096. [CrossRef] [PubMed]
7. Scott, R.L.; Lasiuk, G.; Norris, C. The relationship between sexual orientation and depression in a national population sample. *J. Clin. Nurs.* **2016**, *25*, 3522–3532. [CrossRef]
8. Tarasuk, V.; Mitchell, A.; Dachner, N. *Household Food Insecurity in Canada, 2012*; PROOF: Toronto, ON, Canada, 2014; Available online: http://proof.utoronto.ca/resources/proof-annual-reports/ (accessed on 1 September 2018).
9. Bickel, G.; Nord, M.; Price, C.; Hamilton, W.; Cook, J. *Guide to Measuring Household Food Security*; United States Department of Agriculture Food and Nutrition Services: Alexandria, VA, USA, 2000.
10. Health Canada. Canadian Community Health Survey. Cycle 2.2, Nutrition (2004)—Income-Related Household Food Security in Canada. 2007. Available online: https://www.canada.ca/content/dam/hc-sc/migration/hc-sc/fn-an/alt_formats/hpfb-dgpsa/pdf/surveill/income_food_sec-sec_alim-eng.pdf (accessed on 1 September 2018).
11. Gucciardi, E.; Vogt, J.A.; DeMelo, M.; Stewart, D.E. Exploration of the relationship between household food insecurity and diabetes in Canada. *Diabetes Care* **2009**, *32*, 2218–2224. [CrossRef]
12. Tarasuk, V.; Mitchell, A.; McLaren, L.; McIntyre, L. Chronic physical and mental health conditions among adults may increase vulnerability to household food insecurity. *J. Nutr.* **2013**, *143*, 1785–1793. [CrossRef]
13. Vozoris, N.T.; Tarasuk, V.S. Household food insufficiency is associated with poorer health. *J. Nutr.* **2003**, *133*, 120–126. [CrossRef]
14. Galesloot, S.; McIntyre, L.; Fenton, T.; Tyminski, S. Food insecurity in Canadian adults receiving diabetes care. *Can. J. Pract. Res.* **2012**, *73*, 261–266. [CrossRef] [PubMed]
15. Davison, K.; Kaplan, B. Food insecurity in adults with mood disorders: Prevalence estimates and associations with nutritional and psychological health. *Ann. Gen. Psychiatry* **2015**, *14*, 21. [CrossRef]
16. Heflin, C.M.; Siefert, K.; Williams, D.R. Food insufficiency and women's mental health: Findings from a 3-year panel of welfare recipients. *Soc. Sci. Med.* **2005**, *61*, 1971–1982. [CrossRef] [PubMed]
17. Siefert, K.; Heflin, C.M.; Corcoran, M.E.; Williams, D.R. Food insufficiency and physical and mental health in a longitudinal survey of welfare recipients. *J. Health Soc. Behav.* **2004**, *22*, 171–186. [CrossRef] [PubMed]
18. Leung, C.W.; Epel, E.S.; Willett, W.C.; Rimm, E.B.; Laraia, B.A. Household food insecurity is positively associated with depression among low-income Supplemental Nutrition Assistance Program participants and income-eligible nonparticipants. *J. Nutr.* **2015**, *145*, 622–627. [CrossRef] [PubMed]
19. Whitaker, R.C.; Phillips, S.M.; Orzol, S.M. Food insecurity and the risks of depression and anxiety in mothers and behavior problems in their preschool-aged children. *Pediatrics* **2006**, *118*, 859–868. [CrossRef] [PubMed]
20. Muldoon, K.A.; Duff, P.K.; Fielden, S.; Anema, A. Food insufficiency is associated with psychiatric morbidity in a nationally representative study of mental illness among food insecure Canadians. *Soc. Psychiatry Psychiatr. Epidemiol.* **2013**, *48*, 795–803. [CrossRef]
21. Jessiman-Perreault, G.; McIntyre, L. The household food insecurity gradient and potential reductions in adverse population mental health outcomes in Canadian adults. *SSM Popul. Health* **2017**, *3*, 464–472. [CrossRef]

22. Hadley, C.; Crooks, D.L. Coping and the biosocial consequences of food insecurity in the 21st century. *Am. J. Phys. Anthropol.* **2012**, *149*, 72–94. [CrossRef]
23. Runnels, V.E.; Kristjansson, E.; Calhoun, M. An investigation of adults' everyday experiences and effects of food insecurity in an urban area in Canada. *Can. J. Community Ment. Health* **2011**, *30*, 157–172. [CrossRef]
24. Melchior, M.; Caspi, A.; Howard, L.M.; Ambler, A.P.; Bolton, H.; Mountain, N.; Moffitt, T.E. Mental health context of food insecurity: A representative cohort of families with young children. *Pediatrics* **2009**, *124*, 564–572. [CrossRef] [PubMed]
25. Wehler, C.; Weinreb, L.F.; Huntington, N.; Scott, R.; Hosmer, D.; Fletcher, K.; Goldberg, R.; Gundersen, C. Risk and protective factors for adult and child hunger among low-income housed and homeless female-headed families. *Am. J. Public Health* **2004**, *94*, 109–115. [CrossRef]
26. McIntyre, L.; Officer, S.; Robinson, L.M. Feeling poor: The felt experience of low-income lone mothers. *Affilia* **2003**, *18*, 316–331. [CrossRef]
27. Olson, C. Food insecurity in women: A recipe for unhealthy trade-offs. *Top. Clin. Nutr.* **2005**, *20*, 321–328. [CrossRef]
28. Hamelin, A.-M.; Beaudry, M.; Habicht, J.-P. Characterization of household food insecurity in Quebec: Food and feelings. *Soc. Sci. Med.* **2002**, *54*, 119–132. [CrossRef]
29. Griffith, D.M. An intersectional approach to men's health. *J. Mens Health* **2012**, *9*, 106–112. [CrossRef]
30. Statistics Canada. *User Guide, Public-Use 2007–2008: Microdata File, Canadian Community Health Survey*; Statistics Canada: Ottawa, ON, Canada, 2008.
31. Fram, M.S.; Frongillo, E.A.; Jones, S.J.; Williams, R.C.; Burke, M.P.; DeLoach, K.P.; Blake, C.E. Children are aware of food insecurity and take responsibility for managing food resources. *J. Nutr.* **2011**, *141*, 1114–1119. [CrossRef] [PubMed]
32. Emery, J.C.H.; Fleisch, V.C.; McIntyre, L. Legislated changes to federal pension income in Canada will adversely affect low income seniors' health. *Prev. Med.* **2013**, *57*, 963–966. [CrossRef]
33. Blazer, D.; Burchett, B.; Service, C.; George, L.K. The association of age and depression among the elderly: An epidemiologic exploration. *J. Gerontol.* **1991**, *46*, 210–215. [CrossRef]
34. Inuit Circumpolar Council. Food Security Across the Arctic. 2012. Available online: http://www.inuitcircumpolar.com/uploads/3/0/5/4/30542564/icc_food_security_across_the_arctic_may_2012.pdf (accessed on 1 September 2018).
35. Statistics Canada. *User Guide, Public-Use 2005: Microdata File, Canadian Community Health Survey*; Statistics Canada: Ottawa, ON, Canada, 2006.
36. Statistics Canada. *User Guide, Public-Use 2009–2010: Microdata File, Canadian Community Health Survey*; Statistics Canada: Ottawa, ON, Canada, 2011.
37. Cook, J.T.; Frank, D.A.; Berkowitz, C.; Black, M.M.; Casey, P.H.; Cutts, D.B.; Meyers, A.F.; Zaldivar, N.; Skalicky, A.; Levenson, S.; et al. Community and international nutrition food insecurity is associated with adverse health outcomes among human infants and toddlers. *J. Nutr.* **2004**, *134*, 1432–1438. [CrossRef]
38. Davison, K.M.; Marshall-Fabien, G.L.; Tecson, A. Association of moderate and severe food insecurity with suicidal ideation in adults: National survey data from three Canadian provinces. *Soc. Psychiatry Psychiatr. Epidemiol.* **2015**, *50*, 963–972. [CrossRef] [PubMed]
39. McIntyre, L.; Wu, X.; Fleisch, V.C.; Emery, H.J.C. Homeowner versus non-homeowner differences in household food insecurity in Canada. *J. Hous. Built Environ.* **2015**, *14*, 349–366. [CrossRef]
40. Statistics Canada. *The Consumer Price Index*; Statistics Canada: Ottawa, ON, Canada, 2016.
41. Canadian Institute for Health Information. *Trends in Income-Related Health Inequalities in Canada: Methodology Notes*; Canadian Institute for Health Information: Ottawa, ON, Canada, 2015.
42. Peel Public Health. *Health in Peel: Determinants and Disparities*; Peel Public Health: Mississauga, ON, Canada, 2011.
43. Van Mens-Verhulst, J.; Radtke, L. Intersectionality and Mental Health: A Case Study. 2008. Available online: https://static1.squarespace.com/static/56fd7e0bf699bb7d0d3ff82d/t/593ab6522e69cf01a44b14d4/1497019986918/INTERSECTIONALITY+AND+MENTAL+HEALTH2.pdf (accessed on 1 September 2018).
44. Galdas, P.M.; Cheater, F.; Marshall, P. Men and health help-seeking behaviour: Literature review. *J. Adv. Nurs.* **2005**, *49*, 616–623. [CrossRef] [PubMed]
45. Kartalova-O'Doherty, Y.; Doherty, T.D. Recovering from recurrent mental health problems: Giving up and fighting to get better. *Int. J. Ment. Health Nurs.* **2010**, *11*, 3–15. [CrossRef] [PubMed]

46. Carter, K.N.; Kruse, K.; Blakely, T.; Collings, S. The association of food security with psychological distress in New Zealand and any gender differences. *Soc. Sci. Med.* **2011**, *72*, 1463–1471. [CrossRef]

47. Loopstra, R.; Tarasuk, V. Food bank usage is a poor indicator of food insecurity: Insights from Canada. *Soc. Policy Soc.* **2015**, *14*, 443–455. [CrossRef]

48. Parpouchi, M.; Moniruzzaman, A.; Russolillo, A.; Somers, J.M. Food insecurity among homeless adults with mental illness. *PLoS ONE* **2016**, *11*, e0159334. [CrossRef]

49. Skinner, K.; Hanning, R.M.; Tsuji, L.J. Prevalence and severity of household food insecurity of First Nations people living in an on-reserve, sub-Artic community within the Mushkegowuk Territory. *Public Health Nutr.* **2014**, *17*, 31–39. [CrossRef]

50. St-Pierre, M.; Béland, Y. Mode effects in the Canadian Community Health Survey: A Comparison of CAPI and CATI. In *Proceedings of the American Statistical Association Meeting, Survey Research Methods*; American Statistical Association: Toronto, ON, Canada, 2004.

51. Kirkpatrick, S.I.; Tarasuk, V. Food insecurity and participation in community food programs among low-income Toronto families. *Can. J. Public Health* **2009**, *100*, 135–139.

52. Oleckno, W.A. *Epidemiology: Concepts and Methods*; Waveland Press: Long Grove, IL, USA, 2008.

53. American Psychiatric Association. *Diagnostic and Statistical Manual of Mental Disorders (DSM-5®)*; American Psychiatric Pub: Arlington, VA, USA, 2013.

54. Mawani, F.N.; Gilmour, H. Validation of self-rated mental health. *Health Rep.* **2010**, *21*, 61–75.

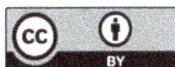

International Journal of
Environmental Research and Public Health

MDPI

Article

The Overlooked Burden of Food Insecurity among Asian Americans: Results from the California Health Interview Survey

Monideepa B. Becerra [1,*] , Salome Kapella Mshigeni [1] and Benjamin J. Becerra [2]

[1] Department of Health Science and Human Ecology, California State University, 5500 University Parkway, San Bernardino, CA 92407, USA; salome.mshigeni@csusb.edu
[2] School of Allied Health Professions, Loma Linda University, 24951 North Circle Drive, Loma Linda, CA 92350, USA; bbecerra@llu.edu
* Correspondence: mbecerra@csusb.edu; Tel.: +1-909-537-5969

Received: 25 June 2018; Accepted: 24 July 2018; Published: 7 August 2018

Abstract: *Objective*: Food insecurity remains a major public health issue in the United States, though lack of research among Asian Americans continue to underreport the issue. The purpose of this study was to evaluate the prevalence and burden of food insecurity among disaggregated Asian American populations. *Methods*: The California Health Interview Survey, the largest state health survey, was used to assess the prevalence of food insecurity among Asian American subgroups with primary exposure variable of interest being acculturation. Survey-weighted descriptive, bivariate, and multivariable robust Poisson regression analyses, were conducted and alpha less than 0.05 was used to denote significance. *Results*: The highest prevalence of food insecurity was found among Vietnamese (16.42%) and the lowest prevalence was among Japanese (2.28%). A significant relationship was noted between prevalence of food insecurity and low acculturation for Chinese, Korean, and Vietnamese subgroups. Language spoken at home was significant associated with food insecurity. For example, among Chinese, being food insecure was associated with being bilingual (prevalence ratio [PR] = 2.51) or speaking a non-English language at home (PR = 7.24), while among South Asians, it was associated with speaking a non-English language at home was also related to higher prevalence (PR = 3.62), as compared to English speakers only. Likewise, being foreign-born also related to being food insecure among Chinese (PR = 2.31), Filipino (PR = 1.75), South Asian (PR = 3.35), Japanese (PR = 2.11), and Vietnamese (PR = 3.70) subgroups, when compared to their US-born counterparts. *Conclusion*: There is an imperative need to address food insecurity burden among Asian Americans, especially those who have low acculturation.

Keywords: Asian Americans; California Health Interview Survey; food security; Supplemental Nutrition Assistance Program (SNAP); acculturation; English language use

---

1. Introduction

The Asian American population is one of the fastest growing minority groups in the United States [1], yet, little research on health disparities exists for the group. One potential reason has been attributed to the model minority myth, which assumes Asians have unparalleled achievements in education and success [2], thus leading to the assumption that the population suffers little health disparities. Yet, studies demonstrate that such a myth has led to internalized racialism, further resulting in negative attitudes towards seeking mental health care and increased psychological distress [3].

Furthermore, Asian American data has been historically aggregated to present a homogeneous representation, resulting in the masking of more vulnerable subpopulations. Recent policy implementations, such as the White House Initiative for Asian Americans and Pacific Islanders [4], and the body of literature, demonstrates the importance of addressing the heterogeneity in the population. For example, Sakamoto, in evaluating the American Community Survey, demonstrated that when compared to whites, Asian Indians, Japanese, and Filipinos were less likely to be living in poverty, while Chinese, Koreans, Vietnamese, and several other Asian American subgroups were more likely to be in poverty [5]; hence contradicting the model minority myth. In an evaluation of hemorrhagic stroke risk among Asian Americans and other ethnic groups, Klatsky et al. [6] noted that while Asian Americans reported a higher risk of such stroke compared to whites, the rate was only explained by Japanese and Filipinos; thus demonstrating the heterogeneity in chronic disease risk among the Asian American population. Similarly, heterogeneity among Asian Americans has been noted in regards to health behaviors and chronic illnesses [7–9]. For example, results from a study addressing physical activity among Asian American subgroups utilizing CHIS data showed Chinese and Vietnamese subgroups who were bilingual were more likely to meet American College of Sport Medicine recommendations of physical activity level, as compared to those who reported only speaking a non-English language at home [10]. Undoubtedly, disaggregated research in the Asian American population is key to ensuring healthier outcomes of the nation's population, as set forth by Healthy People 2020.

In recent years, food insecurity has gained national attention. Food insecurity, defined by the U.S. Department of Agriculture (USDA) as consistent access to and availability of enough food for all members of a household to lead an active and healthy lifestyle. The USDA further defines reduced quality, variety, or desirability of diet as low food security, which was historically called food insecurity without hunger, while the same characteristics with disrupted eating patterns reduction in food intake is considered very low food security, or historically known as food insecurity with hunger [11]. In 2016, 12.3% of U.S. households (42.2 million Americans), were reported to be food insecure. Furthermore, rates of food insecurity were found to be more prevalent among Hispanic and non-Hispanic Black households and those residing below the 185% poverty threshold [12]. Food insecurity has also been associated with negative health outcomes, including poor cognitive development [13,14], poor dietary choices [15,16], and mental illness [17,18]. For example, Weigel and group found higher rate of mental illness (including depression) among food insecure migrant and seasonal farmworkers [19]. Likewise, food insecurity with hunger was found to be substantially related to serious psychological distress among African-Americans [20], while low household food insecurity has been associated with adherence to physical activity guidelines among both children and adults [21]. Despite such empirical evidence, no current research exists on the burden of food insecurity among Asian Americans. As such, in this study we aimed to address this gap in the literature, by evaluating the period prevalence of food insecurity among disaggregation Asian American population using the largest state health survey.

Furthermore, we emphasized the role of acculturation in food insecurity among the population. The literature has identified acculturation, the process by which immigrants adapt to the host nation, as a major determinant of health disparities. For example, Tsunoda et al. [22] demonstrated that while Japanese adults in Japan perceived the time spent with children as appropriate for also drinking alcohol, Japanese Americans in Hawaii and California, on the other hand, perceived such a situation to be inappropriate. Ma and colleagues [23] further noted that cigarette smoking in homes was positively associated with being a new immigrant while less with increasing acculturation to the United States. Likewise, being more acculturated has been associated with higher fast food consumption among South Asian population in California [24]. While studies on the role of acculturation and food insecurity does not exist among Asian Americans, studies among other ethnic groups highlight putative relationship. For example, a study noted among West African refugees [25] noted that low acculturation was substantially related to higher rates of food insecurity, with similar trend noted among Puerto Ricans as well [26]. Despite such empirical evidence, studies on food insecurity and its potential relationship to acculturation is lacking. In fact, a recent study evaluating the burden of food insecurity, excluded Asian Americans from the study due to low sample [27]; thus further limiting the body of literature on the burden of food insecurity among the population. As such, our study addresses this critical gap in the literature. We hypothesize that the prevalence of food insecurity will be substantially different across the Asian American subgroups and less acculturated groups will likely have higher rates, putatively due to their limited knowledge or accessibility to food aid services.

2. Methods

2.1. Data Source

The public-use files of California Health Interview Survey (CHIS) adult section (2001, 2003, 2005, 2007, 2009, and 2011/2012) were used in this study. The study population was limited to Asian American subgroups: Chinese, Filipino, South Asian, Japanese, Korean, and Vietnamese.

2.2. Measures

The primary dependent variable was CHIS-provided variable on food insecurity, categorized in this study as food insecure versus food secure. CHIS provided a combined poverty and food insecurity variable as: at or above 200% federal poverty level (FPL), below 200% FPL and food secure, below 200% FPL and food insecure without hunger, below 200% FPL and food insecure with hunger. CHIS does not ask those at 200% or above their food security status. In this study, to ensure consistency with USDA guidelines, we refer to food insecure without hunger as low food security and food insecure with hunger as very low food secure. To assess food security level, CHIS researchers asked respondents the following questions: [1] "The food that (I/we) bought just didn't last, and (I/we) didn't have money to get more" [2] "(I/We) couldn't afford to eat balanced meals," [3] "In the last 12 months, did you or other adults in your household ever cut the size of your meals or skip meals because there wasn't enough money for food?" [4] "How often did this happen—almost every month, some months but not every month, or only in 1 or 2 months?" [5] "In the last 12 months, did you ever eat less than you felt you should because there wasn't enough money to buy food?" and [6] "In the last 12 months, were you ever hungry but didn't eat because you couldn't afford enough food?", with the last variable assessing hunger. In this study, to ensure adequate sample size, we collapsed low food security and very low food security variables and refer to them as food insecure.

Primary independent variables included acculturation proxies of language spoken at home (Non-English only, English and another, English only) and country of birth (foreign-born vs. U.S.-born). Such measures have shown validity in the literature as proxies of acculturation and thus makes our results comparable to the empirical body of evidence on acculturation among Asian Americans. For example, Van Wieren and others [28] used CHIS data to explore acculturation and cardiovascular behaviors among the Latino population in California, and acculturation was assessed by country of birth. Likewise, An et al. [29] also utilized CHIS to assess how acculturation was related to cigarette smoking behaviors among Asian Americans where acculturation was assessed using language spoken at home.

Control variables included in regression analyses were: age (18–44 years, 45 years or more), sex (male or female), marital status (currently married or not currently married), education (high school or less, some college, bachelor's degree or higher), employment status (currently employed or not currently employed), self-reported general health status (fair or poor vs. excellent, very good, or good), and zip code-based urban or rural residence, as such location may impact food insecurity due to availability of food items. Such variables were categorized based on CHIS-provided groups and/or natural breakpoints in the distribution. Additionally, body mass index (BMI) categories (overweight or obese, not overweight or obese) based on Asian BMI cutoffs [30] and survey year were included as controls. We chose to include BMI, though it is not a commonly utilized sociodemographic characteristics, as some studies have noted that BMI is related to food insecurity status among other populations [31,32]. Given that Supplemental Nutrition Assistant Program (SNAP) may alleviate food insecurity, we further assessed SNAP participation prevalence among the subgroups by citizenship status as a dichotomized variable.

2.3. Data Analysis

STATA v14 (StataCorp; College Station, TX, USA) was used for all analyses. Appropriate CHIS-provided jackknife survey weights were applied using the "svy" command to compute standard errors and obtain weighted prevalence estimates based on California population control totals. Chi-square analyses utilizing survey design-based F values were used to determine if there were significant differences in food insecurity prevalence among aforementioned control variables for each Asian American subgroup, in addition to SNAP participation by such subgroup stratified by citizenship status due to residential requirements for such federal aid programs. Survey-weighted Poisson regression, which utilizes a robust estimator by default in STATA [33], was run to estimate the adjusted prevalence ratios, according to Petersen and Deddens [34], of food insecurity by each Asian American subgroup as well as differences in SNAP participation by such subgroups. Finally, we also compared the food insecurity rates to the overall CHIS population for the study years. An alpha less than 0.05 was set for all analyses. The study was approved by the Institutional Review Board of California State University (approval number: 13086).

3. Results

A total of 24,803 Asian Americans, representing an average annual population estimate of 18,975,978, were included in this study. As displayed in Table 1, the highest period prevalence of food insecurity was noted among the Vietnamese subgroup (16.42%) and lowest among the Japanese subgroup (2.28%). Prevalence of speaking only a foreign language at home (acculturation proxy) was also highest among the Vietnamese subgroups (52.36%) and lowest among the Japanese (4.95%). Similarly, highest percent of foreign-born individuals (acculturation proxy) was noted among Vietnamese households (88.59%), with the lowest rate for foreign-born individuals among Japanese households (27.02%). Additional population characteristics are further displayed in Table 1.

Table 1. Study population characteristics by Asian American subgroup.

	Chinese	Filipino	South Asian	Japanese	Korean	Vietnamese
Food insecure						
No	6859 (92.4)	3506 (91.74)	2443 (96.86)	2325 (97.72)	3887 (93.43)	3732 (83.58)
Yes	488 (7.60)	259 (8.26)	90 (3.14)	52 (2.28)	308 (6.57)	854 (16.42)
Language spoken at home						
Non-English only	3204 (45.93)	563 (13.39)	351 (14.38)	135 (4.95)	2235 (44.3)	2791 (52.36)
English and another	2788 (38.31)	2008 (53.81)	1792 (70.88)	596 (26.51)	1600 (45.1)	1611 (42.22)
English only	1355 (15.76)	1194 (32.8)	390 (14.74)	1646 (68.54)	359 (10.6)	184 (5.424)
Country of birth						
Foreign-born	5790 (78.05)	2945 (72.69)	2289 (86.78)	652 (27.02)	3838 (82.62)	4370 (88.59)
U.S.-born	1557 (21.95)	820 (27.31)	244 (13.22)	1725 (72.98)	357 (17.38)	216 (11.41)
Age (years)						
18–44	3245 (54.39)	1782 (56.45)	1696 (74.79)	653 (33.61)	1760 (57.35)	1881 (56.77)
45 or more	4102 (45.61)	1983 (43.55)	837 (25.21)	1724 (66.39)	2435 (42.65)	2705 (43.23)
Sex						
Male	3103 (45.41)	1484 (45.87)	1352 (57.24)	926 (40.95)	1568 (39.00)	2263 (49.48)
Female	4244 (54.59)	2281 (54.13)	1181 (42.76)	1451 (59.05)	2627 (61.00)	2323 (50.52)
Marital status						
Not currently married	2647 (38.23)	1492 (42.62)	655 (29.42)	1096 (39.68)	1402 (39.67)	1595 (40.93)
Currently married	4700 (61.77)	2273 (57.38)	1878 (70.58)	1281 (60.32)	2793 (60.33)	2991 (59.07)

Table 1. *Cont.*

	Chinese	Filipino	South Asian	Japanese	Korean	Vietnamese
Education						
High school or less	1980 (31.9)	718 (23.58)	274 (12.14)	488 (26.54)	1334 (30.76)	2478 (51.93)
Some college	1162 (15.07)	927 (25.72)	263 (10.55)	632 (25.17)	570 (13.87)	833 (19.89)
Bachelors or higher	4205 (53.03)	2120 (50.7)	1996 (77.31)	1257 (48.3)	2291 (55.37)	1275 (28.18)
Employment status						
Currently employed	4598 (62.74)	2643 (70.07)	1857 (73.87)	1259 (54.34)	2097 (58.93)	2337 (59.20)
Currently unemployed	2749 (37.26)	1122 (29.93)	676 (26.13)	1118 (45.66)	2098 (41.07)	2249 (40.80)
Self-rated general health status						
Fair or poor	1574 (20.03)	605 (15.68)	189 (5.548)	296 (11.91)	1250 (22.89)	2249 (40.43)
Excellent, very good, or good	5773 (79.97)	3160 (84.32)	2344 (94.45)	2081 (88.09)	2945 (77.11)	2337 (59.57)
Asian-specific BMI category						
Not overweight or obese	3814 (53.37)	1272 (32.62)	978 (40.95)	993 (41.11)	2116 (53.97)	2430 (60.1)
Overweight or obese	3533 (46.63)	2493 (67.38)	1555 (59.05)	1384 (58.89)	2079 (46.03)	2156 (39.9)
Urban/rural status						
Urban	7162 (97.57)	3541 (95.12)	2427 (96.4)	2220 (95.04)	4092 (97.37)	4539 (99.27)
Rural	182 (2.43)	224 (4.88)	106 (3.60)	157 (4.96)	95 (2.63)	34 (0.73)

As shown in Table 2, a significant relationship was found between prevalence of food insecurity and acculturation proxies for Chinese, Korean, and Vietnamese subgroups. For example, prevalence of food insecurity was reported to be 13.72% among non-English speaking Chinese households, as compared to 1.04% among English-only speaking households. Likewise, prevalence of food insecurity was higher among foreign-born Chinese households than those born in the United States (8.90% vs. 3.00%). Among Koreans, prevalence of food insecurity was significantly higher among non-English speaking households than their English-speaking counter parts (9.55% vs. 2.41%), with a similar trend noted for Vietnamese subgroup as well (23.46% vs. 4.84%). Similarly, when compared to those born in the U.S., food insecurity was more prevalent among foreign-born Vietnamese households (18.03% vs. 3.93%). As further noted in Table 2, several other characteristics were associated with food insecurity; and thus all variables were included in the full survey weighted multivariable regression analyses.

Table 2. Association between prevalence of food insecurity and study population characteristics, by Asian American subgroups, results of chi-square analysis.

	Chinese	Filipino	South Asian
Language spoken at home	<0.0001	0.316	0.0722
English only	1.04 (0.56, 1.94)	6.55 (4.04, 10.45)	1.12 (0.46, 2.69)
English and another	2.97 (2.19, 4.01)	9.04 (7.20, 11.29)	3.24 (2.35, 4.45)
Non-English only	13.72 (11.26, 16.59)	9.30 (6.59, 12.96)	4.73 (2.37, 9.22)
Country of birth	0.001	0.422	0.2622
U.S.-born	3.00 (1.52, 5.83)	6.91 (3.97, 11.75)	2.20 (1.16, 4.13)
Foreign-born	8.90 (7.40, 10.65)	8.76 (7.26, 10.54)	3.29 (2.42, 4.45)
Age	0.0032	0.1556	0.0428
18–44 years	5.57 (3.87, 7.96)	7.29 (5.30, 9.95)	2.66 (1.90, 3.73)
45 years or more	10.02 (8.42, 11.89)	9.51 (7.80, 11.54)	4.57 (2.94, 7.04)
Sex	0.9977	0.1846	0.3004
Male	7.60 (5.50, 10.43)	9.40 (6.94, 12.61)	2.73 (1.79, 4.17)
Female	7.60 (6.24, 9.22)	7.29 (5.86, 9.04)	3.69 (2.53, 5.36)
Marital Status	0.4084	0.0272	0.0036
Currently married	8.03 (6.38, 10.04)	6.74 (5.18, 8.71)	2.35 (1.62, 3.37)
Not currently married	6.91 (5.24, 9.06)	10.31 (7.84, 13.44)	5.06 (3.37, 7.54)
Education	<0.0001	<0.0001	<0.0001

Table 2. *Cont.*

	Chinese	Filipino	South Asian
Bachelors or higher	2.69 (1.75, 4.11)	4.25 (3.15, 5.71)	1.42 (0.89, 2.25)
High school or less	16.69 (13.57, 20.34)	17.19 (12.80, 22.69)	10.25 (6.28, 16.29)
Some college	5.67 (4.15, 7.70)	7.97 (5.76, 10.91)	7.62 (4.59, 12.39)
Employment status	0.0005	0.0001	0.0899
Currently employed	5.59 (4.08, 7.62)	6.15 (4.83, 7.81)	2.68 (1.89, 3.78)
Currently unemployed	10.98 (8.85, 13.54)	13.19 (9.90, 17.36)	4.46 (2.75, 7.15)
General health status	<0.0001	<0.0001	<0.0001
Excellent, very good, good	5.49 (4.22, 7.12)	6.80 (5.30, 8.69)	2.57 (1.88, 3.50)
Fair or poor	16.01 (12.67, 20.02)	16.11 (12.05, 21.20)	12.93 (7.65, 21.00)
Asian-specific BMI category	0.7872	0.0666	0.1769
Not overweight/obese	7.77 (6.00, 10.00)	6.57 (5.04, 8.53)	2.49 (1.56, 3.93)
Overweight/obese	7.41 (5.86, 9.32)	9.07 (7.19, 11.39)	3.60 (2.58, 5.00)
Urban/rural status	0.0163	0.3464	0.0589
Urban	7.72 (6.46, 9.20)	8.14 (6.71, 9.84)	2.96 (2.21, 3.97)
Rural	3.15 (1.47, 6.60)	10.57 (6.16, 17.54)	7.96 (2.90, 20.04)
	Japanese	**Korean**	**Vietnamese**
Language spoken at home	0.358	0.0005	<0.0001
English only	2.06 (1.22, 3.47)	2.41 (1.08, 5.29)	4.84 (1.66, 13.28)
English and another	2.45 (1.31, 4.54)	4.63 (2.89, 7.35)	9.18 (6.85, 12.19)
Non-English only	4.46 (1.86, 10.29)	9.55 (7.73, 11.75)	23.46 (20.81, 26.33)
Country of birth	0.0863	0.0932	<0.0001
U.S.-born	1.87 (1.08, 3.24)	3.02 (1.04, 8.44)	3.93 (1.74, 8.60)
Foreign-born	3.38 (2.14, 5.32)	7.32 (5.96, 8.97)	18.03 (15.99, 20.26)
Age	0.2102	<0.0001	<0.0001
18–44 years	3.05 (1.68, 5.47)	4.02 (2.72, 5.89)	12.46 (9.96, 15.47)
45 years or more	1.89 (1.15, 3.10)	10.01 (7.92, 12.57)	21.63 (19.09, 24.39)
Sex	0.2766	0.0221	0.0019
Male	2.88 (1.59, 5.17)	4.86 (3.65, 6.45)	13.30 (10.91, 16.11)
Female	1.87 (1.12, 3.10)	7.66 (5.87, 9.94)	19.48 (16.72, 22.56)
Marital Status	0.26	0.0245	0.5668
Currently married	1.87 (1.03, 3.38)	5.32 (4.21, 6.71)	16.88 (14.61, 19.41)
Not currently married	2.91 (1.75, 4.78)	8.47 (6.07, 11.70)	15.76 (12.85, 19.17)
Education	0.0335	<0.0001	<0.0001
Bachelors or higher	1.20 (0.71, 2.02)	2.43 (1.73, 3.41)	6.74 (4.39, 10.20)
High school or less	3.73 (1.97, 6.96)	13.18 (10.17, 16.91)	23.06 (20.57, 25.75)
Some college	2.84 (1.39, 5.72)	8.43 (4.93, 14.03)	12.80 (8.48, 18.86)
Employment status	0.3548	<0.0001	<0.0001
Currently employed	1.91 (1.00, 3.60)	3.99 (2.92, 5.44)	11.65 (9.26, 14.55)
Currently unemployed	2.73 (1.73, 4.29)	10.27 (7.92, 13.21)	23.34 (20.51, 26.43)
General health status	0.2197	<0.0001	<0.0001
Excellent, very good, good	2.10 (1.35, 3.25)	3.93 (2.91, 5.29)	10.22 (8.06, 12.86)
Fair or poor	3.63 (1.65, 7.76)	15.47 (11.89, 19.87)	25.56 (22.50, 28.88)
Asian-specific BMI category	0.7825	0.5507	0.0316
Not overweight/obese	2.42 (1.54, 3.79)	6.21 (4.67, 8.22)	14.72 (12.22, 17.62)
Overweight/obese	2.19 (1.22, 3.89)	7.00 (5.26, 9.25)	18.98 (16.34, 21.92)
Urban/rural status	0.192	0.1162	0.2329
Urban	2.34 (1.57, 3.48)	6.67 (5.42, 8.18)	16.45 (14.54, 18.55)
Rural	1.08 (0.34, 3.38)	2.48 (0.66, 8.84)	6.68 (1.16, 30.43)

As shown in Table 3 (data on prevalence ratio [PR] for control variables is not shown), both acculturation proxies were associated with food insecurity among Asian Americans, though the relationships varied between subgroups. For example, speaking a language other than English at home was associated with 7.24 times higher prevalence of being food insecure, as compared to speaking English only, among the Chinese subgroup. Similarly, speaking English and another language was associated with nearly three times higher prevalence of food insecurity compared to only speaking English in the same population. South Asians speaking a non-English language at home also had over three and a half times higher prevalence of food insecurity, compared to those who reported speaking English only at home. Furthermore, prevalence food insecurity was significantly associated with being foreign-born among Chinese (prevalence ratio [PR] = 2.31), Filipino (PR = 1.75), Japanese (PR = 2.11), South Asian (PR = 3.35), and Vietnamese (PR = 3.70) subgroups.

Table 3. Prevalence ratio of food insecurity by acculturation status, among Asian American subgroup, results of multivariable robust Poisson regression analysis.

	Language Spoken at Home [a] PR (95% CI)			Country of Birth [b] PR (95% CI)	
	English Only (Reference)	English and Another	Non-English only	U.S.-Born (Reference)	Foreign-Born
Chinese	Ref.	2.51 (1.28, 4.94) **	7.24 (3.68, 14.24) ***	Ref.	2.31(1.17, 4.54) *
Filipino	Ref.	1.55 (0.98, 2.47)	1.56 (0.95, 2.55)	Ref.	1.75 (1.06, 2.87) *
South Asian	Ref.	2.53 (0.97, 6.64)	3.62 (1.04, 12.66) *	Ref.	3.35 (1.36, 8.20) **
Japanese	Ref.	1.24 (0.51, 3.00)	1.82 (0.71, 4.70)	Ref.	2.11 (1.09, 4.09) *
Korean	Ref.	1.57 (0.58, 4.23)	2.06 (0.73, 5.78)	Ref.	1.81 (0.67, 4.90)
Vietnamese	Ref.	1.56 (0.56, 4.40)	2.76 (0.99, 7.66)	Ref.	3.70 (1.58, 8.66) **

[a] Poisson regression model includes language spoken at home as the primary exposure variable and control variables of age, sex, martial status, education, employment, self-reported general health status, urban/rural, BMI, and survey year; [b] Poisson regression model includes country of birth as the primary exposure variable and control variables of age, sex, martial status, education, employment, self-reported general health status, urban/rural, BMI, and survey year; PR = prevalence ratio, CI = confidence interval, Ref. = reference category; * $p < 0.05$, ** $p < 0.01$, *** $p < 0.001$.

Table 4 further displays the SNAP participation rate by acculturation status among the six Asian American subgroups.

Table 4. Prevalence of SNAP participation among Asian American subgroups.

	Language Spoken at Home			Country of Birth		Citizenship Status	
	English only	English and Another	Non-English only	U.S.-Born	Foreign-Born	Citizen	Non-Citizen
Chinese	–	2.95	4.77	–	4.28	1.3397	3.4626
Filipino	–	2.88	1.75	–	2.64	0.5794	2.9532
South Asian	–	3.35	–	–	3.48	0.7457	1.0001
Japanese	–	–	–	–	–	–	–
Korean	–	1..85	3.16	–	2.94	1.2389	1.3562
Vietnamese	–	9.02	15.67	3.12	14.33	6.7969	17.4218

– The percent is not reported due to sample size being $n < 10$.

As noted, such participation is substantially low in the population over all. The highest rate based on language spoken at home was noted among Vietnamese who spoke a non-English only (15.67%) and were foreign-born (14.33%). Even when looking at by citizenship status, the prevalence was substantially low for all with the higher rates noted among non-citizens, especially among Vietnamese. For most subgroups, the participation rate was less than n = 10, thus resulting in lack of data reporting to ensure privacy of CHIS participants.

4. Discussion

While evaluation of the burden of food insecurity among minority populations is prevalent in the empirical body of literature, little assessment exists among the Asian American population. We thus studied the period prevalence of food insecurity among disaggregated Asian American subgroups in California, as well as whether acculturation was a determining factor of such disparities. The results of our study highlight several key findings: (1) food insecurity among Asian American subgroups is diverse, with lowest prevalence noted among Japanese (2.28%) and highest among Vietnamese (16.42%), (2) low acculturation is predominantly associated with higher prevalence of food insecurity among most Asian American subgroups, and (3) SNAP participation among the population remains substantially low.

Such results have several implications. In a previous study based in Los Angeles, Furness et al. noted that Whites, African-Americans, and Latinos had a higher prevalence of food insecurity compared to Asian/Pacific Islanders [35]. One plausible difference from such results to what is highlighted in our study is the disaggregation of data. Asian Americans are a diverse population with unique cultural and linguistic characteristics. Thus, the aggregation into one homogenous group can often mask true disparities among subgroups. Furthermore, in our study the highest prevalence of food insecurity was noted among the Vietnamese subgroup (16.42%), which is substantially higher than the other Asian American subgroup population as well as the entire CHIS population (11.80%). As such, consistent with the literature evaluating health disparities among Asian American, our study also demonstrate that Asian Americans remain a diverse population [36] with unique needs and thus disaggregation of data when assessing such social determinants of health are critical for public health efforts.

In addition, we noted that two proxies of acculturation were related to food insecurity among specific Asian American subgroups. This is similar to other studies that have shown Asian Americans who are less acculturated to suffer worse disparities. For instance, Tang et al. [37] noted that less acculturation was associated higher tobacco use while Jang and group [38] noted that alienation from heritage culture was associated with worse physical and mental health among Asian Americans.

One putative explanation for our results could be that less acculturated populations are more likely to adhere to Asian-based traditional food items, which are often more difficult to access due to cost [39], thus making such households more food insecure; however comprehensive assessment of Asian traditional food cost as compared to American food remains limited in the literature. In addition, in our study, we further see a substantially low SNAP participation in each Asian American subgroup, even among citizens. This could be potentially explained by culture-based stigma. For example, a report including Korean-speaking adults noted that most participants would not turn to a food assistance program for help and often considered them as a last option, often due to limitations of culturally appropriate food items [40] and culturally-associated stigma as such opportunities are often considered "handouts" [40]. The lack of any empirical evidence understanding the barriers to food aid participation among the Asian American population and the limitation of the aforementioned report to Korean population only, further highlights the imperative need for further research on understanding the barriers to ensuring food security among the Asian American population.

Finally, given the negative burden of food insecurity on health and behavioral outcomes, as noted in the literature, [18,21], the higher rates of food insecurity among less acculturated Asian American subgroups further shown in our study, the cumulative evidence warrants targeted public health efforts among the most at-risk groups. However, limited studies exist on what such public health efforts should include.

Herein also lies the opportunity for collaborative effort between the healthcare system and the community to ensure more positive outcomes. For example, in a proof of concept assessment of the efficacy of community health workers to improve childhood health outcomes, Martin et al. demonstrated the positive influence of home visitations on asthma control, emergency care utilizations, and inhaler usage [41]. While similar assessment on the efficacy of home visitation techniques on food insecurity remains limited, Tough et al. noted that home visitations improved nutrition counselling attendance among at-risk mothers, including those with language barriers [42]. As such, public health efforts to pilot test the efficacy of community health workers among Asian American subgroups and to create home visitation programs in order to assess food availability and increase participation in food assistance programs may help alleviate the burden of food insecurity among the most vulnerable Asian American populations.

Additionally, a critical point of contact for most populations remain the healthcare system. Means to identify Asian American subgroups at risk of food insecurity at healthcare facilities remains imperative. For example, the American Academy of Pediatrics notes the importance of a screening tool utilized during practice to identify children living in food insecure households; such as the Household Food Security Scale or the in-office 2-item screener [43]. A similar strategy can be utilized when screening adults, especially one tailored to Asian-specific languages.

Finally, as noted by Roncarolo and Potvin [44], simply providing access to food banks or food aid program is analogous to treating diseases with drugs. Instead, there is undoubtedly a need to identify the most at-risk populations early to prevent food insecurity from occurring. As such, to preventing the onset of food insecurity, if it were to be truly treated as a symptom of "social disease" [44], then governmental-level interventions, including that of local initiatives, are needed to improve continued access to healthy food options. For example, while farmers' markets continue to be considered a key component of improving access to food, often they lack culturally appropriate food items. In San Francisco, California, a collaborative effort among food stamp programs and public health and nonprofit organizations demonstrated feasibility of increased access to farmers' markets, especially through payment systems [45]. Similar strategies that incorporate partnerships between Asian American-based organizations and local public health agencies may provide a scope of improved access to food among such at-risk groups.

The results of our study should be interpreted in the context of some limitations inherent to the study design. The study sample is limited to California and thus cannot be generalized outside of the state. Furthermore, the proxies of acculturation utilized in this study may not encompass all feasible operationalization of acculturation. For example, studies note that acculturation can be bidimensional or unidimensional and these domains are not captured by the proxies. The self-report and recall biases inherent to surveys may further posit as limitations to interpretation of results. Nevertheless, such limitations do not negate the diversity in food insecurity prevalence noted in the Asian American subgroups, especially the disproportionately high levels noted among the Vietnamese subgroup.

5. Conclusions

Our study results demonstrate heterogeneity in the burden of food insecurity among the most vulnerable Asian American subgroups, especially those who are less acculturated. There is a significant gap in the literature addressing barriers to food aid among such populations and thus our results not only highlight the need for more comprehensive assessment, but also outreach to increase food aid participation for the most at-risk groups. There are also several strengths to this study. The sampling design of CHIS and survey-weighted analyses allow for generalization to Asian Americans in California, thus increasing the external validity of this study. Furthermore, the results provide one of the first assessments of food insecurity among Asian American subgroups, especially since there remains limited data to assess South Asian health, with CHIS being one of the few to provide public access to such data. As such, this study's results provide a valuable addition by providing the first comprehensive analyses of the burden of food insecurity among disaggregated Asian American populations.

Author Contributions: M.B.B. was the principal investigator of this study. S.K.M. conducted literature review. B.J.B. conducted data analysis. All authors contributed to data interpretation and manuscript development.

Funding: M.B.B. was supported by the faculty professional development mini-grant from California State University, San Bernardino.

Acknowledgments: M.B.B. would also like to thank the Institute for Child Development and Family Relations and Faculty Center for Excellence for providing M.B.B. the time and resources for writing.

Conflicts of Interest: The authors of this study declare no conflict of interest.

References

1. Colby, S.; Ortman, J. *Projections of the Size and Composition of the U.S. Population: 2014 to 2060, Current Population Reports, P25-1143*; U.S. Census Bureau: Washington, DC, USA, 2015.
2. Yi, V.; Museus, S.D. Model Minority Myth. In *The Wiley Blackwell Encyclopedia of Race, Ethnicity, and Nationalism*; John Wiley & Sons, Ltd.: Hoboken, NJ, USA, 2015.
3. Gupta, A.; Szymanski, D.M.; Leong, F.T.L. The 'model minority myth': Internalized racialism of positive stereotypes as correlates of psychological distress, and attitudes toward help-seeking. *Asian Am. J. Psychol.* 2011, 2, 101–114. [CrossRef]

4.   Initiative on Asian Americans and Pacific Islanders. 24 September 2014. Available online: https://www. whitehouse.gov/embeds/footer (accessed on 3 October 2016).

5.   Takei, I.; Sakamoto, A. Poverty among Asian Americans in the 21st Century. *Sociol. Perspect.* **2011**, *54*, 251–276. [CrossRef]

6.   Klatsky, A.L.; Friedman, G.D.; Sidney, S.; Kipp, H.; Kubo, A.; Armstrong, M.A. Risk of hemorrhagic stroke in Asian American ethnic groups. *Neuroepidemiology* **2005**, *25*, 26–31. [CrossRef] [PubMed]

7.   Sarwar, E.; Arias, D.; Becerra, B.J.; Becerra, M.B. Sociodemographic Correlates of Dietary Practices among Asian-Americans: Results from the California Health Interview Survey. *J. Racial Ethn. Health Disparities* **2015**, *2*, 494–500. [CrossRef] [PubMed]

8.   Becerra, M.B.; Becerra, B.J. Disparities in Age at Diabetes Diagnosis among Asian Americans: Implications for Early Preventive Measures. *Prev. Chronic. Dis.* **2015**, *12*, E146. [CrossRef] [PubMed]

9.   Palaniappan, L.; Wang, Y.; Fortmann, S.P. Coronary heart disease mortality for six ethnic groups in California, 1990–2000. *Ann. Epidemiol.* **2004**, *14*, 499–506. [CrossRef] [PubMed]

10.   Becerra, M.B.; Herring, P.; Marshak, H.H.; Banta, J.E. Social Determinants of Physical Activity among Adult Asian-Americans: Results from a Population-Based Survey in California. *J. Immigr. Minor. Health* **2014**, *17*, 1061–1069. [CrossRef] [PubMed]

11.   United States Department of Agriculture. *Definitions of Food Security*; United States Department of Agriculture: Washington, DC, USA, 2017.

12.   United States Department of Agriculture. *Economic Research Service, Key Statistics & Graphics*; United States Department of Agriculture: Washington, DC, USA, 2016.

13.   Wong, J.C.; Scott, T.; Wilde, P.; Li, Y.; Tucker, K.L.; Gao, X. Food Insecurity Is Associated with Subsequent Cognitive Decline in the Boston Puerto Rican Health Study. *J. Nutr.* **2016**, *146*, 1740–1745. [CrossRef] [PubMed]

14.   Alaimo, K.; Olson, C.M.; Frongillo, E.A. Food Insufficiency and American School-Aged Children's Cognitive, Academic, and Psychosocial Development. *Pediatrics* **2001**, *108*, 44–53. [PubMed]

15.   Becerra, M.B.; Hassija, C.M.; Becerra, B.J. Food insecurity is associated with unhealthy dietary practices among US veterans in California. *Public Health Nutr.* **2016**, *20*, 2569–2576. [CrossRef] [PubMed]

16.   Kaiser, L.L.; Lamp, C.L.; Johns, M.C.; Sutherlin, J.M.; Harwood, J.O.; Melgar-Quiñonez, H.R. Food Security and Nutritional Outcomes of Preschool-Age Mexican-American Children. *J. Am. Diet. Assoc.* **2002**, *102*, 924–929. [CrossRef]

17.   Pryor, L.; Lioret, S.; van der Waerden, J.; Fombonne, É.; Falissard, B.; Melchior, M. Food insecurity and mental health problems among a community sample of young adults. *Soc. Psychiatry Psychiatr. Epidemiol.* **2016**, *51*, 1073–1081. [CrossRef] [PubMed]

18.   Becerra, B.J.; Sis-Medina, R.C.; Reyes, A.; Becerra, M.B. Association between Food Insecurity and Serious Psychological Distress among Hispanic Adults Living in Poverty. *Prev. Chronic. Dis.* **2015**, *12*, E206. [CrossRef] [PubMed]

19.   Weigel, M.M.; Armijos, R.X.; Hall, Y.P.; Ramirez, Y.; Orozco, R. The Household Food Insecurity and Health Outcomes of U.S.–Mexico Border Migrant and Seasonal Farmworkers. *J. Immigr. Minor. Health* **2007**, *9*, 157–169. [CrossRef] [PubMed]

20.   Allen, N.L.; Becerra, B.J.; Becerra, M.B. Associations between food insecurity and the severity of psychological distress among African-Americans. *Ethn. Health* **2017**, *23*, 511–520. [CrossRef] [PubMed]

21.   To, Q.G.; Frongillo, E.A.; Gallegos, D.; Moore, J.B. Household food insecurity is associated with less physical activity among children and adults in the U.S. population. *J. Nutr.* **2014**, *144*, 1797–1802. [CrossRef] [PubMed]

22.   Tsunoda, T.; Parrish, K.M. The effect of acculturation on drinking attitudes among Japanese in Japan and Japanese Americans. *J. Stud. Alcohol* **1992**, *53*, 369. [CrossRef] [PubMed]

23.   Ma, G.X.; Shive, S.E.; Tan, Y.; Feeley, R.M. The Impact of Acculturation on Smoking in Asian American Homes. *J. Healthc. Poor Underserved* **2004**, *15*, 267–280. [CrossRef] [PubMed]

24.   Becerra, M.B.; Herring, P.; Marshak, H.H.; Banta, J.E. Generational differences in fast food intake among South-Asian Americans: Results from a population-based survey. *Prev. Chronic. Dis.* **2014**, *11*, E211. [CrossRef] [PubMed]

25.   Hadley, C.; Zodhiates, A.; Sellen, D.W. Acculturation, economics and food insecurity among refugees resettled in the USA: A case study of West African refugees. *Public Health Nutr.* **2007**, *10*, 405–412. [CrossRef] [PubMed]

26. Dhokarh, R.; Himmelgreen, D.A.; Peng, Y-K.; Segura-Perez, S.; Hromi-Fiedler, A.; Perez-Escamilla, R. Food Insecurity is Associated with Acculturation and Social Networks in Puerto Rican Households. *J. Nutr. Educ. Behav.* **2011**, *43*, 288–294. [CrossRef] [PubMed]

27. Strings, S.; Ranchod, Y.K.; Laraia, B.; Nuru-Jeter, A. Race and Sex Differences in the Association between Food Insecurity and Type 2 Diabetes. *Ethn. Dis.* **2016**, *26*, 427–434. [CrossRef] [PubMed]

28. Van Wieren, A.J.; Roberts, M.B.; Arellano, N.; Feller, E.R.; Diaz, J.A. Acculturation and cardiovascular behaviors among Latinos in California by country/region of origin. *J. Immigr. Minor. Health Cent. Minor. Public Health* **2011**, *13*, 975–981. [CrossRef] [PubMed]

29. An, N.; Cochran, S.D.; Mays, V.M.; McCarthy, W.J. Influence of American acculturation on cigarette smoking behaviors among Asian American subpopulations in California. *Nicotine Tob. Res. Off. J. Soc. Res. Nicotine Tob.* **2008**, *10*, 579–587. [CrossRef] [PubMed]

30. WHO Expert Consultation. Appropriate body-mass index for Asian populations and its implications for policy and intervention strategies. *Lancet* **2004**, *363*, 157–163. [CrossRef]

31. Townsend, M.S.; Peerson, J.; Love, B.; Achterberg, C.; Murphy, S.P. Food Insecurity Is Positively Related to Overweight in Women. *J. Nutr.* **2001**, *131*, 1738–1745. [CrossRef] [PubMed]

32. Dinour, L.M.; Bergen, D.; Yeh, M. The Food Insecurity–Obesity Paradox: A Review of the Literature and the Role Food Stamps May Play. *J. Acad. Nutr. Diet.* **2007**, *107*, 1952–1961. [CrossRef] [PubMed]

33. StataCorp LLC. A Stata Press Publication, Stata Survey Data Reference Manual: Release 14, 2015. Available online: https://www.stata.com/manuals14/svy.pdf (accessed on 20 October 2017).

34. Petersen, M.R.; Deddens, J.A. A comparison of two methods for estimating prevalence ratios. *BMC Med. Res. Methodol.* **2008**, *8*, 9. [CrossRef] [PubMed]

35. Furness, B.W.; Simon, P.A.; Wold, C.M.; Asarian-Anderson, J. Prevalence and predictors of food insecurity among low-income households in Los Angeles County. *Public Health Nutr.* **2004**, *7*, 791–794. [CrossRef] [PubMed]

36. Holland, A.T.; Palaniappan, L.P. Problems with the Collection and Interpretation of Asian-American Health Data: Omission, Aggregation, and Extrapolation. *Ann. Epidemiol.* **2012**, *22*, 397–405. [CrossRef] [PubMed]

37. Tang, H.; Shimizu, R.; Chen, M.S. English Language Proficiency and Smoking Prevalence among California's Asian Americans. *Cancer* **2005**, *104*, 2982–2988. [CrossRef] [PubMed]

38. Jang, Y.; Park, N.S.; Chiriboga, D.A.; Kim, M.T. Latent Profiles of Acculturation and Their Implications for Health: A Study with Asian Americans in Central Texas. *Asian Am. J. Psychol.* **2017**, *8*, 200–208. [CrossRef] [PubMed]

39. Mekouar, D. Does Bias Impact Price of U.S. Ethnic Food?—All about America. VOA, 2016. Available online: https://blogs.voanews.com/all-about-america/2016/04/13/why-americans-will-pay-more-for-french-food-than-chinese-cuisine/ (accessed on 20 October 2017).

40. Gabor, V.; Williams, S.; Bellamy, H.; Hardison, B.; Health Systems Research, Inc. *Seniors' Views of the Food Stamp Program and Ways to Improve Participation—Focus Group Findings in Washington State*; Economic Research Service, U.S. Department of Agriculture: Washington, DC, USA, 2002.

41. Martin, M.A.; Rothschild, S.K.; Lynch, E.; Christoffel, K.K.; Pagán, M.M.; Rodriguez, J.L.; Barnes, A.; Karavolos, K.; Diaz, A.; Hoffman, L.M.; et al. Addressing asthma and obesity in children with community health workers: Proof-of-concept intervention development. *BMC Pediatr.* **2016**, *16*, 198. [CrossRef] [PubMed]

42. Tough, S.C.; Johnston, D.W.; Siever, J.E.; Jorgenson, G.; Slocombe, L.; Lane, C.; Clarke, M. Does Supplementary Prenatal Nursing and Home Visitation Support Improve Resource Use in a Universal Health Care System? A Randomized Controlled Trial in Canada. *Birth* **2006**, *33*, 183–194. [PubMed]

43. Council on Community Pediatrics. Commitee on Nutrition, Promoting Food Security for All Children. *Pediatrics* **2015**, *136*, e1431–e1438. [CrossRef] [PubMed]

44. Roncarolo, F.; Potvin, L. Food insecurity as a symptom of a social disease. *Can. Fam. Physician* **2016**, *62*, 291–292. [PubMed]

45. Jones, P.; Bhatia, R. Supporting Equitable Food Systems through Food Assistance at Farmers' Markets. *Am. J. Public Health* **2011**, *101*, 781–783. [CrossRef] [PubMed]

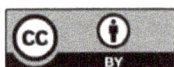

International Journal of
*Environmental Research
and Public Health*

MDPI

Article

The Association between Stressful Events and Food Insecurity: Cross-Sectional Evidence from Australia

Jeromey B. Temple[ORCID]

Demography and Ageing Unit, Melbourne School of Population and Global Health, University of Melbourne, Melbourne 3010, Australia; Jeromey.Temple@unimelb.edu.au; Tel.: +61-3-9035-9900

Received: 1 August 2018; Accepted: 17 October 2018; Published: 23 October 2018

Abstract: A considerable body of empirical evidence exists on the demographic and socio-economic correlates of food insecurity in Australia. An important omission from recent studies, however, is an understanding of the role of stressful life events, or stressors in explaining exposure to food insecurity. Using nationally representative data from the 2014 General Social Survey and multivariable logistic regression, this paper reports on the association between 18 discrete stressors and the likelihood of reporting food insecurity in Australia. The results, adjusted for known correlates of food insecurity and complex survey design, show that exposure to stressors significantly increased the likelihood of experiencing food insecurity. Importantly, stressors related to employment and health approximately doubled the odds of experiencing food insecurity. The results underscore the complex correlates of food insecurity and indicates that conceptually it interacts with many important social and economic problems in contemporary Australia. There is no simple fix to food insecurity and solutions require co-ordination across a range of social and economic policies.

Keywords: food insecurity; stressors; stressful life events; access to food; food equality

1. Introduction

Food insecurity is the "limited or uncertain availability of nutritionally adequate and safe foods or limited or uncertain ability to acquire acceptable foods in socially acceptable ways" [1]. In 1975, Australia ratified the United Nations International Covenant on Economic, Social and Cultural Rights, recognising the fundamental human right for its citizenry to be free from hunger [2]. More recently, in 2015, Australia further ratified the United Nations 2030 Agenda for Sustainable Development and the Sustainable Development Goals which seek to eliminate poverty and inequality, with a target of 'zero hunger' by 2030 [3].

Indeed, it is now widely understood that food insecurity is a problem facing not only low and middle-income countries, but also high-income countries such as the USA, Canada and Australia [4,5]. In Australia, approximately 4–5% of the population are estimated to be food insecure, due to a lack of financial resources, with about 40% of this group (or 2% of the population) going without food consequently [6,7]. However, the experience of food insecurity is not evenly spread throughout the Australian population, with a growing number of studies showing that constellations of socio-economic, demographic and geographic factors are associated with food insecurity. For example, young age, being divorced or separated, low income, low education, low financial resources, a high number of resident children, poor health, not owning your home, being unemployed, being an Aboriginal or Torres Strait Islander and measures of spatial disadvantage are all associated with experiencing food insecurity in Australia [7–23].

One important omission from recent studies, however, is an understanding of the role of stressful life events, or stressors, in explaining exposure to food insecurity. Stressors are events, whether anticipated or not, that can have a deleterious effect on the wellbeing of individuals and their families (e.g., onset of a serious health condition or unanticipated unemployment). Independent of known risk factors of food insecurity, an analysis of the association between stressors and food insecurity may provide evidence as to why some households beyond the bottom quintile of household income experience food insecurity in high income countries such as Australia.

International studies, mostly qualitative, have provided some evidence that stressors are associated with, or are a precursor to experiencing food insecurity. In two qualitative studies of low-income older Americans, major sickness and unexpected expenses and medical bills were key factors explaining food insecurity [24,25]. Moreover, family events such as Christmas were cited as a precursor to food insecurity, due to the financial costs associated with filial obligations such as gift giving [25]. A recent US mixed methods study provides some evidence that exposure to adverse childhood experiences (e.g., abuse, neglect, household instability) was associated with experiencing food insecurity later in adulthood [26]. A further qualitative American study found that stressful events such as those related to health and employment were related to food insecurity, but were also mediated by families 'capabilities' to offset negative consequences [27]. This finding is supported by a recent quantitative study which found that families adjusting to negative life events with low levels of income and social support were at a much greater risk of child hunger [28]. In Canada, both the onset of chronic disease and problem gambling were found to be associated with food insecurity in higher-income households [29].

Within the Australian literature, there have been few studies examining the link between stressors and food insecurity. Australian studies have, however, investigated the coping mechanisms used to avoid hunger when stressors such as homelessness, enduring social disadvantage and exogenous policy changes to welfare payments occur [20,30,31]. Generally, it is widely acknowledged that stressors may be an important determinant of food insecurity. For example, Burns (2004) has suggested "Although most persons living in poverty are at risk of food insecurity, it cannot be assumed that they are, in fact, food insecure. In addition, for many reasons, including factors such as ill health, disability, sudden job loss, and high living expenses, persons above the poverty line cannot be assumed to be food secure" [32], p. 7. Furthermore, in Temple's (2008) study of food insecurity in Australia, it is noted "It may be that in times of sudden unemployment, divorce, death or unexpected illness, greater stress is placed on family resources. The ability to negotiate these stresses is likely to contribute to the prevalence of food insecurity" [7], p. 662.

In this study, nationally representative data were used to examine the association between stressors and food insecurity. Firstly, the likelihood of food insecure persons (relative to the food secure) reporting a stressor in the previous 12 months was examined. Secondly, the prevalence of food insecurity categorised by 18 discrete stressors was calculated. Finally, multivariable logistic regression models were used to examine the association between individual stressors and the odds of food insecurity, once extensive controls were accounted for.

2. Materials and Methods

2.1. Survey Data

Data used in this study were from the 2014 General Social Survey (GSS) conducted by the Australian Bureau of Statistics (ABS) between March and June 2014. Using a face-to-face interview along with prompt cards, the ABS collected information using a Computer Assisted Interviewing (CAI) questionnaire on a range of domains to understand the "multi-dimensional nature of relative advantage and disadvantage across the population, and to facilitate reporting on and monitoring of people's opportunities to participate fully in society" [33]. The GSS was designed to provide nationally and state representative estimates across these domains. From a sample of 18,574 private dwellings, 16,145 dwellings were used due to issues of scope or uninhabited dwellings. In total, 80% fully responded, yielding a sample of 12,932 people aged 15 years and over.

The GSS included persons who were usual residents of private dwellings at the time of the survey. This sampling design meant that several populations were excluded including those living in non-private dwellings (e.g., hostels, hospitals, short-stay caravan parks). Also excluded were diplomatic or defence personnel of overseas governments stationed in Australia, those whose usual place of residence was outside of Australia, or those living in very remote areas of discrete Aboriginal and Torres Strait Islander communities. People experiencing homelessness were also excluded from the survey.

2.2. Measurement

Two questions were included in the GSS instrument to identify exposure to stressors. Firstly, the interviewer asked: "Have any of these been a problem for you or anyone close to you, during the last 12 months?". A prompt card (Card F15) was shown to respondents listing: 1. Serious illness, 2. Serious accident, 3. Death of a family member of close friend, 4. Mental illness, 5. Serious disability. Respondents were than further prompted, repeating the question with a second prompt card (Card F16) listing: 10. Divorce or separation, 11. Not able to get a job, 12. Involuntary loss of job, 13. Alcohol or drug related problems, 14. Witness to violence, 15. Abuse or violent crime, 16. Trouble with police, 17. Gambling problem, 18. Discrimination because of ethnic or cultural background 19. Discrimination for any other reason, 20. Bullying and/or harassment, 21. Removal of children, 22. Other. Using these questions, variables measuring 18 distinct stressors were generated.

Measurement of food insecurity in the GSS is included in the financial stress, resilience and exclusion module. Respondents were asked "In the last 12 months, have any of these happened because you were short of money?" A prompt card (Card K1) was shown to the respondent. Respondents who indicated that they went without meals due to a shortage of money were coded as being food insecure. The measurement of going without a meal due to a shortage of money is considered a measure of considerable financially attributable food insecurity, indicative of both inadequate food intake and food depletion [7].

2.3. Statistical Model

To examine the association between stressors and food insecurity multivariable logistic regression models were fitted. Using the raw logit coefficients, adjusted odds ratios (AOR) were calculated, which measure the change in the odds of experiencing food insecurity given an experience of each stressor, once all other factors in the model are controlled for. Regression models were estimated for each stressor independently. Given that food insecurity attributable to financial constraints is a relatively rare event, the stability of the logit coefficients were compared against those of a Scobit (Skewed Logit), Complementary Log-Log and Log Poisson regression model. The strength, significance and direction of parameter coefficients was highly comparable across all regression models, and the logit results are presented herein for simplicity.

Due to complex survey design, adjustments are necessary to generate correct variance estimates. The GSS includes 60 replicate weights on the data file to adjust for sample design and non-response. Utilizing an algorithm developed by Winter, the delete-one jackknife method was used to make the necessary replicate adjustments [34,35]. All analyses were conducted using Stata via the ABS Remote Access Data Laboratory.

Control Variables

Drawing upon previous Australian research outlined above, variables know to be associated with food insecurity were included in the regressions to control for potentially confounding effects. Specifically, the control variables included:

- Age: 15–29, 30–44, 45–59, 60+.
- Marital Status: Married, not married.

- Equivalised Household Income: The measure of household income available in the GSS is gross household income, adjusted or 'equivalised' using an equivalence scale to account for household size and placed in deciles. The ABS make this adjustment in household income to allow for welfare and financial wellbeing comparisons between households of different sizes and compositions. The categories included in the regression based upon income distribution include: 0 to 20%, 20% to 40%, 40% to 60%, 60% to 80%, 80% to 100%, not reported.
- Self-Rated Health: Poor or fair health, good or excellent health.
- Tenure: Renter, not a renter.
- University educated: Has university education, does not have university education.

Additional variables including gender and measures of geography were also included but were not found to be significant at the 95% critical level. For each stressor model, it would be inappropriate to include all control variables due to concerns regarding multicollinearity and other model misspecification issues. Specifically, for the divorce or separation model, marital status was omitted. For the illness, accident, mental illness and disability stressor models, self-rated health was omitted.

3. Results

3.1. Experiences of Stressors

Except for 'other' stressors, food insecure respondents were more likely to report experiencing each type of stressor, relative to the food secure (Table 1). Over one third of food insecure respondents reported not being able to get a job (40.5%), death of a family member or close friend (35.1%), mental illness (34.9%) and serious illness (33.3%). Large differences in the reporting of stressors between food insecure and secure respondents existed for not being able to get a job (40.5% v 16.8%) and mental illness (34.9% v 13.0%). Other considerable differences between food secure and secure respondents (with a difference in prevalence of greater than 10%) included bullying and harassment, alcohol or drug related problems, death of a family member or close friend, witness to violence, trouble with the police and serious illness. Whereas 38% of food secure persons reported no stressors in the last 12 months, only 14% of food insecure respondents did not experience stressors. In contrast, about half of the food insecure reported three or more stressors, compared with 16% of the food secure.

Table 1. Stressors reported by Food Insecurity Status, Weighted (%), 2014.

	Food Insecure (%)	Food Secure (%)		n [1]
Type of Stressor [2]				
Divorce or Separation	17.6	11.3	***	1467
Death of Family Member/Close Friend	35.1	21.4	***	2957
Serious Illness	33.3	22.3	***	3008
Serious Accident	7.7	4.5	**	612
Alcohol or Drug Related Problems	20.7	6.8	***	988
Mental Illness	34.9	13.0	***	1769
Serious Disability	13.1	6.0	***	914
Not Able to Get a Job	40.5	16.8	***	1952
Involuntary Job Loss	16.5	7.0	***	859
Witness to Violence	15.8	2.2	***	426
Abuse or Violent Crime	12.6	2.5	***	428
Trouble with the Police	14.2	2.8	***	413
Gambling Problem	6.6	2.6	***	308
Discrimination-Ethnic or Cultural Background	5.5	2.1	***	301
Discrimination-Other Reason	7.6	1.6	***	262
Bullying and/or Harassment	20.6	6.4	***	929
Removal of Children	4.8	<1%	***	141
Other	<1%	<1%		88

Table 1. *Cont.*

	Food Insecure (%)	Food Secure (%)		n [1]
Number of Stressors [3]				
None	14.0	38.1	***	4845
1	21.1	30.2	***	3807
2	15.7	15.4		1991
3	15.9	7.4	***	1011
4+	33.4	8.9	***	1278
Total	100	100		
Unweighted (n)	403	12,529		12,932

[1] Unweighted sample size per stressor; [2] Experiencing each stressor in the previous 12 months; [3] Number of stressors reported in previous 12 months. *** $p < 0.001$, ** $p < 0.01$. Significance tests denote test of proportion of exposure to each stressor by food insecurity status.

3.2. Prevalence of Food Insecurity by Stressor Type

Given that food insecure respondents were more likely to experience a range of stressors relative to their food secure peers, it is therefore not unexpected that the prevalence rates of food insecurity were much higher for those experiencing stressors (Table 2). Consistent with previous research using a similar measure, the prevalence of food insecurity with insufficient intake and food depletion was approximately 2% among the general population living in households [7]. The prevalence of food insecurity among those reporting no stressors in the previous 12 months was less than 1%. In strong contrast, the prevalence of food insecurity was very high among those reporting witness to violence (12.6%), removal of children (11.7%), abuse or violent crime (9.3%), trouble with the police (9.3%), discrimination—other reason (8.7%) and bullying or harassment (6.1%). Again, across all categories of stressors with the exception of 'other' stressors, prevalence rates of food insecurity were significantly above those who did not report any stressors or the general population level prevalence.

Table 2. Prevalence of food insecurity by stressor type, 2014.

	Weighted [1] (%)	Unweighted [2] (%)	
Type of Stressor [3]			
Divorce or Separation	3.1	5.7	***
Death of Family Member/Close Friend	3.2	4.9	***
Serious Illness	2.9	5.1	***
Serious Accident	3.4	5.9	**
Alcohol or Drug Related Problems	5.8	9.7	***
Mental Illness	5.2	8.7	***
Serious Disability	4.2	7.9	***
Not Able to Get a Job	4.6	7.7	***
Involuntary Job Loss	4.5	7.3	***
Witness to Violence	12.6	16.4	***
Abuse or Violent Crime	9.3	15.0	***
Trouble with the Police	9.3	12.6	***
Gambling Problem	5.0	9.1	***
Discrimination-Ethnic or Cultural Background	5.1	9.0	***
Discrimination-Other Reason	8.7	14.1	***
Bullying and/or Harassment	6.1	9.0	***
Removal of Children	11.7	15.6	***
Other	2.0	5.7	

Table 2. *Cont.*

	Weighted [1] (%)	Unweighted [2] (%)	
Number of Stressors [4]			
None	<1%	<1%	–
1	1.4	1.7	**
2	2.0	3.9	***
3	4.2	6.2	***
4+	7.1	11.7	***
Full Sample	2.0	3.1	***

[1] Prevalence weighted using ABS survey weights; [2] Unweighted prevalence; [3] Tests of proportions for type of stressor relative to not experiencing each stressor; [4] Tests of proportions for number of stressors relative to those reporting no stressors. 'None' is the comparison category; *** $p < 0.001$, ** $p < 0.01$, + $p < 0.1$.

Although these descriptive results indicate significant differences in the prevalence of food insecurity by exposure to stressors, it is important to control for variables that may indicate spurious statistical relationships. For example, was the prevalence of food insecurity high among those reporting bullying or harassment due to a younger age profile of those reporting this stressor? Similarly, were prevalence rates of food insecurity among those reporting a mental health stressor high because of lower average levels of economic resources available to those with mental health conditions?

3.3. Regression Results

To control for confounding effects, multivariable logistic regression models were fitted to calculate odds ratios to measure the association between each stressor and food insecurity, once extensive controls for socio-economic factors previously shown to be associated with food insecurity in Australia were accounted for. Odds ratios adjusted for control variables (AOR) and unadjusted for control variables (UOR) are presented for transparency (Table 3). Comparing the adjusted and unadjusted results, the higher magnitude of the unadjusted odds ratios indicates the importance of the control factors in explaining food insecurity. This is further discussed below.

Table 3. Odds ratios from multivariable logistic regression models of food insecurity, 2014.

	Odds Ratio (UOR) [1]	Odds Ratio (AOR) [2]	
Stressor Type Models [3]			
Divorce or Separation	1.68	1.53	*
Death of Family Member/Close Friend	1.99	2.01	***
Serious Illness	1.74	1.81	**
Serious Accident	1.78	1.55	
Alcohol or Drug Related Problems	3.58	2.35	***
Mental Illness	3.59	2.87	***
Serious Disability	2.36	2.30	**
Not Able to Get a Job	3.35	2.49	***
Involuntary Job Loss	2.62	2.59	***
Witness to Violence	8.27	4.40	***
Abuse or Violent Crime	5.67	3.26	***
Trouble with the Police	5.75	3.70	***
Gambling Problem	2.69	2.53	*
Discrimination-Ethnic or Cultural Background	2.76	2.17	*
Discrimination-Other Reason	5.04	3.75	***
Bullying and/or Harassment	3.79	2.82	***
Removal of Children	6.79	4.58	**
Other	1.00	0.66	

[1] Unadjusted Odds Ratios with no control variables included. [2] Odds Ratios adjusted for controls including age, marital status, household income, self-rated health, housing tenure and education. [3] Multivariable logistic regression models estimated for each stressor; *** $p < 0.001$, ** $p < 0.01$, * $p < 0.05$; Standard errors calculated using survey replicate weights.

Broadly repeating the descriptive prevalence rates, those reporting witness to violence (AOR = 4.40 $p < 0.001$), removal of children (AOR = 4.58 $p < 0.01$), trouble with police (AOR = 3.70 $p < 0.01$), discrimination-other reason (AOR = 3.75 $p < 0.01$), abuse or violent crime (AOR = 3.26 $p < 0.001$) and bullying/harassment (AOR = 2.82 $p < 0.001$) were approximately three or more times more likely to report food insecurity.

Among the health-related stressors, mental illness (AOR = 2.87 $p < 0.001$), serious disability (AOR = 2.30 $p < 0.01$) and serious illness (AOR = 1.81 $p < 0.01$) approximately doubled the odds of experiencing food insecurity. Similarly, difficulties in the workplace also doubled the odds of experiencing food insecurity: not able to get a job (AOR = 2.49 $p < 0.001$) and involuntary job loss (AOR = 2.59 $p < 0.001$). An experience of a serious accident in the last 12 months was not associated with food insecurity ($p > 0.05$).

Table 4 displays results from a logistic regression model measuring the association between the number of stressors reported by the respondent and food insecurity. The full parameter coefficients measuring the relative role of the control variables are also included for context. The direction, magnitude and significance of the parameter coefficients for the control variables are highly comparable across all models in Tables 3 and 4.

Table 4. Multivariable logistic regression model of number of stressors and food insecurity, 2014.

	Odds Ratio (AOR) [1]	
Number of Stressors [2]		
0	-	
1–2	1.76	*
3–4	3.75	***
5+	8.90	***
Control Variables		
Age		
15–29		
30–44	1.42	+
45–59	1.42	
60+	0.40	**
University Education		
Yes	0.39	*
Married		
Yes	0.39	***
Tenure-Renting		
Yes	3.10	***
Poor Self Rated Health		
Yes	2.28	***
Equivalent Household Income		
0–19%	-	
20–39%	0.81	
40–59%	0.52	*
60–79%	0.28	*
80–100%	0.15	**
Unknown	0.71	

[1] Adjusted Odds Ratios (AOR) with controls for all variables included in the model. [2] Count of the number of stressors reported by the respondent in the previous 12 months; *** $p < 0.001$, ** $p < 0.01$, * $p < 0.05$, + $p < 0.10$; Estimates adjusted using survey replicate weights.

Findings from this analysis showed a slightly non-linear relationship between stressors and the odds of food insecurity. Relative to those reporting no stressors, those reporting one or two stressors were about 1.8 times more likely to be food insecure (OR = 1.76 $p < 0.05$). Those reporting three or four stressors were about 3.8 times more likely (OR = 3.75 $p < 0.05$) and those reporting five or more were approximately nine times more likely to report food insecurity (OR = 8.9 $p < 0.05$). As a proxy for the severity of stressors, these findings indicate that multiple stressors play a significant role in explaining exposure to food insecurity.

Contextualizing the results in Tables 3 and 4, the control variables remain important determinants of food insecurity. Consistent with previous Australian studies, reporting food insecurity was about 60% less likely for university educated respondents (relative to those with no university education) and for those who were married (relative to the unmarried), OR = 0.39 $p < 0.05$ and OR = 0.39 $p < 0.001$, respectively. Reporting poor or fair self-rated health almost doubled the odds of experiencing food insecurity. Again, consistent with Australian studies, renters (as opposed to owners or purchasers of primary residences) were at a considerably greater risk of food insecurity in Australia (OR = 3.10 $p < 0.05$). As expected, household income (specifically equivalized household income) was strongly associated with food insecurity. Those in the top 20% of the income distribution were about 85% less likely to report food insecurity, relative to those in the bottom 20% of the distribution (OR = 0.15 $p < 0.05$).

The increased likelihood of experiencing food insecurity for those reporting multiple stressors raises the question of the composition of stressors experienced in the previous 12 months. Table 5 tabulates the types of stressors experienced by the number of stressors reported. Of those persons reporting 5 or more stressors, over half reported death of a family member or friend (59.8%), serious illness (65.9%), mental illness (60.5%), not able to get a job (67.5%) or bullying and/or harassment (51.7%). These percentages are considerably above those reported by people reporting only 1 or 2 stressors. For example, about 12% of those reporting 1–2 stressors report a mental illness shock, compared with 39% of those reporting 3–4 stressors and 61% of those reporting five or more stressors.

Table 5. Percentage of persons experiencing each stressor by number of stressors reported (%), 2014.

	Number of Stressors [1]		
	1–2	3–4	5+
Stressor Type (%) [2]			
Divorce or Separation	12.0	28.9	48.5
Death of Family Member/Close Friend	29.8	42.6	59.8
Serious Illness	29.0	50.3	65.9
Serious Accident	4.8	9.6	24.4
Alcohol or Drug Related Problems	4.1	23.8	46.3
Mental Illness	12.5	39.5	60.5
Serious Disability	6.2	16.5	26.4
Not Able to Get a Job	19.0	43.8	67.5
Involuntary Job Loss	5.7	19.4	45.3
Witness to Violence	0.7	5.8	28.9
Abuse or Violent Crime	1.0	8.3	24.3
Trouble with the Police	1.4	7.3	30.1
Gambling Problem	1.3	8.8	19.5
Discrimination-Ethnic/Cultural Background	1.0	6.1	18.9
Discrimination-Other Reason	<1%	4.9	17.9
Bullying and/or Harassment	4.2	18.0	51.7
Removal of Children	<1%	2.2	6.7
Other	<1%	<1%	1.4
Unweighted (n)	5804	1566	733

[1] Number of stressors reported in previous 12 months. [2] Percentage of respondents in each category of stressor counts (1–2, 3–4, 5+) reporting each stressor.

4. Discussion

Research in the fields of psychology and behavioural economics has emphasised the importance of stressors in explaining health and wellbeing throughout the life course [36,37]. Public health research too is increasingly recognising the important role that precariousness (through broader economic and political changes) plays in deleterious health and wellbeing outcomes [38]. Indeed, experiencing stressors and precariousness may be tied to experiences of economic and social inequality in Australia, contributing to overall food inequality [39]. Motivated by these broader frameworks, and by a limited number of American and Canadian qualitative studies, this study sought to examine the prevalence and association of 18 types of stressful events, or stressors, with food insecurity in Australia.

This analysis found that respondents reporting food insecurity were more likely to report stressors relative to food secure persons. Across 17 of the 18 stressor domains, food insecure people were significantly more likely to report experiences of a stressor. Moreover, the food insecure were significantly more likely to have encountered multiple stressors within the previous 12 months. Unsurprisingly then, the analysis herein demonstrated that the prevalence of food insecurity was considerably higher among those experiencing stressors. It was further demonstrated that once known determinants of food insecurity were controlled for, the odds of experiencing food insecurity remain highly statistically significant across 16 stressor types. Experiencing multiple stressors was also associated with significantly increased odds of food insecurity.

These findings raise the question of how stressors and precariousness can be built into policy or programs to address food insecurity? Of course, not all people who experience a stressor are at risk of food insecurity. Indeed, beyond individual levels of resilience and vulnerability, support systems from family, friends, the government and the broader community play an important role in managing the potential adverse effects of stressors [36]. However, in the absence of familial or other social-support mechanisms, how can Government support individuals at risk of food insecurity as they face potentially adverse stressors?

Solutions proposed for the broader community to protect financial wellbeing against stressors more generally include financial education, insurance and financial planning and preparedness [40]. However, for many food insecure people, lifelong disadvantage and detachment from the labour market makes such planning complex, if not unfeasible. The ability for policy to support people at risk of food insecurity also depends on the type of stressor. Of particular relevance, stressors related to both health (serious illness, mental illness, serious disability) and the labour market (not able to get a job, involuntary job loss) were strongly associated with food insecurity in this study.

Regarding labour market stressors, consideration should be given to the suitability of extant labour market programs for food insecure people. To assess this, it is necessary to firstly understand the barriers to labour force participation faced by food insecure people? Although much is known about labour market barriers more generally, there are no Australian studies that examine how policy can support unemployed food insecure people specifically. Moreover, it is well understood that higher levels of education are protective against experiences of both food insecurity and unemployment [8,9,41]. What are the barriers to education and training reported by food insecure people? These questions are being considered by the author in a subsequent analysis and underscore the complex policy solutions to food insecurity which must extend beyond food and nutrition programs alone. Relatedly, exogenous labour market shocks (e.g., unanticipated unemployment) raise the issue of the suitability of income support provided through the welfare support system. For example, the main income support payment available to unemployed people in Australia, the Newstart Allowance, has long been criticised for not providing a healthy living allowance, and the problem has compounded over time due to the method of indexation [42–44].

Onset of disability, mental health illness and other serious illness stressors were also strongly associated with food insecurity. The onset of health conditions, particularly multimorbidity and chronic conditions in Australia, has been shown to be associated with deleterious financial wellbeing [45,46]. For some Australians, analysis herein shows that health stressors may translate into a significantly higher likelihood of food insecurity. This however raises the question of the direction of the relationship between health and food insecurity. Is illness a precursor, an outcome or both with respect to food insecurity? For example, a recent scoping paper shows that a number of longitudinal studies find a bidirectional relationship between mental health and food insecurity [47]. Moreover, there is a significant literature on the detrimental mental health effects of unemployment [48]. Thus, there may be a complex relationship *between* and *within* stressors and food insecurity. Further research on the pathways between health and food security using longitudinal data is a priority. More generally, the particularly high odds ratios measuring the association between mental health stressors and food insecurity is also important given reported difficulties accessing and funding mental health care and support programs in Australia [49].

Among the strongest association between stressors and food insecurity identified in this study were for those related to violence and addiction including issues with alcohol or drug related problems and gambling. As noted previously, Canadian studies have noted gambling addiction issues as a possible precursor to food insecurity [29]. An Australian qualitative study of a charity-run soup kitchen noted issues of alcohol and illicit drug use and gambling in food insecure clients [50]. Issues of drug use (both licit and illicit) and gambling are important social problems in Australia with considerable implications for the economy as well as individual wellbeing [51,52]. The complexity of these problems and their solutions again underscore the multidimensional levers that must be employed by governments to address food insecurity.

The association between removal of children and food insecurity was very strong and highly significant. Although this result is not unexpected, interpreting this result requires some caution due to the high prevalence of Aboriginal children in out-of-home care relative to non-Indigenous children [53]. As the Aboriginal and Torres Strait Islander population are at a considerably higher risk of food insecurity in Australia, it may be that the measure of removal of children is confounding this effect [23]. Notwithstanding, just under 3% of the Australian population were Aboriginal and Torres Strait Islanders in the 2016 Census of Population and Housing and it is not clear how many Aboriginal respondents were included in the GSS. Although Aboriginal and Torres Strait Islander people are included in the GSS, variables measuring Indigenous status are not available in the datafile. The National Aboriginal and Torres Strait Islander Social Survey (NATSISS) collects similar measures of food insecurity and stressors to those collected in the GSS and the analysis presented herein could be replicated for the Aboriginal and Torres Strait Islander population.

As a proxy for the severity of stressors, reporting higher numbers of personal stressors was strongly associated with experiencing food insecurity. Descriptive statistics herein further illustrated that almost half of those reporting higher order stressors experienced death of a family member or friend, serious illness, mental illness, trouble finding employment and bullying or harassment. This raises the important point of the intercorrelation between stressors. For example, as noted above, the literature has highlighted the detrimental mental health effects of unemployment [48]. There is also a growing evidence base on experiences of violence by people living with a disability [54]. A further example of the intercorrelation between the various stressors is the relationship between onset of health conditions and difficulties finding or maintaining work and poverty [55,56]. The pathways between these stressors and food insecurity is an area that requires further research. Unfortunately, the GSS data are inappropriate to answer these questions for two reasons. First, the data are cross-sectional and retrospective questions were not asked on the timing of events. Second, the measurement of stressors in the GSS is aggregated so that it is not possible to identify whether the stressor was experienced by (i) the respondent; or (ii) somebody close to them. Detailed longitudinal data are required to disentangle these important questions for future research.

More generally, it is important to note that stressors as a risk factor for food insecurity should not lead to a disregard of other socio-economic factors and food supply characteristics placing individuals at risk. In their analysis of life events on family wellbeing, the Australian Institute of Family Studies (AIFS) notes "sole reliance on life events as indicators of the need for service provision would be unfortunate. The identification of individuals or families who are vulnerable to experiencing adverse events in the future is clearly important, but so too is the identification of families experiencing chronically destructive circumstances" [57]. In the context of food insecurity, the analyses herein should be interpreted as complementary to existing studies and further highlighting at risk population groups. This is further supported by the findings underscoring the relative importance of control variables, such as education, income and marital status, in explaining food insecurity.

Study Strengths and Limitations

The key strength of this study is that it is the first Australian and one of a few internationally that have sought to examine the experiences of a range of stressors and their association with food insecurity. This addresses an important research gap in the extant quantitative literature on food insecurity. A further important strength of this study is that it is nationally representative. Booth and Smith's (2001) key study bringing food insecurity to the fore for Australian dietitians and policy makers pointed to the key at risk populations of food insecurity in Australia [13]. Following this study, most Australian analyses of food insecurity tend to focus on population sub groups. For example, homeless or 'at risk' youth [58], students [10,59], refugees [60,61], children or families with young children [19–21], Aboriginal and Torres Strait Islanders [23,62], older Australians [14,16,22,23,63,64], those living in disadvantaged suburbs [20,65] or middle-income groups [11]. Most Australian studies also focus on cities or states: Adelaide and South Australia [9,58], Sydney and New South Wales [14,20,22,63] Brisbane Queensland [10,17,65] Melbourne and Victoria [11,15] or Tasmania and the Northern Territory [18,19]. There are very few Australian quantitative studies seeking a nationally representative view of the prevalence and correlates of food insecurity [7,16]. This study adds to that list.

Notwithstanding these strengths, there are several limitations of this study. Firstly, as the GSS data are cross-sectional, it is not possible to draw a causal link between stressors and food insecurity. Rather, the analyses show a clear association between the two, once known determinants of food insecurity have been controlled for. Second, and related to the above, due to the cross-sectional nature of the data, it is not possible to measure the complex pathways between the various stressors and food insecurity. It may be that some stressors are a precursor or outcome (or both) of food insecurity. More generally, food insecurity has been shown to be a cyclical phenomenon, varying over time. Longitudinal data are required to measure these complex pathways. A third limitation of this study relates to measurement of the experience of stressors. The GSS instrument asks whether the stressor impacted the individual respondent or someone close to them. The argument that stressors experienced by someone close to you would impact on your likelihood of food insecurity can clearly be made. For example, a spouse losing their job, or a respondent's child becoming seriously ill. Furthermore, qualitative studies provide evidence of how shocks to one person's health can impact on the food insecurity of all household members [66]. However, it may be that when the stressor is experienced by the respondent alone, the effect on the likelihood of experiencing food insecurity is stronger. Unfortunately, the GSS does not enable this disaggregation. However, this analysis would be possible for the Aboriginal and Torres Strait Islander population using NATSISS.

Furthermore, there are a range of exogenous events, such as natural disasters, that may impact exposure to food insecurity and are not measured in the GSS. This study has focussed on personal stressors only, but clearly natural disasters, even in a high-income context, will impact levels of food insecurity. For example, a recent American study found that, even after a recovery phase following Hurricane Katrina, almost one in four people reported food insecurity five years later [67]. Moreover, the personal stressors measured in the GSS exclude potentially positive life events, for example birth of a child or marriage. It may be that for some demographic groups positive life events reduce the likelihood of food insecurity, whereas for other groups it may increase exposure to food insecurity. For example, for some vulnerable populations, positive events such as birth of a child may place greater stress on family resources, leading to a higher likelihood of food insecurity. These data are currently unavailable in the GSS, and this presents an important area for future research.

A fourth limitation of this study is the measurement of food insecurity itself. Going without a meal due to financial constraints is considered a measure of considerable financially attributable food insecurity, indicative of both inadequate intake and food depletion [7]. However, food insecurity exists in circumstances beyond financial considerations alone. Indeed, a number of recent Australian studies have sought to pilot or test more comprehensive measures of food insecurity which include non-financial barriers to food [8,22,68]. These more comprehensive measures show that the prevalence of food insecurity is much higher than when measured based on financial restrictions in accessing food alone. How stressors impact non-financial forms of food insecurity is a priority for future research.

5. Conclusions

Noting these limitations and extensions, to the author's knowledge, this is one of only a few studies to examine the association of a wide range of stressors with food insecurity. Analysis herein showed specific as well as multiple occurrences of stressful events or stressors were associated with food insecurity, independent of known risk factors. These results underscore the complex determinants of food insecurity in Australia and complement existing studies which heretofore have focussed on socio-economic and demographic correlates. Further confirmation of these findings with longitudinal data is a priority, in order to establish the complex pathways in and out of food insecurity and the role of stressors as either precursors or outcomes (or indeed whether a bidirectional relationship exists). Moreover, extending this study to the Aboriginal and Torres Strait Islander population and with more comprehensive measures of food insecurity could provide further insight into stressful events and food insecurity.

Designing policy interventions to support people at risk of food insecurity is key to reducing food insecurity in Australia. Unfortunately, the results from this study suggest that addressing food insecurity is not a straightforward task for policy makers. Many of the stressors interact with important and difficult social problems in Australia, for which there are no straightforward solutions. With further longitudinal research on the pathways within and between stressors and food insecurity, appropriate interventions for those at risk of particularly deleterious stressors, could be designed in tandem with nutrition programs. By addressing food insecurity alongside the related social and economic problems identified in this study, health and economic outcomes for vulnerable populations may be improved and inequalities in health and wellbeing addressed consequently. This approach views food security as a fundamental human right, as recognised by the Australian Governments agreement with key UN accords.

Funding: This research received no external funding. The author is funded by the ARC Centre for Excellence in Population Ageing Research (CE1101029).

Acknowledgments: Data for this study were provided to the author by the Australian Bureau of Statistics (ABS) through the ABS Universities Australia agreement.

Conflicts of Interest: The author declares no conflict of interest.

References

1. American Dietetic Association. Domestic food and nutrition security: Position of the American Dietetic Association. *J. Am. Diet. Assoc.* **1998**, *98*, 337–342. [CrossRef]
2. United Nations. *International Covenant on Economic, Social and Cultural Rights*; United Nations: New York, NY, USA, 2015; Available online: https://treaties.un.org/Pages/ViewDetails.aspx?src=IND&mtdsg_no=IV-3&chapter=4&clang=_en (accessed on 30 June 2018).
3. United Nations. *Transforming Our World: The 2030 Agenda for Sustainable Development*; United Nations: New York, NY, USA, 2015; Available online: http://www.un.org/ga/search/view_doc.asp?symbol=A/RES/70/1&Lang=E (accessed on 30 June 2018).
4. Jones, A.D. Food insecurity and mental health status: A global analysis of 149 countries. *Am. J. Prev. Med.* **2017**, *53*, 264–273. [CrossRef] [PubMed]
5. Smith, M.D.; Rabbitt, M.P.; Coleman-Jensen, A. Who are the world's food insecure? New evidence from the Food and Agriculture Organization's food insecurity experience scale. *World Dev.* **2017**, *31*, 402–412. [CrossRef]
6. Australian Bureau of Statistics. *Australian Health Survey: Nutrition—State and Territory Results, 2011–2012 (Catalogue Number 4364.0.55.009)*; Australian Bureau of Statistics: Canberra, Australia, 2015.
7. Temple, J.B. Severe and moderate forms of food insecurity in Australia: Are they distinguishable? *Aust. J. Soc. Issues* **2008**, *43*, 649–668. [CrossRef]

8. Butcher, L.M.; O'Sullivan, T.A.; Ryan, M.M.; Lo, J.; Devine, A. Utilising a multi-item questionnaire to assess household food security in Australia. *Health Promot. J. Aust.* **2018**. [CrossRef] [PubMed]

9. Foley, W.; Ward, P.; Carter, P.; Coveney, J.; Tsourtos, G.; Taylor, A. An ecological analysis of factors associated with food insecurity in South Australia, 2002–2007. *Public Health Nutr.* **2010**, *13*, 215–221. [CrossRef] [PubMed]

10. Hughes, R.; Serebryanikova, I.; Donaldson, K.; Leveritt, M. Student food insecurity: The skeleton in the university closet. *Nutr. Diet.* **2011**, *68*, 27–32. [CrossRef]

11. Kleve, S.; Davidson, Z.E.; Gearon, E.; Booth, S.; Palermo, C. Are low-to-middle-income households experiencing food insecurity in Victoria, Australia? An examination of the Victorian Population Health Survey, 2006–2009. *Aust. J. Prim. Health* **2017**, *23*, 249–256. [CrossRef] [PubMed]

12. Pollard, C.M.; Landrigan, T.; Ellies, P.; Kerr, D.A.; Lester, M.; Goodchild, S. Geographic factors as determinants of food security: A Western Australian food pricing and quality study. *Asia Pac. J. Clin. Nutr.* **2014**, *23*, 703–713. [CrossRef] [PubMed]

13. Booth, S.; Smith, A. Food security and poverty in Australia-challenges for dietitians. *Aust. J. Nutr. Diet.* **2001**, *58*, 150–156.

14. Quine, S.; Morrell, S. Food insecurity in community-dwelling older Australians. *Public Health Nutr.* **2006**, *9*, 219–224. [CrossRef] [PubMed]

15. Thornton, L.E.; Pearce, J.R.; Ball, K. Sociodemographic factors associated with healthy eating and food security in socio-economically disadvantaged groups in the UK and Victoria, Australia. *Public Health Nutr.* **2014**, *17*, 20–30. [CrossRef] [PubMed]

16. Temple, J.B. Food insecurity among older Australians: Prevalence, correlates and well-being. *Aust. J. Ageing* **2006**, *25*, 158–163. [CrossRef]

17. Radimer, K.L.; Allsopp, R.; Harvey, P.W.; Firman, D.W.; Watson, E.K. Food insufficiency in Queensland. *Aust. N. Z. J. Public Health* **1997**, *21*, 303–310. [CrossRef] [PubMed]

18. Lê, Q.; Auckland, S.; Nguyen, H.B.; Murray, S.; Long, G.; Terry, D.R. Food security in a regional area of Australia: A socio-economic perspective. *Univers. J. Food Nutr. Sci.* **2014**, *2*, 50–59. [CrossRef]

19. McCarthy, L. Household Food Security and Child Health Outcomes in Families with Children Aged 6 Months to 4 Years Residing in Darwin and Palmerston, Northern Territory Australia. Ph.D Thesis, Charles Darwin University, Casuarina, Northern Territory, Australia, 2017.

20. Nolan, M.; Rikard-Bell, G.; Mohsin, M.; Williams, M. Food insecurity in three socially disadvantaged localities in Sydney, Australia. *Health Promot. J. Aust.* **2006**, *17*, 247–253. [CrossRef]

21. Godrich, S.; Lo, J.; Davies, C.; Darby, J.; Devine, A. Prevalence and socio-demographic predictors of food insecurity among regional and remote Western Australian children. *Aust. N. Z. J. Public Health* **2017**, *41*, 585–590. [CrossRef] [PubMed]

22. Russell, J.; Flood, V.; Yeatman, H.; Mitchell, P. Prevalence and risk factors of food insecurity among a cohort of older Australians. *J. Nutr. Health Aging* **2014**, *18*, 3–8. [CrossRef] [PubMed]

23. Temple, J.B.; Russell, J. Food insecurity among older Aboriginal and Torres Strait Islanders. *Int. J. Environ. Res. Public Health* **2018**, *15*, 1766. [CrossRef] [PubMed]

24. Wolfe, W.S.; Olson, C.M.; Kendall, A.; Frongillo, E.A. Understanding food insecurity in the elderly: A conceptual framework. *J. Nutr. Educ.* **1996**, *28*, 92–100. [CrossRef]

25. Frongillo, E.A.; Valois, P.; Wolfe, W.S. Using a concurrent events approach to understand social support and food insecurity among elders. *Fam. Econ. Nutr. Rev.* **2003**, *15*, 25.

26. Chilton, M.; Knowles, M.; Rabinowich, J.; Arnold, K. The relationship between childhood adversity and food insecurity: 'It's like a bird nesting in your head'. *Public Health Nutr.* **2015**, *18*, 2643–2653. [CrossRef] [PubMed]

27. Younginer, N.A.; Blake, C.E.; Draper, C.L.; Jones, S.J. Resilience and hope: Identifying trajectories and contexts of household food insecurity. *J. Hunger Environ. Nutr.* **2015**, *10*, 230–258. [CrossRef]

28. Jones, S.J.; Draper, C.L.; Bell, B.A.; Burke, M.P.; Martini, L.; Younginer, N.; Blake, C.E.; Probst, J.; Freedman, D.; Liese, A.D. Child hunger from a family resilience perspective. *J. Hunger Environ. Nutr.* **2018**, *13*, 340–361. [CrossRef]

29. Olabiyi, O.M.; McIntyre, L. Determinants of food insecurity in higher-income households in Canada. *J. Hunger Environ. Nutr.* **2014**, *9*, 433–448. [CrossRef]

30. Booth, S. Eating rough: Food sources and acquisition practices of homeless young people in Adelaide, South Australia. *Public Health Nutr.* **2006**, *9*, 212–218. [CrossRef] [PubMed]

31. McKenzie, H.J.; McKay, F.H. Food as a discretionary item: The impact of welfare payment changes on low-income single mother's food choices and strategies. *J. Poverty Soc. Justice* **2017**, *25*, 35–48. [CrossRef]

32. Burns, C.A. *Review of the Literature Describing the Link between Poverty, Food Insecurity and Obesity with Specific Reference to Australia*; VicHealth: Melbourne, Australia, 2004. Available online: https://www.vichealth.vic.gov.au/~/media/ResourceCentre/PublicationsandResources/healthy%20eating/Literature%20Review%20Poverty_Obesity_Food%20Insecurity.ashx (accessed on 30 June 2018).

33. Australian Bureau of Statistics. *General Social Survey: Summary Results, Australia, 2014 (Catalogue Number 4159.0)*; Australian Bureau of Statistics: Canberra, Australia, 2015.

34. Winter, N. SVR: Stata Module to Compute Estimates with Survey Replication Based Standard Errors. 2008. Available online: https://ideas.repec.org/c/boc/bocode/s427502.html (accessed on 1 March 2017).

35. Wolfer, K. *Introduction to Variance Estimation*; Springer: New York, NY, USA, 1985.

36. Moloney, L.; Weston, R.; Qu, L.; Hayes, A. *Families, Life Events and Family Service Delivery*; Australian Institute of Family Studies: Canberra, Australia, 2012; pp. 1447–1469.

37. Sharam, A.; Ralston, L.; Parkinson, S. Security in retirement. The impact of housing and key critical life events. In *SISR Working Paper*; Swinburne University of Technology: Melbourne, Australia, 2016.

38. McKee, M.; Reeves, A.; Clair, A.; Stuckler, D. Living on the edge: Precariousness and why it matters for health. *Arch. Public Health* **2017**, *75*, 13. [CrossRef] [PubMed]

39. Pollard, C.; Begley, A.; Landrigan, T. The Rise of Food Inequality in Australia. In *Food Poverty and Insecurity: International Food Inequalities*; Springer: Cham, Switzerland, 2016; pp. 89–103.

40. West, T.; Worthington, A. The impact of major life events on Australian Household Financial Decision-making and portfolio rebalancing. *SSRN Electron. J.* **2016**. [CrossRef]

41. Woessmann, L. The economic case for education. *Educ. Econ.* **2016**, *24*, 3. [CrossRef]

42. Morris, A.; Wilson, S. Struggling on the Newstart unemployment benefit in Australia: The experience of a neoliberal form of employment assistance. *Econ. Labour Relat. Rev.* **2014**, *25*, 202–221. [CrossRef]

43. Saunders, P.; Bedford, M. New minimum healthy living budget standards for low-paid and unemployed Australians. *Econ. Labour Relat. Rev.* **2018**, *29*, 3. [CrossRef]

44. Saunders, P. Using a budget standards approach to assess the adequacy of Newstart allowance. *Aust. J. Soc. Issues* **2018**, *53*, 4–17. [CrossRef]

45. Kemp, A.; Preen, D.B.; Glover, J.; Semmens, J.; Roughead, E.E. Impact of cost of medicines for chronic conditions on low income households in Australia. *J. Health Serv. Res. Policy* **2013**, *18*, 21–27. [CrossRef] [PubMed]

46. McRae, I.; Yen, L.; Jeon, Y.H.; Herath, P.M.; Essue, B. Multimorbidity is associated with higher out-of-pocket spending: A study of older Australians with multiple chronic conditions. *Aust. J. Prim. Health* **2013**, *19*, 144–149. [CrossRef] [PubMed]

47. Maynard, M.; Andrade, L.; Packull-McCormick, S.; Perlman, C.M.; Leos-Toro, C.; Kirkpatrick, S.I. Food Insecurity and Mental Health among Females in High-Income Countries. *Int. J. Environ. Res. Public Health* **2018**, *15*, 1424. [CrossRef] [PubMed]

48. Modini, M.; Joyce, S.; Mykletun, A.; Christensen, H.; Bryant, R.A.; Mitchell, P.B.; Harvey, S.B. The mental health benefits of employment: Results of a systematic meta-review. *Aust. Psychiatry* **2016**, *24*, 331–336. [CrossRef] [PubMed]

49. Meadows, G.N.; Enticott, J.C.; Inder, B.; Russell, G.M.; Gurr, R. Better access to mental health care and the failure of the Medicare principle of universality. *Med. J. Aust.* **2015**, *202*, 190–194. [CrossRef] [PubMed]

50. Wicks, R.; Trevena, L.J.; Quine, S. Experiences of food insecurity among urban soup kitchen consumers: insights for improving nutrition and well-being. *J. Am. Diet. Assoc.* **2006**, *106*, 921–924. [CrossRef] [PubMed]

51. Collins, D.; Lapsley, H.M. *The Costs of Tobacco, Alcohol and Illicit Drug Abuse to Australian Society in 2004/05*; Department of Health and Ageing: Canberra, Australia, 2008.

52. Armstrong, A.R.; Thomas, A.; Abbott, M. Gambling participation, expenditure and risk of harm in Australia, 1997–1998 and 2010–2011. *J. Gambl. Stud.* **2018**, *34*, 255–274. [CrossRef] [PubMed]

53. Productivity Commission. Report on Government Services. Chapter 15: Child Protection; 2016; Productivity Commission: Melbourne, Victoria. Available online: http://www.pc.gov.au/research/ongoing/report-on-

54. Hughes, K.; Bellis, M.; Jones, L.; Wood, S.; Bates, G.; Eckley, L.; McCoy, E.; Mikton, C.; Shakespeare, T.; Officer, A. Prevalence and risk of violence against adults with disabilities: A systematic review and meta-analysis of observational studies. *Lancet* **2012**, *379*, 1621–1629. [CrossRef]

55. Callander, E.; Schofield, D.; Shrestha, R. Multi-dimensional poverty in Australia and the barriers ill health imposes on the employment of the disadvantaged. *J. Socio-Econ.* **2011**, *40*, 736–742. [CrossRef]

56. Schofield, D.; Shrestha, R.; Passe, M.; Earnest, A.; Fletcher, S. Chronic Disease and Labour Force Participation among Older Australians. *Med. J. Aust.* **2008**, *189*, 447–450. [PubMed]

57. Baxter, J.; Qu, L.; Weston, R.; Moloney, L.; Hayes, A. Experiences and effects of life events: Evidence from two Australian longitudinal studies. *Fam. Matters* **2012**, *90*, 6.

58. Crawford, B.; Yamazaki, R.; Franke, E.; Amanatidis, S.; Ravulo, J.; Steinbeck, K.; Ritchie, J.; Torvaldsen, S. Sustaining dignity? Food insecurity in homeless young people in urban Australia. *Health Promot. J. Aust.* **2014**, *25*, 71–78. [CrossRef] [PubMed]

59. Micevski, D.A.; Thornton, L.E.; Brockington, S. Food insecurity among university students in Victoria: A pilot study. *Nutr. Diet.* **2014**, *71*, 258–264. [CrossRef]

60. Gallegos, D.; Ellies, P.; Wright, J. Still there's no food! Food insecurity in a refugee population in Perth, Western Australia. *Nutr. Diet.* **2008**, *65*, 78–83. [CrossRef]

61. McKay, F.H.; Dunn, M. Food security among asylum seekers in Melbourne. *Aust. N. Z. J. Public Health* **2015**, *39*, 344–349. [CrossRef] [PubMed]

62. Pollard, C.M.; Nyaradi, A.; Lester, M.; Sauer, K. Understanding food security issues in remote Western Australian Indigenous communities. *Health Promot. J. Aust.* **2014**, *25*, 83–89. [CrossRef] [PubMed]

63. Russell, J.C.; Flood, V.M.; Yeatman, H.; Wang, J.J.; Mitchell, P. Food insecurity and poor diet quality are associated with reduced quality of life in older adults. *Nutr. Diet.* **2016**, *73*, 50–58. [CrossRef]

64. King, A.C. Food Security and Insecurity in Older Adults: A Phenomenological Ethnographic Study. Ph.D. Thesis, University of Tasmania, Tasmania, Australia, 2014.

65. Ramsey, R.; Giskes, K.; Turrell, G.; Gallegos, D. Food insecurity among Australian children: Potential determinants, health and developmental consequences. *J. Child Health Care* **2011**, *15*, 401–416. [CrossRef] [PubMed]

66. Higashi, R.T.; Lee, S.C.; Pezzia, C.; Quirk, L.; Leonard, T.; Pruitt, S.L. Family and Social Context Contributes to the Interplay of Economic Insecurity, Food Insecurity, and Health. *Ann. Anthropol. Pract.* **2017**, *41*, 67–77. [CrossRef] [PubMed]

67. Clay, L.A.; Papas, M.A.; Gill, K.; Abramson, D.M. Application of a theoretical model toward understanding continued food insecurity post hurricane Katrina. *Disaster Med. Public Health Prep.* **2018**, *12*, 47–56. [CrossRef] [PubMed]

68. Kleve, S.; Gallegos, D.; Ashby, S.; Palermo, C.; McKechnie, R. Preliminary validation and piloting of a comprehensive measure of household food security in Australia. *Public Health Nutr.* **2018**, *21*, 526–534. [CrossRef] [PubMed]

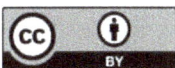

International Journal of
Environmental Research and Public Health

MDPI

Article

Social Assistance Payments and Food Insecurity in Australia: Evidence from the Household Expenditure Survey

Jeromey B. Temple [1,*], Sue Booth [2] and Christina M. Pollard [3]

1   Demography and Ageing Unit, Melbourne School of Population and Global Health,
    University of Melbourne, Melbourne 3010, Australia
2   College of Medicine and Public Health, Flinders University, Adelaide 5000, Australia;
    sue.booth@flinders.edu.au
3   Faculty of Health Sciences, School of Public Health, Curtin University, Perth 6102, Australia;
    C.Pollard@curtin.edu.au
*   Correspondence: Jeromey.Temple@unimelb.edu.au; Tel.: +61-3-9035-9900

Received: 7 January 2019; Accepted: 30 January 2019; Published: 4 February 2019

Abstract: It is widely understood that households with low economic resources and poor labour market attachment are at considerable risk of food insecurity in Australia. However, little is known about variations in food insecurity by receipt of specific classes of social assistance payments that are made through the social security system. Using newly released data from the 2016 Household Expenditure Survey, this paper reports on variations in food insecurity prevalence across a range of payment types. We further investigated measures of financial wellbeing reported by food-insecure households in receipt of social assistance payments. Results showed that individuals in receipt of Newstart allowance (11%), Austudy/Abstudy (14%), the Disability Support Pension (12%), the Carer Payment (11%) and the Parenting Payment (9%) were at significantly higher risk of food insecurity compared to those in receipt of the Age Pension (<1%) or no payment at all (1.3%). Results further indicated that food-insecure households in receipt of social assistance payments endured significant financial stress, with a large proportion co-currently experiencing "fuel" or "energy" poverty. Our results support calls by a range of Australian non-government organisations, politicians, and academics for a comprehensive review of the Australian social security system.

Keywords: food insecurity; access to food; social assistance payments; social security; Newstart allowance

---

1. Introduction

In Australia, conservative estimates show food insecurity attributable to financial constraints is experienced by 4–5% of the population, with the rate significantly higher among Aboriginal and Torres Strait Islander people [1–3]. Addressing food insecurity in high-income countries such as Australia is important because of the deleterious consequences of exposure for individual health and wellbeing. A substantial and growing evidence base shows food insecurity is associated with symptoms of depression and anxiety, multimorbidity, lower levels of self-reported health status, poor nutrition, a greater likelihood of reporting social isolation, long-standing health problems and activity limitations, and a greater likelihood of reporting heart disease, diabetes, high blood pressure, or peripheral arterial disease [4–13]. Food insecurity experienced within households also has implications for the intergenerational transmission of health issues for children living in food-insecure households [14–16] and may also contribute to ongoing economic inequality [17]. Given these significant outcomes of food insecurity, many high-income countries have extensive social welfare safety nets to alleviate poverty which, in turn, reduces food insecurity at a population level.

However, studies have shown that welfare reforms over recent years have had a severe impact on vulnerable populations and increased the likelihood of food insecurity. For example, in the UK, increased sanctioning of unemployment claimants led to an increase in the rate of adults attending food banks [18]. In the U.S., welfare reforms limiting access to immigrant populations had the impact of significantly increasing levels of food insecurity [19]. In Australia, too, evidence from a recent qualitative study showed changes to welfare eligibility by low-income single parents increased the risk of food insecurity [20].

Australian studies have also shown significantly higher levels of food insecurity among the unemployed relative to other Australians [2,21]. Indeed, numerous Australian studies have underscored the strength of economic factors (e.g., income and labour force status) in explaining exposure to food insecurity. Temple's (2008) nationally representative study of food insecurity in Australia concludes that because of this strong association, policies must target improvements to economic wellbeing through revisiting the appropriateness of extant unemployment benefits and labour market programs [2].

Omitted from existing research on food insecurity and social assistance in Australia is an understanding of how the likelihood of food insecurity differs across the range of social assistance payments provided by the Federal Government. In this paper, newly released data from the 2016 ABS Household Expenditure Survey were used to investigate levels of food insecurity and financial wellbeing reported by recipients of a range of social assistance payments, broadly categorised as the Age Pension, Disability and Carer payments, Family Support payments, and Unemployment and Student allowances.

Background to Social Assistance Payments in Australia

The Australian social security system is intended to increase the wellbeing of the population by redistributing Government revenue collected in the tax system to individuals and families [22]. It is a broader part of a social protection system that includes direct expenditure on services and infrastructure (such as health, education, and community services), the superannuation system—which complements the age pension in Australia's retirement income system—and payments, services, and investment to promote the efficient and effective functioning of the economy, which underpins individual and national wellbeing [22].

Relative to other Organisation for Economic Co-Operation and Development (OECD) member countries, Australia's social security system is unique as (1) most social assistance cash payments are flat-rate entitlements funded by direct Government revenue, and (2) most benefits are heavily income- or asset-tested, with payment reducing as individual private resources increase [23]. This design enables Australia to have a relatively broad social safety net encompassing unemployment benefits and universal health care and assistance for vulnerable populations across the life course [24]. Concerns have been raised, however, about the erosion of the safety net and the particularly low levels of income support provided through social assistance payments, such as the Newstart Allowance—the key payment available for unemployed people of working age [25–27].

Previous Australian studies on food insecurity have focused on particularly vulnerable populations, many with an increased higher likelihood of receipt of some form of social benefit payments—for example, homeless or at-risk youth [28,29], students [30,31], refugees [32,33], Aboriginal and Torres Strait Islander peoples [3,34], older Australians [35,36] and those living in disadvantaged suburbs [37]. Despite this significant evidence base, there is a paucity of studies examining variations in food insecurity across a range of social assistance payments. This is important as variations in the prevalence of food insecurity by payment type may uncover populations at particular risk, which could be addressed through the existing social welfare system.

In this study, we examine food insecurity by receipt of social assistance payments, broadly classified at the household level as the Age Pension, Disability and Carer payments, Family Support payments, Unemployment and Student allowances, and other Government pensions and allowances.

At the individual level, we further analyse food insecurity by a number of specific social assistance payments. Among those discussed in this paper include [38]:

- Austudy: Available to persons aged 25 and over undertaking study or a full-time Australian apprenticeship. Basic rates start from $445 per fortnight for a single person with no dependent children.
- Abstudy: Available to persons of Aboriginal or Torres Strait Islander descent, undertaking an approved course on full-time Australian apprenticeship. Basic rates start from $445.80 per fortnight for a single person with no dependent children.
- Age pension: Available to persons aged 65 or over (if born before July 1952) to 67 and over (if born January 1957 and later). Basic rates start from $834.40 per fortnight for a single person. Subject to income and assets test.
- Carer payment: Available to persons providing constant care to 1 or more persons with a disability as determined by specific assessment tools and as a result of the carer role do not work. Basic rates start from $834.40 per fortnight for a single person. Subject to income and assets test.
- Disability support pension (DSP): Available to persons aged 16 or over, but less than Age Pension age, with a disability as defined by an impairment table, and who are unable to work or undertake training within the next two years. Basic rates start from $572.90 per fortnight for a single person (Independent).
- Newstart allowance: Available to Australian residents who are aged 22 or over (but less than age pension age) and unemployed. Basic rates range from $550 per fortnight for a single person depending on circumstances.
- Parenting payment: Available for parents who have a child under 6 (if partnered), or 8 (if single). Once the child is beyond these ages, the parent must enter into a job plan. Subject to stringent income and assets test. Basic rates of up to a maximum of $768 per fortnight, inclusive of a pension supplement.
- Youth allowance: Available to full-time students and Australian apprentices aged 16–24. Basic rates range from $244 to $768 per fortnight depending on household circumstances.

2. Materials and Methods

2.1. Survey Data

Data for this study were from the Household Expenditure Survey (HES) conducted by the Australian Bureau of Statistics (ABS) over the period July 2015 to June 2016. The purpose of the HES was to "facilitate the analysis and monitoring of the social and economic welfare or Australian residents in private dwellings. The main users are government and other social and economic analysts involved in the development, implementation and evaluation of social and economic policies" [39].

The HES is a repeated cross-section design, with nine surveys conducted since 1974–1975. Since 2003–2004, the HES sample was drawn alongside respondents of the ABS Survey of Income and Housing (SIH). Of the 17,768 households recorded in the SIH, 10,046 were included in the HES. Dwellings were sampled using a stratified, multistage cluster design across a 12-month enumeration period to account for seasonality effects on income and expenditure.

As the HES samples private dwellings, a number of populations are excluded from our analyses. These include persons residing in hotels, boarding schools, and institutions. Also excluded are households containing members of non-Australian Defence forces, diplomatic personnel as well as households in very remote areas of Australia. Apart from houses and flats, the ABS consider persons residing in caravans, garages, tents, and other structures used as residences to be private dwellings.

These data were collected by Australia's official statistical agency, and accordingly, the protection of participants and the provision of data to us is enshrined in legislation. Specifically, data for the Household Expenditure Survey were collected by the ABS under the provisions of the *Census and Statistics Act (CSA) 1905*. Prior to field operations, the survey was submitted to the Australian Privacy

Commissioner and tabled in the Australian Parliament. The confidentiality of these data is guaranteed under the Act and information was provided freely from respondents. Confidentialised data were made available to the authors for this study through the ABS and Universities Australia agreement.

2.2. Measurement

The measures of food insecurity used by the ABS have heretofore been confined to measures of financial attributions of running out of food. For example, two item questions in the National Nutrition Survey and National Health Survey ask: "In the past 12 months were there any time(s) when you ran out of food and couldn't afford to buy any more". Those who reported yes to this question are considered food-insecure. The measure used in the HES is comparable but is likely to identify a more at-risk group of food-insecure persons [3]. Respondents in the 2009/10 HES were asked: "Over the past year, have any of the following happened to (you/your household) because of a shortage of money?" Those reporting 'yes' to 'went without meals' are coded as food-insecure.

The HES also included a number of measures of financial wellbeing, consisting of measures of financial stress, income management, standard of living, and access to emergency funds. These measures provide a complimentary view of the financial position of food-insecure households in receipt of social assistance payments. Respondents were sought to identify whether in the previous 12 months, they had undertaken a number of financial stress behaviours, including seeking help from welfare or community organisations, pawning or selling something, seeking financial help from family or friends, or inability to heat their home or pay utility or other bills on time. As a summary measure of self-assessed financial wellbeing, respondents were further asked: "Thinking of your household's situation over the last 12 months, which of the following statements best describes your financial situation?" A prompt card was then displayed listing: Spend more money than we get, just break even most weeks or able to save money most weeks. Furthermore, respondents were prompted: "Which of these statements best describes your household's standard of living compared to 2 years ago?" A prompt card was then shown listing: Better than 2 years ago, the same as 2 years ago or worse than 2 years ago.

Finally, as a measure of financial resilience to unanticipated events, respondents were asked: "If all of a sudden your household had to get two thousand dollars for something important, could the money be obtained within a week"? Following a response, using a prompt card, respondents were asked to nominate the sources of the emergency funds from a list including: Savings, loan from bank/building society, loan from finance company, loan on credit card, loan from family or friends, loan from welfare or community organisation, sell something or from any other source.

In this descriptive study, we calculated the weighted prevalence of food insecurity by payment type with tests of proportions between groups.

3. Results

Table 1 cross-tabulates source of household income and main source of social assistance payments by food insecurity status. The first panel of Table 1 displays the proportion of each group (food-secure by receipt of benefits and food-insecure by receipt of benefits) by the main source of household income. In the second panel, the broad social assistance payment types are tabulated by food security status.

Approximately 80% of Australian households who report food insecurity received some form of social assistance payment in 2015–2016 (82.4%), with 75% of food-insecure households in receipt of social assistance benefits listing this as the main source of household income (74.8%). Food-insecure households receiving social assistance payments are predominately in receipt of Disability and Carer payments (38%) and Unemployment and Student allowances (28.7%)—Table 1. By contrast, food-secure households in receipt of social assistance payments are more likely to receive the Age Pension (36.6%), with less than 10% being in receipt of Unemployment and Student allowances. Approximately 20% of food-insecure and 24% of food-secure households are in receipt of Family benefits. Of households not in receipt of social assistance payments, almost 90% of both food-insecure and -secure households receive wages from employment. Approximately 2.8% of households reported food insecurity (as measured by going without a meal due to financial constraints).

Table 1. Food insecurity and receipt of social assistance, by main source of income and source of social assistance—households, weighted (%), 2016.

Food-Secure:	Yes		No [1]	
Receipt of Social Assistance Benefits:	**No**	**Yes**	**No**	**Yes**
Main Source of Income [2]				
Employee Income	85.7	43.2	89.4	23.8 ***
Own Business Income	4.8	3.5	6.8	0.4 ***
Government Pensions & Allowances	0.0	41.3	0.0	74.8 ***
Other Income	9.5	12.1	3.8	1.0 ***
Main Source of Social Assistance Payments [3]				
No Social Assistance	100	n.a.	100	n.a.
Age Pension	n.a.	36.6	n.a.	9.4 ***
Disability and Carer Payments	n.a.	12.2	n.a.	38.3 ***
Family Support Payments	n.a.	24.1	n.a.	19.7
Unemployment and Student Allowances	n.a.	9.7	n.a.	28.7 ***
Other Government Pensions/Allowances	n.a.	17.4	n.a.	4.0 ***
Unweighted *n* [4]	3855	5884	38	263
Weighted % [5]	43.5	53.7	0.5	2.3

[1] Going without meals due to financial constraints in the previous 12 months; [2] Household main source of income in the previous 12 months; [3] Source of social assistance benefits at the household level; n.a. not applicable for households not in receipt of social assistance payments; [4] number of raw observations; [5] percentages weighted using survey weights to account for non-response. *** $p < 0.001$ for test of proportions. Test of proportions conducted between each social assistance benefit groups. That is, assistance benefit recipients (food-secure) compared with assistance benefit recipients (food-insecure) and for non-assistance benefits also (insignificant differences).

As indicators of financial wellbeing, the HES includes a number of measures of financial stress (Appendix Table A1), income management, standard of living (Appendix Table A2), and access to emergency funds (Appendix Table A3). About 60% of food-insecure households in receipt of social assistance payments reported seeking financial help from friends or family and about 43% had sought assistance from a welfare or community organisation (Appendix Table A1). Sixty per cent could not pay utility bills on time, about 35% had pawned or sold something, and 30% reported being unable to heat their home. Less than one per cent of households who are food-secure and not in receipt of social assistance payments were unable to heat their home or had pawned something, and <6% had difficulty paying for utilities. Almost half of food-insecure households receiving social assistance payments reported spending more money than they receive and just over half reported their standard of living as worse than 2 years ago (Appendix Table A2). By contrast, 82% of food-secure households not receiving benefits reported their standard of living as the same or better than two years ago and 60% of this group were able to save money most weeks.

Seventy three percent of food-insecure households in receipt of social assistance payments could not raise $2000 within a week, with very few options from capital markets with respect to raising funds (Appendix Table A3). The key source of emergency funds for this group was reported as loans from family or friends (20%). By contrast, only 6% of food-secure households with no social assistance payments and 16% of those with social assistance payments could not raise emergency funds, with a much broader range of emergency fund sources across capital markets and personal resources.

When these measures of financial stress (Appendix Table A1), income management, and standard of living (Appendix Table A2) and access to emergency funds (Appendix Table A3) are cross-tabulated by social assistance type, households in receipt of Disability and Carer payments as well as Unemployment and Student allowances are shown to be in a financially precarious position. In comparison, among social assistance recipients, households in receipt of the Age Pension appear to have lower levels of financial stress, higher self-assessed standard of living, and an improved access to emergency funds.

The specific social assistance benefit received by individuals who are members of food-insecure households in the HES is shown in Table 2. The higher prevalence of food insecurity reported by those receiving Unemployment, Student, and Disability payments is highlighted in these data. Prevalence was highest among people receiving Austudy/Abstudy (14%), Disability Support Pension (12%), Newstart Allowance (11%) and the Carer payment (11%). Age pension recipients were significantly less likely to report food insecurity (<1%), as were those receiving the DVA Disability pension.

Table 2. Food insecurity prevalence and percentage receiving social assistance payments—persons, weighted (%), 2016.

Social Assistance Benefit Type	Food Insecurity (%) [3]	Food-Insecure in Receipt of Benefit (%) [2]	n [1] =
Austudy/Abstudy	13.8 **	3.9 *	83
Age Pension	<1 ***	4.6 ***	3733
Carer Allowance	5.0 **	4.8 **	470
Carer Payment	10.9 ***	5.8 ***	255
Carer Supplement	5.9 **	6.9 **	565
Disability Pension (DVA)	<1	<1	101
Disability Support Pension	12.4 ***	18.9 ***	803
Family Tax Benefits	5.5 ***	17.3 ***	1284
Newstart Allowance	11.0 ***	14.6 ***	645
Parenting Payment	9.0 ***	5.7 ***	322
Youth Allowance	6.0 *	4.0 *	233
Any Social Assistance Payment?			
Yes	3.9	64.2	8545
No	1.3	35.8	10,660

[1] Unweighted sample size per benefit; [2] percentage of food-insecure persons in receipt of each social assistance payment. Tests of proportions for proportion of food-insecure in receipt of each benefit compared to food-secure in receipt of each benefit; [3] food insecurity prevalence. Tests of proportions for in receipt of each payment compared to those not in receipt; percentages weighted using survey weights to account for non-response; *** $p < 0.001$ ** $p < 0.01$ * $p < 0.05$ denoting significance tests for tests of proportions.

4. Discussion

International evidence shows that individuals in receipt of social assistance payments are at increased risk of food insecurity [40]. To date, there has been scant evidence on the prevalence of food insecurity by social assistance payment type in Australia. Of the information available, a 2013 study of people accessing Anglicare Australia's emergency relief centres in two states reported that 31% of food-insecure households were reliant upon the Newstart allowance and 44% on the disability support pension [41]. Using nationally representative data, this study confirms the significantly higher prevalence of food insecurity among recipients of Australian government social assistance payments—with about 80% of households reporting food insecurity receiving some form of social assistance payment.

Particularly high levels of food insecurity were found among households in receipt of Unemployment, Student, Carer, and Disability payments, suggesting the inadequacy of these transfers. Specifically, when examined at the level of specific payment types, individuals in receipt of Newstart Allowance (11%), Austudy/Abstudy (14%), Disability Support Pension (12%), the Carer Payment (11%), and Parenting Payment (9%) were at significantly higher risk of food insecurity compared to those in receipt of the Age Pension (<1%) or no payment (1.3%).

In 2018, the Australian Prime Minister indicated that his Government prioritises an increase to the Age Pension above any changes to the Newstart Allowance [42]. This is despite research underscoring the deleterious financial position of those in receipt of unemployment and student payments. For example, the Newstart Allowance has long been criticised for not providing a healthy living allowance, and the problem has compounded over time due to the method of indexation [26,27].

The current study findings are consistent with research showing that the standard of living experienced by older Australians has increased considerably over the past decade, with higher levels of income and wealth relative to previous generations of older persons [43–45]. The basic rate for the Age Pension is currently AUD \$834 per fortnight compared with AUD \$550 per fortnight for Newstart Allowance recipients. Further, the Australian Council of Social Services (2018) reported that the poverty gaps (the average depth of poverty for those living below the poverty line) among people aged 65 years and over in income support households were much lower than those across the whole population [45]. The mismatch between indicated government policy for older and younger and working age people and research evidence is concerning.

Apart from Newstart Allowance recipients, the higher levels of food insecurity reported by those in receipt of Disability Support Pension are consistent with recent research on disabilities, health conditions, and food insecurity in Australia and internationally [46,47]. Temple (2018) found that the onset of serious disability (OR 2.3 $p < 0.01$) or mental illness (OR 2.9 $p < 0.001$) more than doubled the odds of experiencing food insecurity in Australia [21]. Although the Disability Support Pension has a higher basic rate of payment than the Newstart Allowance, almost one in five food-insecure respondents in this current study are in receipt of the disability support pension. The findings are consistent with UK research, which shows that households with a disability are almost three times more likely to be foodbank users [48].

This study also identified those on Parenting and Carer payments were at an increased risk of food insecurity. These findings resonate with previous Australian research that found single parents were more likely to experience food insecurity due to factors such as income and housing instability [49,50]. Australia shifted its welfare policy context to 'Welfare to Work' in 2006, founded on the principle of mutual obligation where recipients must complete compulsory activities in order to access income support. Those receiving parenting benefits were transitioned to the lower-rate Newstart Allowance [50,51]. Single mothers relying on the Newstart Allowance experienced a struggle to buy basics such as food, reliance on foodbanks, and keeping children home from school as they were unable to provide food which met the school lunchbox policy [50]. The higher prevalence of food insecurity among persons in receipt of the Carer payment is consistent with recent evidence showing financial support is the greatest unmet need reported by Australian carers [52].

Our findings pointing to the higher prevalence of food insecurity on these payments is concerning given recent research on intergenerational transfer of disadvantage. Cobb-Clark (2017) has shown that households in receipt of Disability, Carer, and Parenting payments are at a strong risk of intergenerational persistence of disadvantage [53]. Of major concern is that children living in households dependent on these specific payments are more likely themselves to receive more intensive social assistance payments in their early adulthood and more likely to experience unemployment.

Finally, our findings underscore the deleterious financial position experienced by food-insecure households and those on specific social assistance payments in Australia. The high levels of 'fuel or energy poverty' faced by food-insecure Australians is of particular concern. About 30% of food-insecure households in receipt of social assistance payments reported being unable to heat their home, and 60% were unable to pay their utility bills on time.

UK and U.S. research has also drawn attention to the relationship between food insecurity and fuel or energy poverty. Anderson et al. (2012) described the experience of 'cold' homes in the UK where households faced with financial difficulty cut the range and quality of food while simultaneously cutting energy consumption [54]. Large reductions in food expenditure have been reported in low-income households during colder than expected winter conditions [55]. Poor families living in the US reduced their food expenditure commensurate to increases in fuel expenditures when cold-weather shocks occurred, suggesting that existing social programs were ineffectual in buffering against these shocks [56]. Canadian evidence shows energy price shocks at the turn of the century led to an increase in the population at risk of food insecurity [57].

Australia has experienced significant energy price inflation following the deregulation of energy markets [58]. The high levels of concurrent energy poverty facing the food-insecure can lead to further financial burden, for example, the cost of reconnection or default payments [59]. Australian households that were disconnected or at risk of disconnection experienced very difficult financial circumstances, in which they often struggled to afford necessities such as food and housing [59]. In a recent article, Nelson et al. (2019) suggested, among other solutions, increasing income support for particular groups (including those on Newstart) as well as the reform of state-based energy concessions to combat energy poverty [60].

These solutions, by reducing energy costs and increasing income support, would undoubtedly reduce the likelihood of vulnerable populations experiencing food insecurity. International evidence suggests that increases to social assistance payments reduce the prevalence and severity of food insecurity at a population level. For example, in Newfoundland and Labrador in Canada, the prevalence of food insecurity reduced dramatically from 2007–2011 due to welfare reforms [61]. Another Canadian study found that a one-off increase in social assistance benefits led to a significant decline in moderate and severe food insecurity among households on social assistance [62].

Study Limitations

In interpreting results from this study, it is important to recognise the limitations. Firstly, the measure of food insecurity in Australia comprising of measures of 'going without meals due to financial constraints' captures neither temporality nor severity [2]. However, currently, these are the only population-based measures available. Our study, however, does raise the question of the use of household expenditure data to improve measurement and understanding of food insecurity. Future research on this issue is currently underway by the authors.

The measurement issue is also important given the differences in food insecurity prevalence experienced by those of working age or younger populations compared to older persons in receipt of the age pension. Previous studies have note that food insecurity attributable to financial constraints tends to decrease in older age in Australia [2,35]. Part of this may reflect a measurement issue. Herein, we focus only on financially attributable food insecurity, but international studies show that storage, transportation, and functional barriers are all important in explaining food insecurity in older populations [63]. Thus, we are likely to be biasing downward the prevalence of food insecurity among older Australians. Moreover, the prevalence of food insecurity may be higher for age pension recipients who rent rather than own their home. Secondly, there is the role of selective mortality in these cross-sectional data. As individuals with higher economic and social resources are more likely to exhibit higher survival prospects relative to their financially disadvantaged peers, in cross-sectional data we may be observing these individuals in later life.

More generally, the HES data are cross-sectional, and it is not possible to draw any type of causal relationship between receipt of certain payments and food insecurity. Specifically, we do not know if prior to receipt of certain payments, they were food-insecure, or only insecure once on payments. However, recent evidence shows that experience of involuntary job loss (OR 2.6 $p < 0.001$) or difficulty finding employment (OR 2.5 $p < 0.001$) within the past 12 months increases the odds of food insecurity by about 2.5 times [21]. The purpose of this paper has been to present prevalence rates of food insecurity across a range of social benefit payment types. Further multivariable analyses, ideally with longitudinal data, should be conducted to provide further detail on the experiences of food insecurity faced by social assistance payment recipients in Australia.

5. Conclusions

This is the first Australian study to examine the differences in the prevalence of food insecurity across a wide range of social assistance payments. We found a high prevalence of food insecurity among those receiving Australian Government social assistance payments, including the Newstart Allowance, Austudy/Abstudy, Disability Support Pension, the Carer payment, and Parenting payment. The relatively higher levels of income support through the Age Pension payment may have had a protective effect on food insecurity and financial wellbeing, demonstrating the benefits of addressing income inadequacy that has been found in the international literature. Due to differences in indexing the respective payments, the level of the Newstart Allowance as a percentage of the age pension has fallen from 90% in the 1990s to 60% today [64].

Australian advocates for action to reduce poverty and inequality have called for the Government to 'raise the rate' of Newstart and related payments, noting that Newstart has not increased in real terms for 24 years [65]. Recent Australian modelling indicates that an increase in the Newstart Allowance to $800 per fortnight in Australia would significantly decrease the poverty gap in Australia by about 11% [66]. Our results support calls by a range of Australian non-government organisations, politicians, and academics calling for a comprehensive review of the Australian social security system [67]. Our findings, when combined with others in the Australian literature, suggest well designed increases in the Newstart, Disability, Student, Carer, and disability payments may improve the material resources of food-insecure households and thus ameliorate their food insecurity experience and potentially offset health and economic risks [4–17].

Author Contributions: Conceptualization, J.B.T., C.M.P., and S.B.; Formal Analysis, J.B.T.; Writing—Original Draft Preparation, J.B.T., S.B., and C.M.P.

Funding: This research received no external funding. J.B.T. is funded by the ARC Centre for Excellence in Population Ageing Research (CE1101029).

Acknowledgments: Data for this study were provided to the authors by the Australian Bureau of Statistics (ABS) through the ABS Universities Australia agreement.

Conflicts of Interest: The authors declare no conflict of interest.

Appendix A

Table A1. Indicators of Financial Stress (%) by Food Insecurity Status and Receipt of Social Assistance, Households 2015/2016.

Receives Social Assistance Benefits:	Food Insecure				Main Source of Household Social Assistance Benefits in Cash					
	No		Yes		None	Age Pension	Disability and Carer Payments	Family Support Payments	Unemployment and Student Allowances	Other Pensions and Allowances
	No	Yes	No	Yes						
Sought assistance from welfare/community organisation	<1	2.7	1.1	42.7	<1	1.6	10.4	5.4	9.6	<1
Pawned or sold something	<1	2.3	12.9	34.7	1.1	<1	7.8	5.2	8.8	1
Sought financial help from friends or family	3.9	6.9	57.6	59.7	4.5	2.5	14.2	14	21.5	4.2
Unable to heat home	<1	2.1	22.8	30.4	1	1.9	6.9	2.6	8.3	1.1
Could not pay gas/electricity/telephone	5.6	10.5	55.9	59.3	6.1	4	19.6	22	20.9	6.1
Could not pay registration / insurance on time	2.3	3.8	35.2	31.6	2.7	1	6.7	8.6	12.1	2.3
Unweighted (n)	3855	5884	38	263	3894	2680	836	1177	528	926
Weighted (%)	43.5	53.7	0.5	2.3	44.0	19.9	7.4	13.4	5.9	9.5

Table A2. Management of Household Income and Standard of Living (%) by Food Insecurity Status and Receipt of Social Assistance, Households 2015/2016.

Receives Social Assistance Benefits:	Food Insecure				Main Source of Household Social Assistance Benefits in Cash					
	No		Yes		None	Age Pension	Disability and Carer Payments	Family Support Payments	Unemployment and Student Allowances	Other Pensions and Allowances
	No	Yes	No	Yes						
Management of Household Income										
Spend more money than we get	10	13.6	22	46.1	10.1	8.9	21	19.8	20.9	12.3
Just break even most weeks	33.2	49.6	60.2	48.8	33.5	49.5	50.1	52.3	55.1	41.1
Able to save money most weeks	56.8	36.8	17.8	5.1	56.4	14.6	28.9	27.4	24	46.6
Present Standard of Living										
Better than 2 years ago	41	22.3	15.2	22.9	40.7	13.1	22.9	31.6	27.9	25.1
The same as 2 years ago	40.9	50.6	32.5	24.9	40.8	62.6	43.6	39.3	30.6	50.6
Worse than 2 years ago	18.1	27.1	52.4	52.1	18.5	23.4	33.5	29.1	41.5	24.4
Unweighted (n)	3855	5884	38	263	3894	2680	836	1177	528	926
Weighted (%)	43.5	53.7	0.5	2.3	44.0	19.9	7.4	13.4	5.9	9.5

Table A3. Access to Emergency Funds (%) by Food Insecurity and Receipt of Social Assistance, Households 2015/2016.

| | Food Insecure | | | | Main Source of Household Social Assistance Benefits in Cash | | | | | |
| | No | | Yes | | | | | | | |
Receives Social Assistance Benefits:	No	Yes	No	Yes	None	Age Pension	Disability and Carer Payments	Family Support Payments	Unemployment and Student Allowances	Other Pensions and Allowances
Access to Emergency Funds										
Could not raise $2000 within a week	6.3	16.1	32.5	73.2	6.6	11.3	34.7	21.5	33.9	6.7
Source(s) of Emergency Funds										
Own Savings	77.9	65.1	19	10.4	77.3	74.5	45.4	51.9	41.9	78.6
Loan from a Bank, Building Society	14.3	9.9	8.9	<1	14.3	5.8	9.3	13.3	9	12.4
Loan from a Finance Company	4.3	1.8	0	1.1	4.2	<1	2.6	2.3	1.2	3.3
Loan on Credit Card	19.5	11.8	25.1	2.2	19.6	8.1	9.5	15.9	11.2	13.4
Loan from Family or Friends	19.4	15.9	26.7	19.7	19.5	8.5	15.3	25.3	20.5	16.6
Loan from Welfare or Community Organisation	<1	<1	<1	4.3	<1	<1	2.4	1	<1	<1
Sell Something	9.1	4.9	6.7	<1	9.1	1.7	3.8	7.8	7.1	6.7
Other Sources	2.4	2.8	3.1	<1	2.5	2.7	1.9	2.3	3.9	3.1
Unweighted (n)	3855	5884	38	263	3894	2680	836	1177	528	926
Weighted (%)	43.5	53.7	0.5	2.3	44.0	19.9	7.4	13.4	5.9	9.5

References

1. Australian Bureau of Statistics. *Australian Health Survey: Nutrition—State and Territory Results, 2011–2012 (Catalogue Number 4364.0.55.009)*; Australian Bureau of Statistics: Canberra, Australia, 2015.
2. Temple, J.B. Severe and moderate forms of food insecurity in Australia: Are they distinguishable? *Aust. J. Soc. Issues* **2008**, *43*, 649–668. [CrossRef]
3. Temple, J.B.; Russell, J. Food insecurity among older Aboriginal and Torres Strait Islanders. *Int. J. Environ. Res. Public Health* **2018**, *15*, 1766. [CrossRef]
4. Kendall, A.; Olson, C.; Frongillo, E. Relationship of hunger and food insecurity to food availability and consumption. *J. Am. Diet. Assoc.* **1996**, *96*, 1019–1024. [CrossRef]
5. Rose, D.; Oliveria, D. Nutrient intakes of individuals from food insufficient households in the United States. *Am. J. Public Health* **1997**, *87*, 1956–1961. [CrossRef] [PubMed]
6. Heflin, C.; Siefert, K.; Williams, D. Food insufficiency and women's mental health: Findings from a 3 year panel of welfare recipients. *Soc. Sci. Med.* **2005**, *61*, 1971–1982. [CrossRef] [PubMed]
7. Sharkey, J. Risk and presence of food insufficiency are associated with low nutrient intakes and multimorbidity among housebound older women who receive home-delivered meals. *J. Nutr.* **2003**, *133*, 3485–3491. [CrossRef]
8. Stuff, J.; Casey, P.; Szeto, K.; Gossett, G.; Robbins, J.; Simpson, P.; Connell, C.; Bogle, M. Household food insecurity is associated with adult health status. *J. Nutr.* **2004**, *134*, 2330–2335. [CrossRef]
9. Tarasuk, V. Household food insecurity with hunger is associated with women's food intakes, health and household circumstances. *J. Nutr.* **2001**, *131*, 2670–2676. [CrossRef]
10. Vozoris, N.; Tarasuk, V. Household food insufficiency is associated with poorer health. *J. Nutr.* **2003**, *133*, 120–126. [CrossRef]
11. Laraia, B.; Siega-Riz, A.; Gundersen, C.; Dole, N. Psychosocial factors and socioeconomic indicators are associated with household food insecurity among pregnant women. *J. Nutr.* **2006**, *136*, 177–182. [CrossRef]
12. German, L.; Kahana, C.; Rosenfeld, V.; Zabrowsky, I.; Wiezer, Z.; Fraser, D.; Shahar, D. Depressive symptoms are associated with food insufficiency and nutritional deficiencies in poor community-dwelling elderly people. *J. Nutr. Health Aging* **2011**, *15*, 3–8. [CrossRef] [PubMed]
13. Redmond, M.; Dong, F.; Goetz, J.; Jacobson, L.; Collins, T. Food insecurity and peripheral arterial disease in older adult populations. *J. Nutr. Health Aging* **2016**, *20*, 989–995. [CrossRef] [PubMed]
14. Cook, J.; Frank, D.; Berkowitz, C.; Black, M.; Casey, P.; Cutts, D.; Meyers, A.; Zaldivar, N.; Skalicky, A.; Levenson, S.; et al. Food insecurity is associated with adverse health outcomes among human infants and toddlers. *J. Nutr.* **2004**, *134*, 1432–1438. [CrossRef] [PubMed]
15. Jyoti, D.; Frongillo, E.; Jones, S. Food insecurity affects children's academic performance, weight gain, and social skills. *J. Nutr.* **2005**, *135*, 2831–2839. [CrossRef] [PubMed]
16. Alaimo, K.; Olson, C.; Frongillo, E. Family food insufficiency, but not low family income, is positively associated with dysthymia and suicide symptoms in Adolescents. *J. Nutr.* **2002**, *132*, 719–725. [CrossRef] [PubMed]
17. Hamelin, A.; Habicht, J.; Beaudry, M. Food insecurity: Consequences for the household and broader social implications. *J. Nutr.* **1999**, *129*, 525s–528s. [CrossRef] [PubMed]
18. Loopstra, R.; Fledderjohann, J.; Reeves, A.; Stuckler, D. Impact of welfare benefit sanctioning on food insecurity: A dynamic cross-area study of food bank usage in the UK. *J. Social Policy* **2018**, *47*, 437–457. [CrossRef]
19. Borjas, G.J. Food insecurity and public assistance. *J. Public Econ.* **2004**, *88*, 1421–1443. [CrossRef]
20. McKenzie, H.J.; McKay, F.H. Food as a discretionary item: The impact of welfare payment changes on low-income single mother's food choices and strategies. *J. Poverty Soc. Just.* **2017**, *25*, 35–48. [CrossRef]
21. Temple, J.B. The association between stressful events and food insecurity: Cross-sectional evidence from Australia. *Int. J. Environ. Res. Public Health* **2018**, *15*, 2333. [CrossRef]
22. Harmer, J. *Pension Review Report*; Department of Families, Housing, Community Services and Indigenous Affairs: Canberra, Austria, 2009.
23. Davidson, P.; Whiteford, P. *An Overview of Australia's System of Income and Employment Assistance for the Unemployed*; OECD Social, Employment and Migration Working Papers, No. 129; OECD: Paris, France, 2012.

24. Pollard, C.; Begley, A.; Landrigan, T. The Rise of Food Inequality in Australia. In *Food Poverty and Insecurity: International Food Inequalities*; Caraher, M., Coveney, J., Eds.; Springer: Cham, Switzerland, 2016.
25. Friel, S. A fair go for health? Not at the moment. *Aust. N. Z. J. Public Health* **2014**, *38*, 302–303. [CrossRef] [PubMed]
26. Saunders, P.; Bedford, M. New minimum healthy living budget standards for low-paid and unemployed Australians. *Econ. Labour Rel. Rev.* **2018**. [CrossRef]
27. Saunders, P. Using a budget standards approach to assess the adequacy of Newstart allowance. *Aust. J. Soc. Issues* **2018**, *53*, 4–17. [CrossRef]
28. Crawford, B.; Yamazaki, R.; Franke, E.; Amanatidis, S.; Ravulo, J.; Steinbeck, K.; Ritchie, J.; Torvaldsen, S. Sustaining dignity? Food insecurity in homeless young people in urban Australia. *Health Prom. J. Aust.* **2014**, *25*, 71–78. [CrossRef] [PubMed]
29. Booth, S. Eating rough: Food sources and acquisition practices of homeless young people in Adelaide, South Australia. *Public Health Nutr.* **2006**, *9*, 212–218. [CrossRef] [PubMed]
30. Hughes, R.; Serebryanikova, I.; Donaldson, K.; Leveritt, M. Student food insecurity: The skeleton in the university closet. *Nutr. Diet* **2011**, *68*, 27–32. [CrossRef]
31. Micevski, D.A.; Thornton, L.E.; Brockington, S. Food insecurity among university students in Victoria: A pilot study. *Nutr. Diet* **2014**, *71*, 258–264. [CrossRef]
32. Gallegos, D.; Ellies, P.; Wright, J. Still there's no food! Food insecurity in a refugee population in Perth, Western Australia. *Nutr. Diet.* **2008**, *65*, 78–83. [CrossRef]
33. McKay, F.H.; Dunn, M. Food security among asylum seekers in Melbourne. *Australian and New Zealand. J. Public Health* **2015**, *39*, 344–349. [CrossRef]
34. McCarthy, L.; Chang, A.; Brimblecombe, J. Food insecurity experiences of Aboriginal and Torres Strait Islander Families with young children in an urban setting: Influencing factors and coping strategies. *Int. J. Environ. Res. Public Health* **2018**, *15*, 2649. [CrossRef]
35. Temple, J.B. Food insecurity among older Australians: Prevalence, correlates and well-being. *Aust. J. Ageing* **2006**, *25*, 158–163. [CrossRef]
36. Russell, J.; Flood, V.; Yeatman, H.; Mitchell, P. Prevalence and risk factors of food insecurity among a cohort of older Australians. *J. Nutr. Health Aging* **2014**, *18*, 3–8. [CrossRef] [PubMed]
37. Nolan, M.; Rikard-Bell, G.; Mohsin, M.; Williams, M. Food insecurity in three socially disadvantaged localities in Sydney, Australia. *Health Prom. J. Aust.* **2006**, *17*, 247–253. [CrossRef]
38. DHS. *A Guide to Australian Government Payments*; Department of Human Services: Canberra, Australia, 2018. Available online: https://www.humanservices.gov.au/organisations/about-us/publications-and-resources/guide-australian-government-payments (accessed on 1 November 2018).
39. ABS. *Household Expenditure Survey and Survey of Income and Housing, User Guide, Australia, 2015–2016*; Catalogue Number 6503.0; Australian Bureau of Statistics: Canberra, Australia, 2017.
40. Tarasuk, V.; Mitchell, A.; Dachner, N. *Household Food Insecurity in Canada*; PROOF: Toronto, ON, Canada, 2014; Available online: https://proof.utoronto.ca/ (accessed on 1 November 2018).
41. King, S.; Bellamy, J.; Kemp, B.; Mollenhauer, J. Hard Choices—Going without in a Time of Plenty. A Study of Food Insecurity in NSW and the ACT. 2013. Available online: https://www.anglicare.org.au/media/2850/anglicaresydney_hardchoicesfoodinsecurity_2013.pdf (accessed on 1 December 2018).
42. Banger, M.; McCulloch, D. Increase Pension before Newstart: Morrison. Australian Associated Press. 2 November 2018. Available online: https://www.news.com.au/national/breaking-news/morrison-ridicules-raising-newstart-rate/news-story/04df1d4237f9e609435362de5153c15b (accessed on 1 November 2018).
43. Temple, J.B.; Rice, J.M.; McDonald, P.F. Mature age labour force participation and the life cycle deficit in Australia: 1981–82 to 2009–10. *J. Econ. Ageing* **2017**, *10*, 21–33. [CrossRef]
44. Temple, J.B.; McDonald, P.F.; Rice, J.M. Net assets available at age of death in Australia: An extension of the National Transfer Accounts methodology. *Popul. Rev.* **2017**, *56*. [CrossRef]
45. Davidson, P.; Saunders, P.; Bradbury, B.; Wong, M. *Poverty in Australia*; ACOSS/UNSW Poverty and Inequality Partnership Report No. 2; ACOSS: Sydney, Australia, 2018.
46. Gorton, D.; Bullen, C.R.; Mhurchu, C.N. Environmental influences on food security in high-income countries. *Nutr Rev.* **2010**, *68*, 1–29. [CrossRef] [PubMed]

47. Huang, J.; Guo, B.; Kim, Y. Food insecurity and disability: Do economic resources matter? *Soc. Sci. Res.* **2010**, *39*, 111–124. [CrossRef]

48. Loopstra, R.; Lalor, D. *Financial Insecurity, Food Insecurity, and Disability: The Profile of People Receiving Emergency Food Assistance from The Trussell Trust Foodbank Network in Britain*; The Trussell Trust, University of Oxford, King's College London: London, UK, 2017.

49. Stevens, C.A. Exploring food insecurity among young mothers (15–24 years). *J. Spec. Pediatric Nurs.* **2010**, *15*, 163–171. [CrossRef]

50. Good Shepherd Australia New Zealand. Outside Systems Control My Life: Single Mothers' Stories of Welfare and Work. 2018. Available online: https://goodshep.org.au/media/2188/outside-systems-control-my-life_single-mothers-stories-of-welfare-to-work.pdf (accessed on 1 December 2018).

51. Brady, M. Targeting single mothers? Dynamics of contracting Australian employment services and activation policies at the street level. *J. Soc. Policy* **2018**, *47*, 827–845. [CrossRef]

52. Temple, J.B.; Dow, B. The unmet support needs of carers of older Australians: Prevalence and mental health. *Int. Psychoger.* **2018**. [CrossRef]

53. Cobb-Clark, D.; Dahman, S.; Salamanca, N.; Zhu, A. *Intergenerational Disadvantage: Learning about Equal Opportunity from Social Assistance Receipt*; IZA Discussion Paper No. 11070; IZA Institute of Labour Econmics: Bonn, Germany, 2017.

54. Anderson, W.; White, V.; Finney, A. Coping with low incomes and cold homes. *Energy Policy* **2012**, *49*, 40–52. [CrossRef]

55. Beatty, T.; Blow, L.; Crossley, T. Is there a 'heat-or-eat' trade-off in the UK? *J. R. Stat. Soc. A* **2014**, *177*, 281–294. [CrossRef]

56. Bhattacharya, J.; DeLeire, T.; Haider, S.; Currie, J. Heat or eat? Cold-weather shocks and nutrition in Poor American Families. *Am. J. Public Health* **2003**, *93*, 1149. [CrossRef] [PubMed]

57. Emery, J.; Bartoo, A.; Matheson, J.; Ferrer, A.; Kirkpatrick, S.; Tarasuk, V.; McIntyre, L. Evidence of the association between household food insecurity and heating cost inflation in Canada 1998–2001. *Can. Public Policy* **2012**, *38*, 181–215. [CrossRef]

58. Valadkhani, A.; Nguyen, J.; Smyth, R. Consumer electricity and gas prices across Australian capital cities: Structural breaks, effects of policy reforms and interstate differences. *Energy Econ.* **2018**, *72*, 365–375. [CrossRef]

59. Urbis. South Australian Disconnection Project: Final Report. 2014. Available online: https://www.sacoss.org.au/sites/default/files/public/140828_South%20Australian%20Disconnection%20Project.pdf (accessed on 1 December 2018).

60. Nelson, T.; McCracken-Hewson, E.; Sundstrom, G.; Hawthorne, M. The drivers of energy-related financial hardship in Australia–understanding the role of income, consumption and housing. *Energy Policy* **2019**, *124*, 262–271. [CrossRef]

61. Loopstra, R.; Dachner, N.; Tarasuk, V. An exploration of the unprecedented decline in the prevalence of household food insecurity in Newfoundland and Labrador, 2007–2012. *Can. Public Policy* **2015**, *41*, 191–206. [CrossRef]

62. Li, N.; Dachner, N.; Tarasuk, V. The impact of changes in social policies on household food insecurity in British Columbia, 2005–2012. *Prev. Med.* **2016**, *93*, 151–158. [CrossRef]

63. Wolfe, W.; Frongillo, E.; Valois, P. Understanding the experience of food insecurity by elders suggests ways to improve its measurement. *J. Nutr.* **2003**, *133*, 2762. [CrossRef]

64. Phillips, B.; Gray, M.; Webster, R. Cut the Pension, Boost Newstart. What Our Algorithm Says I the Best Way to Get Value for Our Welfare Dollars. *The Conversation.* 2018. Available online: https://theconversation.com/cut-the-pension-boost-newstart-what-our-algorithm-says-is-the-best-way-to-get-value-for-our-welfare-dollars-108417 (accessed on 10 December 2018).

65. ACOSS. Raise the Rate. 2018. Available online: https://www.acoss.org.au/raisetherate/ (accessed on 10 December 2018).

66. Phillips, B.; Webster, R.; Gray, M. Optimal Policy Modelling: A Microsimulation Methodology for Setting the Australian Tax and Transfer System. CSRM Working Paper N. 10/2018, Centre for Social Research and Methods; The Australian National University. 2018. Available online: http://csrm.cass.anu.edu.au/sites/default/files/docs/2018/12/Optimal-policy-modelling-setting-Australian-tax-and-transfer-system-10-2018-CSRM-working-paper_0.pdf (accessed on 10 December 2018).

67. Whiteford, P.; Phillips, B.; Bradbury, B. It's Not Just Newstart. Single Parents Are $271 per Fortnight Worse off. *Labor Needs an Overarching Welfare Review. The Conversation.* 2018. Available online: https://theconversation.com/its-not-just-newstart-single-parents-are-271-per-fortnight-worse-off-labor-needs-an-overarching-welfare-review-107521 (accessed on 10 December 2018).

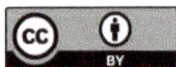

International Journal of
Environmental Research and Public Health

MDPI

Article

Walking the Food Security Tightrope—Exploring the Experiences of Low-to-Middle Income Melbourne Households

Sue Kleve [1,*], Sue Booth [2], Zoe E. Davidson [1] and Claire Palermo [1]

1   Department of Nutrition, Dietetics and Food, School of Clinical Sciences, Faculty of Medicine, Nursing and
    Health Sciences, Monash University, Level 1, 264 Ferntree Gully Road, Notting Hill 3168, Australia;
    zoe.davidson@monash.edu (Z.E.D.); claire.palermo@monash.edu (C.P.)
2   College of Medicine and Public Health, Flinders University, GPO Box 2100, Adelaide 5000, Australia;
    sue.booth@flinders.edu.au
*   Correspondence: suzanne.kleve@monash.edu; Tel.: +61-3-9902-4268

Received: 12 September 2018; Accepted: 6 October 2018; Published: 10 October 2018

Abstract: There is limited evidence of how Australian low-to-middle income (AUD $40,000–$80,000) households maintain food security. Using a sequential explanatory mixed methods methodology, this study explored and compared the food security (FS) and insecurity (FIS) experiences of these households. An initial quantitative survey categorised participants according to food security status (the 18-item United States Department of Agriculture Household Food Security Survey Module) and income level to identify and purposefully select participants to qualitatively explore food insecurity and security experiences. Of the total number of survey participants (n = 134), 42 were categorised as low-to-middle income. Of these, a subset of 16 participants (8 FIS and 8 FS) was selected, and each participant completed an in-depth interview. The interviews explored precursors, strategies to prevent or address food insecurity, and the implications of the experience. Interview data were analysed using a thematic analysis approach. Five themes emerged from the analysis: (i) food decision experiences, (ii) assets, (iii) triggers, (iv) activation of assets, and (v) consequences and emotion related to walking the food security tightrope. The leverage points across all themes were more volatile for FIS participants. Low-to-middle income Australians are facing the challenges of trying to maintain or improve their food security status, with similarities to those described in lower income groups, and should be included in approaches to prevent or address food insecurity.

Keywords: food insecurity; low-to-middle income; experience; mixed methodology research

---

1. Introduction

Food insecurity—the limited or uncertain availability of individuals' and households' physical, social, and economic access to sufficient, safe, nutritious, and culturally relevant food—is a complex, persistent, and multidimensional phenomenon [1]. Irrespective of an abundance of food and relative wealth, the issue of food insecurity is one experienced amongst high income countries, including Australia. The 2011–2012 National Health Survey, using a single-item tool, indicated that 4% of Australians, or approximately one million, were living in a household that was food insecure [2]. Utilising different valid multi-item tools, the prevalence of food insecurity in other high income countries was found to be 15% in New Zealand [3], 12.3% in Canada [4], 8% in England, Wales, and Northern Ireland (U.K.) [5], and 14% in the United States (U.S.) [6].

Food insecurity has a temporal dimension, and households may transition between episodic or chronic experiences [7]. The core characteristics of food insecurity have been described at both an individual and household level to include anxiety, concern, compromise to the quantity and nutritional quality of food, and social isolation [8,9]. The food insecurity experience may vary in severity along a continuum [10]. At one end of the continuum are initial indicators, such as anxiety and concern about an adequate food budget or food supply, and, at the other extreme end, the more severe indicators, perturbations in diet quality and quantity of food intake and hunger, become apparent [7,8,10,11]. Numerous negative implications of food insecurity have been reported, including physical, social, and emotional health impacts across the lifespan [12–16] and developmental and educational impacts in children [17]. Food insecurity is a serious public health issue.

Regardless of households' geographic location, food insecurity is influenced by the interactions of a range of factors as described by the four dimensions of food security—food availability, supply, utilisation, and stability [1]—and the socio-demographic characteristics of households [3,18–22]. The major predictor of food insecurity is a low income or limited available economic resources for purchasing food or general resources in a household [18,19,23–27]. Although an inverse relationship between income and food insecurity exists [19,24,28], not all very-low-income households are food insecure, nor are households progressing up the income gradient food secure [28–30]. While the prevalence of food insecurity is greater in very-low-income groups, evidence from high-income countries indicates that households beyond this income group are experiencing food insecurity [19,26,31–36]. Categorisation of food insecurity based on the static measure of annual income may be problematic as this measure is insensitive to sudden economic changes within a household [28].

Whilst the existence of food insecurity in higher-income groups has been reported, there has been limited research examining the factors that contribute to food insecurity in these groups. Additional factors for Canadian and U.S. higher-income households include a fluctuating income, a sudden change in employment, a change in household composition, illness, disability, increased housing costs, and housing tenure [34,36,37]. Further significant predictors reported from Victoria, Australia in low-to-middle income households include an inability to raise money in an emergency, housing tenure, support from friends, and the cost of food [32].

There is a limited understanding of the nature of the experience of food insecurity in low-to-middle income Australian households. This may hinder the development of approaches to address the determinants of food insecurity more broadly across income groups. Furthermore, the factors that protect people from food insecurity and the coping strategies of households need to be explored. Approaches to address food insecurity need to consider the complex range of determinants that trigger food insecurity in households; and, consequently, a measurement of food insecurity must capture these determinants.

This study had three aims. The first was to identify low-to-middle income Melbourne participants who are food secure and food insecure. The second was to explore and compare food security and insecurity experiences; specifically, the precursors to, and strategies for preventing or addressing, food insecurity. The third was to examine the implications of the experience of food insecurity for those experiencing it to inform policy and practice.

2. Materials and Methods

2.1. Study Design

The study employed a pragmatic approach and positioning. The researchers were interested in understanding the experience of food insecurity from the perspective of participants from low-to-middle income households and the implications of this on their lives for policy and practice. An explanatory sequential mixed methods research design approach of collecting, analysing, and integrating both quantitative and qualitative data in the research process was employed [38–40]. Typically, the emphasis in this design is on the quantitative phase; however, in this study, the research emphasis was on the qualitative phase to explore the experience of food security and food insecurity within low-to-middle income households. The initial quantitative results were used to identify and purposefully select participants to qualitatively examine the food insecurity phenomenon [38,41].

The study was conducted according to guidelines in the Declaration of Helsinki, and all procedures were approved by the Monash University Human Research Ethics Committee (CF14/1382-201400647). Informed consent was implied for the quantitative phase, and written informed consent was obtained for the qualitative phase.

2.2. Participants

A cross-sectional convenience sample was recruited from metropolitan Melbourne, Victoria. Suburbs were selected according to the 'Vulnerability Assessment for Mortgage, Petrol, and Inflation Risks and Expenditure' (VAMPIRE) 2008 Index [42]. The VAMPIRE index is based on Census data and calculates suburb vulnerability based on three socio economic stressors: mortgage, car, and income, providing a ranking from minimal to very high vulnerability. Those with high levels of car ownership, who journey to work by car, who have mortgage tenure, and/or who have low incomes are considered 'more vulnerable'. A higher vulnerability VAMPIRE rating is likely to impact on finances available for food [43]; thus, all Melbourne suburbs with medium to very high ratings were selected for inclusion. These suburbs provided a varied sample in which food insecurity is likely to occur in some households due to characteristic stressors [44].

The convenience sample aimed to identify information-rich participants to interview as part of the qualitative phase, rather than be representative of the population. Eligibility for study inclusion was conducted in two stages. In the quantitative phase, participants were over 18 years of age and residing in metropolitan Melbourne, living in or adjacent to VAMPIRE suburbs. In the qualitative phase, participants from the quantitative phase were included as low-to-middle income if they had a gross household income of AUD $40,000–$80,000 per annum before tax. This income categorisation was based on Australian Bureau of Statistics quintiles of gross Victorian household income [45]. Respondent anonymity was preserved by a unique code that was assigned for survey responses, and all interview participants were provided with a pseudonym. Figure 1 summarises the study design procedures.

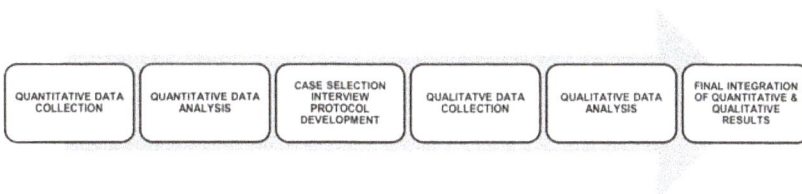

| QUANTITATIVE DATA COLLECTION | QUANTITATIVE DATA ANALYSIS | CASE SELECTION INTERVIEW PROTOCOL DEVELOPMENT | QUALITATVE DATA COLLECTION | QUALITATIVE DATA ANALYSIS | FINAL INTEGRATION OF QUANTITATIVE & QUALITATIVE RESULTS |

Figure 1. Summary of Sequential Explanatory Mixed Methods research design.

2.3. Quantitative Phase: Data Collection and Analysis

The quantitative survey, 'Food Security in Melbourne Households Survey' (FSiMH survey), was designed by the researchers using a mix of validated questions and instruments. Demographic questions were developed to gather information on factors that are associated with food insecurity in the literature and support categorisation based on income [19,32,46]. Food security status was determined using the validated 18-item United States Department of Agriculture Household Food Security Survey Module (USDA-HFSSM) [7]. The survey was promoted across a diverse range of community organisations and websites located in, or in close proximity to, the VAMPIRE suburbs. The main household shopper or food preparer was asked to complete the survey. The FSiMH survey was administered in both an electronic (Qualtrics, Provo UT, US platform) and paper format between September 2014 and February 2015.

The USDA-HFSSM was selected for determination of food security status because of its reliability across populations and population subgroups and its ability to capture the severity level and continuum of experience of food insecurity [7,47–49]. The USDA-HFSSM categorises households as food secure or food insecure with varying severity levels of experience. Households with affirmative scores of 0–2 are classified as food secure; those with an affirmative score of 0 are classified as food secure at the high food security (no reported indications of food-access limitations) severity level, whereas those with affirmative scores of 1 or 2 are classified as food secure at the marginal food security (anxiety over food sufficiency or a shortage of food in the house) severity level. Scores of 3 or greater are classified as food insecure at the low food security (reduced quality and variety of food with little or no indication of reduced intake) and very low food security (multiple indications of a disrupted eating pattern and reduced food intake) severity levels [7]. Studies from the United States and Canada report an increase in marginally food secure households that display greater health outcomes and similar characteristics to food insecure households [4,10,24,50]. Those who are marginally food secure may also be at greater risk of progressing to more severe forms of food insecurity. Consequently, using the philosophical pragmatic approach that guides this research, the modified Canadian food security categorisation was applied [4]. Respondents that were classified as experiencing marginal food security with a score of 1 or 2 were included in the food insecure category. The severity categorisations and scores are consistent with the USDA-HFSSM classifications [7,51].

Data were analysed using the statistical software package IBM SPSS Statistics for Windows, Version 22.0 (SPSS INC., Chicago, IL, USA). For the purpose of this analysis, respondents were dichotomised as food secure or food insecure, and demographic characteristics were explored descriptively and reported as counts and percentages.

2.4. Qualitative Phase: Data Collection and Analysis

The results from the quantitative phase supported the case selection and the interview protocol's development. The logic underpinning the interview protocol and questions was informed by both the existing literature [9,25,52–54] and the quantitative analysis, in particular the responses to the USDA-HFSSM items that described the experiences and consequences of food insecurity. The USDA-HFSSM assesses food security status based on an inability to access food due to a lack of financial resources; however, additional factors beyond this may impact upon food security status [47,55]. Consequently, the interviews allowed for elaboration and exploration beyond these economic factors and a deeper understanding and extension of the experiences of food insecurity that are measured by the USDA-HFSSM questions. The interviews explored low-to-middle income participants' experiences of accessing food (physical and economic), factors that influenced and impacted this, and the consequences of these factors. Four key areas were explored in the interviews: (i) accessing food and food choices for the household, (ii) factors impacting on food for the household, (iii) consequences when sufficient food quantity and preferred foods cannot be accessed, and (iv) coping and protective strategies: asset exploration (Supplementary Table S1). The researcher used a semi-structured interview format whereby the key areas were used to construct the main questions that were asked of participants and a series of prompting questions that were subsequently asked based on participants' initial response. The interviewer continued probing the participants until they were satisfied that responses of an adequate breadth and depth in each of the four interview areas were obtained.

All interviews were individually undertaken between June 2015 and September 2015 by the first author with each participant at a mutually suitable time in interview rooms at local community centres. The interviews were digitally recorded and transcribed, and field notes were kept after each interview. The interview duration ranged from 45 to 90 min. The NVivo qualitative software (QSR International, Version 10.3, Melbourne, Australia) was used to manage, store, and support the data analysis. A thematic data analysis was chosen, as the researchers acknowledged the complexities of food security and the need for more than one theoretical framework to explain the data and the emergence of new concepts. Braun and Clarke (2006) describe the benefits of a thematic analysis as 'providing a flexible and useful research tool, which can potentially provide a rich and detailed, yet complex account of data' [56]. The qualitative analysis approach included familiarisation with a transcript's content, open content coding with coding nodes, and inter-coder agreement. The codes were grouped into themes and subthemes in light of the research questions with the verification of themes amongst the researchers. A constant comparison approach to analysis was performed to describe patterns in the data to inform the initial formation of categories, where a content comparison within each category enabled the description of categories to evolve [57,58]. The constant comparison approach was implemented at three levels: for individual participants regardless of food security status; within food secure and food insecure groups; and between food secure and food insecure groups [57]. This analysis approach allowed for exploration of similarities and differences across and between groups.

3. Results

3.1. Quantitative Phase: Demographic Characteristics and Food Security Status

One hundred and thirty-four participants completed the FSiMH survey. Thirteen participants declined to indicate their income level, reducing the participant income data to $n = 121$. Forty-two participants were classified as low-to-middle income (food secure (FS), $n = 26$ and food insecure (FIS), $n = 16$), including 12 households with children.

The majority of participants were female and Australian-born. FIS participants ($n = 16$) included participants that were homeowners with a mortgage ($n = 8$), participants living with their spouse/partner and children ($n = 11$), and participants that had some form of paid employment ($n = 11$) (Table 1). In comparison, FS participants ($n = 26$) included participants that were homeowners ($n = 19$), of which nine were mortgage free, participants living with their spouse/partner and children ($n = 10$), and participants that had some form of paid employment ($n = 10$).

Table 1. Characteristics of low-to-middle income survey respondents ($n = 42$) and in-depth interview participants ($n = 16$) according to food security status.

Demographic Characteristics	Quantitative Survey Respondents $n = 42$		Respondents Selected for Qualitative Interview $n = 16$	
	Food Insecure $n = 16$(%)	Food Secure $n = 26$(%)	Food Insecure $n = 8$(%)	Food Secure $n = 8$(%)
Gender				
Male	1(6.2)	4(15.4)	0	1(12.5)
Female	15(93.8)	21(80.8)	8(100.0)	7(87.5)
Prefer not to say	0	1(3.9)	-	-
Age				
18–25	2(12.5)	2(7.7)	1(12.5)	1(12.5)
26–35	6(37.5)	4(15.4)	2(25.0)	2(25.0)
36–45	5(31.3)	7(26.9)	3(37.5)	1(12.5)
46–55	1(6.2)	6(23.0)	0	3(37.5)
56–65	2(12.5)	3(11.5)	2(25.0)	0
Over 65	0	4(15.4)	0	1(12.5)
Country of Birth				
Australia	11(69.0)	16(61.5)	5(62.5)	4(50.0)
Other	5(31.0)	10(38.5)	3(37.5)	4(50.0)
Housing Tenure				
Homeowner, mortgage	8(50.0)	10(38.5)	4(50.0)	3(37.5)
Homeowner, no mortgage	0	9(34.6)	1(12.5)	3(37.5)
Renting, privately	8(50.0)	4(15.4)	3(37.5)	1(12.5)
Other	0	3(11.5)	0	1(12.5)
Household Structure/Composition				
Living alone	1(6.2)	1(3.9)	2(25.0)	0
With parents/family	0	3(11.5)	1(12.5)	1(12.5)
With spouse/partner	1(6.2)	11(42.3)	1(12.5)	3(37.5)
With spouse/partner and children <18 years	10(62.5)	10(38.5)	4(50)	3(37.5)
With spouse/partner and children >18 years	1(6.2)	0	0	1(12.5)
With my children <18 years	2(12.5)	1(3.9)	0	0
Living in a share house	1(6.2)	0	0	0

Table 1. *Cont.*

Demographic Characteristics	Quantitative Survey Respondents $n = 42$		Respondents Selected for Qualitative Interview $n = 16$	
	Food Insecure $n = 16(\%)$	Food Secure $n = 26(\%)$	Food Insecure $n = 8(\%)$	Food Secure $n = 8(\%)$
Number of children in household				
0	4(25.0)	14(53.9)	3(37.5)	4(50.0)
1	3(18.8)	3(11.5)	1(12.5)	1(12.5)
2	8(50)	4(15.4)	3(37.5)	3(37.5)
3	1(6.2)	5(19.2)	1(12.5)	0
Education Level Attained				
Completed some school	4(25.0)	7(26.9)	2(25.0)	2(25.0)
Completed school	1(6.2)	2(7.7)	2(25.0)	1(12.5)
TAFE [1], diploma, or trade	6(37.5)	5(19.2)	0	1(12.5)
Any completed tertiary study	5(31.3)	12(46.2)	4(50.0)	4(50.0)
Employment				
Full-time paid work	4(25.0)	3(11.5)	2(25.0)	2(25.0)
Part-time paid work	3(18.8)	4(15.4)	0	1(12.5)
Casual paid work	3(18.8)	2(7.7)	1(12.5)	0
Work without pay (family business)	1(6.2)	1(3.9)	1(12.5)	3(37.5)
Home duties	3(18.8)	7(26.9)	1(12.5)	0
Unemployed	0	2(7.7)	0	0
Studying	2(12.5)	1(3.9)	0	0
Studying + casual/part time work	*	*	3(37.5)	1(12.5)
Studying + house duties	*	*	1(12.5)	0
Carer	0	1(3.9)	0	0
Retired	0	5(19.2)	0	1(12.5)
Income source				
Salary	*	*	5(62.5)	4(50)
Salary and Government benefit	*	*	3(37.5)	2(25.0)
Savings and Superannuation	*	*	0	1(12.5)
Savings and Government benefit	*	*	0	1(12.5)
Main Transport				
Car/Motor Bike	14(87.5)	24(92.3)	6(75.0)	8(100.0)
Walking/Bike	2(12.5)	0	1(12.5)	0
Public Transport	0	2(7.7)	1(12.5)	0

* Not collected in the Food Security in Melbourne Households (FSiMH) survey. [1] TAFE, Technical and Further Education.

Twenty-four low-to-middle-income participants, FS ($n = 12$) and FIS ($n = 12$), consented in the FSiMH survey to be contacted to participate in the qualitative phase. Eight participants declined due to an illness, a work commitment, or no longer being interested in further participation. Sixteen in-depth interviews, FS ($n = 8$) and FIS ($n = 8$), were completed, 13 face-to-face and 3 by telephone. A key emphasis of qualitative research is the focus on the quality and not the quantity of interviews; so, sampling for the qualitative interviews in this study continued until theoretical data saturation was achieved. Theoretical data saturation in this study meant that the researcher was satisfied with the quality of the information that was obtained to be able to answer the research questions [54]. The majority of interview participants were female ($n = 15$), and nine were living in households with children. The most common housing tenure included mortgage holders ($n = 11$), and four participants were privately renting.

The severity of food insecurity experienced by the qualitative interview participants ($n = 16$) varied: marginal food security ($n = 4$, two with children), low food security ($n = 2$, one with children), and very low food security ($n = 2$, both with children).

3.2. Qualitative Results

The qualitative interview data analysis yielded 5 interacting themes and 10 subthemes. Table 2 summarises the key similarities and differences between and across the food-secure and food-insecure participants. The five main themes are presented below.

Table 2. Summary of theme and subtheme comparison between and across the food-secure and food-insecure participants.

Themes and Sub Themes	Both Food-Secure & Food-Insecure Participants	Food-Secure Participants	Food-Insecure Participants
	Theme 1: Food decisions are complex, dynamic, and multi-factorial		
Roles and values that shape food decisions	Food provision is a priority especially if children are present but money available for food challenges this.	Greater freedom for social eating but less likely to eat out with children due to cost.	Food is the priority but this is a challenge when the budget is pressured
	Food provides a connection to a community.		Stress related to social eating; budget manipulation required. Dilemmas created and potential ramifications.
Other forces that shape household food decisions	Nutrition/health priority: Quality and variety	Cognisant of food ethics: supermarket duopoly. Some households' greater financial capacity: able to respond	Budget tightrope: constant compromises to food choices
	Time available to cook and shop		
	Theme 2: Multiple protective assets: financial, social, physical, human, natural		
Strength in food literacy capabilities and resources	Food literacy skills/resourcefulness		Amplification of resourcefulness and food literacy skills. Budget assets are highly refined, creative, time-consuming, and may be unique to the household but are in a constant state of play at greater intensity.
	Budgeting skills and strategies are defined but have a differing intensity level across all households		
	Highly refined planning, food preparation, shopping assets	*	Food cost literacy: developed capabilities to monitor food costs; with product knowledge
	Knowledge of food alternatives: supporting modifications to food for the household.		
	Resourcefulness present and developed based on life experiences.		
Strength in social capital capabilities and resources	Connection to community/agencies that is required to know what broader financial resources are possible.		Connections to the broader community and social support from family and friends; these relationship assets support other assets or may facilitate them to action.
	Communities look out for each other		
	Relationships to support food literacy skills within and external to households: role models	*	Greater sense of resilience drawn from within based on personal experiences and at times less reliance on social relationships
	Growing food facilitates relationships with neighbours/community		

Table 2. *Cont.*

Themes and Sub Themes	Both Food-Secure & Food-Insecure Participants	Food-Secure Participants	Food-Insecure Participants
	Theme 3: Food insecurity triggers act alone or are cumulative and may be beyond household control		
Internal triggers	Time available to shop and cook can manifest in households in different ways	Episodic nature of triggers. Households may have experienced triggers in past life stages that increase the risk of food insecurity; these were recalled along with stress or anxiety. These triggers mirrored those described by food insecure (FIS) participants Financial resources may be available, but physical access is challenged e.g., moving to an area with limited public transport infrastructure/no car	Triggers/trigger risks are constantly in the background. Budget/financial/income triggers: shocks Cost of Living expenses and bill shocks: utilities and seasonal fluctuations. E.g., an increase in child care fees and unresponsive government support Changes to household composition: these may be short or long-term but consequential impacts are felt. E.g., addition of a child or family member (adult child/sibling) Change in relationship status: divorce Budget stress of trying to shop in bulk or shop for specials: trying to plan ahead.
External triggers	Perceived fluctuations in cost of food Physical access to food shops, availability beyond the Coles/Woolworths-type supermarkets, the preference for local shopping	*	Households may not have the financial resources to weather food cost changes, especially when this is added to other internal triggers.
	Theme 4: Assets amplified: juggling and applying management strategies as required		
Households transform	Assets are enacted in both households but at different levels (amplification effect)	Budget/shopping management assets are present, but are not or are rarely amplified to the extent of food insecure households.	Asset pooling and juggling across the households. Often, it is just the assets from the household gatekeeper wearing the stress and strain. Amplification of transformation of assets
assets into action			Assets used in all situations at home: day-to-day, entertaining at home, and eating out/purchase of takeaway food

Table 2. *Cont.*

Themes and Sub Themes	Both Food-Secure & Food-Insecure Participants	Food-Secure Participants	Food-Insecure Participants
Transform and adapt assets with external support	Both may receive financial support from Government benefits: Family Tax Benefit, Child Care Rebate, study assistance. Households attend community-based activities: gardens, farmers markets, or similar (food source, social) but often for a different purpose.	May have the social support assets but serve a different purpose than in FIS households. Not used as a food access means.	Households may require the assets that are transformed through social/financial support: community, family, or friends, and not through welfare/food relief agencies. Issues of inability to access, and pride; there are those who are in greater need. Households rely on grandparents to pay for activities, bring food, or 'shout' lunch in food court
Theme 5: The consequences and emotional rollercoaster of food access and provision			
Stress and strain matched with give and take	Attempts to protect children if food is scarce Frustrations in both households: cost of food, availability of food, marketing of food	Some food-secure households that have experienced food insecurity or have been at risk of food security in their lifetime reflected on the level of impact of the experience and the strain, and how this has shaped their desire to not experience this again: stress, embarrassment.	Often significant compromise on food quality, quantity, and nutrition: these are constantly amplified across households compared to food secure (FIS) households. Compromises may be limited to one person in the household: the food gatekeeper. Guilt associated with compromises, especially if other household members (children) are affected. The relentless, constant stresses of making ends meet: the load of this, the potential for allostatic load, and impacts on physical, social, and emotional wellbeing. This is amplified in these households. Social consequences: the compromise that is made to these opportunities and potential repercussions to self and household budgets.
4R's: Resilience, Respect, Resourceful, and Responsible	Pride/respect in strategies and skills that a household may possess, especially relating to food procurement, cooking, and sharing. Resilience/Respect/Resourcefulness Responsibility present in all households, but greater in FIS households	Present and in action, but the intensity may vary across and within households	Present in FIS households, but is greatest for the food/household gatekeeper: amplification effect

* No additional difference noted.

3.2.1. Theme 1: Food Decisions are Complex, Dynamic, and Multi-Factorial

Irrespective of food security status, food decisions were complex, often interconnected, dynamic, and multifactorial in nature, with an array of influencing factors. The role and values that were associated with food, and internal factors, such as food budgets, were impacting factors. External factors, such as cost of food and food availability, also contributed to the dynamic nature of food decisions.

Food was a priority, as described by a FS participant, Amelia, who had experienced food insecurity growing up and stated that she *'would go without anything to make sure that food was on the table'* for her children. For those experiencing, or were at risk of, food insecurity, there were additional, often constant, pressures on food decisions for the household, where the complexity and interaction of deciding factors were magnified.

Both participant groups identified food as a social conduit that provided a connection to a community. However, this was described with some preoccupation by FIS participants, who detailed a more stressed approach to eating out or entertaining that impacted on their enjoyment of the social interaction when compared to FS participants:

'I try to avoid it. Most I'll have is a coffee from uni … if they (Uni friends) buy lunch …. you miss out, but—there are times when I was really hungry and I didn't have my lunch, so I had to buy it. That would mean … , 'what am I going to do about that money when I shop on the weekend?' Ann (FIS)

In contrast, FS participants described food as a medium to socialise over, with a greater sense of 'freedom' that enables social situations. This in part was reported to be influenced by a greater available budget that provided flexibility, the participant's life stage, and the presence of children in the household.

Importance was placed on the quality and variety of nutritious foods. This value was often challenged for FIS participants, especially when the budget was tight, creating competing demands for the food dollar. Both groups of participants described a hierarchy of food decision drivers in which household bills were prioritised, impacting on the available food budget:

'meet my expenses first, and then what money I have left over is what I would do the shopping with. I think I've just stayed that way.' Maureen (FIS)

Time was an important resource in food decisions for all participants, particularly when the main food gatekeeper worked, studied, and/or cared for children. Shopping and food preparation tasks were often time-consuming and labour-intensive. These tasks required high levels of organisation, and often impacted on decisions that were associated with foods that were purchased for convenience (for example, the use of pre-prepared vegetables) and the question of where to shop (for example, a supermarket versus a mix of shops). FIS participants reported investing a large amount of time and energy in shopping routines. A trade-off and compromise was described:

'one of the biggest things that I think a lot of people have trouble with; is time … So it might be saving a little bit of money, but then it's costing time, and time is probably more expensive now than that' Ava (FS) and *'it's not easy to be able to spend money on whatever you want kind of thing, so I had to invest time to look around and shop around.'* Ann (FIS).

This highlights the difference in how each of the two participant types perceived time as a resource.

3.2.2. Theme 2: Multiple Protective Assets

The participants described an array of skills and strategies that were used to both protect and support food security. Food literacy and social connections were assets that could be enacted, especially in times of greater need. For FIS participants, assets (financial, human, social, physical, and natural) were of greater intensity, well-developed, and varied. All participants described these food literacy 'life skills' as invaluable, with their development varying over each participant's lifespan.

All participants described an array of financial management assets that were employed to manage food. The intensity of these skills was greatest for FIS participants. Some FS participants recalled life stages when fiscal resources were constrained. The management strategies that they used closely mirrored those that were used by FIS participants. FS participants described the importance of an overall budget to their household. However, how it was used varied significantly in FIS participants, where the budget was closely scrutinized, as Clara explains:

> 'depends on robbing Peter to pay Paul with the food budget ... it goes down to the last $10 by the end of the week... what level of food we get for the week' Clara (FIS)

Both FS and FIS participants described a range of practical strategies; for example, planning for and organisation of food to support money saving and to have pantry staples. Aspects of Theme 1 overlay this range of practical strategies.

Broader connections to community were evident across both FIS and FS participants, and were reported to be protective against food insecurity. An example is neighbours looking out for each other and sharing home grown produce. Social support that was provided by family and friends was evident. This was often in the form of general groceries and food, including meals.

3.2.3. Theme 3: Food Insecurity Triggers Act Alone or Are Cumulative and May Be beyond Household Control

The food insecurity 'triggers' were often unforeseen events or experiences that impacted on food security status and were either internal or external to the participant's household. Internal triggers included income changes, expected and unexpected expenses, and household composition changes. External triggers often reflected the broader system, economic situation, and food supply. All participants reported that these triggers acted alone or in unison, magnifying their effect on each other. Triggers, real or potential, were perceived to hover in the background of day-to-day life for FIS participants and were commonly reported. Triggers impacting on the household budget and/or total finances were points of stress and heightened the risk of food insecurity. However, participants from FS households, especially those with children, said that they were often still *'walking a budget tightrope'* Ava (FS). Those classified as food secure reported previous episodes where they had difficulties accessing food as a result of the reported food insecurity triggers. These experiences were detailed with evidence of anxiety and *'not wanting to go back there (being food insecure)'* Amelia (FS).

The financial triggers described by both FS and FIS participants were reported to manifest in a number of forms, from a sudden and unexpected reduction in household income or a change in household composition (birth of a child) to unexpected household expenses, including an increase living and medical expenses. These impacted on the financial stability and well-being of households, and influenced decisions on the question of whether the main caregiver should return to employment to relieve the financial load:

> 'No longer did we have additional income, bills kept coming plus the mortgage things were very tight.' Ann (FIS) and 'When my wife stopped working, we nearly went broke. We were down to our last dollar.' Eric (FS)

Two FS participants without a car identified difficulties in easily accessing food due to limited public transport infrastructure in their area despite adequate financial resources.

3.2.4. Theme 4: Assets Amplified: Juggling and Applying Management Strategies as Required

Whilst the assets described in Theme 2 were ever-present for all participants, it was not until one or more of the triggers (Theme 3) occurred that the assets were transformed and amplified into coping strategies. For FIS participants, there was a distinct difference in the rate and urgency of transformation of these assets. Often, these management strategies did not occur in isolation but in unison or in a staged format. This process of putting these assets into action could occur with or without support from the participant's immediate household.

Saving money was recognised as an important strategy for all participants. For FIS participants, this was invariably difficult; it meant that there was never a reserve or buffer to draw upon. In contrast, most FS participants had at least one option as a backup plan if finances were limited, including savings, credit cards, and loan redraws. This was a key point of difference when compared to FIS participants who did not have these options:

'There are times when we have had to redraw on our home loan to have more money to live off...
to buy food but sometimes the usual savings account may be down so we use Visa—that's how we
manage our money—then pay the card off at the end of the month so we never have to pay interest.'
Rowena (FS)

When finances were limited, alternative funding for shopping was enacted, including supermarket reward and loyalty schemes that allow cash/credit for shopping, by both FS and FIS participants:

'We have [Loyalty scheme name], quite often, it will be, 'Do I need to convert my [Loyalty] points to
[Loyalty] dollars, and can we go to [named Supermarket] and spend $10 getting what we need?' I
always leave that as my backup of the backup plan.' Clara (FIS)

Both participant types discussed how such strategies often meant spending more on food or other household items that impact on food budgets in the short term. However, the long-term benefit of credit towards future shopping outweighed this short-term risk.

3.2.5. Theme 5: The Consequences and Emotional Rollercoaster of Food Access and Provision

The consequences and emotions that were associated with food access and provision varied considerably. For FIS participants, the experience was often fraught with relentless emotional lows. The reported consequences of not being able to access food ranged from worry to compromises on food choices and amounts. Food-secure participants reflected on a significant past experience that was related to financial difficulties that impacted on food access and provision and instigated a range of emotions. Whilst stress and anxiety were evident for some FS participants, it was not to the extent described by FIS participants. However, the impact of these past experiences was significant enough for FS participants to reflect and articulate why they wanted things to be different:

'The juggle and stress to make ends meet was too much I deferred for a year, worked fulltime, earnt
money, then went back the following year and completed my degree. I don't want to go back to that
stress.' Lucy (FS)

Whilst the stress of food provision often dominated participants' stories, there were also elements of triumph that were centred on respect, resilience, responsibility, and resourcefulness.

For both FIS and FS participants, respect, resilience, and resourcefulness grew from difficult experiences during childhood and adolescence:

'I'm a ... stronger person because of my childhood: a person with a different upbringing may look at
things differently.' Clara (FIS) and

'It was really hard growing up and moving around all the time. Family is everything to me; it
means stability, and I'm the rock for the family now ... having them over for a meal helps this ... '
Amelia (FS)

These experiences often shaped their current food access and provision life skills.

4. Discussion

The purpose of this study was to identify low-to-middle income food secure and food insecure households from Melbourne and explore and compare food security and insecurity experiences and implications. The results highlight the precarious nature of achieving food security in lower-income groups and the resourcefulness, resilience, and array of assets or strengths that participants use when facing triggers that threaten their food security. Furthermore, they indicate that those who were categorised as food secure using the USDA-HFSSM may be at risk due to the existence of additional factors beyond those of a financial origin, such as a lack of physical access to, or a limited supply of, culturally appropriate foods. To our knowledge, this is the first study to explore the experience of food insecurity of low-to-middle income households in Australia.

4.1. Low-to-Middle Income Households' Experiences: Assets, Resourcefulness, Resilience, and Emotions

The food insecurity triggers that were described by both groups of participants, such as a change in income, increased cost of living expenses, and changes in household composition, are consistent with those reported for low-to-middle income households in Canada and the U.S. [34,36] and lower-income U.S. and Australian households [25,59,60]. The key differences between food-secure and food-insecure participants were the number and complexity of factors and the cumulative and relentless nature of the triggers.

The interviews allowed for the exploration of the range of assets possessed by both FS and FIS low-to middle income participants. At the core of these assets was food literacy and social connection, which supported both the capabilities and resources of the household. The existence of assets and skills inclusive of, but not limited to, budgeting and planning for food, and purchasing and preparing food, have been reported in food-insecure, lower-income households [52,61–63]. A key difference between FS and FIS participants in this study was the amplification of these assets and their ability to provide a crucial buffer to the food insecurity experience, but only up to a certain point. This is consistent with the limited capacity of food literacy skills to ameliorate the food insecurity experience because of the complex range of food insecurity determinants [64,65]. The range of assets was found to support the high degree of resourcefulness with food acquisition and (food and financial) management that was demonstrated by FS and FIS participants. The resourcefulness of individuals facing food insecurity has been reported previously, and should be considered in approaches to prevent or address food insecurity [63,64].

The asset of support was important to both FS and FIS participants. Social support in the food security literature has been described in the contexts of emotional, instrumental (child care, food, or material items), and informational support (advice and factual information) [66]. Consistent with this literature, the social support that is reported in this study was described as arising from two sources: (1) networks of family and friends, and (2) networks in the broader environment, such as community agencies and government benefits systems. Both FS and FIS participants described sourcing support predominately from friends and family and limited interaction with community welfare. This was driven by the potential shame and stigma, and confirms that reported in some low-income groups [63].

The associated emotions and experiences of trying to achieve or maintain food security were evident in both participant groups. Despite previous and current food insecurity experiences, its impacts were felt both psychologically and physically. Participants detailed the stress, shame, embarrassment, and concern due to the stigma of not being able to pay for food and/or feed children. The emotional experiences of these low-to-middle income participants are consistent with those reported principally by women in Australian and Canadian low-income, food-insecure households [9,25,63]. Often, counteracting these emotions was the high degree of resilience present in many participants. Resilience is a dynamic concept influenced by life-course events, and has been believed to contain two key elements: adversity and positive adaptation [67,68]. The level of resilience evident in both FS and FIS participants was shaped through life experiences that were often adverse in nature [69].

4.2. Categorisation of Food Security and Examining Etiology

The USDA HFSSM classification of food insecurity is based on a lack of money available to purchase food, and the interviews confirmed that financial factors/stressors were the main food insecurity trigger in the participant groups. While this finding supports the association with financial factors that has been described in the literature, it is important to reflect upon this trigger more broadly in the context of both financial constraints and assets [52,70]. The finding provides a rationale for examining the financial causes of food insecurity beyond household annual income, which is a static, insensitive measure and may not reflect sudden household economic changes that can temporarily lead to bouts of food insecurity [28,71]. Of note is that all low-to-middle income participants' main income sources were from salaries alone, in some cases supplemented with Government assistance payments, such as the Family Tax Benefit. This is supported by previous studies that found that those who are employed also experience food insecurity [24,50,72,73]. Employment status, in particular having multiple part-time jobs rather than full-time work, has been associated with an increased risk of food insecurity [73]. Additionally, having more than one income earner in a household has been shown to reduce the odds of experiencing food insecurity [72]. In this study, 12 of the 16 interviewed participants indicated that the primary income earner in the household was employed at a full-time or near full-time level. Furthermore, in seven of these households, another member was employed full-time, part-time, or casually.

The participants discussed the need for sufficient income or financial resources to meet the rising cost of living expenses. The capacity to have savings available when needed was described by both FS and FIS participants as a crucial strategy to buffer against the impact of unexpected expenses, but one that some FIS participants described as being difficult to implement. The evidence for savings as a protective factor against food insecurity is recognised both internationally [74] and nationally [22,75]. Australian evidence on the association between the capacity to save and food insecurity is limited. Foley (2010) reported that those Australians who were unable to save were 6.5 times more likely to have experienced food insecurity in the last 12 months [75].

This research highlights two points related to food security status classification that warrant further consideration.

4.2.1. Marginal Food Security Severity Categorisation

This study modified the food security classification from that of the original USDA-HFSSM protocol, where one or two affirmative responses were classified as food insecure at the severity level of marginally food secure, and allowed for exploration of their experience [10,14,24]. Understanding the marginally food secure experience has importance from epidemiological, public health, and public policy perspectives [14]. The decision to categorise those participants that were experiencing marginal food security as food insecure was supported by the findings, particularly by those stories that portrayed the experience of anxiety and stress regarding food provision. Despite two FIS participants being classified as marginally food insecure, their stories revealed a history of more severe forms of food insecurity over their lifetime and described rapid transitions between severity levels. As suggested by Loopstra (2013), those experiencing marginal food security may experience poorer health outcomes and increased forms of material hardship when compared to food-secure individuals [50].

4.2.2. Classification of Food Security Status beyond Financial Resource Constraints

Whilst financial resource challenges may be the primary determinant of food security status, there may be circumstances where other determinants beyond this are challenged. The USDA-HFSSM is based on economic access to food; it does not take into consideration other reasons for the existence of food insecurity. A recent systematic literature review indicated that there is an absence of multi-item tools that can assess food security beyond the one dimension of financial access [47]. Both FS and FIS participants described additional experiences beyond those of financial resources that challenged their food security status and constituted limitations in their physical access to a food supply. For FS participants, this was despite having adequate financial resources. One FS participant described her recent move from interstate to an area that had poor public transport infrastructure, and, as she did not have a car, this resulted in a limited capacity to source culturally relevant foods. Despite being able to access some food in a small but more expensive food outlet, her food choices were compromised. A lack of access to a car has been associated with an increased difficulty of accessing food outlets [19,76]. This experience highlights the importance of all dimensions of food security, including an adequate supply, physical and economic access, and the resources to utilise food, to achieve and maintain food security [1], and supports the need for a food security measurement tool that is inclusive of these dimensions. Such a measurement tool, the Household Food and Nutrition Security Survey (HFNSS), which is based on the USDA-HFSSM, has been developed and undergone preliminary validation in Australia [77,78].

4.3. Strengths, Limitations, and Further Research

This study is the first Australian study to examine the existence and experience of FS and FIS in low-to-middle income Australian households. Additionally, the focus of the research in the qualitative phase provides an important contribution to the literature, particularly in Australia, as it provides the first exploration of the experience of food insecurity within this income group. The mixed-methods approach allowed for detailed exploration of the experiences of food insecurity and food security. The methodology supported the understanding of the construct and experience of food insecurity in this income group more than a quantitative or qualitative methodology alone. The constant comparison approach to the analysis supported the interpretation of the findings. An additional strength was the case selection method for the interviews, which supported the transferability of the qualitative findings. Selecting participants from those that had participated in the quantitative survey allowed for further interpretation of the findings when supported by the stories of participants.

A potential limitation is the gender-biased nature of the recruitment. This resulted from the main food provider completing the survey, which resulted in a higher number of women participants (88%). Fifteen women and one male were interviewed, which potentially may impact on the credibility and dependability of the interview data. The inclusion of only one male voice provided a narrow view of how men may perceive food insecurity. However, this response rate is reflective of gender food provision roles, where women predominantly have the responsibility of being the principal food provider [79], which may subsequently affect how they report these experiences. While a theoretical gender lens was not applied in this study, the findings on the physical, social, and emotional food insecurity experiences of women have been previously described in food-insecure households [80].

Further exploration of the experiences of, and the role of the extensive range of assets in, these low-to-middle income participants can better inform responses to food insecurity. In addition, more research is needed to explore the experience of food insecurity in different contexts, including: geographic locations of rural and metropolitan areas of Australia, sub-population groups, and both lower- and higher-income groups. This should include the exploration of determinants inclusive of a range of financial indicators, such as capacity to save, but also additional determinants of food insecurity. The use of mixed methods in future research efforts is crucial to provide a more detailed and rich understanding of the true and precarious nature of this phenomenon.

5. Conclusions

This study reveals novel and important findings on the existence of food insecurity amongst low-to-middle income Melbourne households, an income group that would not necessarily be considered food insecure within the context of a high-income country. Additionally, these findings support the precarious nature and balancing act of achieving food security for some low-to-middle income households. The experiences of those classified as marginally food secure confirm the need for further research within this severity-level group regardless of income.

While limited financial resources are a primary determinant of food security status, this research confirmed that there are multiple additional determinants that must be considered to maintain food security.. The results revealed the constant balancing act, especially of a range of financial, social, physical, and personal assets, that must be undertaken to prevent or alleviate the experiences of food insecurity. The findings of this work may be used to support policies and practices to prevent or alleviate food insecurity in low-to-middle income groups in urban Australia.

Supplementary Materials: The following are available online at http://www.mdpi.com/1660-4601/15/10/2206/s1, Table S1: Quantitative United States Department of Agriculture Food Security Survey Module (18 items) and Qualitative Question Logic.

Author Contributions: Conceptualization, S.K., S.B., Z.E.D., and C.P.; Methodology, S.K., S.B., Z.E.D., and C.P.; Software, S.K.; Formal Analysis, S.K.; Investigation, S.K.; Data Curation, S.K.; Writing (Original Draft Manuscript Preparation), S.K.; Writing (Review & Editing), all authors.

Funding: This research received no external funding.

Acknowledgments: The authors thank the Department of Nutrition, Dietetics, and Food vacation scholarship students Emma Chappell and Tracey Nau for their support in identifying community agencies in VAMPIRE suburbs. The authors also thank Steph Ashby, dietitian and honours student, for her assistance with the implementation of the 'Food Security in Melbourne Households' survey.

Conflicts of Interest: The authors declare no conflict of interest.

References

1. Food and Agriculture Organization. An Introduction to the Basic Concepts of Food Security. Available online: www.fao.org/docrep/013/al936e/al936e00.pdf (accessed on 2 August 2018).

2. Australian Bureau of Statistics. Australian Health Survey: Nutrition State and Territory Results 2011–2012 Cat No. 4364.0.55.009. Available online: http://www.abs.gov.au/AUSSTATS/abs@.nsf/DetailsPage/4364.0.55.0092011-12?OpenDocument (accessed on 10 August 2018).

3. Carter, K.N.; Lanumata, T.; Kruse, K.; Gorton, D. What are the determinants of food insecurity in New Zealand and does this differ for males and females? *Aust. N. Z. J. Public Health* **2010**, *34*, 602–608. [CrossRef] [PubMed]

4. Tarasuk, V.; Mitchell, A.; Dachner, N. Household Food Insecurity in Canada, 2012. Available online: http://nutritionalsciences.lamp.utoronto.ca/Research (accessed on 19 August 2018).

5. Bates, B.; Roberts, C.; Lepps, H.; Porter, L. *The Food and Your Survey Wave 4. Combined Report for England, Wales and Northern Ireland*; Food Standards Agency: London, UK, 2017; pp. 26–29.

6. United States Department of Agriculture. Food Security Status of U.S. Households in 2014. Available online: http://www.ers.usda.gov/topics/food-nutrition-assistance/food-security-in-the-us.aspx (accessed on 1 September 2018).

7. Bickel, G.; Nord, M.; Price, C.; Hamilton, W.; Cook, J. *Guide to Measuring Household Food Security, Revised 2000*; U.S. Department of Agriculture: Alexandria, VA, USA, 2013; pp. 1–75.

8. Radimer, K.L.; Olson, C.M.; Campbell, C.C. Development of Indicators to Assess Hunger. *J. Nutr.* **1990**, *120*, 1544–1548. [CrossRef] [PubMed]

9. Hamelin, A.-M.; Beaudry, M.; Habicht, J.-P. Characterization of household food insecurity in Québec: Food and feelings. *Soc. Sci. Med.* **2002**, *54*, 119–132. [CrossRef]

10. Coleman-Jensen, A.U.S. Food Insecurity Status: Toward a Refined Definition. *Soc. Indic. Res.* **2010**, *95*, 215–230. [CrossRef]

11. Radimer, K.L. Measurement of household food security in the USA and other industrialised countries. *Public Health Nutr.* **2002**, *5*, 859–864. [CrossRef] [PubMed]

12. Vozoris, N.T.; Tarasuk, V.S. Household food insufficiency is associated with poorer health. *J. Nutr.* **2003**, *133*, 120–126. [CrossRef] [PubMed]

13. Stuff, J.E.; Casey, P.H.; Szeto, K.L.; Gossett, J.M.; Robbins, J.M.; Simpson, P.M.; Connell, C.; Bogle, M.L. Household food insecurity is associated with adult health status. *J. Nutr.* **2004**, *134*, 2330–2335. [CrossRef] [PubMed]

14. Cook, J.T.; Black, M.; Chilton, M.; Cutts, D.; Ettinger de Cuba, S.; Heeren, T.C.; Rose-Jacobs, R.; Sandel, M.; Casey, P.H.; Coleman, S.; et al. Are food insecurity's health impacts underestimated in the U.S. population? Marginal food security also predicts adverse health outcomes in young U.S. children and mothers. *Adv. Nutr.* **2013**, *4*, 51–61. [CrossRef] [PubMed]

15. Tarasuk, V.; Cheng, J.; de Oliveira, C.; Dachner, N.; Gundersen, C.; Kurdyak, P. Association between household food insecurity and annual health care costs. *Can. Med. Assoc. J.* **2015**, *187*, E429–E436. [CrossRef] [PubMed]

16. Adams, D.; Galvin, L. *Institutional Capability. Food Security and Local Government in Tasmania*; Heart Foundation: Tasmania, Australia, 2015; pp. 1–29.

17. Winicki, J.; Jemison, K. Food insecurity and hunger in the kindergarten classroom: Its effect on learning and growth. *Contemp. Econ. Policy* **2003**, *21*, 145–157. [CrossRef]

18. Bartfeld, J.; Dunifon, R. State-level predictors of food insecurity among households with children. *J. Policy Anal. Manag.* **2006**, *25*, 921–942. [CrossRef]

19. Gorton, D.; Bullen, C.R.; Mhurchu, C.N. Environmental influences on food security in high-income countries. *Nutr. Rev.* **2010**, *68*, 1–29. [CrossRef] [PubMed]

20. Chilton, M.M.; Rabinowich, J.R.; Woolf, N.H. Very low food security in the USA is linked with exposure to violence. *Public Health Nutr.* **2014**, *17*, 73–82. [CrossRef] [PubMed]

21. McIntyre, L.; Wu, X.; Fleisch, V.C.; Emery, H.J.C. Homeowner versus non-homeowner differences in household food insecurity in Canada. *J. Hous. Built Environ.* **2016**, *31*, 349–366. [CrossRef]

22. Nolan, M.; Williams, M.; Rikard-Bell, G.; Mohsin, M. Food insecurity in three socially disadvantaged localities in Sydney, Australia. *Health Promot. J. Aust.* **2006**, *17*, 247–254. [CrossRef]

23. Kirkpatrick, S.I.; Tarasuk, V. Assessing the relevance of neighbourhood characteristics to the household food security of low-income Toronto families. *Public Health Nutr.* **2010**, *13*, 1139–1148. [CrossRef] [PubMed]

24. Gunderson, C.; Kreider, B.; Pepper, J. The economics of food insecurity in the United States. *AEPP* **2011**, *33*, 281–303. [CrossRef]

25. King, S.; Moffitt, A.; Bellamy, J.; Carter, S.; McDowell, C.; Mollenhauser, J. *When There's Not Enough to Eat. A National Study of Food Insecurity among Emergency Relief Clients*; Anglicare, Diocese of Sydney: Sydney, Australia, 2012; pp. 1–138.

26. Ramsey, R.; Giskes, K.; Turrell, G.; Gallegos, D. Food insecurity among adults residing in disadvantaged urban areas: Potential health and dietary consequences. *Public Health Nutr.* **2012**, *15*, 227–237. [CrossRef] [PubMed]

27. Langellier, B.A.; Chaparro, M.P.; Sharp, M.; Birnbach, K.; Brown, E.R.; Harrison, G.G. Trends and Determinants of Food Insecurity among Adults in Low-Income Households in California. *J. Hunger Environ. Nutr.* **2012**, *7*, 401–413. [CrossRef]

28. Rose, D. Economic determinants and dietary consequences of food insecurity in the United States. *J. Nutr.* **1999**, *129* (Suppl. 2), S517–S520. [CrossRef] [PubMed]

29. Tarasuk, V. Household food insecurity in Canada. *Top. Clin. Nutr.* **2005**, *20*, 299–312. [CrossRef]

30. Guo, B. Household Assets and Food Security: Evidence from the Survey of Program Dynamics. *J. Fam. Econ. Issues* **2011**, *32*, 98–110. [CrossRef]

31. Martin-Fernandez, J.; Grillo, F.; Parizot, I.; Caillavet, F.; Chauvin, P. Prevalence and socioeconomic and geographical inequalities of household food insecurity in the Paris region, France, 2010. *BMC Public Health* **2013**, *13*, 486. [CrossRef] [PubMed]

32. Kleve, S.; Davidson, Z.E.; Gearon, E.; Booth, S.; Palermo, C. Are low-to-middle-income households experiencing food insecurity in Victoria, Australia? An examination of the Victorian Population Health Survey, 2006–2009. *Aust. J. Prim. Health* **2017**, *23*, 249–256. [CrossRef] [PubMed]

33. Tarasuk, V.; Vogt, J. Household food insecurity in Ontario. *Can. J. Public Health* **2009**, *100*, 184–188. [PubMed]

34. Olabiyi, O.M.; McIntyre, L. Determinants of Food Insecurity in Higher-Income Households in Canada. *J. Hunger Environ. Nutr.* **2014**, *9*, 433–448. [CrossRef]

35. Nord, M. *Food Spending Declined and Food Insecurity Increased for Middle-Income and Low-Income Households from 2000 to 2007*; 61; United States Department of Agriculture: Washington, DC, USA, 2009; pp. 1–25.

36. Nord, M.; Brent, C. *Food Insecurity in Higher Income Households*; United States Department of Agriculture: Washington, DC, USA, 2002.

37. Huang, J.; Guo, B.; Kim, Y. Food insecurity and disability: Do economic resources matter? *Soc. Sci. Res.* **2010**, *39*, 111–124. [CrossRef]

38. Creswell, J.W.; Piano Clark, V.L. *Designing and Conducting Mixed Methods Research*, 2nd ed.; Sage Publications Inc.: Thousand Oaks, CA, USA, 2011; pp. 1–443.

39. Tashakkori, A.; Teddlie, C. *Handbook of Mixed Methods in Social & Behavioral Research*, 1st ed.; Sage Publciations: Thousand Oak, CA, USA, 2003; pp. 1–768.

40. Tashakkori, A.; Teddlie, C. *Handbook of Mixed Methods in Social & Behavioral Research*, 2nd ed.; Sage: Thousand Oak, CA, USA, 2010.

41. Morgan, D. Practical strategies for combining qualitatve and quantitative methods. Applications in health research. *Qual. Health Res.* **1998**, *8*, 362–376. [CrossRef] [PubMed]

42. Dodson, J.; Sipe, N. *Unsettling Suburbia the New Landscape of Oil and Mortgage Vulnerability in Australian Cities*; 17; Griffith University: Queensland, Australia, 2008; pp. 1–42.

43. Webber, C.B.; Rojhani, A. Rise In Gasoline Price Affects Food Buying Habits of Low-Income, Ethnically-Diverse Families Enrolled In Southwest Michigan WIC Program. *J. Nutr. Educ. Behav.* **2009**, *41* (Suppl. 4), S1. [CrossRef]

44. Rossimel, A.; Han, S.S.; Larsen, K.; Palermo, C. Access and affordability of nutritious food in metropolitan Melbourne. *Nutr. Diet.* **2016**, *73*, 13–18. [CrossRef]

45. Australian Bureau of Statistics. Household Income and Income Distribution Australia Detailed Tables Table 2011 Table 2012. Available online: www.abs.gov.au?AUSSTATS/abs@.nsf/DetailsPage/6523.02011-12?OpenDocument (accessed on 25 August 2018).

46. Victorian Department of Health. Victorian Population Health Survey 2008. Available online: www.health.vic.gov.au/healthstatus/vphs.htm (accessed on 3 February 2014).

47. Ashby, S.; Kleve, S.; McKechnie, R.; Palermo, C. Measurement of the dimensions of food insecurity in developed countries: A systematic literature review. *Public Health Nutr.* **2016**, *19*, 2887–2896. [CrossRef] [PubMed]

48. Ramsey, R.; Giskes, K.; Turrell, G.; Gallegos, D. Food insecurity among Australian children: Potential determinants, health and developmental consequences. *J. Child Health Care* **2011**, *15*, 401–416. [CrossRef] [PubMed]

49. Marques, E.S.; Reichenheim, M.E.; de Moraes, C.L.; Antunes, M.M.; Salles-Costa, R. Household food insecurity: A systematic review of the measuring instruments used in epidemiological studies. *Public Health Nutr.* **2015**, *18*, 877–892. [CrossRef] [PubMed]

50. Loopstra, R.; Tarasuk, V. What does increasing severity of food insecurity indicate for food insecure families? Relationships between severity of food insecurity and indicators of material hardship and constrained food purchasing. *J. Hunger Environ. Nutr.* **2013**, *8*, 337–349. [CrossRef]

51. Economic Research Service. Ranges of Food Security and Food Insecurity. USDA Labels Describe Range of Food Security. 2006. Available online: www.ers.usda.gov/topics/food-nutrition-assistance/food-security-in-the-us/definitions-of-food-security/#ranges (accessed on 1 September 2017).

52. Hamelin, A.-M.; Mercier, C.; Bédard, A. Discrepancies in households and other stakeholders viewpoints on the food security experience: A gap to address. *Health Educ. Res.* **2010**, *25*, 401–412. [CrossRef] [PubMed]

53. Hamelin, A.-M.; Mercier, C.; Bédard, A. Needs for food security from the standpoint of Canadian households participating and not participating in community food programmes. *Int. J. Consum. Stud.* **2011**, *35*, 58–68. [CrossRef]

54. Liamputtong, P. *Qualitative Research Methods*, 4th ed.; Oxford University Press: Melbourne, Australia, 2013; pp. 1–379.

55. Committee on World Food Security. *Coming to Terms with Terminology*; CFS 2012/39/4; Food and Agriculture Organisation: Rome, Italy, 2012; pp. 1–33.

56. Braun, V.; Clarke, V. Using thematic analysis in psychology. *Qual. Res. Psychol.* **2006**, *3*, 77–101. [CrossRef]

57. Boeije, H. A Purposeful Approach to the Constant Comparative Method in the Analysis of Qualitative Interviews. *Qual. Quant.* **2002**, *36*, 391–409. [CrossRef]

58. Liamputtong, P. *Research Methods in Health. Foundations for Evidence-Based Practice*, 2nd ed.; Oxford University Press: Melbourne, Australia, 2013.

59. De Marco, M.; Thorburn, S.; Kue, J. "In a Country as Affluent as America, People Should be Eating": Experiences With and Perceptions of Food Insecurity Among Rural and Urban Oregonians. *Qual. Health Res.* **2009**, *19*, 1010–1024. [CrossRef] [PubMed]

60. King, S.; Bellamy, J.; Kemp, B.; Mollenhauer, J. *Hard Choices. Going Without in a Time of Plenty a Study of Food Insecurity in NSW and the ACT*; Prepared on behalf of ANGLICARE Sydney, the Samaritans Foundation and Anglicare NSW South, NSW West & ACT; ANGLICARE Diocese of Sydney Social Policy & Research Unit: Parramatta, Australia, 2013.

61. Loopstra, R.; Tarasuk, V. Perspectives on community gardens, community kitchens and the good food box program in a community-based sample of low-income families. *Can. J. Public Health* **2013**, *104*, e55–e59. [PubMed]

62. Tarasuk, V. A Critical Examination of Community-Based Responses to Household Food Insecurity in Canada. *Health Educ. Behav.* **2001**, *28*, 487–499. [CrossRef] [PubMed]

63. Buck-McFadyen, E. Rural food insecurity: When cooking skills, homegrown food, and perseverance aren't enough to feed a family. *Can. J. Public Health* **2015**, *106*, 140–146. [CrossRef] [PubMed]

64. Gallegos, D. The nexus between food literacy. Food security and disadvantage. In *Food Literacy: Key Concepts for Health and Education*, 1st ed.; Vidgen, H., Ed.; Routledge: London, UK, 2016; pp. 134–150.

65. Collins, P.A.; Power, E.M.; Little, M.H. Municipal-level responses to household food insecurity in Canada: A call for critical, evaluative research. *Can. J. Public Health* **2014**, *105*, e138–e141. [CrossRef] [PubMed]

66. Davis, B.L.; Grutzmacher, S.K.; Munger, A.L. Utilization of Social Support among Food Insecure Individuals: A Qualitative Examination of Network Strategies and Appraisals. *J. Hunger Environ. Nutr.* **2016**, *11*, 162–179. [CrossRef]

67. Fletcher, D.; Sarkar, M. Psychological Resilience: A Review and Critique of Definitions, Concepts, and Theory. *Eur. Psychol.* **2013**, *18*, 12–23. [CrossRef]

68. Rutter, M. Resilience as a dynamic concept. *Dev. Psychopathol.* **2012**, *24*, 335–344. [CrossRef] [PubMed]

69. Younginer, N.A.; Blake, C.E.; Draper, C.L.; Jones, S.J. Resilience and Hope: Identifying Trajectories and Contexts of Household Food Insecurity. *J. Hunger Environ. Nutr.* **2015**, *10*, 230–258. [CrossRef]

70. Coleman-Jensen, A.; Gregory, C.; Singh, A. *Household Food Security in the United States in 2013*; United States Department of Agriculture, Economic Research Service: Washington, DC, USA, 2014.

71. Chang, Y.; Chatterjee, S.; Kim, J. Household Finance and Food Insecurity. *J. Fam. Econ. Issues* **2014**, *35*, 499–515. [CrossRef]

72. McIntyre, L.; Bartoo, A.C.; Emery, J.H. When working is not enough: Food insecurity in the Canadian labour force. *Public Health Nutr.* **2012**, *17*, 49–57. [CrossRef] [PubMed]

73. Coleman-Jensen, A.J. Working for Peanuts: Nonstandard Work and Food Insecurity across Household Structure. *J. Fam. Econ. Issues* **2011**, *32*, 84–97. [CrossRef]

74. Olson, C.M.; Rauschenbach, B.S.; Frongillo, E.A., Jr.; Kendall, A. Factors contributing to household food insecurity in a rural upstate New York county. *Fam. Econ. Nutr. Rev.* **1997**, *10*, 2–17.

75. Foley, W.; Ward, P.; Carter, P.; Coveney, J.; Tsourtos, G.; Taylor, A. An ecological analysis of factors associated with food insecurity in South Australia, 2002–2007. *Public Health Nutr.* **2010**, *13*, 215–221. [CrossRef] [PubMed]

76. Burns, C.; Bentley, R.; Thornton, L.; Kavanagh, A. Reduced food access due to a lack of money, inability to lift and lack of access to a car for food shopping: A multilevel study in Melbourne, Victoria. *Public Health Nutr.* **2011**, *14*, 1017–1023. [CrossRef] [PubMed]

77. Archer, C.; Gallegos, D.; McKechnie, R. Developing measures of food and nutrition security within an Australian context. *Public Health Nutr.* **2017**, *20*, 2513–2522. [CrossRef] [PubMed]

78. Kleve, S.; Gallegos, D.; Ashby, S.; Palermo, C.E.; McKechnie, R. Preliminary validation and piloting of a comprehensive measure of household food security in Australia. *Public Health Nutr.* **2018**, *21*, 526–534. [CrossRef] [PubMed]

79. DeVault, M.L. *Feeding the Family: The Social Organization of Caring as Gendered Work*; University of Chicago Press: Chicago, IL, USA, 1991.

80. Matheson, J.; McIntyre, L. Women respondents report higher household food insecurity than do men in similar Canadian households. *Public Health Nutr.* **2014**, *17*, 40–48. [CrossRef] [PubMed]

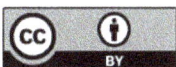

International Journal of
*Environmental Research
and Public Health*

MDPI

Article

Using Cross-Sectional Data to Identify and Quantify the Relative Importance of Factors Associated with and Leading to Food Insecurity

Alison Daly [1,*], Christina M. Pollard [1], Deborah A. Kerr [1], Colin W. Binns [1], Martin Caraher [2] and Michael Phillips [3]

1   Faculty of Health Science, School of Public Health, Curtin University, GPO Box U1987, Perth 6845, Western Australia, Australia; C.Pollard@curtin.edu.au (C.M.P.); D.Kerr@curtin.edu.au (D.A.K.); C.Binns@curtin.edu.au (C.W.B.)
2   Centre for Food Policy, City University of London, Northampton Square, London EC1V 0HB, UK; m.caraher@city.ac.uk
3   Harry Perkins Institute for Medical Research, University of Western Australia, Perth 6009, Western Australia, Australia; michael.phillips@perkins.uwa.edu.au
*   Correspondence: alison.daly@curtin.edu.au; Tel.: +61-8-9266-9266

Received: 10 August 2018; Accepted: 16 November 2018; Published: 22 November 2018

Abstract: Australian governments routinely monitor population household food insecurity (FI) using a single measure—'running out of food at least once in the previous year'. To better inform public health planning, a synthesis of the determinants and how they influence and modify each other in relation to FI was conducted. The analysis used data from the Health & Wellbeing Surveillance System cross-sectional dataset. Weighted means and multivariable weighted logistic regression described and modelled factors involved in FI. The analysis showed the direction and strength of the factors and a path diagram was constructed to illustrate these. The results showed that perceived income, independent of actual income was a strong mediator on the path to FI as were obesity, smoking and other indicators of health status. Eating out three or more times a week and eating no vegetables more strongly followed FI than preceded it. The analysis identified a range of factors and demonstrated the complex and interactive nature of them. Further analysis using propensity score weighted methods to control for covariates identified hypothetical causal links for investigation. These results can be used as a proof of concept to assist public health planning.

Keywords: food insecurity; monitoring; surveillance; determinants; path diagram

1. Introduction

Food security exists "when all people, at all times, have physical, social and economic access to sufficient safe and nutritious food that meets their dietary needs and food preferences for an active and healthy life" [1]. Conversely, food insecurity (FI) is the "limited or uncertain availability of nutritionally adequate and safe foods or the limited or uncertain ability to acquire acceptable food in socially acceptable ways" [2], and is increasing in developed countries [3]. FI is adversely related to diet quality [4–10] and has been associated with the double burden of malnutrition, including undernourishment and obesity [11–13] and additionally it has been associated with poor mental health and socioeconomic disadvantages [14–20].

The complexity and impact of FI has been acknowledged and there is an growing amount of attention being directed to its determinants and how they influence and modify each other, calling for a systemic food system response [21]. FI is a problem of social and economic disadvantage, of which 'running out of food' due to insufficient money is only one component [22]. The complex nature of decisions about food is constrained by both physical access and choice [23], underpinned by the Food and Agricultural Organization's four pillars of availability: Access, utilization, stability and sustainability [24–26]. There is growing consensus regarding the need to focus on and better integrate social and structural factors when developing policies and interventions to improve public health in high income countries [27,28]. Evidence that is accessible to policy makers in the increasingly interrelated and complicated health policy area requires new approaches to research types and analyses [29].

The prevalence of FI in Australia, based on a 2001 review of the literature, showed that the rates were higher among the following groups: Families living with low or unstable incomes, those in remote areas, Aboriginal and Torres Strait Islander people, the unemployed, those living in rental households, single parents, those who were never married, separated or divorced, young adults and the elderly, asylum seekers and migrants, and people with disabilities [30]. FI directly impacts short and long-term health status, contributing to poor physical and psychological health outcomes and Australian health care costs [30]. The paradoxical relationship between FI and obesity has also been demonstrated, also significantly contributing to increasing health care costs [31–34].

Governments are increasingly encouraged to monitor FI, its determinants, mitigating actions, and their effectiveness [35]. Some countries, including Australia, do measure and report the prevalence of FI, including its severity and/or its determinants [36–39], but not routinely. While FI measures are continuously being evaluated and validated to come up with more accurate estimates of FI, the evaluation of the measures generally only contain limited references to determinants [5,40–42]. The severity of FI's effects, as well as its determinants and associated factors are important information used to inform public health planning. Currently there is little recognition among health or social services policy makers regarding the extent of the problem among some population sub-groups, nor the impact of sociodemographic determinants.

This study uses a cross-sectional self-reported dataset (the Western Australian Department of Health's *Health & Wellbeing Surveillance System* 2009–2013, *(HWSS))* to construct a path diagram of variables leading to 'running out of food' at least once in the previous year because of insufficient money. The analysis evaluates the relative importance of variables associated with FI. Specifically, the study aims to: Conduct an analysis to evaluate the relative importance of a range of associated variables with FI; use the results of the analysis to construct a path diagram to FI; propose hypothetical causal paths to and from FI; and suggest how future research and policy can be developed more effectively.

2. Materials and Methods

2.1. Sample and Measures

The HWSS cross-sectional computer-assisted telephone interview survey has measured health and wellbeing indicators (including risk factors) since 2002. Stratified samples by area were drawn from the statewide telephone book *Electronic White Pages* with geocoded addresses. The average participation rate was 90.2%. The 2009 to 2013 dataset, with a total of 21,710 adults aged 18–64 years was analysed. Data were pooled and weighted for probability of selection using iterative proportional fitting with marginal totals for the distribution of Western Australia (WA) residents in 2011 by age, sex and geographic area. The Department of Health in Western Australia datasets are not publicly available. The HWSS was granted ethics approval from the Western Australia Department of Human Research Ethics Committee (HREC 2011/65).

The sociodemographic variables used in this study were: Age, gender, highest level of education attained, living arrangements, area of residence, annual household income (AUD$), perceived discretional income, country of birth employment status and the geographic area based index that reflects socioeconomic advantage and disadvantage (SEIFA) [43]. Self-reported body weight and height, using a correction for over-reported height and under-reported weight [44], was used to estimate the Body Mass Index (BMI) of each respondent. Health-related variables included the self-assessment of: General health, comparison of health with a year prior, psychological distress (using the Kessler 10 index) [45], health risk factors and whether or not the respondent had these variables diagnosed by a doctor. The indicators of self-reported dietary behaviour included daily fruit, vegetable, and low-fat milk intake, as well as weekly take-away food consumption.

2.2. Analysis

The strategy adopted for this analysis was to develop a path diagram to describe a hypothetical model for the network of associations that describe running out of food and its consequences. This method has been used previously [46]. Usually this approach would use a structural equation model (SEM) but the outcome (running out of food or not) was dichotomous, meaning that SEM could not be used. Logistic regression analyses were conducted with a reference group of respondents who did not run out of food. The variables listed in Table 1 were statistically significant at $p \leq 0.1$ and were entered into weighted multivariable logistic regression analyses. While some variables were collected as continuous (e.g., age, K10, fruit, vegetables and physical activity estimates) values, we grouped them based upon accepted guidelines for Australian adults where possible. This was done to avoid assumptions of linearity. Both two way and three way interaction terms between the variables were tested on the final multivariable regression models. Bootstrapping (100 repetitions) produced final model estimates with robust measures used to estimate standard errors for the regression analyses. Results at $p < 0.05$ were considered to be statistically significant and kept in the model. Goodness of fit was assessed using the Hosmer–Lemeshow test. Diagnostic post-estimation tests, including tests for multicollinearity were conducted. The regression results were used to conduct a path diagram where the Bayesian Information Criteria (BIC) [47] was used to determine whether or not an association preceded or came after 'running out of food'. The ordering with the lowest BIC was used to determine the direction of the association. A difference in BIC of 10 or more (considered a very strong indicator) was the minimum value when deciding upon direction of effect. This corresponded to a p value of <0.0004 [48]. The multivariable model was modified to incorporate this information and the path diagram was constructed to reflect the results of the final model. Propensity scores were used to control for potential confounding from the covariates in iterative propensity score weighted logistic regression analyses for four variables. The four variables tested were income, discretional income, eating fast food three or more times a week and eating no vegetables. These four independent variables were operationally defined as variables in the path leading to the outcome of either 'running out of food' or not [49]. Each of these variables were tested for hypothetical causality. All analysis was conducted using Stata 13.1 [50].

3. Results

A total of 709 respondents reported 'running out of food' at least once in the previous twelve months and couldn't afford more (unweighted prevalence = 3.3%; weighted prevalence = 4.0%). The prevalence of variables associated with running out of food at $p < 0.1$ are shown in Table 1. The table presents both the unweighted and weighted prevalences with 95% confidence limits and p values for 'running out of food'. A total of 17,682 correspondents had information for all the variables on Table 1 and this was the sample used to run the multivariable weighted logistic regressions.

Table 2 presents the primary multivariable weighted logistic regression that was used as a basis to create the path analysis. The odds ratios for interaction terms that are presented in the path are estimates based on the results of the regression which either attenuates the effect or enhances the effect. This model showed good fit with the data ($\chi^2 = 11.02$, $p = 0.27$) and was used as the basis of the path diagram.

Table 1. The unweighted and weighted prevalences of 'running out of food' by sample characteristics, HWSS 2009–2013 (n = 21,705 [a]).

Demographic Variables	Unwght %	Wght %	95% CI	p
18–24	7.8	8.0	[6.5, 9.9]	
25–34	5.1	4.9	[3.8, 6.2]	
35–44	3.6	3.2	[2.6, 4.0]	
45–54	2.8	2.4	[1.9, 2.9]	
55–64	2.0	1.6	[1.3, 2.0]	<0.0001
Tertiary education	1.4	1.9	[1.3, 2.6]	
Less than tertiary education	3.8	4.7	[4.1, 5.3]	<0.0001
Employed	2.2	2.9	[2.5, 3.4]	
Unemployed	11.4	12.6	[9.0, 17.7]	
Home duties	4.3	5.2	[4.0, 6.7]	
Retired	2.3	2.0	[1.3, 3.0]	
Student	7.5	7.1	[4.8, 10.3]	
Unable to work	17.3	17.6	[13.2, 23.0]	<0.0001
Annual household income: over AUD $40,000	1.7	2.4	[2.0, 2.9]	
Annual household income: AUD $20,001–$40,000	7.0	9.6	[7.6, 12.2]	
Annual household income: up to AUD $20,000	15.0	17.8	[14.2, 22.2]	<0.0001
Spend left over money or save some per pay	1.1	1.7	[1.4, 2.0]	
Just enough money to get by per pay	10.6	12.5	[10.7, 14.5]	
Not enough money to get by per pay	17.5	19.0	[15.1, 23.6]	<0.0001
Not aboriginal	3.1	3.8	[3.4, 4.2]	
Aboriginal	12.5	15.0	[9.8, 22.1]	<0.0001
Adults living with others	2.8	3.7	[3.3, 4.2]	
Adults living alone	6.0	6.4	[5.2, 7.8]	<0.0001
Born outside Australia	2.8	2.9	[2.3, 3.7]	
Born in Australia	3.5	4.4	[3.9, 5.0]	0.002
Rents or pays mortgage	4.1	4.6	[4.3, 5.0]	
No mortgage or Government subsidized housing	2.5	3.1	[2.7, 3.4]	0.0003
SEIFA [b] Quintile 5 (least disadvantaged area)	2.4	2.9	[2.3, 3.6]	
SEIFA Quintiles 3,4 (less disadvantaged areas)	3.4	4.5	[3.9, 5.3]	
SEIFA Quintiles 1,2 (most disadvantages areas)	4.0	5.2	[4.2, 6.4]	<0.0001
Has a health care card	10.3	11.3	[9.7, 13.2]	<0.0001
Doesn't have private health insurance	7.0	8.3	[7.2, 9.6]	<0.0001
Has asthma	5.7	6.3	[4.7, 8.4]	0.0011
Some cardiovascular condition	5.8	7.4	[4.9, 11.0]	0.0022
Has cancer	4.5	7.0	[4.3, 11.3]	0.0167
Current mental health (depression/anxiety/other)	9.1	9.7	[8.3, 11.4]	<0.0001
Health rated as fair/poor	8.8	8.9	[7.2, 11.0]	<0.0001
Always or often feel a lack of control over health	12.8	13.9	[11.0, 17.3]	<0.0001
Health rated worse than 12 months ago	7.3	9.4	[7.6, 11.6]	<0.0001
High/very high Kessler 10 score	14.1	14.8	[12.4, 17.6]	<0.0001
BMI 30 or more (in obese range)	4.3	5.2	[4.4, 6.1]	<0.0012
Currently smoking	7.1	8.5	[7.0, 10.3]	<0.0001
Does no leisure time physical activity	4.4	5.5	[4.0, 7.5]	0.0447
Spends four or more hours sitting in leisure time	6.4	7.6	[5.8, 9.8]	<0.0001
Eats 'fast food' [c] three or more times a week	9.1	11.9	[8.3, 17.0]	<0.0001
Uses full fat milk	4.6	5.7	[4.9, 6.7]	<0.0001
Doesn't eat any fruit	6.3	6.4	[4.5, 9.1]	
Eats less than two serves of fruit daily	3.4	4.2	[3.6, 4.9]	
Eats two or more serves of fruit daily	2.7	3.3	[2.8, 4.0]	0.0030
Doesn't eat any vegetables	15.0	14.9	[6.5, 30.4]	
Eats less than five serves daily	3.3	4.0	[3.6, 4.5]	
Eats five or more serves daily	2.3	2.6	[1.7, 3.9]	<0.0012

[a] Sample with no missing values for each sociodemographic variable: Age (n = 21,705); education (n = 21,659); employment status (21,556); income (n = 17,964); perceived spending power (n = 20,959); aboriginal or not (n = 21,694); born in Australia or not (n = 21,704); living arrangements (n = 21,687); own or mortgage/rent (n = 21,705) SEIFA (n = 21,705); [b] SEIFA is an index of relative social disadvantage by area of residence [43] usually presented as quintiles which have been grouped into three levels of social disadvantage for this study; [c] Fast food is operationally defined as take away food such as burgers, pizza, chicken or chips from places like McDonalds, Hungry Jacks, Pizza Hut or Red Rooster.

Table 2. Weighted multivariable logistic regression for associations with running out of food including interaction terms, HWSS 2009–2013 (n = 17,638 [a]) [b].

Main Effects	Odd Ratio (95% CI)	p
35 over	Ref	
18–34 years	5.29 (3.65, 7.65)	0.000
Has tertiary education	Ref	
Does not have tertiary education	1.87 (1.38, 2.54)	0.000
Not Aboriginal	Ref	
Aboriginal	2.07 (1.34, 3.2)	0.001
Household income over $40,000	Ref	
Household income $20,000 to $40,000	1.65 (1.29, 2.1)	0.000
Household income under $20,000	5.28 (3.91, 7.13)	0.000
Can save a bit of money	Ref	
Just enough money to get by	1.08 (0.69, 1.71)	0.730
Not enough money to get by	3.11 (2.17, 4.46)	0.000
Has private health insurance	Ref	
Has no private health insurance	1.80 (1.46, 2.22)	0.000
Does not have doctor diagnosed mental health problem	Ref	
Has a doctor diagnosed mental health problem	2.56 (1.96, 3.35)	0.000
Low or moderate Kessler 10 score	Ref	
High or very high Kessler 10 score	1.65 (1.31, 2.06)	0.000
Health same or better than same time previous year	Ref	
Health worse or much worse than same time previous year	1.70 (1.37, 2.09)	0.000
Does not smoke	Ref	
Smokes	1.58 (1.29, 1.93)	0.000
Is not in Body Mass Index obese range	Ref	
Is in Body Mass Index obese range	1.44 (1.18, 1.76)	0.000
Eats some vegetables daily	Ref	
Eats no vegetables daily	2.40 (1.34, 4.3)	0.003
Eats fast foods less than three times a week	Ref	
Eats fast foods three or more times a week	1.83 (1.11, 3.01)	0.018
Interaction terms		
Has just enough money to get by [#] age 18–24 years	0.56 (0.35, 0.91)	0.019
Has a mental health problem [#] age 18–24 years	0.52 (0.31, 0.86)	0.010
Housing whether or not owned or rented [#] Not enough or just enough money to get by	3.35 (2.41, 4.65)	0.000
Household income under $20,000 [#] Not enough or just enough money to get by	3.05 (1.94, 4.80)	0.000

[a] Logistic reduced the estimation sample as it ran with post stratification adjustment (accounting for new weighted estimation sample); [b] This is the basic model used to determine the direction of effect. Two further models were then produced: One for associations preceding running out of food and one for associations following running out of food. The odd ratios in the path diagram were taken from these two models; [#] Denotes interaction terms between variables: Odds ratios less than 1 attenuate the effect and odds ratios greater than 1 enhance the effect.

The path to 'running out of food' and the associations between variables are shown in Figure 1. The path diagram shows both the main effects and the interaction terms that directly or indirectly influence the primary outcome of 'running out of food'. The models showed a good fit with the data, both for the variables that are associated with 'running out of food' (χ^2 = 12.75; p = 0.17) and the possible consequences of 'running out of food' (fast food consumption χ^2 = 5.48; p = 0.71; not eating vegetables χ^2 = 8.82; p = 0.31).

In Figure 1, the red box represents the outcome measure, demonstrating food insecurity, i.e., 'running out of food' at least once in the previous twelve months. The blue boxes represent sociodemographics that are not able to be changed or are not easily changed. The yellow boxes represent associations which modify other variables on the path to food insecurity as well as being directly associated with food insecurity. The grey boxes represent the hypothesised consequences of food insecurity as informed by the BIC analysis.

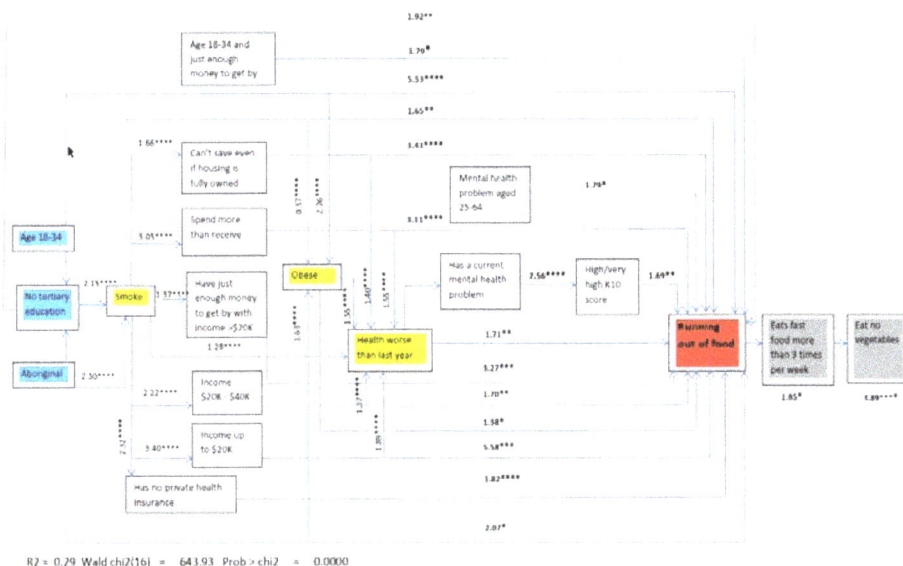

Figure 1. Estimate of probability of eating fast food more than twice a week and eating no vegetables by 'running out of food', adjusted using propensity scores: Showing probable outcomes of 'running out of food', HWSS 2009–2013. * $p < 0.05$; ** $p < 0.01$; *** $p < 0.001$; **** $p < 0.0001$.

3.1. Direct Associations with Food Insecurity

Of the variables regarded as fixed, only three were directly associated with food insecurity: Age group (18–34 years compared to 35–64 years, odds ratio (OR) = 5.53, $p < 0.0001$), prior education level (no tertiary education compared with tertiary education, OR = 1.92, $p < 0.01$) and Aboriginality (of Aboriginal or Torres Strait Islander origin compared with not, OR = 2.07, $p < 0.05$). With the exception of two variables (which are dependent on 'running out of food') all other variables predicted FI. The two variables that were dependent on 'running out of food' were frequent fast food consumption, which subsequently predicted eating no vegetables.

3.2. Effect Modifiers in the Food Insecurity Path

Three variables acted as powerful effect modifiers in the path, shown in the yellow boxes: Smoking, obesity and the perception of worsening health over time (direct association). The size of the effects is shown on the chart as odds rations. To illustrate: Smoking, which is influenced by Aboriginality (OR = 2.30, $p < 0.0001$) and education (OR = 2.15, $p < 0.0001$), has a main effect on 'running out of food' (OR = 1.65, $p < 0.01$) and also acts as an effect modifier for perceived spending power and income (OR = 1.65, $p < 0.01$), income (AUD$20–40K OR = 2.22, $p < 0.0001$; up to AUD$20K OR = 3.40, $p < 0.0001$), private health insurance (OR = 1.65, $p < 0.01$) and worsening health status (OR = 1.65, $p < 0.01$).

Obesity influenced by smoking, where aboriginality and younger age has a main effect (OR = 1.38, $p < 0.05$) acts as an effect modifier for worsening health (OR = 1.55 $p < 0.0001$). Worsening health is influenced by smoking, obesity, low income, discretional income, and money problems, which are defined here as any income perceived to be less than needed. It has a main effect (OR = 1.71, $p < 0.01$) and acts as an effect modifier on mental health (OR = 1.71, $p < 0.01$).

Independent associations between younger age and spending power, low income and spending power, money problems, and mental health problems for older respondents are all directly associated with 'running out of food'. Other direct effects include not having private health insurance, having a low income, discretional income and mental health. Mental health also has an indirect effect mediated by high psychological distress, with the score measured by the K10 scale.

Respondents who are younger or who have very low incomes are more than five times as likely to report 'running out of food' compared with older age respondents and those with higher incomes. Respondents with money problems, low discretional income, and those with both low income and low discretional income are more than three times as likely to report 'running out of food' compared with respondents who don't have money problems and higher income as well as higher discretional spending power.

3.3. Adjustment for Covariates and Indicators of Hypothetical Causality

Using iterative propensity score weighted analyses, three areas of the path were tested for hypothetical causality with regard to food insecurity: Having a low annual household income, an inadequate perceived discretional income and obesity. Additionally, two areas were tested for possible causality due to food insecurity: Eating fast food more than twice a week and not eating any vegetables. Table 3 shows the results for the link between food insecurity and having an annual household income of up to AUD$20,000, being able to save versus other discretional income categories and being obese versus not.

Table 3. Estimate of probability of food insecurity ('running out of food' and not being able to afford more) by income, discretional income and obesity, adjusted using propensity scores: Showing probable antecedent factors of 'running out of food', HWSS 2009–2013.

Outcome: 'Running out of Food' at Least Once in the Previous Twelve Months	Coef.	95%	CI	Robust Std. Err	Z	*p*
Annual household income						
Average effect when income <$20,000	0.038	0.013	0.063	0.013	3.02	0.003
Probability if income is >$20,000	0.028	0.025	0.03	0.001	19.33	<0.001
Discretional income						
Difference between spend left over vs. able to save	0.023	0.014	0.033	0.005	4.85	<0.001
Difference between just enough vs. able to save	0.056	0.046	0.067	0.005	10.48	<0.001
Difference between not enough vs. able to save	0.066	0.048	0.083	0.009	7.38	<0.001
Average probability of outcome for those able to save	0.012	0.009	0.014	0.001	9.05	<0.001
Obesity						
Difference in probability when obese	0.008	0.003	0.013	0.003	3.15	0.002
Average probability of outcome if not obese	0.029	0.026	0.032	0.002	17.88	<0.001

vs = versus.

The first line of Table 3 shows the difference in the probability of 'running out of food' for the population with low income compared with those with a higher income. The second line of the table shows the probability for a reference higher income group 'running out of food'. The overall probability of 'running out of food' for the low income group is the sum of the two coefficients (e.g., 0.038 + 0.028 = 0.066). The next lines of Table 3 show the difference between the population and the reference category(ies) with which they are being compared for the independent variables: Perceived discretional income and obesity. The Supplementary Table S1 shows the full model for incomes above and below $20,000.

Table 4 shows the difference between the population and the reference category(ies) with which they are being compared for eating fast food three or more times a week and not eating vegetables. Eating fast food three or more times a week precedes eating no vegetables (as assessed using BIC in the path analysis).

Table 4. Estimate of probability of eating fast food more than twice a week and eating no vegetables by 'running out of food', adjusted using propensity scores: Showing probable outcomes of 'running out of food', HWSS 2009-2013.

Outcome:	Coef.	95%	CI	Robust Std. Err	Z	*p*
Eats fast food more than three times a week						
Difference in probability of 'running out of food' vs. not	−0.007	−0.013	−0.0002	0.003	−2.03	0.042
Average probability of outcome when didn't run out	0.019	<0.001	0.017	0.001	17.83	<0.001
Eats no vegetables						
Difference in probability of fast food >2 times weekly	0.029	0.007	0.051	0.011	2.61	0.009
Average probability of FI when fast food <3 times weekly	0.006	0.005	0.007	0.001	10.32	<0.001

4. Discussion

This analysis using a population-based survey resulted in the description of a plausible and quantified pathway to food insecurity, as well as measurement of its dietary impacts. The findings support the hypothesis that food insecurity, measured by whether or not a household ran out of food in the last year, appears to more strongly precede the poor diet indicators of eating fast food three or more times a week and eating no vegetables. While this hypothesis has been proposed previously [51], this proof-of-concept study is the first to quantify both the relative importance of the factors within the feedback loop to food insecurity and the complex nature of the factors leading to it.

The odds of 'running out of food' were higher for younger adults, those without tertiary education and Aboriginal people (odds ratios of 5.53, 2.15 and 2.3 respectively). These findings are consistent with the findings of the Australian national dietary survey which found that the prevalence of food insecurity was higher in Aboriginal populations compared to non-Indigenous Australians (22% compared to 3.7%) [52]. A UK study of 10,452 adults found that different socioeconomic indicators predicted dietary intake, for example, economic access to food, educational attainment and age were related to fruit and vegetable intake and diet costs [53]. The study also showed that dietary costs were not equally important in the causal pathway between socioeconomic position, suggesting that health and diet may be a factor when allocating funding for food [53].

The risk of running out of money for food has been associated with one-off financial stressors such as medical or other expenses due to unexpected events [54] and the price of food has been shown to contribute to food stress among low income families [55]. This current research highlights many other interrelated and potentially changeable factors. Saving ability, at any income level, appears to protect against food insecurity. Financial over-commitment is particularly relevant during times of economic downturn, as has occurred in Western Australia over recent years. The financial stress of housing costs may contribute to food insecurity as people can no longer afford their mortgage or rent, leading to money for food, a discretionary expense, potentially being sacrificed and instead put towards covering housing costs.

Attitudes toward income inequality and how poor people manage their money and cope in stressful situations are underpinned by cultural beliefs, related to blame, plight and privilege [56]. Although most Canadians were willing to accept differences in income related health inequalities such as food insecurity, they were less willing to attribute health inequalities to differences in personal health practices and coping skills [56]. The current study found increased odds of smoking, eating fast food and obesity associated with running out of money to buy food, independent of income level. Similar associations with food insecurity, perceived financial difficulty, smoking, lower fruit and vegetable intake and higher discretionary food intake were found in a representative sample of French households [57].

There are significant associations with not having private health insurance and feeling a lack of control over one's own health, both of which have adjusted odds ratios of 1.9. There is also an increased likelihood of food insecurity associated with social, mental and physical disadvantage as noted in other studies [58]. The number of factors on the path support the notion of deprivation amplification [59]. The results also show that quantification of the degree and direction of effects associated with food insecurity is possible. This quantification lends support to the concept that there may be causality between some of the variables on the path.

According to the theory underlying propensity score methodology as developed by Rosenbaum and Rubin [60], adjustment for propensity scoring removes the influence of confounding by multiple covariates and provides plausible evidence for causation for cross-sectional studies, even though one cannot ascribe any statistical significance to the findings [61]. The results from this current study suggest evidence of a hypothetical causal relationship within the path for the variables presented. The direction of effect is the relative strength of the association, so for example, while obesity may follow FI, it more strongly precedes it. The same applies to eating no vegetables and fast food consumption, which also precede but more strongly follow FI as shown in the path diagram. This is one possible path to FI which provides opportunities to investigate the mechanisms underlying its effects and the mediation illustrated in the path diagram. Other paths to FI can further investigate latent effects such as dietary eating patterns [10]. Unhealthy eating patterns are associated with similar sociodemographics found in the FI pathway of this study [62].

There is value for policy decision makers in quantifying both the relative importance of a range of associations with food insecurity and constructing a path to food insecurity. The path diagram uses a population dataset with enough statistical power to allow for a subsequent investigation of possible causal links, highlighting the need to address the determinants of food insecurity as well as considering the consequences. The complex nature of the path also adds weight to the need for inter-sectoral collaborations to address the various determinants of food security. The results from the path diagram support the need for a system level policy to address this [63,64]. For example, obesity, which in the path diagram more strongly precedes FI has been shown also to follow it [62,65], suggesting the need for a policy that addresses both obesity as well as FI in tandem rather than as a separate policy for each.

The strength of this analysis is that the population survey and large sample size enabled the complex analysis to establish a proof-of-concept study to be undertaken. As with all survey data, there are limitations associated with this research, including some level of non-response and the self-reported nature of the data. The use of sample design weights incorporated in iterative proportional fitting (IFP), also known as 'raking', allowed for adjustment of over and under representation of age, gender and area of residence within the sample. This weighting was also incorporated into the multivariable regression models. The one question measure of food insecurity, based on 'running out of food' and not being able to afford more, does not measure the extent and experience of food insecurity, nor did the self-reported brief diet questions measure actual dietary intake. However, that was not the purpose of this investigation, which was to explore the complex mix of influences leading to FI. A further limitation was the omission of questions relating to attitudinal and lifestyle behaviours which would have allowed for the creation of a model that included these modifiable attributes.

5. Conclusions

The findings support evidence that decisions about food insecurity are complex and interactive, with a variety of factors contributing to the issue. While the single measure of FI cannot be considered adequate to fully estimate the prevalence of FI, the proof-of-concept using this single measure showed expected associations and quantified the effects of 'running out of food' over a range of determinants, such as income and physical and mental wellbeing. The path diagram presented suggests that a wider approach to bringing about change in access and use of food needs to be considered. The findings highlight the need to focus policy effort on mitigating the social determinants of food insecurity and the potential complexity of the pathways to food insecurity. This requires a system approach to policy development for FI and we could encourage policy makers and researchers to use this methodology to explore and quantify the complex relationships leading to food insecurity.

Supplementary Materials: The following are available online at http://www.mdpi.com/1660-4601/15/12/2620/s1, Table S1: Illustrating the full model of propensity scoring for incomes above and below $20,000.

Author Contributions: A.D. was involved in the conception and design of the HWSS; A.D. and C.P. were involved in the conception and design of the NMSS; A.D. and M.P. conceived the approach and analyzed the data; A.D. wrote the first draft of the paper; A.D., C.P., D.K., M.C., C.B., M.P. reviewed and agreed with final drafts of the paper.

Funding: This research was funded by Healthway, the Western Australian Health Promotion Foundation (Grant number 19986).

Acknowledgments: The Department of Health, Western Australia owns, conducts and funds the Health and Wellbeing Surveillance System (HWSS). The authors are grateful for the ongoing monitoring of nutrition relating attitudes and behaviours and encourage ongoing execution of the survey. Healthway, the Western Australian Health Promotion Foundation, funded the *Food Law, Policy and Communications to Improve Public Health Project (Grant 19986)* to assist the translation of research into practice. The funder had no role in study design, data collection and analysis, decision to publish, or preparation of the manuscript. All sources of funding of the study should be disclosed. A.D. undertook this work as part of her Doctor of Philosophy and received a Healthway Health Promotion Research Scholarship (23342) part of which is being used to support publication.

Conflicts of Interest: The authors declare no conflict of interest. A.D. and C.P. worked for the Department of Health, Western Australia. The founding sponsors had no role in the design of the study; in the analyses or interpretation of data; in the writing of the manuscript, and in the decision to publish the results.

References

1. Food and Agriculture Organization. *Rome Declaration on World Food Security and World Food Summit Plan of Action: World Food Summit 13–17 November*; FAO: Rome, Italy, 1996.

2. Anderson, S.A. Core indicators of nutritional state for difficult-to-sample populations. *J. Nutr.* **1990**, *120*, 1555–1600. [CrossRef] [PubMed]

3. Riches, G. *Food Bank Nations: Poverty, Corporate Charity and the Right to Food*; Routledge: New York, NJ, USA, 2018.

4. Hanson, K.L.; Connor, L.M. Food insecurity and dietary quality in us adults and children: A systematic review. *Am. J. Clin. Nutr.* **2014**, *100*, 684–692. [CrossRef] [PubMed]

5. Jones, A.D.; Ngure, F.M.; Pelto, G.; Young, S.L. What are we assessing when we measure food security? A compendium and review of current metrics. *Adv. Nutr.* **2013**, *4*, 481–505. [CrossRef] [PubMed]

6. Robaina, K.A.; Martin, K.S. Food insecurity, poor diet quality, and obesity among food pantry participants in hartford, ct. *J. Nutr. Educ. Behav.* **2013**, *45*, 159–164. [CrossRef] [PubMed]

7. Dowler, E. Symposium on 'intervention policies for deprived households' policy initiatives to address low-income households' nutritional needs in the uk. *Proc. Nutr. Soc.* **2008**, *67*, 289–300. [CrossRef] [PubMed]

8. Mook, K.; Laraia, B.A.; Oddo, V.M.; Jones-Smith, J.C. Food security status and barriers to fruit and vegetable consumption in two economically deprived communities of oakland, california, 2013–2014. *Prev. Chronic Dis.* **2016**, *13*, E21. [CrossRef] [PubMed]

9. Tingay, R.S.; Tan, C.J.; Tan, N.C.; Tang, S.; Teoh, P.F.; Wong, R.; Gulliford, M.C. Food insecurity and low income in an english inner city. *J. Public Health Med.* **2003**, *25*, 156–159. [CrossRef] [PubMed]

10. Thornton, L.E.; Pearce, J.R.; Ball, K. Sociodemographic factors associated with healthy eating and food security in socio-economically disadvantaged groups in the uk and victoria, australia. *Public Health Nutr.* **2013**, *17*, 20–30. [CrossRef] [PubMed]

11. Metallinos-Katsaras, E.; Must, A.; Gorman, K. A longitudinal study of food insecurity on obesity in preschool children. *J. Acad. Nutr. Diet.* **2012**, *112*, 1949–1958. [CrossRef] [PubMed]

12. Larson, N.I.; Story, M.T. Food insecurity and weight status among u.S. Children and families: A review of the literature. *Am. J. Prev. Med.* **2011**, *40*, 166–173. [CrossRef] [PubMed]

13. Crawford, P.B.; Webb, K.L. Unraveling the paradox of concurrent food insecurity and obesity. *Am. J. Prev. Med.* **2011**, *40*, 274–275. [CrossRef] [PubMed]

14. Hernandez, D.C.; Marshall, A.; Mineo, C. Maternal depression mediates the association between intimate partner violence and food insecurity. *J. Womens Health* **2014**, *23*, 29–37. [CrossRef] [PubMed]

15. Young, S.L.; Plenty, A.H.; Luwedde, F.A.; Natamba, B.K.; Natureeba, P.; Achan, J.; Mwesigwa, J.; Ruel, T.D.; Ades, V.; Osterbauer, B.; et al. Household food insecurity, maternal nutritional status, and infant feeding practices among hiv-infected ugandan women receiving combination antiretroviral therapy. *Matern. Child Health J.* **2014**, *18*, 2044–2053. [CrossRef] [PubMed]

16. Whitaker, R.C.; Phillips, S.M.; Orzol, S.M. Food insecurity and the risks of depression and anxiety in mothers and behavior problems in their preschool-aged children. *Pediatrics* **2006**, *118*, E859–E868. [CrossRef] [PubMed]

17. Melchior, M.; Chastang, J.F.; Falissard, B.; Galera, C.; Tremblay, R.E.; Cote, S.M.; Boivin, M. Food insecurity and children's mental health: A prospective birth cohort study. *PLoS ONE* **2012**, *7*, e52615. [CrossRef] [PubMed]

18. Muldoon, K.A.; Duff, P.K.; Fielden, S.; Anema, A. Food insufficiency is associated with psychiatric morbidity in a nationally representative study of mental illness among food insecure canadians. *Soc. Psychiatry Psychiatr. Epidemiol.* **2013**, *48*, 795–803. [CrossRef] [PubMed]

19. Pobutsky, A.M.; Baker, K.K.; Reyes-Salvail, F. Investigating measures of social context on 2 population-based health surveys, hawaii, 2010–2012. *Prev. Chron. Dis.* **2015**, *12*, E221.

20. Friel, S. Climate change, food insecurity and chronic diseases: Sustainable and healthy policy opportunities for australia. *N. S. W. Public Health Bull.* **2010**, *21*, 129–133. [CrossRef] [PubMed]

21. Ashe, L.M.; Sonnino, R. At the crossroads: New paradigms of food security, public health nutrition and school food. *Public Health Nutr.* **2013**, *16*, 1020–1027. [CrossRef] [PubMed]

22. Tarasuk, V. Implications of a Basic Income Guarantee for Household Food Insecurity. Northern Policy Institute, 2017. Available online: https://proof.utoronto.ca/wp-content/uploads/2017/06/Paper-Tarasuk-BIG-EN-17.06.13-1712.pdf (accessed on 22 November 2018).

23. Lang, T.; Barling, D.; Caraher, M. Food, social policy and the environment: Towards a new model. *Soc. Policy Adm.* **2001**, *35*, 538–558. [CrossRef]

24. Food and Agriculture Organisation. *Declaration of the World Summit on Food Security 16–18 November*; Food and Agriculture Organisation: Rome, Italiy, 2009.

25. Carletto, C.; Zezza, A.; Banerjee, R. Towards better measurement of household food security: Harmonizing indicators and the role of household surveys. *Glob. Food Secur.* **2013**, *2*, 30–40. [CrossRef]

26. Ecker, O.; Breisinger, C. The Food Security System: A New Conceptual Framework. International Food Policy Research Institute, 2012. Available online: http://ebrary.ifpri.org/cdm/ref/collection/p15738coll2/id/126837 (accessed on 22 November 2018).

27. Rideout, K.; Seed, B.; Ostry, A. Putting food on the public health table: Making food security relevant to regional health authorities. *Can. J. Public Health* **2006**, *97*, 233–236. [PubMed]

28. Bastian, A.; Coveney, J. Local evidenced-based policy options to improve food security in south australia: The use of local knowledge in policy development. *Public Health Nutr.* **2012**, *15*, 1497–1502. [CrossRef] [PubMed]

29. Bell, E. *Research for Health Policy*; Oxford University Press: Oxford, UK, 2009.

30. Caraher, M.; Coveney, J. Public health nutrition and food policy. *Public Health Nutr.* **2004**, *7*, 591–598. [CrossRef] [PubMed]

31. Booth, S.; Smith, A. Food security and poverty in australia-challenges for dietitians. *Aust. J. Nutr. Diet.* **2001**, *58*, 150–156.

32. Tarasuk, V. Health implications of food insecurity. *Soc. Déterm. Health Can. Perspect.* **2004**, 187–200.

33. Dinour, L.M.; Bergen, D.; Yeh, M.-C. The food insecurity–obesity paradox: A review of the literature and the role food stamps may play. *J. Am. Diet. Assoc.* **2007**, *107*, 1952–1961. [CrossRef] [PubMed]

34. Franklin, B.; Jones, A.; Love, D.; Puckett, S.; Macklin, J.; White-Means, S. Exploring mediators of food insecurity and obesity: A review of recent literature. *J. Commun. Health* **2012**, *37*, 253–264. [CrossRef] [PubMed]

35. HLPE, Nutrition and Food Systems. *A Report by the High Level Panel of Experts on Food Security and Nutrition of the Committee on World Food Security*; HLPE: Rome, Italy, 2017.

36. Foley, W.; Ward, P.; Carter, P.; Coveney, J.; Tsourtos, G.; Taylor, A. An ecological analysis of factors associated with food insecurity in south australia, 2002–2007. *Public Health Nutr.* **2010**, *13*, 215–221. [CrossRef] [PubMed]

37. Quine, S.; Morrell, S. Food insecurity in community-dwelling older australians. *Public Health Nutr.* **2006**, *9*, 219–224. [CrossRef] [PubMed]

38. Russell, J.; Flood, V.; Yeatman, H.; Mitchell, P. Prevalence and risk factors of food insecurity among a cohort of older australians. *J. Nutr. Health Aging* **2014**, *18*, 3–8. [CrossRef] [PubMed]

39. Kleve, S.; Davidson, Z.; Gearon, E.; Booth, S.; Palermo, C. Are low-to-middle-income households experiencing food insecurity in victoria, australia? An examination of the victorian population health survey, 2006–2009. *Aust. J. Prim. Health* **2017**, *23*, 249–256. [CrossRef] [PubMed]

40. Marques, E.S.; Reichenheim, M.E.; de Moraes, C.L.; Antunes, M.M.L.; Salles-Costa, R. Household food insecurity: A systematic review of the measuring instruments used in epidemiological studies. *Public Health Nutr.* **2015**, *18*, 877–892. [CrossRef] [PubMed]

41. McKechnie, R.; Turrell, G.; Giskes, K.; Gallegos, D. Single-item measure of food insecurity used in the national health survey may underestimate prevalence in australia. *Aust. N. Z. J. Public Health* **2018**, *42*, 389–395. [CrossRef] [PubMed]

42. Butcher, L.M.; O'Sullivan, T.A.; Ryan, M.M.; Lo, J.; Devine, A. Utilising a multi-item questionnaire to assess household food security in australia. *Health Promot. J. Aust.* **2018**. [CrossRef] [PubMed]

43. Australian Bureau of Statistics. *Socio-Economic Indexes for Areas (Seifa) 2011*; Australian Bureau of Statistics: Canberra, Australia, 2013.

44. Hayes, A.J.; Kortt, M.A.; Clarke, P.M.; Brandrup, J.D. Estimating equations to correct self-reported height and weight: Implications for prevalence of overweight and obesity in australia. *Aust. N. Z. J. Public Health* **2008**, *32*, 542–545. [CrossRef] [PubMed]

45. Andrews, G.; Slade, T. Interpreting scores on the kessler psychological distress scale (k10). *Aust. N. Z. J. Public Health* **2001**, *25*, 494–497. [CrossRef] [PubMed]

46. Gill, T.K.; Price, K.; Dal Grande, E.; Daly, A.; Taylor, A.W. Feeling angry about current health status: Using a population survey to determine the association with demographic, health and social factors. *BMC Public Health* **2016**, *16*, 588. [CrossRef] [PubMed]

47. Burnham, K.P.; Anderson, D.R. Multimodel inference-understanding aic and bic in model selection. *Sociol. Methods Res.* **2004**, *33*, 261–304. [CrossRef]

48. Raftery, A.E. Bayesian model selection in social research. *Sociol. Methodol.* **1995**, *25*, 111–163. [CrossRef]

49. Little, R.J.; Rubin, D.B. Causal effects in clinical and epidemiological studies via potential outcomes: Concepts and analytical approaches. *Annu. Rev. Public Health* **2000**, *21*, 121–145. [CrossRef] [PubMed]

50. StataCorp. *Stata Statistical Software: Release 13*; StataCorp LP: College Station, TX, USA, 2013.

51. Ramsey, R.; Giskes, K.; Turrell, G.; Gallegos, D. Food insecurity among adults residing in disadvantaged urban areas: Potential health and dietary consequences. *Public Health Nutr.* **2012**, *15*, 227–237. [CrossRef] [PubMed]

52. Australian Bureau of Statistics. *4727.0.55.005-Australian Aboriginal and Torres Strait Islander Health Survey: Nutrition Results-Food and Nutrients, 2012-13*; Australian Bureau of Statistics: Canberra, Australia, 2015.

53. Mackenbach, J.D.; Brage, S.; Forouhi, N.G.; Griffin, S.J.; Wareham, N.J.; Monsivais, P. Does the importance of dietary costs for fruit and vegetable intake vary by socioeconomic position? *Br. J. Nutr.* **2015**, *114*, 1464–1470. [CrossRef] [PubMed]

54. King, S.; Moffitt, A.; Bellamy, J.; Carter, S.; McDowell, C.; Mollenhauer, J. When there not enough to eat: A national study of food insecurity among emergency relief clients. *State Family Report* **2012**, *2*, 137–161. [CrossRef]

55. Landrigan, T.J.; Kerr, D.A.; Dhaliwal, S.S.; Savage, V.; Pollard, C.M. Removing the australian tax exemption on healthy food adds food stress to families vulnerable to poor nutrition. *Aust. N. Z. J. Public Health* **2017**, *41*, 591–597. [CrossRef] [PubMed]

56. Lofters, A.; Slater, M.; Kirst, M.; Shankardass, K.; Quinonez, C. How do people attribute income-related inequalities in health? A cross-sectional study in ontario, canada. *PLoS ONE* **2014**, *9*, e85286. [CrossRef] [PubMed]

57. Bocquier, A.; Vieux, F.; Lioret, S.; Dubuisson, C.; Caillavet, F.; Darmon, N. Socio-economic characteristics, living conditions and diet quality are associated with food insecurity in france. *Public Health Nutr.* **2015**, *18*, 2952–2961. [CrossRef] [PubMed]

58. Stuff, J.E.; Casey, P.H.; Szeto, K.L.; Gossett, J.M.; Robbins, J.M.; Simpson, P.M.; Connell, C.; Bogle, M.L. Household food insecurity is associated with adult health status. *J. Nutr.* **2004**, *134*, 2330–2335. [CrossRef] [PubMed]

59. Macintyre, S. Deprivation amplification revisited; or, is it always true that poorer places have poorer access to resources for healthy diets and physical activity? *Int. J. Behav. Nutr. Phys. Activ.* **2007**, *4*, 32. [CrossRef]

60. Rosenbaum, P.R.; Rubin, D.B. The central role of the propensity score in observational studies for causal effects. *Biometrika* **1983**, *70*, 41–55. [CrossRef]

61. Habicht, J.P.; Victora, C.G.; Vaughan, J.P. Evaluation designs for adequacy, plausibility and probability of public health programme performance and impact. *Int. J. Epidemiol.* **1999**, *28*, 10–18. [CrossRef] [PubMed]

62. Daly, A.; Pollard, C.M.; Kerr, D.A.; Binns, C.W.; Phillips, M. Using short dietary questions to develop indicators of dietary behaviour for use in surveys exploring attitudinal and/or behavioural aspects of dietary choices. *Nutrients* **2015**, *7*, 6330–6345. [CrossRef] [PubMed]

63. Caraher, M.; Furey, S. *The Economics of Emergency Food Aid Provision: A Financial, Social and Cultural Perspective*; Palgrave Macmillan: Basingstoke, UK, 2018.

64. Steiner, J.F.; Stenmark, S.H.; Sterrett, A.T.; Paolino, A.R.; Stiefel, M.; Gozansky, W.S.; Zeng, C. Food insecurity in older adults in an integrated health care system. *J. Am. Geriat. Soc.* **2018**, *66*, 1017–1024. [CrossRef] [PubMed]

65. Kaiser, M.L.; Cafer, A. Understanding high incidence of severe obesity and very low food security in food pantry clients: Implications for social work. *Soc. Work Public Health* **2018**, *33*, 125–139. [CrossRef] [PubMed]

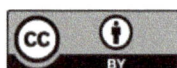

International Journal of
Environmental Research and Public Health

MDPI

Article

Food Insecurity among Older Aboriginal and Torres Strait Islanders

Jeromey B. Temple [1,*] and Joanna Russell [2]

[1] Demography and Ageing Unit, Melbourne School of Population and Global Health, University of Melbourne, Melbourne 3010, Australia

[2] School of Health and Society, University of Wollongong, Wollongong 2522, Australia; jrussell@uow.edu.au

* Correspondence: Jeromey.Temple@unimelb.edu.au; Tel.: +61-3-9035-9900

Received: 27 June 2018; Accepted: 10 August 2018; Published: 17 August 2018

Abstract: It is well established that Indigenous populations are at a heightened risk of food insecurity. Yet, although populations (both Indigenous and non-Indigenous) are ageing, little is understood about the levels of food insecurity experienced by older Indigenous peoples. Using Australian data, this study examined the prevalence and correlates of food insecurity among older Aboriginal and Torres Strait Islanders. Using nationally representative data, we employed ordinal logistic regression models to investigate the association between socio-demographic characteristics and food insecurity. We found that 21% of the older Aboriginal and Torres Strait Islander population were food insecure, with 40% of this group exposed to food insecurity with food depletion and inadequate intake. This places this population at a 5 to 7-fold risk of experiencing food insecurity relative to their older non-Indigenous peers. Measures of geography, language and low socio-economic status were highly associated with exposure to food insecurity. Addressing food insecurity offers one pathway to reduce the disparity in health outcomes between Aboriginal and Torres Strait Islanders and non-Indigenous Australians. Policies that consider both remote and non-remote Australia, as well as those that involve Aboriginal people in their design and implementation are needed to reduce food insecurity.

Keywords: food insecurity; food security; Indigenous population; ageing; Indigenous

1. Introduction

Like many Indigenous populations, the Aboriginal and Torres Strait Islander population in Australia has considerably poorer health outcomes when compared to their non-Indigenous peers, experiencing a range of health conditions at an earlier age of onset and considerably lower life expectancy [1–4]. The health issues facing many older people is an issue of increasing importance given persisting inequalities in socio-economic outcomes, as well as the ageing of this population [5]. In the 10 years to 2026, the population of Aboriginal and Torres Strait Islanders aged 45 and over is projected to increase by 35%, accounting for 22% of this population [6].

Importantly, many of the health conditions prevalent among older Aboriginal and Torres Strait Islanders are preventable, notwithstanding the levels of socio-economic disadvantage faced by this population. The Australian Institute of Health and Welfare (2016) estimates that the burden of disease in the Aboriginal population is 2.3 times of that experienced by non-Indigenous Australians [2]. Through reducing exposure to modifiable risk factors, such as tobacco and alcohol use and poor dietary behaviors, they estimate that about half of the difference in disease burden between Aboriginal and non-Indigenous Australians could be removed. In total, poor dietary behaviors were estimated to account for 10% of the total burden of disease faced by Aboriginal and Torres Strait Islanders.

An important proximate determinant and risk factor of poor nutrition outcomes is food insecurity. Food insecurity refers to the "limited or uncertain availability of nutritionally adequate and safe foods or limited or uncertain ability to acquire acceptable foods in socially acceptable ways" [7]. A growing number of studies have shown that Indigenous populations around the world are at a heightened risk of food insecurity [8–12]. For example, Canadian research has shown that Aboriginal people living on reservations were at 2.6 times the risk of being food insecure when compared to their non-Indigenous peers [8]. Research from the USA shows that levels of food insecurity experienced by American Indians are double that reported by non-Indigenous people [9]. Within the American population, food insecurity rates among the Navajo Nation were the highest reported within the USA to date, with just under 80% of this population experiencing some form of food insecurity [10]. Evidence from Australia shows that about 22% of Aboriginal and Torres Strait Islanders were exposed to food insecurity compared with 4% of non-Indigenous Australians [13].

Despite evidence of heightened risk of food insecurity within Indigenous populations, little is known about the prevalence and correlates of food insecurity in the older Aboriginal and Torres Strait Islander population. However, studies have examined food insecurity among the older non-Indigenous population, concluding the strength of socio-economic factors in explaining food insecurity in later life [14–16]. The aim of this study is to address this research gap through an examination of food insecurity among older Aboriginal and Torres Strait Islanders. Firstly, we assess the prevalence of food insecurity in Aboriginal and Torres Strait Islander older adults and secondly, we examine the risk factors for food insecurity in this population. We conclude with a discussion of the implications of our findings.

2. Materials and Methods

2.1. Survey Data

Data for this study are from the 2012–2013 Australian Aboriginal and Torres Strait Islander Nutrition and Physical Activity Survey (NATSINPAS) conducted by the Australian Bureau of Statistics (ABS) from August 2012 to July 2013 [17]. The survey is based on a sample of 2900 private dwellings across Australia, with a response rate of 79% (3661 households were approached). Within each dwelling, one adult (aged 18 and over) and one child (where applicable) were randomly selected for interview. The survey excluded those living in non-private dwellings such as hospitals, nursing homes and hotels. The survey also excluded all non-Indigenous persons including non-Indigenous born Australians, non-Australian diplomats, and overseas visitors.

An important advantage of the NATSINPAS is the geographic coverage of the survey, including remote and non-remote areas as well as discrete Aboriginal and Torres Strait Islander communities. Remote areas include very remote Australia and remote Australia under the Australian Statistical Geography Standard [18]. Non-remote areas include those residing in major cities, inner or outer regional Australia. The final sample included data on 1792 individuals living in non-remote areas and 2317 individuals in remote areas in Australia. ABS interviewers conducted face to face interviews, collecting information on health, nutrition and characteristics of the household and dwelling.

NATSINPAS was part of the larger Australian Aboriginal and Torres Strait Islander Health Survey (AATSIHS). The sampling design of NATSINPAS sought to provide reliable estimates at the national level, as well as for remote and non-remote Australia. The in-scope population was divided into two broad populations. The first group included those living in discrete Aboriginal and Torres Strait Islander communities in remote Australia, defined as the 'community frame'. The second group included the remainder of the in-scope population, referred to as the 'non-community frame'. The Indigenous Community Frame (ICF) was used to target respondents for the community frame, and was built from a combination of Census data as well as data from the Discrete Indigenous Communities Database. The non-community frame was formed using Census data at a low geographic level (SA1). For some States and Territories, the non-community sample was disaggregated into non-remote and remote non-community areas. Survey weights at the person level were calculated by the ABS to calibrate the probability of selection into the survey relative to estimated resident population counts (less those in non-private dwellings).

Data from NATSINPAS were collected under the Census and Statistics Act 1905. As NATSINPAS included a biomedical component, ethics approvals were sought at both the national level (by the Australian Government Department of Health and Ageing) and at the state and Territory level (by a range of medical and Aboriginal ethics committees). Data for this study were made available by the ABS through the Universities of Australia agreement. NATSINPAS survey data are available to registered users of ABS microdata.

2.2. Measurement

In this study, we consider the prevalence and risk factors for food insecurity among older Aboriginal and Torres Strait Islanders aged 45 years and over ($n = 1062$). Defining the sample aged 45 years and over as 'older' is common in studies of ageing among Aboriginal and Torres Strait Islander people for several reasons [4,19,20]. Firstly, there is a considerable gap in life expectancy of about one decade between Aboriginal and non-Indigenous Australians, reducing the proportion of the population living into advanced old age [3,21]. Second, many conditions and comorbidities as well as frailties commonly associated with aging are early onset in this population [2,3,22]. Third, in recognition of the above two points, government programs such as those governing access to specific aged care services are available to Aboriginal and Torres Strait Islanders from earlier ages when compared to non-Indigenous Australians.

The measurement of food insecurity in NATSINPAS consists of two questions. The household spokesperson (adult aged 18 or over) was asked, "In the last 12 months was there any time when you (or members of this household) ran out of food and couldn't afford to buy more?" A follow up question was asked, "When this happened, did you (or members of this household) go without food?" Following other Australian studies, we use these two questions to create a variable which views food insecurity on a continuum [23]. Those answering 'no' to the first question are coded as 'food secure'. Those who answer 'yes' to the first question, but 'no' to the second are coded as 'food insecure—food depletion'. That is, they ran out of money for food, but did not go without food. The final group, 'food insecure—food depletion and inadequate intake' are those who ran out of money for food and went without food consequently. Although there are a number of limitations to this measure (as discussed in Section 4.4), this is the most detailed measure of financially attributable food insecurity that is collected by the ABS on an irregular basis.

2.3. Statistical Model

To model the association between socio-economic characteristics and food insecurity, we utilized Stata 14.0. As the dependent variable is ordinal, standard logistic regression is inappropriate. We utilized ordered logistic regression fitted by maximum likelihood [24]. Initial variable selection was informed by the growing literature on food insecurity among older Australians [14–16]. Variables entered the regression model and improvement to model fit assessed using the Bayesian Information Criteria following Raftery's (1995) procedure [25]. With the full model specified, we check the conditioning of the matrix of independent variables to investigate any collinearity influence [26]. The condition numbers were very small providing support for the model specification. An important assumption underlying ordinal logistic regression is the parallel lines or proportional odds assumption. This assumption states that the coefficients of variables associated with the probability of food security versus food insecurity with depletion and food security versus depletion and inadequate intake are constant. We follow Brant's (1990) procedure and the non-significant test result provides strong support for modeling the severity of food insecurity within an ordinal framework [27].

Independent Variables

Informed by the literature on food insecurity in Australia and using model selection techniques outlined above, variations in food insecurity were identified by a range of socio-economic characteristics. The final variables included in the model were:

- Age: Measured in aggregate categories (45–54, 55–64, 65–74, 75+).
- Marital Status: Married or not married. Unfortunately, more detailed items such as widowed, never married or separated were unavailable on the data set.
- Gender: Male or Female.
- Household Size: Categorized as 1, 2, 3 or 4, 5 or more.
- Household Composition: Whether the household includes Aboriginal and Torres Strait Islander members only, or with non-Indigenous members also present.
- Indigenous Language Speaking: Whether the persons speaks an Australian Indigenous language.
- Remoteness: Whether the household resides in remote or non-remote parts of Australia, as defined by the Australian Statistical Geography Standard (ASGS).
- Household Income: The measure of household income provided by the ABS was equivalized household income (adjusted or equivalized using an equivalence scale) and collapsed into deciles. This adjusted form of household income allows for welfare and financial wellbeing comparisons between households of different sizes and compositions.
- Self-Reported Health: A dichotomous variable indicating whether the person self-reported their health as being excellent or good versus fair or poor.

3. Results

3.1. Prevalence of Food Insecurity

Table 1 displays the weighted estimates of the severity of food insecurity among Aboriginal and Torres Strait Islanders aged 45 and over. In 2012–2013, approximately 21% of this population reported being food insecure. Of this group of food insecure persons, about 41% reported both food depletion and inadequate intake, that is, they ran out of money and went without food consequently. This group accounted for about 8% of the Aboriginal and Torres Strait Islander population aged 45 years and over.

There is considerable socio-economic and demographic variation in exposure to food insecurity among older people (Table 1). Important to this analysis of food insecurity among older Aboriginal and Torres Strait Islanders is Indigenous language speaking, living in a remote area, and Indigenous household composition. Interestingly, we observe differences in exposure to food insecurity by discrete categories of English language speaking and geography. In this sample, almost all respondents in non-remote areas speak English in the household. Approximately 19% of this group were food insecure, as were those who spoke English in remote areas of Australia. However, for those who speak Indigenous languages residing in remote areas, the prevalence of food insecurity was almost double (about 37%). Indeed, 12% of Indigenous language speakers in remote areas were severely food insecure (or one third of all food insecure people).

Similarly, strong differences in food insecurity by Aboriginal household composition are observed. Those living in a household with both Aboriginal and non-Indigenous members have a food insecurity prevalence of about 7%, compared with 28% of those in Aboriginal only households. Overall, we identify several population sub-groups with a food insecurity prevalence rate of around 30%: Indigenous speakers in remote communities (37%), Aboriginal and Torres Strait Islander only households (28%), smokers (31%), persons in households with a large number of occupants (32%), non-married females (35%), and income earners in the lowest centile (31%).

Although these descriptive results indicate significant differences in exposure to food insecurity by socio-economic characteristics, it is important to control for confounding effects to measure the association between each covariate and the probability of food insecurity.

Table 1. Food Insecurity (%) by Socio-Economic Characteristics, 2012–2013.

	Food Secure		Insecure: Depletion		Insecure: Depletion & Intake		Food Insecure [1]	Unweighted n =
Age		-		-		-		
45–54	76.3		14.2		9.5		23.7	435
55–64	82.6		9.8		7.6		17.4	356
65–74	80.6		11.0		8.4		19.4	200
75+	89.7		8.7		1.6		10.3	71
Self-Reported Health								
Excellent or Good	81.4	-	9.9	-	8.7	-	18.6	667
Fair or Poor	76.1	*	16	*	7.9	*	23.9	395
Language & Remoteness								
Non-remote	81.3	-	10.6	-	8.1	-	18.7	451
Remote-English	80.9		11.6		7.4		19.0	374
Remote-Indigenous [2]	62.7	***	25.1	***	12.2	***	37.3	236
Household Income [3]								
Lowest 20%	69.1	-	16.7	-	14.3	-	31.0	472
20–40%	86.9	**	7.9	*	5.2	*	13.1	215
40–60%	90.5	***	5.0	**	4.5	*	9.5	109
60–80%	84.1	***	7.1	***	8.8	***	15.9	77
80–100%	94.7	***	5.3	***	0.0	***	5.3	57
Unknown	77.1		18.9		3.9		22.8	132
Household Composition								
Aboriginal only	72.1	-	15.6	-	11.9	-	27.5	779
Aboriginal and Non [4]	92.6	***	5.4	***	2.0	***	7.4	283
Smoker Status								
Yes	68.8	-	16.1	-	15.1	-	31.2	420
No	86.9	***	9.4	*	3.7	**	13.1	642
Household Size								
1	75.1	-	14.6	-	10.3	-	24.9	422
2	88.3	**	7.5	*	4.2	*	11.7	413
3–4	72.8		14.1		13.2		27.3	176
5+	68.1	*	24.0	*	7.9		31.9	51
Marital Status								
Female, Unmarried	65.4	-	17.7	-	16.9	-	34.6	393
Female, Married	90.5	***	5.7	***	3.7	**	9.4	225
Male, Unmarried	79.3	*	13.6	*	7.0		20.6	247
Male, Married	87.3	***	9.7	***	9.7	***	19.4	197

Table 1. *Cont.*

	Food Secure		Insecure: Depletion	Insecure: Depletion & Intake	Food Insecure [1]	Unweighted *n* =
Non-school Qual [5]						
Yes	79.2	-	11.4	9.4	20.8	370
No	79.6	*	12.7	7.7	20.4	692
Weighted 45+ (%)	79.5		12.2	8.4	20.6	
Unweighted 45+ (%)	78.2		13.5	8.3	21.8	
Unweighted (n)	831		143	88	231	1062

[1] Includes respondents indicating food insecurity with food depletion and those indicating food insecurity with food depletion and inadequate intake; [2] Indigenous language; [3] Equivalized household income (to allow for welfare comparisons across households of different sizes) placed into quintiles; [4] Non-Indigenous household members present; [5] Has received post-school education or training; *** $p < 0.001$, ** $p < 0.01$, * $p < 0.05$; - omitted category for tests of proportions. Weighted estimates.

3.2. Regression Results

With a range of demographic and economic controls, English speaking and remoteness remain strong predictors of food insecurity (Table 2). Those speaking Indigenous languages were about 57% more likely to experience food insecurity compared with those in non-remote areas (OR 1.57 95% CI: 1.01–2.44). Again, there was no difference in food insecurity between English speakers in remote and non-remote areas (OR = 0.99 $p < 0.10$). In a similarly sized effect, households with both Aboriginal and non-Indigenous residents were about 60% less likely to experience food insecurity compared with Aboriginal only households, even with controls for geography (OR 0.4 95% CI: 0.22, 0.69).

Table 2. Ordered Logistic Regression Model of Food Insecurity, 2012–2013.

Covariate	Odds Ratio (OR)	95% CI [1]	
Age			
45–54	1.00		
55–64	0.81	0.56, 1.16	
65–74	0.61	0.39, 0.96	*
75+	0.46	0.23, 0.91	*
Marital Status			
Female, Unmarried	1.00		
Female, Married	0.52	0.30, 0.89	*
Male, Unmarried	0.73	0.49, 1.08	
Male, Married	0.62	0.36, 1.05	+
Labor Force Status			
Employed	1.00		
Unemployed	1.58	1.05, 2.36	*
Smoker Status			
Yes	1.00		
No	0.61	0.44, 0.84	***
Self-Reported Health			
Excellent or Good	1.00		
Fair or Poor	1.53	1.10, 2.11	*
Household Income [2]			
Lowest 20%	1.00		
20–40%	0.69	0.45, 1.06	+
40–60%	0.62	0.32, 1.19	
60–80%	0.24	0.08, 0.71	**
80–100%	0.12	0.02, 0.95	*
Unknown	0.89	0.56, 1.42	
Language & Remoteness			
Non-Remote	1.00		
Remote-English	0.99	0.68, 1.47	
Remote-Indigenous [3]	1.57	1.01, 2.44	*
Household Composition			
Aboriginal only	1.00		
Aboriginal and Non [4]	0.40	0.22, 0.69	***
Household Size			
1	1.00		
2	1.27	0.80, 2.01	
3–4	1.95	1.17, 3.25	**
5+	2.64	1.28, 5.46	**

[1] 95% Confidence Interval for the Odds Ratio; [2] Equivalized household income (to allow for welfare comparisons across households of different sizes) placed into quintiles; [3] Indigenous language; [4] Non-Indigenous household members present; *** $p < 0.001$, ** $p < 0.01$, * $p < 0.05$, + $p < 0.1$.

Non-smokers remained 39% less likely to experience food insecurity (OR 0.61 95% CI: 0.44, 0.84) and persons in large households were at a high risk, particularly those in household with 5 or more occupants (OR 2.64 95% CI: 1.28, 5.46). Those in the top 20% of the income distribution were about

88% less likely (OR 0.12 95% CI: 0.02, 0.95) to suffer food insecurity and those in the 60–80 percentile were about 76% less likely (OR 0.24 95% CI: 0.08, 0.71) when compared to lowest income earners.

Gender and social marital status also remains significant in the regression models. Compared to unmarried females, married females were about 48% less likely to experience food insecurity (OR 0.52 95% CI: 0.30, 0.89). Married males were 38% less likely to experience food insecurity relative to non-married females, but the estimate is only significant at the 90% level.

4. Discussion

Although several Australian studies have examined food insecurity in the older population, little is known about the prevalence and risk factors of food insecurity among older Aboriginal and Torres Strait Islanders specifically. In this paper, we have used nationally representative survey data to measure the prevalence and correlates of food insecurity among Aboriginal and Torres Strait Islanders aged 45 and over.

4.1. High Prevalence of Food Insecurity among Older Aboriginal and Torres Strait Islanders

Firstly, we find the prevalence of food insecurity among older Aboriginal and Torres Strait Islanders is high with about 21% reporting exposure, and 41% of this group reporting food depletion and inadequate intake. These estimates are in line with published results from the ABS showing that about 22% of Aboriginal and Torres Strait Islanders experience food insecurity compared to 4% of non-Indigenous Australians (ABS, 2015). The prevalence of food insecurity among older non-Indigenous Australians using a similar measure has previously been reported at 3% [14,28]. That is, older Aboriginal and Torres Strait Islanders are at about a 5–7 fold risk of food insecurity relative to their non-Indigenous peers.

This finding is important for several reasons. There is now a significant body of evidence on the implications of food insecurity for individual health and wellbeing. International studies show exposure to food insecurity is associated with symptoms of depression and anxiety, multimorbidity, lower levels of self-reported health status, lower nutrient diets, a greater likelihood of reporting social isolation, long standing health problems and activity limitations, and a greater likelihood of reporting heart disease, diabetes, and high blood pressure [29–37]. Among non-Indigenous Australians, food insecurity has also been shown to be associated with self-reported depression, reduced quality of life and poor diet quality [14,23,38]. More broadly, food insecurity may be related to decreased productivity and social interaction and contribute to increased economic inequality [39].

The high prevalence of food insecurity among older Aboriginal and Torres Strait Islanders is also important in the context of the gap in health outcomes that persists between Aboriginal and non-Indigenous Australians. 'Closing the Gap' is an Australian Government strategy whereby a key goal is to improve the health outcomes of Aboriginal and Torres Strait Islander populations. Specifically, the strategy seeks to reduce mortality by 2030 to levels experienced by the non-Indigenous population [40]. Addressing food insecurity among Aboriginal and Torres Strait Islanders by providing appropriate access to safe and nutritious foods has the potential to improve dietary behaviors that ultimately would contribute to increased life expectancy.

The 'Closing the Gap' strategy recognizes that the likelihood of co-morbidities is higher in the Aboriginal population when compared to the non-Indigenous population [41]. For example, about 38% of Aboriginal adults with either cardiovascular disease (CVD), diabetes or chronic kidney disease (CKD) had two or more health conditions compared to 26% of non-Indigenous people [2,41]. Coronary heart disease and diabetes are major contributors to the disease burden in Indigenous populations aged 45 years and over [2]. Poor dietary habits are known risk factors for poor health outcomes, with poor dietary habits contributing 50.1% towards the burden of CVD in Aboriginal populations [2,41]. Improving access to food is one factor that could affect the ability to choose a nutritious diet and improve dietary behaviors thereby improving health outcomes in Aboriginal and Torres Strait Islander population.

4.2. Socio-Economic Characteristics Are Strongly Associated with Food Insecurity

The prevalence of food insecurity is not evenly spread throughout the population and we find socio-economic factors are strongly associated with food insecurity and that specific demographic groups report higher rates of food insecurity. In the model of food insecurity formulated here, socio-economic factors are viewed as moderating food insecurity through the degree of resource-constrained access to the food supply.

Specifically, we identify a number of population sub-groups with a food insecurity prevalence rate of around 1 in 3: Indigenous speakers in remote communities (37%), Aboriginal and Torres Strait Islander only households (28%), smokers (31%), persons in households with a large number of occupants (32%), non-married females (35%) and income earners in the lowest centile (31%).

Differences in food insecurity status by socio-economic factors is consistent with studies in community dwelling non-Indigenous older Australians showing food insecurity differs by a range of socio-demographic risk factors, such as income, marital status, and smoker status [14–16]. The strength of socio-economic factors in explaining heightened food insecurity among Indigenous populations has also been noted elsewhere. For example, Pardilla et al. (2013), in their study of the Navajo Nation, note "Low socio-economic status, which is highly prevalent on the Navajo Nation and which we found to be significantly associated with food insecurity, must be considered in future endeavors to improve food security and decrease the risk of chronic disease" ([10] p. 64).

The strength of socio-economic factors as risk factors in experiencing food insecurity is concerning given the continued economic deprivation experienced by many Aboriginal and Torres Strait Islanders. For example, considerable disparities in socio-economic outcomes persist between non-Indigenous and Aboriginal persons across all age groups through lower levels of education, employment and living in areas with greater socio-economic disadvantage, while also being at considerable risk of experiencing interpersonal racism [5,42]. Not only do socio-economic factors provide greater access to the food supply (e.g., due to greater resources with which to purchase food), but these resources may also enable families to better cope with unexpected shocks (e.g., unexpected unemployment or disability) that could be a precursor to food insecurity.

4.3. Food Insecurity is High in Both Urban and Remote Settings

Results presented here also underscore differences in food insecurity risks between remote and non-remote areas of Australia. Interestingly, we find that non-English speaking persons in remote areas (37.3%) are at double the risk of exposure to food insecurity than English speakers in either remote (19%) or non-remote (18.7%) Australia.

Part of this disparity may reflect the lack of detailed geographical measures on NATSINPAS due to confidentialization. That is, non-English speakers are more likely to be resident in particularly isolated areas of remote Australia—with limited access to affordable food sources and health facilities. Notwithstanding, a considerable literature has emerged on the disparity in food prices between urban, regional, and remote regions in Australia. In one study, a 47% difference in prices was reported between remote and urban supermarkets for healthier foods [43]. Solutions to this complex problem include improvements to freight and transport costs, as well as improving low levels of demand for nutritious foods [44]. Indeed, one of the key drivers of food choice in remote Aboriginal communities is poverty [45]. These transport and demand issues are exacerbated by the lack of availability and variety of healthier food choices and lack of locally grown food in remote areas of Australia [45,46]. Combining the high cost of food and high poverty levels in remote regions likely explains the increased likelihood of being food insecure for non-English speaking Aboriginal and Torres Strait Islanders.

However, it was interesting to note that the likelihood of being food insecure did not differ between non- remote and remote English-speaking Aboriginal and Torres Strait Islanders with about 1 in 5 at risk of exposure to food insecurity. This is important as 75% of the Aboriginal and Torres Strait Islander population live in urban and regional areas [47]. Furthermore, projections of the Aboriginal and Torres Strait Islander population indicate future growth of the older population to be more prevalent in cities and regional areas. Between 2016 and 2026, the population aged 45 years and over is projected to grow by 36% in major cities, 39% in Inner and Outer regional areas and by 24% in remote and very remote areas of Australia [6]. These findings suggest that solutions to addressing food insecurity in older Aboriginal and Torres Strait Islander populations need to focus on all geographical locations. Indeed, recent efforts have tended to focus on food insecurity in remote areas, with less focus given to people living in urban areas [48,49].

Despite the focus of recent programs, a greater awareness of the linguistic and cultural needs in remote areas is required for effective solutions to food insecurity. In a systematic review of Aboriginal food and nutrition programs, Browne and colleagues (2018) conclude that "the most important factor determining success of Aboriginal and Torres Strait Islander food and nutrition programs is community involvement in (and ideally, control of) program development and implementation" [50]. As further argued by Bramwell et al. (2017), "given the sensitivity and shame often associated with food insecurity, more needs to be known about how health professionals can broach the issue to ensure dignity and cultural safety" ([48] p. 7). Herein lies a major problem for the implementation of food insecurity programs, as there is a considerable underrepresentation of Aboriginal and Torres Strait Islander people in the health sector—including at the programmatic design level [51].

4.4. Study Limitations

In interpreting our results, it is important to consider the study's limitations. Our findings potentially underestimate the degree of food insecurity in this population for several reasons. Firstly, the NATSINPAS population is limited to Aboriginal and Torres Strait Islanders residing in private dwellings and excludes a range of other vulnerable populations such as the homeless, those in poor health living in care facilities or hospitals. Indeed, there is a considerable need for further research on food insecurity risk in non-community based settings, among both Indigenous and non-Indigenous populations [52]. Secondly, the measure of food insecurity we employ is primarily an indicator of food insecurity as it only addresses access to food by economic means and does not include physical or mobility access. For example, research has shown that along with financial barriers, storage, transportation, health, and functional barriers are associated with experiencing food insecurity [53,54]. Using a more comprehensive tool that addressed issues of anxiety, quality and quantity of food suggested the prevalence of food insecurity in non-Indigenous older adults was 13% compared to 2% resulting from responses to the single item tool [16]. Furthermore, qualitative research suggests that many older people engage in "precarious nutritional self-management strategies" that are important indicators of food insecurity, and are not captured in the measures used herein [55]. Specific to this population, access to and availability of skills to use traditional foods or 'bush tucker' is also likely to be an important component of overall food security [12]. The food insecurity of older Aboriginal and Torres Strait Islanders would undoubtedly be higher according to these broader definitions. Finally, the prevalence and severity of food insecurity may be cyclical and cannot be captured in cross sectional data [56,57]. Longitudinal data are necessary to measure complex movements in and out of food insecurity and unfortunately this data is not collected. Moreover, as these data are cross sectional, we cannot and do not draw a causal relationship between the independent variables and food insecurity.

5. Conclusions

Noting these limitations, this paper was the first to examine food insecurity among older Aboriginal and Torres Strait Islanders. We found that food insecurity is experienced by a sizeable minority of older persons (1 in 5), that 41% of this group go without food consequently and that specific demographic groups are at a considerably heightened risk. In total, older Aboriginal and Torres Strait Islanders are at about a 5–7 fold risk of experiencing food insecurity relative to their non-Indigenous peers.

These findings offer information with which to identify food insecure persons and to inform nutrition programs in place to improve health and wellbeing. Existing studies note the importance of involving Aboriginal and Torres Strait Islander people in the management, design, and implementation of such programs and considerably more needs to be done in this area. However, nutrition programs alone are likely to be ineffective. The strength of socio-economic factors in explaining the prevalence of food insecurity, suggest that policies must improve economic and social wellbeing (through the 'Closing the Gap' strategy) in tandem with targeted nutrition programs and policies aimed at providing an affordable, healthy food supply. Recent evaluation studies, unfortunately, show slow progress with the 'Closing the Gap' strategy, with improvements in some but not all health and economic outcomes for Aboriginal and Torres Strait Islanders over the past decade [58,59].

Our findings further suggest solutions to addressing food insecurity in older Aboriginal and Torres Strait Islander populations need to focus on all geographical locations—not just on remote Australia, which has been the focus to date. In both remote and non-remote Australia, greater awareness of linguistic and cultural needs as well as the involvement and management of programs for and by Aboriginal and Torres Strait Islanders is required to improve levels of food security. Addressing food insecurity through these means offers one pathway for reducing nutrition related disease and co-morbidities, thereby assisting the 'Closing the Gap' strategy to achieve its aim of improving health outcomes for Aboriginal and Torres Strait Islanders.

Author Contributions: J.B.T. and J.R. jointly conceived the study and authored the manuscript. J.B.T. completed the data analysis. Both authors read and approved the final manuscript.

Funding: This research received no external funding. Temple is funded by the ARC Centre for Excellence in Population Ageing Research (CE1101029).

Acknowledgments: Data for this study were provided to the authors by the Australian Bureau of Statistics (ABS) through the ABS Universities Australia agreement.

Conflicts of Interest: The authors declare no conflict of interest.

References

1. Valeggia, C.R.; Snodgrass, J.J. Health of Indigenous People. *Annu. Rev. Anthropol.* **2015**, *44*, 117–135. [CrossRef]

2. Australian Institute of Health and Welfare. *Australian Burden of Disease Study: Impact and Causes of Illness and Death in Aboriginal and Torres Strait Islander People 2011*; Australian Burden of Disease Study Series No. 6. (Cat. no. BOD 7); Australian Institute of Health and Welfare: Canberra, Australia, 2016.

3. Australian Institute of Health and Welfare. *Trends in Indigenous Mortality and Life Expectancy, 2001–2015: Evidence from the Enhanced Mortality Database*; Cat. No. AIHW 174; Australian Institute of Health and Welfare: Canberra, Australia, 2017.

4. Gubhaju, L.; McNamara, J.; Banks, E.; Joshy, G.; Raphael, B.; Williamson, A.; Eades, S. The overall health and risk factor profile of Australian Aboriginal and Torres Strait Islander participants from the 45 and up study. *BMC Public Health* **2013**, *13*, 661. [CrossRef] [PubMed]

5. Cunningham, J.; Paradies, Y. Socio-demographic factors and psychological distress in Indigenous and non-Indigenous Australian adults aged 18–64 years: Analysis of national survey data. *BMC Public Health* **2012**, *12*, 95. [CrossRef] [PubMed]

6. Australian Bureau of Statistics. *Estimates and Projections, Aboriginal and Torres Strait Islander Australians, 2001 to 2026*; Catalogue Number 3238.0; Australian Bureau of Statistics: Canberra, Australia, 2014.

7. American Dietetic Association. Domestic food and nutrition security: Position of the American Dietetic Association. *J. Am. Diet. Assoc.* **1998**, *98*, 337–342. [CrossRef]

8. Willows, N.D.; Veugelers, P.; Raine, K.; Kuhle, S. Prevalence and sociodemographic risk factors related to household food security in Aboriginal peoples in Canada. *Public Health Nutr.* **2009**, *12*, 1150–1156. [CrossRef] [PubMed]

9. Gundersen, C. Measuring the extent, depth and severity of food insecurity: An application to American Indians in the USA. *J. Popul. Econ.* **2007**, *21*, 191–215. [CrossRef]

10. Pardilla, M.; Prasad, D.; Suratkar, S.; Gittelsohn, J. High levels of food insecurity on the Navajo Nation. *Public Health Nutr.* **2013**, *17*, 58–65. [CrossRef] [PubMed]

11. Skinner, K.; Hanning, R.; Tsuji, L.J.S. Prevalence and severity of household food insecurity of First Nations people living in an on-reserve, sub-Arctic community within the Mushkegowuk Territory. *Public Health Nutr.* **2014**, *17*, 31–39. [CrossRef] [PubMed]

12. Skinner, K.; Pratley, E.; Burnett, K. Eating in the city: A review of the literature on food insecurity and Indigenous people living in urban spaces. *Societies* **2016**, *6*, 7. [CrossRef]

13. Australian Bureau of Statistics. *Australian Aboriginal and Torres Strait Islander Health Survey: Nutrition Results—Food and Nutrients (Catalogue Number 4727.0.55.005)*; Australian Bureau of Statistics: Canberra, Australia, 2015.

14. Temple, J. Food insecurity among older Australians: Prevalence, correlates and well-being. *Aust. J. Ageing* **2006**, *25*, 158–163. [CrossRef]

15. Quine, S.; Morrell, S. Food insecurity in community-dwelling older Australians. *Public Health Nutr.* **2006**, *9*, 219–224. [CrossRef] [PubMed]

16. Russell, J.; Flood, V.; Yeatman, H.; Mitchell, P. Prevalence and risk factors of food insecurity among a cohort of older Australians. *J. Nutr. Health Aging* **2014**, *18*, 3–8. [CrossRef] [PubMed]

17. Australian Bureau of Statistics. Microdata. In *National Aboriginal and Torres Strait Islander Nutrition and Physical Activity Survey (Catalogue Number 4715.0.30.002)*; Australian Bureau of Statistics: Canberra, Australia, 2015.

18. Australian Bureau of Statistics. *Australian Standard Geographical Classification (ASGC) 2011 (Catalogue Number 1216.0)*; Australian Bureau of Statistics: Canberra, Australia, 2011.

19. Cotter, P.; Anderson, I.; Smith, L.R. Indigenous Australians: Ageing without longevity. In *Longevity and Social Change in Australia*; Borowski, A., Encel, S., Ozanne, E., Eds.; University of New South Wales Press Ltd.: Sydney, Australia, 2007; pp. 65–98.

20. Waugh, E.; Mackenzie, L. Ageing well from an urban Indigenous Australian perspective. *Aust. Occup. Ther. J.* **2011**, *58*, 25–33. [CrossRef] [PubMed]

21. Australian Bureau of Statistics. *Life Tables for Aboriginal and Torres Strait Islander Australians, 2010–2012 (Catalogue Number 3302.0.55.003)*; Australian Bureau of Statistics: Canberra, Australia, 2013.

22. Hyde, Z.; Flicker, L.; Smith, K.; Atkinson, D.; Fenner, S.; Skeat, L.; Lo Giudice, D. Prevalence and incidence of frailty in Aboriginal Australians, and association with mortality and disability. *Maturitas* **2016**, *87*, 89–94. [CrossRef] [PubMed]

23. Temple, J. Severe and moderate forms of food insecurity in Australia: Are they distinguishable? *Aust. J. Soc. Issues* **2008**, *43*, 649–668. [CrossRef]

24. McCullagh, P. Regression models for ordinal data. *J. R. Stat. Soc. Ser. B (Methodological)* **1980**, *42*, 109–142.

25. Raftery, A. Bayesian model selection in social research. *Sociol. Methodol.* **1995**, *25*, 111–163. [CrossRef]

26. Belsley, D.; Kuh, E.; Welsch, R. *Regression Diagnostics: Identifying Influential Data and Sources of Collinearity*; John Wiley & Sons, Inc.: New York, NY, USA, 1980.

27. Brant, R. Assessing proportionality in the proportional odds model for ordinal logistic regression. *Biometrics* **1990**, *46*, 1171–1178. [CrossRef] [PubMed]

28. Radimer, L.; Allsopp, R.; Harvey, P.; Friman, D.; Watson, E. Food insufficiency in Queensland. *Aust. N. Zeal. J. Public Health* **1997**, *21*, 303–310. [CrossRef]

29. Kendall, A.; Olson, C.; Frongillo, E. Relationship of hunger and food insecurity to food availability and consumption. *J. Am. Diet. Assoc.* **1996**, *96*, 1019–1024. [CrossRef]

30. Rose, D.; Oliveria, D. Nutrient intakes of individuals from food insufficient households in the United States. *Am. J. Public Health* **1997**, *87*, 1956–1961. [CrossRef] [PubMed]

31. Heflin, C.; Siefert, K.; Williams, D. Food insufficiency and women's mental health: Findings from a 3 year panel of welfare recipients. *Soc. Sci. Med.* **2005**, *61*, 1971–1982. [CrossRef] [PubMed]

32. Sharkey, J. Risk and presence of food insufficiency are associated with low nutrient intakes and multimorbidity among housebound older women who receive home-delivered meals. *J. Nutr.* **2003**, *133*, 3485–3491. [CrossRef] [PubMed]

33. Stuff, J.; Casey, P.; Szeto, K.; Gossett, G.; Robbins, J.; Simpson, P.; Connell, C.; Bogle, M. Household food insecurity is associated with adult health status. *J. Nutr.* **2004**, *134*, 2330–2335. [CrossRef] [PubMed]

34. Tarasuk, V. Household food insecurity with hunger is associated with women's food intakes, health and household circumstances. *J. Nutr.* **2001**, *131*, 2670–2676. [CrossRef] [PubMed]

35. Vozoris, N.; Tarasuk, V. Household food insufficiency is associated with poorer health. *J. Nutr.* **2003**, *133*, 120–126. [CrossRef] [PubMed]

36.	Laraia, B.; Siega-Riz, A.; Gundersen, C.; Dole, N. Psychosocial factors and socioeconomic indicators are associated with household food insecurity among pregnant women. *J. Nutr.* **2006**, *136*, 177–182. [CrossRef] [PubMed]

37.	German, L.; Kahana, C.; Rosenfeld, V.; Zabrowsky, I.; Wiezer, Z.; Fraser, D.; Shahar, D. Depressive symptoms are associated with food insufficiency and nutritional deficiencies in poor community-dwelling elderly people. *J. Nutr. Health Aging* **2011**, *15*, 3–8. [CrossRef] [PubMed]

38.	Russell, J.C.; Flood, V.M.; Yeatman, H.; Wang, J.J.; Mitchell, P. Food insecurity and poor diet quality are associated with reduced quality of life in older adults. *Nutr. Diet.* **2016**, *73*, 50–58. [CrossRef]

39.	Hamelin, A.; Habicht, J.; Beaudry, M. Food insecurity: Consequences for the household and broader social implications. *J. Nutr.* **1999**, *129*, 525s–528s. [CrossRef] [PubMed]

40.	Council of Australian Governments. *Closing the Gap in Indigenous Health Outcomes*; Council of Australian Governments: Canberra, Australia, 2009.

41.	Australian Institute of Health and Welfare. *Cardiovascular Disease, Diabetes and Chronic Kidney Disease—Australian Facts: Aboriginal and Torres Strait Islander People*; Cardiovascular, Diabetes and Chronic Kidney Disease Series No. 5. (Cat. No. CDK 5); Australian Institute of Health and Welfare: Canberra, Australia, 2015.

42.	Cunningham, J.; Paradies, Y. Patterns and correlates of self-reported racial discrimination among Australian Aboriginal and Torres Strait Islander adults, 2008–09: Analysis of national survey data. *Int. J. Equity Health* **2013**, *12*, 47. [CrossRef] [PubMed]

43.	Ferguson, M.; King, A.; Brimblecombe, J.K. Time for a shift in focus to improve food afford ability for remote customers. *Med. J. Aust.* **2016**, *204*, 409. [CrossRef] [PubMed]

44.	Pollard, C.; Nyaradi, A.; Lester, M.; Sauer, K. Understanding food security issues in remote Western Australian Indigenous communities. *Health Prom. J. Aust.* **2014**, *25*, 83–89. [CrossRef] [PubMed]

45.	Brimblecombe, J.K.; Ferguson, M.M.; Libert, S.C.; O'Dea, K. Characteristics of the community-level diet of Aboriginal people in remote northern Australia. *Med. J. Aust.* **2013**, *198*, 380–384. [CrossRef] [PubMed]

46.	Pollard, C. Selecting interventions for food security in remote indigenous communities. In *Food Security in Australia: Challenges and Prospects for the Future*; Farmar-Bowers, Q., Higgins, V., Millar, J., Eds.; Springer: New York, NY, USA, 2013; ISBN 978-1-4614-4484-8.

47.	Browne, J.; Laurence, S.; Thorpe, S. Acting on Food Insecurity in Urban Aboriginal and Torres Strait Islander Communities: Policy and Practice Interventions to Improve Local Access and Supply of Nutritious Food. 2009. Available online: http://www.healthinfonet.ecu.edu.au/health-risks/nutrition/other-reviews (accessed on 1 October 2017).

48.	Bramwell, L.; Foley, W.; Shaw, T. Putting urban Aboriginal and Torres Strait Islander food insecurity on the agenda. *Aust. J. Primary Health* **2017**, *23*, 415–419. [CrossRef] [PubMed]

49.	Browne, J.; Hayes, R.; Gleeson, D. Aboriginal health policy: Is nutrition the 'gap' in 'Closing the Gap'? *Aust. N. Zeal. J. Public Health* **2014**, *38*, 362–369. [CrossRef] [PubMed]

50.	Browne, J.; Adams, K.; Atkinson, P.; Gleeson, D.; Hayes, R. Food and nutrition programs for Aboriginal and Torres Strait Islander Australians: An overview of systematic reviews. *Aust. Health Rev.* **2018**. [CrossRef] [PubMed]

51.	LoGiudice, D. The health of older Aboriginal and Torres Strait Islander peoples. *Aust. J. Ageing* **2016**, *35*, 82–85. [CrossRef] [PubMed]

52.	Vahabi, M.; Martin, L. Food insecurity: Who is being excluded? A case of older people with dementia in long-term care homes. *J. Nutr. Health Aging* **2014**, *18*, 685–691. [CrossRef] [PubMed]

53.	Radermacher, H.; Feldman, S.; Bird, S. Food security in older Australians from different cultural backgrounds. *J. Nutr. Educ. Behav.* **2010**, *42*, 328. [CrossRef] [PubMed]

54.	Wolfe, W.; Frongillo, E.; Valois, P. Understanding the experience of food insecurity by elders suggests ways to improve its measurement. *J. Nutr.* **2003**, *133*, 2762. [CrossRef] [PubMed]

55.	Quandt, S.; Arcury, T.; McDonald, J.; Bell, R.; Vitolins, M. Meaning and management of food security among rural elders. *J. Appl. Gerontol.* **2001**, *10*, 356–376. [CrossRef]

56.	Bhargava, V.; Lee, J. Food insecurity and health care utilization among older adults. *J. Appl. Gerontol.* **2017**, *36*, 1415–1432. [CrossRef] [PubMed]

57.	Wolfe, W.; Olson, C.; Kendall, M.; Frongillo, E. Understanding food insecurity in the elderly: A conceptual framework. *J. Nutr. Educ.* **1996**, *28*, 92–100. [CrossRef]

58. Department of Prime Minister and Cabinet. *Closing the Gap: Prime Ministers Report 2018*; Department of Prime Minister and Cabinet: Canberra, Australia, 2018.
59. Biddle, N.; Gray, M.; Schwab, J. *Measuring and analyzing success for Aboriginal and Torres Strait Islander Australians (CAEPR Working Paper 122/2017)*; Centre for Aboriginal Economic Policy Research ANU: Canberra, Australia, 2017.

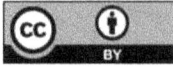

International Journal of
*Environmental Research
and Public Health*

MDPI

Article

Factors Associated with Continued Food Insecurity among Households Recovering from Hurricane Katrina

Lauren A. Clay [1,3,4,*] , Mia A. Papas [2], Kimberly B. Gill [3] and David M. Abramson [4]

1   Health Services Administration, D'Youville College, Buffalo, NY 14201, USA
2   Christiana Care Health System, Value Institute, Wilmington, DE 19899, USA; mia.papas@christianacare.org
3   Disaster Research Center, University of Delaware, Newark, DE 19716, USA; kgill@udel.edu
4   College of Global Public Health, New York University, New York, NY 10012, USA;
    david.abramson@nyu.edu
*   Correspondence: clayl@dyc.edu; Tel.: +1-716-829-8101

Received: 18 June 2018; Accepted: 25 July 2018; Published: 3 August 2018

Abstract: In 2010, 14.5% of US households experienced food insecurity, which adversely impacts health. Some groups are at increased risk for food insecurity, such as female-headed households, and those same groups are often also at increased risk for disaster exposure and the negative consequences that come with exposure. Little research has been done on food insecurity post-disaster. The present study investigates long-term food insecurity among households heavily impacted by Hurricane Katrina. A sample of 683 households participating in the Gulf Coast Child and Family Health Study were examined using a generalized estimation model to determine protective and risk factors for food insecurity during long-term recovery. Higher income (Odds Ratio (OR) 0.84, 95% Confidence Interval (CI) 0.77, 0.91), having a partner (OR 0.93; 95% CI 0.89, 0.97), or "other" race were found to be protective against food insecurity over a five-year period following disaster exposure. Low social support (OR 1.14; 95% CI 1.08, 1.20), poor physical health (OR 1.08; 95% CI 1.03, 1.13) or mental health (OR 1.13; 95% CI 1.09, 1.18), and female sex (OR 1.05; 95% CI 1.01, 1.10) were risk factors. Policies and programs that increase access to food supplies among high-risk groups are needed to reduce the negative health impacts of disasters.

Keywords: food insecurity; disaster; family health; Hurricane Katrina; mental health; physical health; social support

1. Introduction

In 2010, 14.5 percent of households in the United States experienced food insecurity, an increase from 11.0 percent in 2005 and 10.9 percent in 2006. Furthermore, 9.8 percent of households with children experienced food insecurity at some point during 2010, affecting 3.9 million households [1].

Food insecurity is higher than the national average for households with children, headed by a single adult, with low income, in rural or urban areas, for minorities, and those residing in the South region of the US [1,2]. The United States Department of Agriculture (USDA) reports that food insecurity is three times more prevalent in single-female-headed households compared to households headed by married couples [3,4]. Furthermore, food insecurity is more than twice as likely in households headed by Hispanic or Black individuals than those households headed by non-Hispanic whites [2]. Food insecurity in the South in 2010 was 10.4 percent, higher than the West (9.4 percent), Midwest (8.1 percent) and Northeast (7.7 percent) regions [1]. In addition to socio-economic factors, a caregiver with poor physical and mental health, disability, weaker social ties and emotional support, and changes in housing or income stability are risk factors for child food insecurity [5–9].

Many research studies have demonstrated that children in food insecure households are at risk for adverse physical and mental health consequences, such as behavioral problems, lower educational achievement, psychosocial dysfunction, depressive symptoms, suicidal symptoms, anxiety, and chronic health conditions [10–16]. A recent literature review completed by Gunderson and colleagues found that food-insecure children are more likely to experience "anemia, lower nutrient intake, cognitive problems, higher levels of aggression and anxiety, poorer general health, poorer oral health, and higher risk of being hospitalized, having asthma, having some birth defects, or experiencing behavioral problems" [17].

Even though there are a number of assistance programs to increase nutritious food intake among those at risk, such as the Special Supplemental Feeding Program for Women, Infant, and Children (WIC), the Supplemental Nutrition Assistance Program (SNAP), and the National School Lunch Program (NSLP), food insecurity remains high in the United States, due at least in part to the lack of understanding about the causes of food insecurity and lack of evidence for effective policy and program solutions [17]. Gaps in research on food insecurity remain. While research shows that disability influences food security, for example, little research has investigated how disability is associated with food insecurity risk. Many studies of risk and protective factors use nationally representative samples in the United States; little research has focused on overlooked groups or special populations outside of traditional demographic groups. Policy solutions are likely to look different for specific populations, such as those that have experienced a significant disaster event. Long-term data collection has also been called for to better understand how food insecurity changes over time, as well as studies that incorporate qualitative methods and the voices of children to more fully tell the story of food insecurity in the U.S. [17–19].

Few studies have focused on food insecurity post-disaster in the United States. Programs have been implemented to aid food-insecure populations after disaster, such as modifications to allowable purchases for Supplemental Nutrition Assistance Program (SNAP) beneficiaries after Superstorm Sandy in New Jersey so families were able to repurchase lost food supplies [20], however little is understood about those that are living on the cusp of food insecurity that may be pushed into insecurity due to the disruption of a disaster or other change in circumstance, such as changes in housing or decline in mothers' mental health [9].

We know that vulnerability to disaster exposure and negative consequences vary based on resource access, age, physical ability, sex, race and ethnicity, and living conditions [21–23]. We also know that single women, single mothers, and caregivers, in addition to experiencing increased risk of food insecurity, are also more vulnerable following disasters [3,4,24], and race, ethnicity, disability, functional and access needs, and mental health contribute to decreased disaster preparedness and may impede or slow disaster recovery [25–31]. Following disaster exposure, resources are lost, including material (personal property), social (social support), and neighborhood-based resources due to relocation, and food insecurity is common or the odds of food insecurity increase [32–36]. Resource loss contributes to psychological distress, such as anxiety, depression, and post-traumatic stress disorder (PTSD) [33,34,37]. This loops back to the influence of caretaker mental health on child food security.

Factors contributing to food insecurity and disaster risk are complex, and the impact from each influences health outcomes. However, few studies have explored food insecurity in a post-disaster setting. In summary, prior research has established the impact of food insecurity on health and well-being, the noted risk factor of changes in housing and economic circumstance on food insecurity risk, the need for longitudinal study of food insecurity, and the evidence of increased food insecurity risk post-Hurricane Katrina. Given this, the present study examines long-term food insecurity in a sample of households heavily impacted by Hurricane Katrina, taking into account resource loss and demographic characteristics.

2. Materials and Methods

2.1. Sample and Data Collection

Households were surveyed as part of the Gulf Coast Child and Family Health (G-CAFH) Study, a longitudinal study of household disaster recovery following Hurricane Katrina in Louisiana and Mississippi. Households were recruited in 2006 and participated in an annual follow up. Households were randomly sampled from census blocks classified by Federal Emergency Management Agency (FEMA) assessments as moderately to extensively damaged, and from FEMA subsidized housing. The current analysis examined data from households that participated in waves two, three, and four of the G-CAFH Study. Wave two was collected between May and July 2007 (*n* = 803), wave three was collected between June and August 2008 (*n* = 777), and wave four was collected between October 2009 and March 2010 (*n* = 844), resulting in a four-year observation period for 683 households. A bias analysis conducted by the G-CAFH Study team demonstrated that there are no significant differences due to attrition between the cohort at wave one and at wave four. Additional information on study design and methodology has been published elsewhere [38,39].

2.2. Measures

Food insecurity was assessed in waves two, three, and four of the study by asking participants to think about their basic needs over the past three to six months. In wave two, respondents were asked to report on the past six months, "How well has your need for food for the household been met?" (not met, somewhat met, or met completely), and in waves three and four, respondents were asked, "In the past three months, how often it has happened there was not enough money in the household for food that you (the family) should have?" (never, once in a while, fairly often, or very often). Respondents were classified as food insecure in each wave if they answered that the need was not met or they fairly or very often did not have enough money in the household for food. The United States Department of Agriculture defines food insecurity as "a household-level economic and social condition of limited or uncertain access to adequate food [40]." The G-CAFH study questions are intended to capture social and economic limitations to access adequate food. Although not validated against the USDA measure for food insecurity, these questions provide a starting point to understand food insecurity in a disaster-affected population.

Social support was assessed by asking respondents if they had someone they could count on for everyday favors, such as borrowing a little money, to care for you if you were confined to a bed for several weeks, to lend you money for a medical emergency, to talk to about family relationship troubles, or to help you find housing if you had to move. Respondents were categorized as having low social support if they responded yes to fewer than two of these statements.

Physical and mental health were self-reported by respondents using the Short Form (SF)-12 Health Survey [41]. The Mental Component Score (MCS) and Physical Component Score (PCS) were computed. A PCS score of less than 45 was classified as Physical Health Distress, and an MCS score of less than 42 was classified as Mental Health Distress, consistent with past research [41,42]. Respondents were classified as having a disability if they responded "disabled" when reporting on characteristics of the household.

Demographic variables included in this analysis included income (<$10 K, $10–20 K, $20–35 K, $35–50 K, >$50 K), age (18–34, 35–49, 50–65, 66+), race and ethnicity (Black, White, Latino, other), and sex (male, female) and were self-reported by G-CAFH participants.

2.3. Statistical Analysis

Generalized estimating equations were used to determine bivariate associations between each exposure variable and our outcome over time. In addition, this longitudinal modeling strategy was employed to examine multivariate associations between exposures and food insecurity after adjustment for confounding. Models utilized wave of data collection as the family variable and study identification number as the link variable. Generalized estimating equations enable analysis of repeated measures over time and take into account the dependent structure of the data, given within-person correlation. The benefits of this approach include accounting for within-subject and within-group correlation and accommodating inconsistent intervals between data points [43]. Factors that were independently associated with food insecurity over time were included in a multivariate longitudinal model that utilized a generalized estimating equation. Stata 13 version 1 was used for analyses (StataCorp LP, College Station, TX, USA) [44].

3. Results

Table 1 presents demographic characteristics of the sample (*n* = 683) at each wave. Changes in age, sex, partnership status, and race/ethnicity composition over time were assessed, and findings show there was stability in characteristics over the three time periods (all *p*-values for change >0.05). The sample was 51.5 percent Black, 43 percent White and 2.7 percent Latino. Over 60% of respondents were female. Changes in employment status, income level, and number of moves since Hurricane Katrina were statistically significant over the three waves of data collection. Employment dropped in the fourth wave of follow up, and income and number of moves increased over time.

Table 1. Sample Characteristics and significance of change over time.

Sample Characteristics	Wave 2 (2007)	Wave 3 (2008)	Wave 4 (2009–2010)
	n (within col %)	*n* (within col %)	*n* (within col %)
Employed (20+ h per week) **	335 (45.6)	349 (45.5)	328 (40.0)
Partnered (married, living as married)	341 (42.5)	344 (44.5)	372 (44.2)
Income *			
<$10 K	274 (34.3)	224 (29.1)	241 (28.7)
$10–20 K	258 (32.3)	214 (27.8)	265 (31.5)
$20–35 K	126 (15.8)	157 (20.39)	149 (17.7)
$35–50 K	71 (8.9)	88 (11.4)	87 (10.3)
>$50 K	58 (7.3)	68 (8.8)	84 (10.0)
Don't know/refused	12 (1.5)	19 (2.5)	15 (1.8)
Age			
18–34	154 (19.2)	129 (16.7)	142 (16.8)
35–49	272 (34.0)	266 (34.4)	272 (32.2)
50–65	271 (33.8)	271 (35.0)	305 (36.1)
66+	104 (13.0)	108 (14.0)	125 (14.8)
Number of moves since Katrina [Mean (SD)] ***	3.79 (2.00)	3.81 (2.04)	4.59 (2.95)
Race/Ethnicity			
Black	420 (51.5)		
White	351 (43.0)		
Latino	22 (2.7)	Constant variables	
Other	23 (2.8)		
Sex			
Male	305 (39.3)		
Female	471 (60.7)		

* *p* < 0.05, ** *p* < 0.01, *** *p* < 0.001.

Food insecurity, disability, mental health, and social support prevalence in the study sample changed significantly over time (Table 2). Food insecurity ranged from 30.4 percent in wave two to 20.1 percent in wave three. In wave four, food insecurity prevalence increased slightly to 23.1 percent. Disability prevalence increased with each subsequent wave of data collection, from 13.4 percent in wave two to 20.5 percent in wave four. Poor mental health and low social support prevalence decreased with each subsequent wave of data collection (47.9 to 38.5 and 24.2 to 15.3 percent, respectively).

Table 2. Sample Health Characteristics and significance of change over time ˆ.

Health Characteristics	Wave 2	Wave 3	Wave 4
	n (within col %)	*n* (within col %)	*n* (within col %)
Food insecurity ***	244 (30.4)	163 (21.0)	194 (23.1)
Disabled ***	98 (13.4)	121 (15.8)	173 (20.5)
Poor physical health	405 (50.7)	397 (51.2)	435 (51.7)
Poor mental health ***	383 (47.9)	300 (38.7)	324 (38.5)
Low social support ***	186 (24.2)	129 (18.4)	125 (15.3)

*** $p < 0.001$. ˆ p-values from chi2 statistic reported for at least one difference between waves.

Examination of bivariate associations among health, demographic characteristics, and the outcome food insecurity indicated employment, partnership, income, older age (66+), and white race are statistically significant and inversely associated with food insecurity, while female sex, moves since Katrina, disability, poor physical and mental health, and low social support were statistically significant and positively associated with food insecurity (Table 3).

Table 3. Bivariate association between demographic characteristics and health status with food insecurity over time ˆ.

Demographic and Health Characteristics	Beta Coefficient	Standard Error
Employed (20+ h per week) ***	−0.08	0.02
Partnered (married, living as married) ***	−0.10	0.02
Income (<$10 K)		
$10–20 K **	−0.06	0.02
$20–35 K ***	−0.16	0.03
$35–50 K ***	−0.24	0.03
>$50 K ***	−0.30	0.03
Don't know/refused	−0.11	0.06
Age (18–34)		
35–49	0.02	0.03
50–65	−0.03	0.03
66+ **	−0.11	0.04
Race/Ethnicity (Black)		
White **	−0.06	0.02
Latino	0.07	0.07
Other	−0.12	0.07
Sex (Male)		
Female ***	0.08	0.02
Moves since Katrina *	0.01	0.004
Disabled ***	0.13	0.02
Poor physical health ***	0.10	0.02
Poor mental health ***	0.17	0.02
Low social support ***	0.17	0.02

* $p < 0.05$, ** $p < 0.01$, *** $p < 0.001$. ˆ xtgee models run for each independent variable and the dichotomous outcome food insecurity.

These factors were included in a generalized estimation equation model for panel data to determine associations with food insecurity two to five years after initial exposure to Hurricane Katrina (Table 4). Respondents who reported having a partner (OR 0.93; 95% CI 0.89, 0.97), higher income ($35–50 K OR 0.89; 0.83, 0.96; >$50 K OR 0.84; 0.77, 0.91), and being White (OR 0.95; 0.91, 1.10) or "other" race (OR 0.84; 0.73, 0.97) were less likely to report food insecurity over a five-year time frame post-disaster. Respondents who were female (OR 1.05; 1.01, 1.10), reported poor physical health (OR 1.08; 1.03, 1.13) or mental health (OR 1.13; 1.09, 1.18), or low social support (OR 1.14; 1.08, 1.20) were more likely to report food insecurity over time.

Table 4. Odds of reporting food insecurity by demographic and health characteristics of respondents over time.

Demographic and Health Characteristics	Odds Ratio	95% CI
Employed (20+ h per week)	1.00	(0.94, 1.04)
Partnered (married, living as married) *	0.93	(0.89, 0.97)
Income (<$10 K)		
$10–20 K	0.99	(0.94, 1.04)
$20–35 K **	0.92	(0.86, 0.98)
$35–50 K **	0.89	(0.83, 0.96)
>$50 K ***	0.84	(0.77, 0.91)
Don't know/refused	1.01	(0.85, 1.19)
Age (18–34)		
35–49	1.03	(0.97, 1.10)
50–65	0.96	(0.90, 1.02)
66+	0.90	(0.83, 0.98)
Race/Ethnicity (Black)		
White *	0.95	(0.91, 0.99)
Latino	1.06	(0.93, 1.21)
Other *	0.84	(0.73, 0.97)
Sex (Male)		
Female *	1.05	(1.01, 1.10)
Moves since Katrina	1.01	(0.997, 1.01)
Disabled ^	1.06	(1.00, 1.13)
Poor physical health **	1.08	(1.03, 1.13)
Poor mental health ***	1.13	(1.09, 1.18)
Low social support ***	1.14	(1.08, 1.20)

* $p < 0.05$, ** $p < 0.01$, *** $p < 0.001$. ^ $p = 0.05$.

4. Discussion

According to the USDA, average food insecurity prevalence in 2007–2009 in Louisiana and Mississippi was 10.0 percent and 17.1 percent, respectively [45]. We would expect baseline rates of food insecurity in this sample to be similar. We found food insecurity prevalence was 30.4, 21.0, and 23.1 percent in waves two, three, and four of data collection in the present sample, much higher than average state prevalence rates over a similar time frame. However, caution is warranted in comparing food insecurity rates from our study to the National average, since a standardized, validated measure of food insecurity was not included in the G-CAFH study, as the purpose of the study was to more broadly understand child and family health during long-term disaster recovery and it was not focused specifically on food insecurity. However, the high rate of food access issues described in this population make it increasingly important to examine the food environment post-disaster as it is not well understood, and there is little in the literature on the impact of disasters on those families that experience food insecurity during the year or may be living on the edge, and the disruption due to a disaster creates greater household strain.

In this sample of households heavily impacted by Hurricane Katrina, being female, having poor physical and mental health, and low social support were risk factors for food insecurity during long-term disaster recovery, and having a partner, greater income, and being non-Hispanic white or "other" race were protective against food insecurity. This is consistent with food insecurity research that demonstrates that female-headed households, individuals with poor physical or mental health, decline in mothers' physical or mental health and weaker social ties and emotional support are associated with increased food insecurity [3–5,8,9]. It is also consistent with the disaster literature that shows that certain populations are more vulnerable to increased disaster risk and adverse consequences following disasters, such as those with poor physical or mental health, women, and individuals with low social support [21,22,24,28–30,34]

The research question and analyses were planned after data collection was completed for waves one through four of the G-CAFH study, therefore the limitations of secondary analysis apply to the present investigation. There was no pre-event data on food insecurity prevalence for this sample due to the unpredictable nature of disasters, therefore we were not able to determine whether food insecurity was a pre-existing issue for families recovering from Hurricane Katrina or a new situation. For this analysis, the inconsistent wording of the food insecurity question may have resulted in different interpretations by the study participants from wave one to waves two and three. Data on this cohort, however, provide a number of distinct benefits that contribute to the existing literature. It was noted earlier that much of the food insecurity research has been conducted with nationally representative samples [17]. This investigation examined a sample of households heavily impacted by a disaster, and starts to tell the story of household food insecurity in a new population. Another strength of this study is in showing a picture of longer-term recovery and food insecurity through a longitudinal study design, which are costly and rare in the disaster literature [46,47]. The study was also carefully designed and executed to enable longitudinal analysis on a cohort, with an 87.6 percent retention rate at wave four of data collection.

To improve disaster outcomes and reduce recovery time, efforts to mitigate, prepare for, and respond to disasters should focus on engagement with vulnerable groups, such as those with physical and mental health distress, female-headed households, and socially isolated populations, to ensure adequate food access and availability. Following disasters, transportation lines may be interrupted, causing access issues for people with physical disabilities and mobility impairments. Further compounding access issues, supply chains may be interrupted, reducing the availability of foods in some areas following disasters [48,49]. Individuals with low social support may lack people to rely on for rides or other help to access foods. For individuals with poor mental health, the additional stress of the disaster experience may exacerbate conditions and result in lower self-efficacy and reduced functioning.

To reduce food insecurity during long-term recovery from disasters, programs and policies should be implemented to increase access to financial support for food or to ensure access to food supplies. One example of such an intervention is the re-issuance of SNAP or WIC benefits to replace spoiled or soiled food supplies and the expansion of benefits to include prepared foods, to enable families living without kitchen facilities to use benefits for meals, as was done following Superstorm Sandy in New Jersey to meet community needs [20]. Systematically adjusting these programs and making the policy known to the end user may reduce uncertainty following disasters and increase utilization. Furthermore, programs that are targeted to reach single-headed, female-headed, low-income, and minority households during non-disaster times with information about securing food in a disaster may reduce vulnerability. Such programs might include educational sessions on food provisions and programs following disasters, facilitation of neighborhood block or community based bulk purchasing of non-perishable foods, or availability of disaster preparedness kits including non-perishable foods through food banks or other food programs. Communicating and building a rapport with community organizations and high risk populations in non-disaster times may also enable more effective post-disaster communication about resources, programs, and services available to affected households. Additional research is needed to determine the effectiveness of policy interventions, such as the re-issued SNAP benefits, for reducing food insecurity post-disaster.

It is also interesting to note that number of moves post-Katrina was not a statistically significant predictor of food insecurity during long-term recovery. The food insecurity literature shows that a change in housing or income stability increases the risk of food insecurity [9]. The present study includes a sample of households heavily impacted by Hurricane Katrina, with families moving an average of 4.59 times at five years post-Katrina. However, in the present analysis, this was not associated with increased food insecurity risk. Additional research on households experiencing food and housing insecurity post-disaster is needed to better understand this circumstance.

This sample was part of a longitudinal study of child and family health following Hurricane Katrina, a group of households heavily impacted or displaced by Hurricane Katrina. This analysis is only a first step towards understanding food insecurity in a post-disaster setting among displaced families, but is not generalizable to all disaster affected populations or the general U.S. population. Additional research is needed on a representative sample of households impacted by disaster and in other geographic locations and hazard types.

5. Conclusions

Populations at increased risk for food insecurity also experience increased disaster risk and consequences. Disaster managers and public health practitioners working in these two spheres may be able to find synergy in non-disaster times, as well as when preparing for, responding to, and supporting recovery from disasters. Mitigation of food insecurity in the absence of a disaster may increase resilience to disasters for vulnerable households. Additional research on the experience of households that are food insecure at times during the year and those living with marginal food security, where exposure to a disaster leads them to have low or very low food security, is needed to better understand the health impacts of disaster and how to better meet the needs of this population. A better understanding of the role of housing disruption in a post-disaster setting is also needed to inform policies and programs to mitigate food insecurity for families recovering from disaster.

Author Contributions: Conceptualization, L.A.C., M.A.P., K.B.G., D.M.A.; Methodology, L.A.C., M.A.P., D.M.A.; Formal Analysis, L.A.C., M.A.P.; Investigation, L.A.C., M.A.P., K.B.G., D.M.A.; Data Curation, L.A.C., D.M.A.; Writing—Original Draft Preparation, L.A.C., M.A.P.; Writing—Review & Editing, L.A.C., M.A.P., K.B.G., D.M.A.

Funding: This research received no external funding.

Acknowledgments: The authors would like to acknowledge the original research team that conducted the Gulf Coast Child and Family Health Study at the National Center for Disaster Preparedness, the Children's Health Fund for funding the research, and the families that participated in the study for generously sharing their experiences in Hurricane Katrina so that we may learn about and work to improve the disaster recovery process.

Conflicts of Interest: The authors declare no conflict of interest.

References

1.   Coleman-Jensen, A.; Nord, M.; Andrews, M.; Carlson, S. *Household Food Security in the United States in 2011*; ERR-141, United States Department of Agriculture, Economic Research Service: Washington, DC, USA, September 2012.
2.   Nord, M.; Andrews, M.; Carlson, S. *Household Food Security in the United States, 2008*; ERR-83, United States Department of Agriculture, Economic Research Service: Washington, DC, USA, November 2009.
3.   Hill, S.A. Cultural images and the health of African American women. *Gender Soc.* **2009**, *23*, 733–746. [CrossRef]
4.   Schulz, A.J.; Mullings, L. *Gender, Race, Class, and Health: Intersectional Approaches*; Jossey-Bass: San Francisco, CA, USA, 2006.

5. Kaushal, N. *Income and Food Insecurity: New Evidence from the Fragile Families and Child Wellbeing Study*; Columbia University: New York, NY, USA, 2013.
6. Balistreri, K. *Family Structure, Work Patterns and Time Allocations: Potential Mechanisms of Food Insecurity among Children*; University of Kentucky Center for Poverty Research Discussion Paper Series, DP2012-07; Available online: http://www.ukcpr.org/Publications/DP2012-07.pdf (accessed on 3 May 2018).
7. Noonan, K.; Corman, H.; Reichman, N.E. Effects of Maternal Depression on Family Food Insecurity. *Econ. Hum. Biol.* **2016**, *22*, 201–215. [CrossRef] [PubMed]
8. Anderson, P.M.; Butcher, K.; Hoynes, H.; Schanzenbach, D.W. Beyond Income: What Else Predicts Very Low Food Security among Children? *South. Econ. J.* **2016**, *82*, 1078–1105. [CrossRef]
9. Jacknowitz, A.; Morrisey, T. *Food Insecurity across the First Five Years: Triggers of Onset and Exit*; University of Kentucky Center for Poverty Research Discussion Paper Series, DP2012-08; Available online: http://www.ukcpr.org/Publications/DP2012-08.pdf (accessed on 3 May 2018).
10. Bronte-Tinkew, J.; Zaslow, M.; Capps, R.; Horowitz, A.; McNamara, M. Food insecurity works through depression, parenting, and infant feeding to influence overweight and health in toddlers. *J. Nutr.* **2007**, *137*, 2160–2165. [CrossRef] [PubMed]
11. Casey, P.H.; Szeto, K.L.; Robbins, J.M.; Stuff, J.E.; Connell, C.; Gossett, J.M.; Simpson, P.M. Child health-related quality of life and household food security. *Arch. Pediatr. Adolesc. Med.* **2005**, *159*, 51–56. [CrossRef] [PubMed]
12. Jyoti, D.F.; Frongillo, E.A.; Jones, S.J. Food insecurity affects school children's academic performance, weight gain, and social skills. *J. Nutr.* **2005**, *135*, 2831–2839. [CrossRef] [PubMed]
13. Winicki, J.; Jemison, K. Food insecurity and hunger in the kindergarten classroom: Its effect on learning and growth. *Contemp. Econ. Policy* **2003**, *21*, 145–157. [CrossRef]
14. Kleinman, R.E.; Murphy, J.M.; Little, M.; Pagano, M.; Wehler, C.A.; Regal, K.; Jellinek, M.S. Hunger in children in the United States: Potential behavioral and emotional correlates. *Pediatrics* **1998**, *101*, e3. [CrossRef] [PubMed]
15. Weinreb, L.; Wehler, C.; Perloff, J.; Scott, R.; Hosmer, D.; Sagor, L.; Gundersen, C. Hunger: Its impact on children's health and mental health. *Pediatrics* **2002**, *110*, e41. [CrossRef] [PubMed]
16. Whitaker, R.C.; Phillips, S.M.; Orzol, S.M. Food insecurity and the risks of depression and anxiety in mothers and behavior problems in their preschool-aged children. *Pediatrics* **2006**, *118*, e859–e868. [CrossRef] [PubMed]
17. Gundersen, C.; Ziliak, J.P. Childhood food insecurity in the US: Trends, causes, and policy options. *Future Child.* **2014**, *24*, 1–19. [CrossRef]
18. Huang, J.; Guo, B.; Kim, Y. Food insecurity and disability: Do economic resources matter? *Soc. Sci. Res.* **2010**, *39*, 111–124. [CrossRef]
19. Coleman-Jensen, A.; Nord, M.; Singh, A. *Household Food Security in the United States in 2012*; ERR-155; United States Department of Agriculture, Economic Research Service: Washington, DC, USA, September 2013.
20. USDA Offers Food Assistance to Those Affected by Hurricane Sandy. Available online: https://www.fns.usda.gov/pressrelease/2012/034012 (accessed on 10 May 2018).
21. Comfort, L.; Wisner, B.; Cutter, S.; Pulwarty, R.; Hewitt, K.; Oliver-Smith, A.; Wiener, J.; Fordham, M.; Peacock, W.; Krimgold, F. Reframing disaster policy: The global evolution of vulnerable communities. *Environ. Hazards* **1999**, *1*, 39–44.
22. Wisner, B.; Blaikie, P.; Cannon, T.; Davis, I. *At Risk: Natural Hazards, People's Vulnerability and Disasters*, 2nd ed.; Psychology Press: New York, NY, USA, 2004.
23. Klinenberg, E. *Heat Wave. A Social Autopsy of Disaster in Chicago*; The University of Chicago Press: Chicago, IL, USA, 2002.
24. Enarson, E.; Fothergill, A.; Peek, L. Gender and disaster: Foundations and directions. In *Handbook of Disaster Research*; Rodríguez, H., Quarantelli, E.L., Dynes, R., Eds.; Springer: New York, NY, USA, 2007; pp. 130–146.
25. Ablah, E.; Konda, K.; Kelley, C.L. Factors Predicting Individual Emergency Preparedness: A Multi-state Analysis of 2006 BRFSS Data. *Biosecur. Bioterror.* **2009**, *7*, 317–330. [CrossRef] [PubMed]
26. Bethel, J.W.; Foreman, A.N.; Burke, S.C. Disaster preparedness among medically vulnerable populations. *Am. J. Prev. Med.* **2011**, *40*, 139–143. [CrossRef] [PubMed]
27. Eisenman, D.P.; Zhou, Q.; Ong, M.; Asch, S.; Glik, D.; Long, A. Variations in disaster preparedness by mental health, perceived general health, and disability status. *Disaster Med. Public Health Prep.* **2009**, *3*, 33–41. [CrossRef] [PubMed]

28. Bolin, R.; Jackson, M.; Crist, A. Gender inequality, vulnerability, and disaster: Issues in theory and research. In *The Gendered Terrain of Disaster: Through Women's Eyes*; Enarson, E., Hearn Morrow, B., Eds.; Praeger: Westport, CT, USA, 1998; pp. 27–44.

29. Fothergill, A.; Maestas, E.G.; Darlington, J.D. Race, ethnicity and disasters in the United States: A review of the literature. *Disasters* **1999**, *23*, 156–173. [CrossRef] [PubMed]

30. Phillips, B.D. *Disaster Recovery*; Taylor and Francis: Boca Raton, FL, USA, 2009.

31. Clay, L.A.; Goetschius, J.B.; Papas, M.A.; Kendra, J. Influence of Mental Health on Disaster Preparedness: Findings from the Behavioral Risk Factor Surveillance System, 2007–2009. *J. Homel. Secur. Emerg. Manag.* **2014**. [CrossRef]

32. Hobfoll, S.E. Conservation of resources: A new attempt at conceptualizing stress. *Am. Psychol.* **1989**, *44*, 513–524. [CrossRef] [PubMed]

33. Freedy, J.R.; Shaw, D.L.; Jarrell, M.P.; Masters, C.R. Towards an Understanding of the Psychological Impact of Natural Disasters: An Application of the Conservation Resources Stress Model. *J. Trauma. Stress* **1992**, *5*, 441–454. [CrossRef]

34. Zwiebach, L.; Rhodes, J.; Roemer, L. Resource loss, resource gain, and mental health among survivors of Hurricane Katrina. *J. Trauma. Stress* **2010**, *23*, 751–758. [CrossRef] [PubMed]

35. Clay, L.A.; Papas, M.; Gill, K.; Abramson, D. Food Insecurity during Long-term Recovery from Hurricane Katrina: A Longitudinal Analysis. *Ann. Epidemiol.* **2017**, *27*, 527–528. [CrossRef]

36. Hutson, R.A.; Trzcinski, E.; Kolbe, A.R. Features of child food insecurity after the 2010 Haiti earthquake: Results from longitudinal random survey of households. *PLoS ONE* **2014**, *9*, e104497. [CrossRef] [PubMed]

37. Arata, C.M.; Picou, J.S.; Johnson, G.D.; McNally, T.S. Coping with technological disaster: An application of the conservation of resources model to the Exxon Valdez oil spill. *J. Trauma. Stress* **2000**, *13*, 23–39. [CrossRef] [PubMed]

38. Abramson, D.M.; Stehling-Ariza, T.; Park, Y.S.; Gruber, D.; Wilson, C.; Sury, J.; Banister, A.N. *Second Wind: The Impact of Hurricane Gustav on Children and Families Who Survived Katrina*; Columbia University: New York, NY, USA, 2009.

39. Abramson, D.M.; Stehling-Ariza, T.; Park, Y.S.; Walsh, L.; Culp, D. Measuring Individual Disaster Recovery: A Socioecological Framework. *Disaster Med. Public Health Prep.* **2010**, *4*, S46. [CrossRef] [PubMed]

40. United States Department of Agriculture, Definitions of Food Insecurity. 2017. Available online: https://www.ers.usda.gov/topics/food-nutrition-assistance/food-security-in-the-us/definitions-of-food-security/ (accessed on 10 May 2018).

41. Ware, J.E., Jr.; Kosinski, M.; Keller, S.D. A 12-Item Short-Form Health Survey: Construction of scales and preliminary tests of reliability and validity. *Med. Care* **1996**, *34*, 220–233. [CrossRef] [PubMed]

42. Abramson, D.; Stehling-Ariza, T.; Garfield, R.; Redlener, I. Prevalence and predictors of mental health distress post-Katrina: Findings from the Gulf Coast Child and Family Health Study. *Disaster Med. Public Health Prep.* **2008**, *2*, 77–86. [CrossRef] [PubMed]

43. Fitzmaurice, G.M.; Laird, N.M.; Ware, J.H. *Applied Longitudinal Analysis*, 2nd ed.; Wiley-Interscience: Hoboken, NJ, USA, 2011.

44. StataCorp. *Stata Statistical Software*; StataCorp: College Station, TX, USA, 2013.

45. Nord, M.; Coleman-Jensen, A.; Andrews, M.; Carlson, S. *Household Food Security in the United States, 2009*; ERR-108; United States Department of Agriculture, Economic Research Service: Washington, DC, USA, November 2010.

46. Riad, J.K.; Norris, F.H. The influence of relocation on the environmental, social, and psychological stress experienced by disaster victims. *Environ. Behav.* **1996**, *28*, 163–182. [CrossRef]

47. Shrubsole, D. *Natural Disasters and Public Health Issues: A Review of the Literature with a Focus on the Recovery Period*; ICLR Research Paper Series; Institute for Catastrophic Loss Reduction: Toronto, ON, Canada, 1999.

48. Holguín-Veras, J.; Pérez, N.; Ukkusuri, S.; Wachtendorf, T.; Brown, B. Emergency logistics issues affecting the response to Katrina: A synthesis and preliminary suggestions for improvement. *Transp. Res. Rec.* **2007**, *2022*, 76–82. [CrossRef]

49. Holguín-Veras, J.; Jaller, M.; Van Wassenhove, L.N.; Pérez, N.; Wachtendorf, T. On the unique features of post-disaster humanitarian logistics. *J. Oper. Manag.* **2012**, *30*, 494–506. [CrossRef]

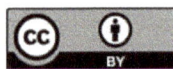

International Journal of
*Environmental Research
and Public Health*

MDPI

Article

The German Food Bank System and Its Users—A Cross-Sectional Study

Anja Simmet [1],*, Peter Tinnemann [2] and Nanette Stroebele-Benschop [1]

[1]   Institute of Nutritional Medicine, University of Hohenheim, 70593 Stuttgart, Germany;
      N.Stroebele@uni-hohenheim.de

[2]   Institute for Social Medicine, Epidemiology, and Health Economics at the Charité University Medical Center
      Berlin, 10117 Berlin, Germany; peter.tinnemann@charite.de

*   Correspondence: Anja.Simmet@uni-hohenheim.de; Tel.: +49-176-2288-9784

Received: 12 June 2018; Accepted: 12 July 2018; Published: 13 July 2018

Abstract: Although food banks are a well-known resource for low-income people struggling to meet their food needs, they have rarely been investigated on a large scale. This study aims to contribute to the actual debate about the potential and limitations of food banks to decrease the prevalence of food insecurity by providing a representative picture of the German food bank system and its users. Publicly accessible data were used to map residents, public welfare recipients, and food banks. In addition, a comprehensive survey was distributed to all 934 "Tafel" food banks. The results show that nearly all residents and welfare recipients have access to at least one food bank located in the districts in which they reside. Differences in the density of food banks exist between eastern and western Germany. Food banks provide mainly healthy fresh food, but they heavily rely on food donations from local retailers and on volunteer labor. Although changes in the number of user households by income seem to mirror trends in the number of welfare recipients, food bank users appear to represent only a fraction of the food-insecure population in Germany. Food banks might have the potential to improve users' diet and food security, but they are not able to reach all food-insecure residents in Germany.

Keywords: food bank; food insecurity; welfare recipients; poverty; food supply; food aid

---

1. Introduction

Over the last decades, food banks have become a critical food source for people with low income in many high-income countries including the USA [1], Canada [2], Australia [3], and in several European countries [4–7]. Although operation and organization of food banks differ widely between and even within countries, food banks are generally operated by charitable organizations that collect, store, and distribute food donated by retailers, the food industry, and farmers to needy people or to other charitable organizations [8].

Despite the differences in the social security systems across high-income countries, there seem to be commonalities in the characterization of food bank users. For instance, food banks initially aimed to provide temporary emergency assistance to people with financial hardships, whereas users today tend to visit food banks regularly for many years [2,6].

In Germany, the food bank system is called "Tafel" (table) and was initiated in 1993 to help homeless people in Berlin. To date, over 930 local branches of the Tafel food banks have been established throughout the country and they no longer limit assistance to homeless people but assist people with a very low or no income. Food banks usually apply eligibility criteria such as an income at or below the federal unemployment pay (Arbeitslosengeld II) and residence in the coverage area of the food bank [9,10], but in contrast to food banks in other countries such as in the UK [11] and the Netherlands [12], there is no referral system and social workers do not need to be involved.

Most food banks in Germany collaborate as members under the umbrella of the federal association "Tafel Deutschland" (Table Germany). Member food banks are solely financed by donations and receive no public financing [13]. As defined by the European Food Banks Federation, a member of which Tafel Deutschland just recently became [14], food banks serve as charitable organizations that help the poor. In this paper we use the expression "food bank" to describe all Tafel entities.

One of the few studies undertaken among food bank users in Germany showed that 70% of over 1000 participating food bank users in three German cities suffered from food insecurity [15]. Thus, food bank users in Germany seem to be less food insecure compared with food bank users in the USA [1], Canada [16], and the Netherlands [7], but they are seven to ten times more often food insecure than the general population [17]. In accordance with studies conducted in other countries [4,6,7], the study found a high prevalence of overweightness and obesity among food bank users (around 68%) [15], in particular among users born outside of Germany [18]. In another study, Depa et al. also revealed that the proportion of people who reported consuming fruit at least daily was lower among the 276 food bank users enrolled than among the representative population with a low socioeconomic status [6]. In addition, around 60% of participating food bank users reported suffering from at least one chronic disease including hypertension, diabetes, or mental illnesses [6]. In summary and in line with international results [4,7,19,20], food bank users in Germany seem to be a very vulnerable population group at high risk of having unfavorable health behaviors and health conditions.

Food banks may serve as an important civil societal resource through their low-threshold services and their nationwide structure. Although the German welfare system is considered more generous compared with those of other countries [21], the Tafel food bank system is the only nationwide immediate food assistance for people struggling to meet their food needs. However, in Germany there is no legal claim to a food bank's assistance and the nationwide distribution of food banks in relation to the general population and welfare recipients is unknown. Information on food banks' activities as well as user characteristics are missing on the national level. Studies on the food bank movement have only included samples from few regions or cities [6,9,15,22,23]. The evolution of food banks and rough estimates of the number of users have been illustrated through reports by Tafel Deutschland [24], but a scientific approach to characterize and describe the food bank system and its users on a national level is still missing.

This study aims to provide a representative overview of the German food bank system and its users by

- presenting the coverage rate of food banks in relation to the proportion of welfare recipients in German districts;
- illustrating food banks' structures, activities, and resources;
- counting and characterizing food bank users by source of household income;
- investigating the association of the number of food bank users and food bank resources and the proportion of welfare recipients in the district the food bank is located in, as well as between the main challenges of food banks and resources and demands of the food banks.

To do this, an explorative cross-sectional study was conducted. Freely accessible data of Tafel Deutschland and the Federal Office of Statistics were used and a comprehensive survey was distributed among all food banks associated with Tafel Deutschland. Illustrating the resources and demands of the food bank system will help to evaluate the potential of food banks to improve the users' food security level and dietary quality.

2. Materials and Methods

The study area included the entire country of Germany consisting of 432 districts and district-free cities (counties, "Landkreise, kreisfreie Städte") and of 11,437 municipalities ("Gemeinden") [25]. Tafel Deutschland provided a current list of all registered member food banks [26].

The cross-sectional survey took place from 13 September until 5 December 2017. All food banks received an email containing information about the study, its aims, the voluntary basis of participation, and data protection. The email included a link to a comprehensive online survey, which took approximately 60 min to complete. The link to the survey was also available as a bulletin posted on the intranet of Tafel Deutschland, which is accessible to all member food banks. The person responsible for the local food bank was requested to respond to the survey. Nine fuel vouchers (three of each, valued at €500, €300, and €100) were raffled among all participating food banks. By 23 October 2017, 281 of the 934 food banks had participated in the survey. In order to increase participation amongst food banks, a shorter version of the survey was developed and all food banks that had not yet participated received a reminder email containing the link to the shortened survey, which took approximately 30 min to complete. Additionally, food banks were contacted by telephone and encouraged to participate by answering the survey over the phone. This increased participation in the survey by another 273 additional food banks.

The study was approved by the Ethics Committee of the University of Hohenheim, Stuttgart.

2.1. Measures

The addresses of all food banks associated to Tafel Deutschland were received from Tafel Deutschland [26]. The most recent publicly available data on recipients of social welfare at district level is from the end of 2015 [27]. Publicly available shape files of German districts and district-free cities as well as of municipalities with the number of residents were retrieved from the Service Center of the Federal Government for Geo-Information and Geodesy [25].

The development of the survey questionnaire was guided by intense literature research [1,8,28,29] and through consultations with staff from Tafel Deutschland. It contained questions of the following domains: distribution schemes, services and projects of the food bank, food bank users, distributed food, food donors, food bank staff, and perceived challenges of the food bank in 2017. In addition, the long version of the questionnaire included questions on food bank's facilities including storage space, waiting room(s) and transportation vehicles, organic waste accrued at the local food banks, and use of materials of the umbrella organization Tafel Deutschland. Due to reasons of clarity, these latter topics will not be included in the present analyses. Since the majority of the local food banks were not able to state the exact change in weight of food distributed or the number of users per month in 2017 compared to 2016, they were asked to rank possible changes from −2 (more than 20% less in 2017 compared to 2016), −1 (1–20% less), 0 (equal), +1 (1–20% more), +2 (more than 20% more) for both number of users and donated food weight.

The shortened questionnaire also covered all of the domains presented by this article, but in less detail (e.g., by asking for only the number of users rather than for the number of users and the number of visits). A selection of the questionnaire content is provided in the Supplementary File 1.

2.2. Geographical and Statistical Analyses

Addresses of all food banks were geocoded using MMQGIS [30] in the freely available GIS (geographic information system) application QGIS (version 2.18.16) [31].

Districts and municipalities with and without at least one food bank available were identified by using the point-in-polygon function in QGIS [31].

The coverage rate of the food banks was determined by calculating the number of districts and municipalities with at least one food bank located in them. Moreover, the number and proportion of residents and of residents receiving welfare benefits living in a district or district-free city with at least one food bank was calculated. Differences in the number of residents between municipalities with and without at least one food bank and differences in the number of residents, the number of welfare recipients, and the proportion of welfare recipients between districts with and without at least one food bank were tested by the *t*-test for independent samples.

Descriptive statistics (mean, standard deviation, median, sum, percentage) were calculated to illustrate the basic characteristics of the participating food banks, the food bank users as well as changes in the number of food bank users per month in 2017 compared to 2016, the food distributed as well as changes in the weight of food distributed per month in 2017 compared to 2016, the food donors, the food bank workers, and the challenges of the participating food banks.

Differences in the central tendencies of ordinal data or data not normally distributed were tested with the Mann–Whitney test for two groups; the Kruskal–Wallis test was used for more than two groups. Differences in continuous data were tested with t-tests for two groups.

Multivariate linear regression models were applied to identify resources of local food banks and the percentage of welfare recipients in the district the food bank was located in that predicted the number of users per month. Variables included in the regression analyses were the number of programs offered, the weight of food distributed per month, the number of workers, the number of services related to food, the number of services unrelated to food, the weight of food each user received per month, the percentage of volunteers of all workers, and the number of welfare recipients in percentage of the population in the district the food bank was located in. Backward selection based on Akaike information criterion was applied to receive a parsimonious model.

To examine the associations of both major challenges of participating food banks (lack of volunteers, lack of food) with the resources and demands of the food bank, logistic regressions were conducted. In the first logistic model, the variables of resources and demands in 2017 were included in the analyses. In the second logistic model, ranked possible changes in the number of users and the weight of food distributed in 2017 compared to in 2016 were included.

Since the number of users per month and the weight of food distributed per month were highly skewed, these variables were log-transformed before conducting regression analyses.

A p-value of <0.05 was considered to be significant. Data cleaning, preparation, and visualization were performed using Microsoft Excel 2007 (Microsoft Corporation, Redmond, WA, USA). Statistical analyses were performed using R, version 3.4.3 (R Foundation for Statistical Computing, Vienna, Austria) [32].

3. Results

At first, results of the geographic analyses will be shown before presenting the descriptive survey results including services provided by food banks, food bank users, food distributed by food banks, food bank workers, and challenges of food banks. Finally, results of multiple regression analyses will be shown.

3.1. Geographic Analyses

There was at least one food bank in 6.89% ($n = 779$) of all German municipalities in 2015, but 53.02% of residents lived in municipalities with at least one food bank. Municipalities with at least one food bank had a significantly larger number of residents (M = 55,935) than municipalities without a food bank ((M = 3667), t(778.23) = -8.4648, $p < 0.0001$). When considering the municipalities with at least 10,000 residents, which correspond to a so-called "big town" ("große Kleinstadt") or larger, the percentage of municipalities with at least one food bank increased to 41.18% ($n = 649$).

At the next level of administrative units, 88.81% of districts had a least one food bank. The districts with at least one food bank had a larger number of residents (M = 214,983) than districts without a food bank ((M=120,592), t(280.58) = -5.9377, $p < 0.0001$). Districts with and without at least one food bank, however, did not differ in the number of welfare recipients as a percentage of the population (t(52.797) = -1.5547, $p = 0.13$). Overall, 93.40% of all residents and 94.52% of welfare recipients lived in districts in which they had access to at least one food bank.

As illustrated by Figure 1, the number of food banks per 10,000 welfare recipients was larger in districts of western Germany (M = 2.12) than in districts of eastern Germany ((M = 1.37), t(162.54) = 4.2424, $p < 0.0001$).

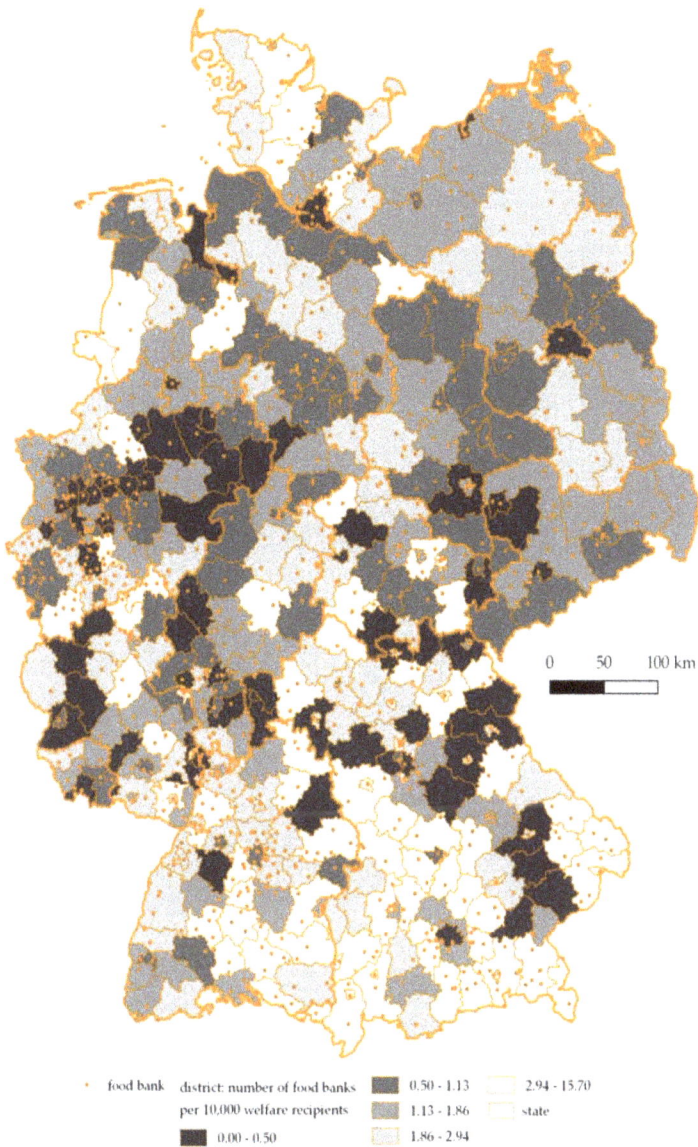

Figure 1. Number of food banks per 10,000 welfare recipients per district in Germany, 2014/2017.

3.2. Survey

A total of 554 questionnaires—329 from the comprehensive online survey, 130 from the survey by phone, and 95 from the short online survey—were analyzed. Due to missing values and invalid data, fewer participating food banks were included in most of the further analyses. Food banks participating in the survey and those not participating in the survey did not differ in the type of community ($\chi(5) = 9.8542$, $p = 0.079$), in the number of residents living in the district the food bank was located in ($t(780.26) = -0.094$, $p = 0.93$), or in the number of welfare recipients living in the district the food bank was located in ($t(660.29) = -0.33$, $p = 0.74$).

3.2.1. Services Provided by Food Banks

The schemes for the distribution of the foods largely varied between participating food banks. The large majority of them distributed foods in more or less predetermined quantities based on household size for a small fee or at no cost at distribution points (84.85% of participating food banks). In contrast, food banks in the Southern state of Germany Baden-Württemberg (state-specific data not shown) tended to operate as "social supermarkets" where eligible individuals can purchase food at a greatly reduced price (18.25%). The difference between a distribution point and a "social supermarket" is that in the latter the clients pay for each food product they want to buy, whereas in a distribution point they pay a predetermined small fee. Whether clients are allowed to choose the food items they want differs between distribution points. On average, each food bank managed 2.21 (SD 3.0) distribution points and/or social supermarkets. Overall, 7.48% of the participating food banks delivered food to other organizations such as women's shelters, youth centers, and drug rehabilitation facilities and served as so-called delivery food banks. In addition to these schemes, 10.40% of participating food banks also regularly supplied warm soups or other meals, whereas only a few of the participating food banks (3.28%) offer children a warm lunch at a so-called "Kinder Tafel" cafeteria. On average, each food bank managed 2.26 (SD 2.81) service programs (distribution points, social supermarkets, delivery food banks, soup kitchens, and/or children's food banks).

The majority of the distribution points (75.50%) and delivery food banks (56.67%) allowed users to collect food once per week, whereas supermarket-like shops (37.14%), soup kitchens (71.15%), and children's food banks (62.50%) tended to be open every day.

In addition to these standard schemes, 45% of participating food banks offered at least one additional service related to food, nutrition, or cooking such as a delivery service for home-dwelling elderly or disabled clients, offerings of coffee and cake during the hours of food distribution, and/or offerings of food recipes; 50% of them provided at least one additional service unrelated to food such as a thrift store, school supplies and toys, and/or social counseling.

3.2.2. Food Bank Users

Descriptive statistics of food bank users are presented in Table 1. Initially, data of 415 food banks were available. Since data of 49 food banks were inconsistent (number of child recipients aged less than 18 years and of adult users did not equal the overall number of users), data of 366 food banks were included in the analyses. As indicated by the large standard deviations, very large variations in the number of users were observed between participating food banks.

There were no significant differences in the number of users between food banks located in western or eastern Germany (U = 5090, p = 0.82).

For 89 districts, all available food banks participated in the survey. On average, 179 (SD = 137) welfare recipients per 1000 welfare recipients and 17 (SD = 17) residents of 1000 residents used a food bank in the district.

For 152 food banks, data of user households by source of household income were available (Table 1).

As illustrated in Figure 2, more than half of the participating food banks reported that the number of users per month had increased in 2017 compared with in 2016. The weighted mean of reported scale points indicated an increase of the number of users per month in 2017 compared with 2016 (Figure 3). The ranked increase was higher among child recipients than among adult users, but the difference was not statistically significant (U = 62,648, p = 0.20).

Participating food banks reported most changes for households receiving support according to the Asylum Seekers Benefit Act (Figure 2). The Kruskal–Wallis test revealed that there was a significant difference in the ranks indicating changes in the number of households per month in 2017 compared with 2016 between the household groups by income (H(7) = 16.949, p = 0.018). A posthoc test using Mann–Whitney tests with Bonferroni correction showed that the ranks for households receiving a low retirement or minimum social security benefits for the elderly was significantly higher than the ranks for households receiving student grants ($p = 0.007$), for households with labor income ($p = 0.022$), and for households with other income ($p = 0.022$).

Table 1. Sociodemographic characteristics of food bank users in Germany, 2017.

Characteristics of Food Bank Users	Mean	Standard Deviation	Median	% of Users
Users	1559	3126	726	100
Adult users	1120	2684	480	72
Child recipients	440	724	209	28
Households	696	952	300	/
Characteristics of Households of Food Bank Users	**Mean**	**Standard Deviation**	**Median**	**% of Households [2]**
Households receiving unemployment pay II [1]	260	436	115	49
Households receiving social security for asylum seekers	139	255	80	26
Senior households receiving low pension or minimum social security	83	131	40	16
Households receiving minimum security or disability benefits	37	63	18	7
Households with low labor income	10	25	0	2
Households with other income/no income	6	19	0	1

Note: For the characteristics of food bank users, data of 366 participating food banks were available and for the characteristics of households of food bank users, data of 152 participating food banks were available; excl. individuals who receive food from other noncharitable organizations such as women's shelters, schools, youth clubs, etc. that are delivered by delivery food banks; [1] unemployment pay II is a basic security benefit for job-seekers; [2] in rounded percent of the overall sum of households for which the source of household income was available.

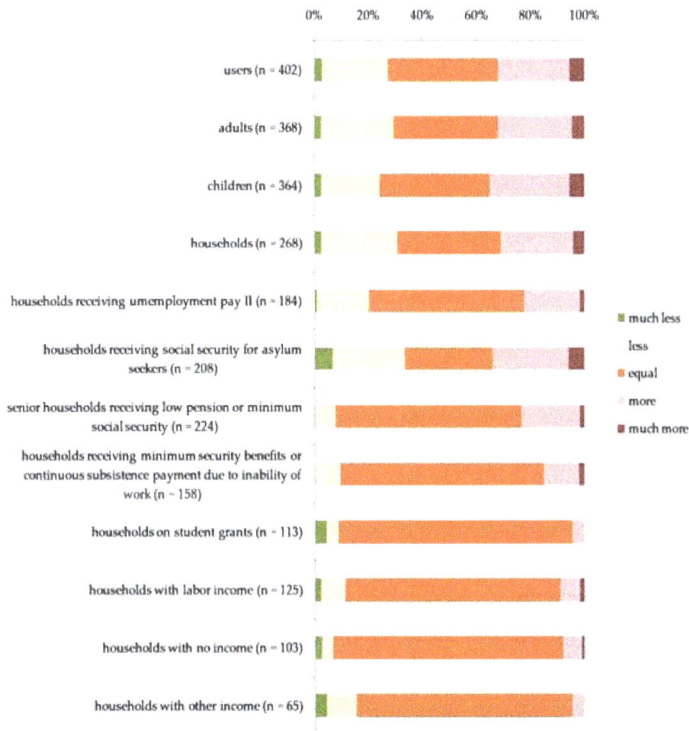

Figure 2. Comparison of the number of users of participating food banks per month in 2017 and 2016 in percent of participating food banks.

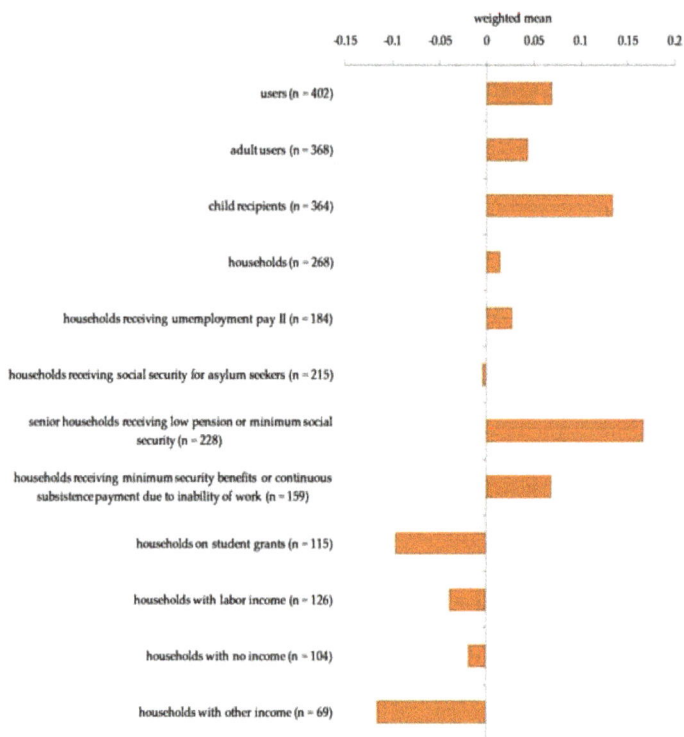

Figure 3. Number of users of participating food banks per month in 2017 compared with 2016 on a five-point scale.

3.2.3. Food Distributed by Food Banks

The mean weight of the food distributed monthly by each of the 328 food banks for which data were available amounted to 25.97 t (SD = 51.59). However, large variations could be observed and the distribution was highly skewed (median= 8.00 t). The mean weight of food per user per month was 23.92 kg (SD = 77.58 kg) and the median was 11.28 kg. There were no significant differences in the weight of the distributed food per month (U = 4647, p = 0.24) or in the weight of food per user per month between food banks in western and eastern Germany (U = 4547, p = 0.16).

The large majority of distributed food (82.29%) came from regular donors such as retailers. Less than 20% of distributed food came from single events or irregular donors (8.02%), the federal association Tafel Deutschland, state associations, and/or local distribution centers (7.68%), and/or from other sources (2.72%). Types of regular food donors are shown in Figure 4. Food banks reported receiving food from an average of 32.32 (SD = 34.25) regular donors.

As seen in Figure 5, the majority of food distributed per month was fruits and vegetables, followed by baked goods such as bread and pastries, milk products, and meat and meat products. Dry and frozen food, beverages, and sweets were distributed only in relatively small amounts. With the exception of baked goods, the amounts of almost all food groups were reported to have decreased in 2017 compared with 2016, as illustrated by Figure 6.

Overall, 47.45% of participating food banks reported that they infrequently (25.12%), sometimes (defined as once per four distribution days; 12.56%), often (defined as twice to thrice per four distribution days; 6.05%), or always (3.72%) had supply constraints, i.e., not enough food to cover demand in the months prior to the survey. Nearly 75% (74.51%) of them responded with a reduction in the amount of distributed food per household, 29.41% attempted to acquire more food from donors, 11.76% of them limited the membership and turned people seeking assistance away, and 7.48% implemented other measures to restrict access or to increase supply.

In contrast, 49.25% of participating food banks reported that they infrequently (32.84%), sometimes (11.94%), or always (4.48%) collected more food than they needed in the months before the survey. The majority of them (79.80%) distributed food they did not need to other nearby food banks, 51.52% of them froze or preserved food, 41.41% distributed excess food to other charitable organizations, 40.40% supplied users with more food, 13.13% threw excess food away, and 21.21% implemented other measures such as delivering the food to farmers for animal feed.

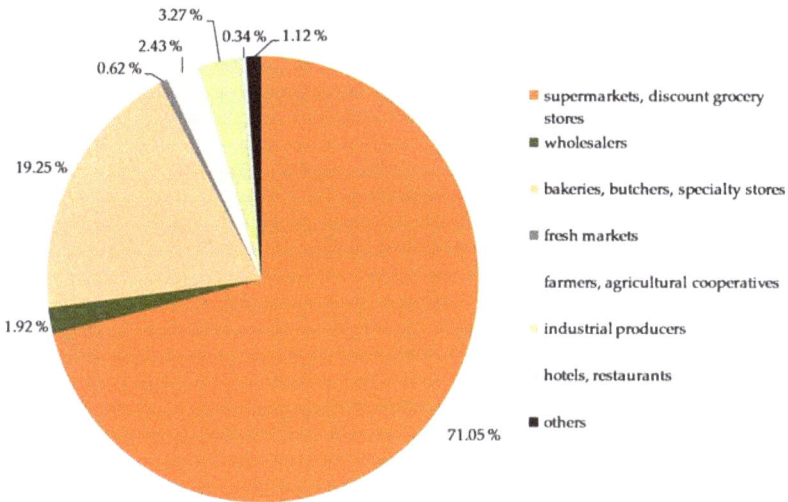

Figure 4. Types of regular food donors of participating food banks in percent, 2017.

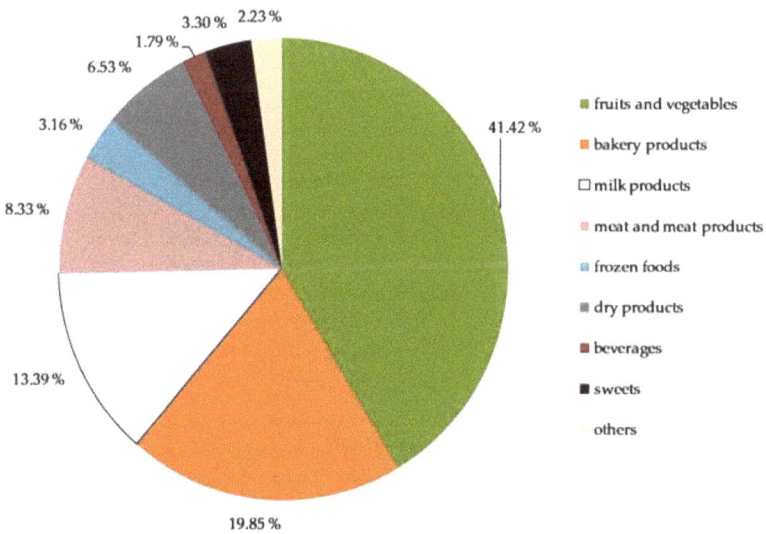

Figure 5. Categories of food distributed by participating food banks in percent, 2017.

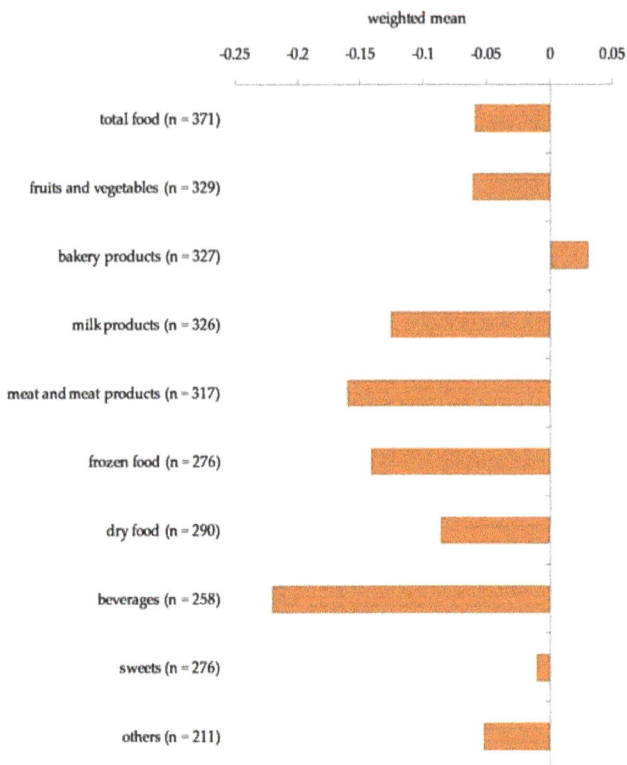

Figure 6. Weight of food distributed monthly by participating food banks in 2017 compared with 2016 on a five-point scale.

3.2.4. Food Bank Workers

The large majority (89.97%) of people working in the 387 participating food banks for which data were available were volunteers. On average, every participating food bank had 59 (SD = 56) volunteers with large variations being observed. Volunteers were mostly 65 years or older (68.46% of volunteers) and female (61.52%).

Overall, 64.16% of the participating food banks had some paid staff, of which the mean number (M = 7, SD = 21) was much lower than that of volunteers. The majority of paid workers were participating in a government-subsidized employment scheme, the so-called One-Euro-Jobs (42.01% of paid workers). Only a few amongst the paid staff were permanent employees (0.67% of paid workers). The number of workers (M = 33.02, SD = 33.90) as well as the number of volunteers as a percent of the total number of workers (M = 65.69, SD = 28.47) were significantly lower for food banks located in eastern Germany than for those located in western Germany (number of workers: M = 82.00, SD = 74.01, t(183.51) = 6.96, $p < 0.0001$; number of volunteers in percent of total number of workers: M = 91.48, SD = 14.47, t(58.01) = 6.32, $p < 0.0001$).

Nearly 20% of all workers (volunteers and paid staff) were eligible to use a Tafel food bank and approximately 2% of all workers were refugees.

On average, volunteers worked 33.23 h (SD = 38.02) and paid workers worked 79.55 h (SD = 47.80) per month in a food bank with large variations observed among food banks.

3.2.5. Challenges of Food Banks

Overall, 34.27% of the 321 participating food banks for which data were available stated that they had no challenges or problems in the last months. If problems were reported, the most frequent problem was a lack of volunteers (33.96% of participating food banks), in particular of volunteers with driver licenses who could pick up the food from retailers, followed by a lack of food (19.63%), in particular of milk products, meat, and sausages, and a lack of financial resources as well as lack of appropriate space (16.51% each).

3.2.6. Associations

Results of multiple linear regression of the log-transformed number of Tafel users on predictors are shown in Table 2. The predictors accounted for 39.44% of the explained variance in the number of users.

Table 2. Association between the log-transformed number of food bank users and food bank resources and district character. Results of multiple linear regression analyses.

	β	*p* Value	95% CI
Intercept	5.23	<0.0001	4.93, 5.53
Number of service programs [a]	0.044	0.05	−0.0007, 0.090
Weight of distributed food per month [b]	0.197	<0.0001	0.13, 0.26
Number of workers [c]	0.005	<0.0001	0.003, 0.006
Number of additional services unrelated to food	0.065	0.13	−0.020, 0.15
Number of welfare recipients in percent of the population	0.070	<0.0001	0.038, 0.010

[a] including distribution points, social supermarkets, delivery food banks, soup kitchens, and children's food banks; [b] log-transformed; [c] including volunteers and paid workers; β: unstandardized regression coefficient; CI: confidence interval.

The odds of having a lack of volunteers were significantly associated with working time per month per volunteer (b = 0.011, 95% CI 0.001, 0.020, OR 1.01, *p* = 0.026), but not with the log-transformed number of users per month, the weight of food distributed per month, or the number of volunteers in percent of the total number of workers. The model analyzing the association of a lack of volunteers and ranked possible changes in the weight of food distributed and the number of people served revealed that the odds of having a lack of volunteers decreased with an increase of food distributed per month in 2017 compared with 2016 (b = −0.57, 95% CI −1.04, −0.12, OR 0.57, *p* = 0.015).

The odds of having a lack of food was not significantly associated with the log-transformed number of users, the log-transformed weight of food distributed per month, the number of workers, the number of programs, or the number of food donors.

However, in the models analyzing the association of a lack of food and ranked possible changes in the weight of food per month and in the number of users per month in 2017 compared with 2016, the odds of having a lack of food significantly increased with a decrease of food per month in 2017 compared with in 2016 (Table 3).

Table 3. Association between the log of having a lack of food and the ranked possible changes in the number of users and the distributed food. Results of logistic regression analyses.

	β	*p* Value	95% CI	OR
Intercept	−1.82	<0.0001	−2.27, −1.42	0.16
Ranged possible changes in the weight of food per month in 2017 compared with 2016	−1.16	0.0001	−1.78, −0.60	0.31
Ranged possible changes in the number of users per month in 2017 compared with 2016	0.31	0.16	−0.12, 0.76	1.37

β: unstandardized regression coefficient; CI: confidence interval; OR: odds ratio.

4. Discussion

This study revealed that a Tafel food bank was in operation in more than every second "big town" and nearly all residents and welfare recipients had access to at least one food bank in the district they lived in. Thus, Tafel Deutschland appears to provide a comprehensive net of local food banks throughout the country. In addition to the regular supply of mainly fresh produce, many food banks provided additional services such as social counseling and meal recipes, which may directly or indirectly impact users' food security. However, the density of food banks per 10,000 welfare recipients differed between parts of former East and West Germany with a lower density in eastern parts.

An analysis of the roots of this pattern is beyond the scope of this paper, but an explanation might be that the total number of workers as well as the number of volunteers as a percentage of all workers was significantly lower among participating food banks located in eastern compared with western Germany. Differences in volunteer engagement between eastern and western Germany were also observed in the German representative volunteer survey of 2014 and have been explained by the long history of Germany's separation, differences in unemployment rate, economic performance, and demographic change [33]. Given that food banks' assistance was largely based on volunteer labor, the number of available volunteers is a main pillar in the establishment of a food bank. The odds of reporting a lack of volunteers increased with increasing working time per volunteer, indicating that the workload of volunteers rather than the sole number of volunteers seems to be one of the limiting factors in balancing the supply and demand of existing food banks.

The volunteer-driven nature of the German Tafel is similar to food banks in other high-income countries such as Canada [28], the USA [1], and Spain [5]. In contrast to food banks in these countries, the German food banks neither involve the public sector nor receive food or other subsidies from the European Union or other national or international political organizations. German food banks heavily rely on surplus food donated from retailers and bakeries, whereas goods from producers or other wholesale donors constitute only a small part of the overall amount of food. This system shapes the quantity, quality, and reliability of the food to be distributed. On one side, it allows local food banks to supply fresh food such as fruits and vegetables, which are food products that food-insecure people tend to consume in particularly low amounts [29], although its health impacts are well known [34]. Moreover, it helps to prevent food being thrown away. According to a study under the authority of the Federal Ministry of Food and Agriculture from 2012, food waste from retailers accounts for 490,000 tons per year, of which around 38% are donated to charitable organizations such as Tafel food banks [35]. On the other side, the dependency of local food banks on donations of surplus food by local retailers makes the quantity, variety, and quality of available food highly unpredictable. Variations have also been observed in the nutritional quality of food distributed by food banks in other high-income countries even if they received government funding, such as U.S. food banks for The Emergency Food Assistance Program [36], but they tend to provide less fresh food [8]. Although this study is not able to evaluate the food donation systems of food banks in other high-income countries, it seems that donations from government programs might not necessarily make the amount of food more predictable.

Food banks participating in the survey reported not only a temporary lack of food but also an irregular surplus of food. More than 40% of food banks that reported this occasional surplus passed this food on to its users even if the amount was likely more than the user household could consume. Although the types of surplus food were unknown and it remained unclear whether users consumed this food or shared it with neighbors or friends, this practice forced the users to solve the problem and potentially might have unfavorable impacts on users' diet and health, e.g., if the surplus food consists of bread and pastries. This holds particular truth given that the association between food insecurity and obesity, the food insecurity–obesity paradox, is well known [37,38]. A diet heavily reliant on food bank types of food may exacerbate existing chronic conditions such as diabetes [39]. Most of the research on the relationship between food insecurity and obesity has, however, been conducted in the USA, where a so called monthly food stamp cycle was identified [10]. At least among subgroups of recipients of the Supplemental Nutrition Assistance Program or residents with low income, food intake and food expenditures were shown to dramatically increase after food assistance [40,41] or after transferred income [42] and then to decrease over time before the next assistance/income. A similar monthly variability has also been observed in the use of soup kitchens [43]. Tafel users tend to visit the food bank every week [15] and this study is not able to reveal whether similar weekly cycles also exist among food bank users in Germany, but an infrequent oversupply of food approaching its best-before date for people already at high risk of being overweight or obese and food insecure [6,15] may be contraproductive and could unintentionally support periods of overeating.

Given that the odds of reporting a lack of food were neither related to the weight of total food distributed per month nor to the weight of food a user received per month, but to a decrease in the total weight of food distributed per month in 2017 compared with 2016, it appears that participating food banks tended to evaluate the quantity of the available food based on their experiences rather than on objective measures. This might contain the risk of dramatic miscalculation. Therefore, food banks and their users might benefit from reliable, user-friendly tools to assess the quantity and quality of the food distributed and from national guidelines regarding the amount and quality of distributed food. Food banks in other countries such as the USA have already applied diverse instruments to assess the nutritional quality of distributed foods by, e.g., nutrition profiling [44–46]. The impact of the implementation of such tools depends, however, on the willingness of food bank managers and of food donors to accept restrictions in the quantity and quality of food and on the limited personnel capacity of the food banks.

Just recently, public and political debate about the role of the Tafel food banks in the German welfare system has increased again [47]. Similar to other European countries [11,48,49], the Tafel movement is considered a seismograph for social developments [50,51] and changes in the number of food banks or its users have been interpreted to indicate changes in the food security rate [52]. The results of this study challenge these interpretations. Most user households relied on public welfare, but only a small part of eligible welfare recipients used a food bank. In 79 districts for which all available food banks participated in the survey, on average, 179 welfare recipients per 1000 welfare recipients and 17 residents per 1000 residents used a food bank. These numbers of usage were larger than the numbers revealed by a study in Berlin [9], but much lower than the prevalence rate of food insecurity of 4.3% (i.e., 43 per 1000 residents; margin of error at 90% confidence ±1.44%) reported by the Food and Agriculture Organization of the United Nations for Germany [17]. Thus, the majority of food-insecure individuals do not appear to use a food bank. One of the possible manifold reasons for this mismatch might be that more than every tenth food bank participating in the survey reported limiting access to its assistance due to a lack of food. In addition, as reported by Tafel users as well as food bank workers, shame and fear of stigmatization associated with food bank use [53,54] might potentially prevent food-insecure people from seeking a food bank's assistance. Although motives for not using a food bank were not assessed by this study, participants reported that shame was a significant barrier, in particular among older people, to seeking assistance from a food bank. Furthermore, compared with other high-income countries, grocery prices in Germany are among the lowest, with budget supermarkets significantly undercutting other chains and driving down prices [55].

Nevertheless, a previous study showed that the distribution of food pantries mirrored the distribution of welfare recipients in Berlin [9], and the present study revealed that the number of food bank users was at least partly a function of the percentage of welfare recipients in the district the food bank was located in. Among all user household groups, user households receiving a low retirement or minimum social security benefits for senior citizens increased highest from 2016 to 2017. Actually, in Germany the rate of older people being at risk of falling into poverty has steadily increased over the last few years [56], whereas the unemployment rate has decreased [57].

Limitations

One of the major limitations of this study is the limited reliability of participants' responses. All data collected by the survey relied on self-reports. Given that food banks focus on the distribution of food and are driven by volunteers, some food banks were not able to provide detailed records, for instance, of the weight of food or the number of users. Additionally, there are no national standard procedures of data collection, and the data presented here might be subject to estimation errors.

Potential changes in the number of users and the weight of distributed food per month were retrospectively requested, which increases the risk of memory bias. The cross-sectional design of the study precludes the drawing of causal relationships.

Given that food banks participating and those not participating in the survey did not differ in location characteristics, it can be assumed that the results are representative for all food banks in the federal umbrella organization Tafel Deutschland. Due to the heterogeneity of food banks in many other characteristics, however, some uncertainty about the representativeness of any food bank sample remains.

Results of the additional services provided by the participating food banks might also give an incomplete picture of services offered in the context of the Tafel, since a service was only recorded if it was administered by the participating Tafel itself. However, there were services located in the same facility as the food bank but being provided by other organizations, which were not recorded.

Lastly, the latest data of the number of welfare recipients per district were available from 2015, whereas the data collected by the survey were from 2017. Although changes in the number of welfare recipients as a percent of the population were presumably small [58], the differences in the years the data were collected should be considered carefully when interpreting the results.

5. Conclusions

The German Tafel system provides a wide range of food assistance schemes supplying food of high nutritional value and additional services with the potential to impact individuals' diet and food insecurity. It appears that changes in the number of food bank users and their source of income partly mirror changes in the at-risk-of-poverty rate and social welfare in Germany, but there obviously are unknown factors influencing the usage of food banks. The number of food bank users seems to be an inappropriate indicator of the food insecurity rate, which can be taken as a sign of the need for implementing a regular food security monitoring system.

Due to the dependency of food banks on volunteers and food donations, they are hardly a reliable food source for parts of the population who are vulnerable to food insecurity due to their socio-economically disadvantaged situation. The obvious strain between the reliance on food donations and the response to the shifting needs of food bank users entails the risk of volunteer overload and inappropriate short-term solutions such as providing users more food than needed. One solution could be collaborations with dieticians and other public health and nutrition professionals to receive support regarding the dietary needs of food bank users. However, this will only be effective if food bank users are able to use the food bank to supplement their usual diet (as is the claim of Tafel Deutschland) rather than to rely on food banks as their primary or even only source of food.

To understand contributing factors as to which individuals use a food bank and why, further research is needed. Moreover, the impact of a food bank's food assistance on an individual's diet and food security level needs to be investigated.

In general, food banks' growth and assistance should be accompanied by vigilant coalitions of the charitable food organizations, the social sector, and professionals of social, nutritional, and health sciences in order to have a working system that supports those in need and contributes to the reduction of food waste.

Supplementary Materials: The following are available online at http://www.mdpi.com/1660-4601/15/7/1485/s1, Table S1: Questionnaire content, developed for a representative survey among German food banks: questions, answer options, variables (selection).

Author Contributions: Conceptualization, A.S. and N.S.-B.; Formal analysis, A.S.; Methodology, A.S. and N.S.-B.; Supervision, P.T. and N.S.-B.; Writing—original draft, A.S.; Writing—review & editing, A.S., P.T. and N.S.-B.

Funding: This research received no external funding.

Acknowledgments: The authors would like to thank all food bank managers and other food bank workers for participating in the survey and the federal association Tafel Deutschland for their administrative support.

Conflicts of Interest: A.S. supported the evaluation of one of Tafel Deutschland's other projects for which she received a small honorarium. This had no role in the design of this study; in the collection, analyses, and interpretation of data; in the writing of the manuscript; nor in the decision to publish the results.

References

1. Weinfield, N.S.; Mills, G.; Borger, C.; Gearing, M.; Macaluso, T.; Montaquila, J.; Zedlewski, S. *Hunger in America 2014. National Report*; Feeding America: Chicago, IL, USA, 2014.

2. Tarasuk, V.; Dachner, N.; Loopstra, R. Food banks, welfare, and food insecurity in Canada. *Br. Food J.* **2014**, *116*, 1405–1417. [CrossRef]

3. Booth, S.; Whelan, J. Hungry for change: The food banking industry in Australia. *Br. Food J.* **2014**, *116*, 1392–1404. [CrossRef]

4. Castetbon, K.; Mejean, C.; Deschamps, V.; Bellin-Lestienne, C.; Oleko, A.; Darmon, N.; Hercberg, S. Dietary behaviour and nutritional status in underprivileged people using food aid (ABENA study, 2004–2005). *J. Hum. Nutr. Diet. Off. J. Br. Diet. Assoc.* **2011**, *24*, 560–571. [CrossRef] [PubMed]

5. González-Torre, P.L.; Coque, J. How is a food bank managed? Different profiles in Spain. *Agric. Hum. Values* **2015**, *33*, 89–100. [CrossRef]

6. Depa, J.; Hilzendegen, C.; Tinnemann, P.; Stroebele-Benschop, N. An explorative cross-sectional study examining self-reported health and nutritional status of disadvantaged people using food banks in Germany. *Int. J. Equity Health* **2015**, *14*, 141. [CrossRef] [PubMed]

7. Neter, J.E.; Dijkstra, S.C.; Visser, M.; Brouwer, I.A. Food insecurity among Dutch food bank recipients: A cross-sectional study. *BMJ Open* **2014**, *4*, e004657. [CrossRef] [PubMed]

8. Simmet, A.; Depa, J.; Tinnemann, P.; Stroebele-Benschop, N. The Nutritional Quality of Food Provided from Food Pantries: A Systematic Review of Existing Literature. *J. Acad. Nutr. Diet.* **2017**, *117*, 577–588. [CrossRef] [PubMed]

9. Simmet, A.; Stroebele-Benschop, N.; Tinnemann, P. Area characteristics associated with food pantry use in Berlin—A cross-sectional ecological study. *Appl. Geogr.* **2017**, *89*, 87–99. [CrossRef]

10. Bundesverband Deutsche Tafel e.V. *Die Tafeln nach Zahlen: Migration und Integration. Ergebnisse der Tafel-Umfrage 2016*; Bundesverband Deutsche Tafel e.V.: Berlin, Germany, 2016.

11. Lambie-Mumford, H. Every Town Should Have One: Emergency Food Banking in the UK. *J. Soc. Policy* **2013**, *42*, 73–89. [CrossRef]

12. Galli, F.; Hebinck, A.; Arcuri, S.; Brunori, G.; Carrol, B.; Connor, D.O.; Oostindie, H. The Food Poverty Challenge: Comparing Food Assistance across EU Countries. A Transformative Social Innovation perspective. In Proceedings of the SIDEA Conference, San Michele, Italy, 22 September 2016.

13. Tafel Deutschland English Information. Available online: https://www.tafel.de/english-information/ (accessed on 24 April 2018).

14. European Federation of Food Banks What's New? FEBA. Available online: https://www.eurofoodbank.org/en/what-s-new/2018-04-03-tafel-is-a-feba-member (accessed on 5 April 2018).

15. Depa, J.; Gyngell, F.; Müller, A.; Eleraky, L.; Hilzendegen, C.; Stroebele-Benschop, N. Prevalence of food insecurity among food bank users in Germany and its association with population characteristics. *Prev. Med. Rep.* **2018**, *9*, 96–101. [CrossRef] [PubMed]

16. Holben, D.H. Food Bank Users in and Around the Lower Mainland of British Columbia, Canada, Are Characterized by Food Insecurity and Poor Produce Intake. *J. Hunger Environ. Nutr.* **2012**, *7*, 449–458. [CrossRef]

17. Cafiero, C.; Nord, M.; Viviani, S.; Del Grossi, E.; Ballard, T.; Kepple, A.; Miller, M.; Nwosu, C. *Voices of the Hungry. Methods for Estimating Comparable Prevalence Rates of Food Insecurity Experienced by Adults throughout the World*; FAO: Rome, Italy, 2016.

18. Stroebele-Benschop, N.; Depa, J.; Gyngell, F.; Müller, A.; Eleraky, L.; Hilzendegen, C. Migration Background Influences Consumption Patterns Based on Dietary Recommendations of Food Bank Users in Germany. *J. Immigr. Minor. Health* **2018**, 1–9. [CrossRef] [PubMed]

19. Martin, K.S.; Wu, R.; Wolff, M.; Colantonio, A.G.; Grady, J. A novel food pantry program: Food security, self-sufficiency, and diet-quality outcomes. *Am. J. Prev. Med.* **2013**, *45*, 569–575. [CrossRef] [PubMed]

20. O'Reilly, S.; O'Shea, T.; Bhusumane, S. Nutritional vulnerability seen within asylum seekers in Australia. *J. Immigr. Minor. Health Cent. Minor. Public Health* **2012**, *14*, 356–360. [CrossRef] [PubMed]

21. Börsch-Supan, A.; Schnabel, R. Social security and retirement in Germany. In *Social Security and Retirement around the World*; Gruber, J., Wise, D.A., Eds.; University of Chicago Press: Chicago, IL, USA, 2008; ISBN 978-0-226-30999-6.

22. Tinnemann, P.; Pastätter, R.; Willich, S.N.; Stroebele, N. Healthy action against poverty: A descriptive analysis of food redistribution charity clients in Berlin, Germany. *Eur. J. Public Health* **2012**, *22*, 721–726. [CrossRef] [PubMed]

23. Sedelmeier, T. *Armut und Ernährung in Deutschland. Eine Untersuchung zur Rolle und Wirksamkeit der Tafeln bei der Lebensmittelausgabe an Bedürftige*, 1st ed.; Mensch und Buch Verlag: Berlin, Germany, 2011; ISBN 3783863870140.

24. Tafel Deutschland Jahresbericht (Annual Report). Available online: https://www.tafel.de/ueber-uns/downloads-und-publikationen/jahresbericht/ (accessed on 5 April 2018).

25. GeoBasis-DE/BKG Open Data—Freie Daten und Dienste des BKG. Verwaltungsgebiete. Available online: http://www.geodatenzentrum.de/geodaten/gdz_rahmen.gdz_div?gdz_spr=deu&gdz_akt_zeile=5&gdz_anz_zeile=1&gdz_unt_zeile=0&gdz_user_id=0 (accessed on 26 February 2018).

26. Tafel Deutschland Tafel-Suche (Locations). Available online: https://www.tafel.de/ueber-uns/die-tafeln/tafel-suche/ (accessed on 5 April 2018).

27. Statistische Ämter des Bundes und der Länder Regionaldatenbank Deutschland. Sozialberichterstattung (Regional Database. Social Reporting). Available online: https://www.regionalstatistik.de/genesis/online/data;jsessionid=F0116E70ADC9302EF8CFFDAB440B5BE8.reg1?operation=statistikenVerzeichnisNextStep&levelindex=0&levelid=1520947704795&index=10&structurelevel=3 (accessed on 10 March 2018).

28. Tarasuk, V.; Dachner, N.; Hamelin, A.-M.; Ostry, A.; Williams, P.; Bosckei, E.; Poland, B.; Raine, K. A survey of food bank operations in five Canadian cities. *BMC Public Health* **2014**, *14*, 1234. [CrossRef] [PubMed]

29. Simmet, A.; Depa, J.; Tinnemann, P.; Stroebele-Benschop, N. The Dietary Quality of Food Pantry Users: A Systematic Review of Existing Literature. *J. Acad. Nutr. Diet.* **2017**, *117*, 563–576. [CrossRef] [PubMed]

30. Minn, M. MMQGIS for QGIS Geographic Information System; Open Source Geospatial Foundation Project. Available online: http://michaelminn.com/linux/mmqgis/ (accessed on 17 May 2018).

31. QGIS Development Team. QGIS Geographic Information System. Open Source Geospatial Foundation Project. Available online: https://www.qgis.org/de/site/ (accessed on 17 May 2018).

32. R Development Core Team. R: A Language and Environment for Statistical Computing. Available online: https://www.r-project.org/ (accessed on 2 February 2018).

33. Kausmann, C.; Simonson, J. Freiwilliges Engagement in Ost-und Westdeutschland sowie den 16 Ländern (Volunteer engagement in eastern and western Germany and 16 states). In *Freiwilliges Engagement in Deutschland. Der Deutsche Freiwilligensurvey 2014*; Simonson, J., Vogel, C., Tesch-Römer, C., Eds.; Springer: Wiesbaden, Germany, 2017; pp. 573–600.

34. Boeing, H.; Bechthold, A.; Bub, A.; Ellinger, S.; Haller, D.; Kroke, A.; Leschik-Bonnet, E.; Müller, M.J.; Oberritter, H.; Schulze, M.; et al. Critical review: Vegetables and fruit in the prevention of chronic diseases. *Eur. J. Nutr.* **2012**, *51*, 637–663. [CrossRef] [PubMed]

35. Kranert, M.; Hafner, G.; Barabosz, J.; Schuller, H.; Leverenz, D.; Kölbig, A.; Schneider, F.; Lebersorger, S.; Scherhaufer, S. *Ermittlung der Weggeworfenen Lebensmittelmengen und Vorschläge zur Verminderung der Wegwerfrate bei Lebensmitteln in Deutschland*; Institut für Siedlungswasserbau, Wassergüte—Und Abfallwirtschaft: Stuttgart, Germany, 2012.

36. Feeding America. *2017 Feeding America Annual Report. A Hunger for a Brighter Tomorrow*; Feeding America: Chicago, IL, USA, 2017.

37. Dinour, L.M.; Bergen, D.; Yeh, M.-C. The food insecurity-obesity paradox: A review of the literature and the role food stamps may play. *J. Am. Diet. Assoc.* **2007**, *107*, 1952–1961. [CrossRef] [PubMed]

38. Franklin, B.; Jones, A.; Love, D.; Puckett, S.; Macklin, J.; White-Means, S. Exploring mediators of food insecurity and obesity: A review of recent literature. *J. Commun. Health* **2012**, *37*, 253–264. [CrossRef] [PubMed]

39. Seligman, H.K.; Lyles, C.; Marshall, M.B.; Prendergast, K.; Smith, M.C.; Headings, A.; Bradshaw, G.; Rosenmoss, S.; Waxman, E. A Pilot Food Bank Intervention Featuring Diabetes-Appropriate Food Improved Glycemic Control Among Clients in Three States. *Health Aff. Proj. Hope* **2015**, *34*, 1956–1963. [CrossRef] [PubMed]

40. Wilde, P.E.; Ranney, C.K. The Monthly Food Stamp Cycle: Shopping Frequency and Food Intake Decisions in an Endogenous Switching Regression Framework. *Am. J. Agric. Econ.* **2000**, *82*, 200–213. [CrossRef]

41. Shapiro, J.M. Is there a daily discount rate? Evidence from the food stamp nutrition cycle. *J. Public Econ.* **2005**, *89*, 303–325. [CrossRef]

42. Tarasuk, V.S.; McIntyre, L.; Li, J. Low-income women's dietary intakes are sensitive to the depletion of household resources in one month. *J. Nutr.* **2007**, *137*, 1980–1987. [CrossRef] [PubMed]

43. Thompson, F.E.; Taren, D.L.; Andersen, E.; Casella, G.; Lambert, J.K.; Campbell, C.C.; Frongillo, E.A.; Spicer, D. Within month variability in use of soup kitchens in New York State. *Am. J. Public Health* **1988**, *78*, 1298–1301. [CrossRef] [PubMed]

44. Seidel, M.; Laquatra, I.; Woods, M.; Sharrard, J. Applying a nutrient-rich foods index algorithm to address nutrient content of food bank food. *J. Acad. Nutr. Diet.* **2015**, *115*, 695–700. [CrossRef] [PubMed]

45. Hoisington, A.; Manore, M.M.; Raab, C. Nutritional quality of emergency foods. *J. Am. Diet. Assoc.* **2011**, *111*, 573–576. [CrossRef] [PubMed]

46. Rambeloson, Z.J.; Darmon, N.; Ferguson, E.L. Linear programming can help identify practical solutions to improve the nutritional quality of food aid. *Public Health Nutr.* **2008**, *11*, 395–404. [CrossRef] [PubMed]

47. DPA. No One in Germany Would Go Hungry If Food Banks Didn't Exist. Available online: https://www.thelocal.de/20180312/no-one-in-germany-would-go-hungry-if-food-banks-didnt-exist (accessed on 31 May 2018).

48. Armiño, K.P. De Erosion of Rights, Uncritical Solidarity and Food Banks in Spain. In *First World Hunger Revisited*; Palgrave Macmillan: London, UK, 2014; pp. 131–145, ISBN 978-1-137-29872-0.

49. Silvasti, T. Food Aid—Normalising the Abnormal in Finland. *Soc. Policy Soc.* **2015**, *14*, 471–482. [CrossRef]

50. Assig, A.; Seewald, S. *Seismograf für das Soziale. Etwa 720 Tafeln gibt es in Deutschland. Von Berlin Breitete sich die Idee aus (Seismograph for Social Developments)*; Berliner Morgenpost: Berlin, Germany, 5 September 2007.

51. Deutscher Caritasverband eV. Kein Grund zum Feiern (No Cause for Celebration). Available online: https://www.caritas.de/neue-caritas/kommentare/kein-grund-zum-feiern (accessed on 28 May 2017).

52. Pfeiffer, S.; Ritter, T.; Oestreicher, E. Food Insecurity in German households: Qualitative and Quantitative Data on Coping, Poverty Consumerism and Alimentary Participation. *Soc. Policy Soc.* **2015**, *14*, 483–495. [CrossRef]

53. Selke, S. *Fast Ganz Unten: Wie Man in Deutschland Durch Die Hilfe von Lebensmitteltafeln Satt Wird*, 2nd ed.; Westfälisches Dampfboot: Münster, Germany, 2009; ISBN 978-3-89691-754-6.

54. Bergt, H. *Das Schlimmste ist die Scham*; MAZ—Märkische Allg: Potsdam, Germany, 3 March 2018.

55. European Union Comparative Price Levels for Food, Beverages and Tobacco—Statistics Explained. Available online: http://ec.europa.eu/eurostat/statistics-explained/index.php/Comparative_price_levels_for_food,_beverages_and_tobacco (accessed on 24 May 2018).

56. Statistisches Bundesamt (Destatis) EU-SILC—Erfasste Personen, Hochgerechnete Personen, Nettoäquivalenzeinkommen, Armutsgefährdungsquote: Deutschland, Jahre, Geschlecht, Altersgruppen. Available online: https://www-genesis.destatis.de/genesis/online;jsessionid=60013C2EE852D7E8D999733AED7F0AA0.tomcat_GO_1_2?operation=previous&levelindex=2&levelid=1522837663497&step=2 (accessed on 4 April 2018).

57. Bundesagentur für Arbeit Arbeitslose, Unterbeschäftigung und Arbeitsstellen (Unemployed People, Underemployment, Jobs). Available online: https://statistik.arbeitsagentur.de/Navigation/Statistik/Statistik-nach-Themen/Arbeitslose-und-gemeldetes-Stellenangebot/Arbeislose-und-gemeldetes-Stellenangebot-Nav.html (accessed on 4 April 2018).
58. Statistische Ämter des Bundes und der Länder Armut und Soziale Ausgrenzung: B1: Mindestsicherungsleistungen (Poverty and Social Exclusion. Minimum Social Security). Available online: http://www.amtliche-sozialberichterstattung.de/B1mindestsicherungsquote.html (accessed on 28 March 2018).

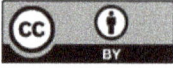

International Journal of
*Environmental Research
and Public Health*

MDPI

Article

Food Security Experiences of Aboriginal and Torres Strait Islander Families with Young Children in An Urban Setting: Influencing Factors and Coping Strategies

Leisa McCarthy [1,*], Anne B. Chang [1,2,3] and Julie Brimblecombe [1,4]

1   Menzies School of Health Research, 0870 Darwin, Australia; anne.chang@menzies.edu.au (A.B.C.);
    julie.brimblecombe@monash.edu.au (J.B.)
2   Department of Respiratory Medicine, Queensland Children's Hospital, 4101 Brisbane, Australia
3   Children's Centre for Health Research, Queensland University of Technology; 4101 Brisbane, Australia
4   Department of Nutrition, Dietetics and Food, School of Clinical Sciences, Monash University,
    3168 Melbourne, Australia
*   Correspondence: leisa.mccarthy@menzies.edu.au; Tel.: +61-088-959-5389

Received: 26 October 2018; Accepted: 21 November 2018; Published: 26 November 2018

Abstract: Evidence on Aboriginal and Torres Strait Islander peoples' food security experiences and coping strategies used when food insecurity occurs is limited. Such evidence is important to inform policies that can reduce the consequences of food insecurity. This study investigated factors perceived by Aboriginal and Torres Strait Islander families with young children to influence household food security, and coping strategies used, in an urban setting. A qualitative research inductive approach was used. Data were collected through an iterative process of inquiry through initial interviews with 30 primary care-givers, followed by in-depth interviews with six participants to further explore emerging themes. Major topics explored were: influencing factors, food insecurity experiences, impact on food selection, and coping strategies. Food affordability relating to income and living expenses was a major barrier to a healthy diet with large household bills impacting food choice and meal quality. Access to family support was the main reported coping strategy. Food insecurity is experienced by Aboriginal and Torres Strait Islander families, it is largely intermittent occurring especially when large household bills are due for payment. Family support provides an essential safety net and the implications of this are important to consider in public policy to address food insecurity.

Keywords: food security; food insecurity; Aboriginal and Torres Strait Islander population; children; urban; experiences; coping strategies

---

1. Introduction

Food security is "access by all people, at all times to sufficient food for an active and healthy life. Food security includes at a minimum: the ready availability of nutritionally adequate and safe foods, and an assured ability to acquire acceptable foods in socially acceptable ways" [1] (p. 337). Irrespective of a country's affluence status, some population groups within high income countries experience food insecurity and varying degrees of hunger. For these groups, strategies to overcome or alleviate food insecurity have been employed, but most measures are thought to be short-lived and a 'stop gap' to temporarily relieve problems [2–11]. Evidence that can inform longer-term solutions are required. Availability of such evidence is important to inform possible practice and policy interventions.

However, literature about people's experiences with household food insecurity is limited, particularly within Indigenous populations of affluent countries, the group most at risk of household food insecurity and poor health [2,7,12–14]. Among families with young children in the United States and Canada, studies reported that although families access food assistance programs, food shortages and hunger are still experienced [2–11]. A study in six Inuit communities of Nunavut, Canada, focused on the availability and accessibility of traditional and market foods (i.e., foods purchased from a shop), found inconsistencies between perceived food security status and experiences in obtaining enough food to eat [7]. In contrast, another study undertaken with a Nunavut Inuit population, found participants who reported food insecurity also reported regular use of community food programs to assist with alleviating hunger [2]. The variance in results likely reflects the different sampling frame of these studies, as one [7] recruited from the broader community and the other [2] through food assistance programs [2,7].

To mitigate household food insecurity, coping strategies (i.e., the mechanisms families have in place to cope with food and money problems) are used [4,5,10,11,15]. A Canadian Quebec-based study described several coping strategies used by participants to overcome household food insecurity: adults reduced size of meals or forwent food so children could eat; modified lifestyle (e.g., forgoing purchases of less essential items and payment of bills to free up money for food); purchased sale item foods and foods close to use by date; and visited a food bank when desperate [10]. An Australian study undertaken in South Western Sydney investigated coping strategies [15]. The most frequent responses of nine coping strategies to select from were, cutting down on the variety of household foods (59.1%); a parent or guardian skipping meals or eating less (58.8%); and putting off paying bills (57.4%) [15]. Other coping strategies reported (among a multicultural group of 90 food pantry users in Washington, USA) include using leftover food, cooking food in bulk and freezing food for later use [11]; and among Latino immigrant families in North Carolina, USA, limiting food purchases considered expensive, e.g., meats and fruits and; shopping for specials and bulk-buying [5].

To alleviate household food insecurity, social support systems are important and include assistance from food programs, food charity organisations, faith communities, neighbours and friends [2–11,13]. Extended family as a social support system is also important [2–4,8,9,11] One study reported support from friends and neighbours as a main coping mechanism in response to food insecurity [5]. Within an Inuit population, living with family as a temporary coping strategy until housing was obtained was identified [2]. Another study, highlighted reciprocity where young mothers would rely on family members for food assistance and then 'return the favour' when other family members experienced difficulties [4].

Among Aboriginal and Torres Strait Islander peoples, the concept of reciprocity is an important component of the social connectedness [16]. This cultural sharing practice is important in maintaining and reinforcing individual and group social bonds and imparting knowledge about good food as related to balance—life, resources, food, knowledge [16,17]. Studies undertaken in Inuit populations have also noted reciprocity has a place in maintaining and reinforcing family and broader community relationship obligations as well as cultural identity and practice [2,7]. 'Cultural sharing' and 'sharing networks' ensure that excess traditional food is provided to the more vulnerable members of the community who cannot obtain these foods [2,7]. Identified in these studies, was that money or other services were exchanged for traditional foods to keep with continuing cultural practices for those who could not hunt [2,7]. Similarly, in a study undertaken with Latino Immigrant Families in North Carolina, USA, money was sent home to families to support food security. This action was justifiable from the belief family back home were in a worse situation to their own and a cultural obligation to look after ones' parents [8].

Despite the importance of knowing coping mechanisms used when household food insecurity occurs within families, there is little to no such data among Aboriginal and Torres Strait Islander people. Obtaining such data provides knowledge on enablers that can inform policies to enhance existing coping strategies and support families. Therefore, this qualitative study explores the experiences of household food insecurity and coping strategies used among Aboriginal and Torres Strait Islander families residing in Darwin and Palmerston, two cities of remote Northern Australia.

2. Materials and Methods

A qualitative research inductive approach was used, where data collection involved an iterative process of inquiry through initial interviews and subsequent in-depth interviews. All interviews were undertaken by the primary author, an Aboriginal woman and nutritionist. An iterative process of data collection and analysis was undertaken. Thematic analysis was applied. The inductive method used was not confined to existing theoretical frameworks [18] or pre-determined categories and allowed for the creation of categories or codes during data collection to arise. These codes were then combined into themes which were mapped to reveal relationships between them. This process of qualitative data collection and analysis makes it particularly suitable to exploring an under-investigated study area.

This qualitative study was part of a larger study that aimed to investigate food security among families with use of a modified study version of the United States Department of Agriculture 18-item Household Food Security Module (mUS 18-item Module). It was during the administration of the mUS 18-item Module, that the initial interviews occurred and were initiated by the participants.

Human Research Ethics approval was obtained from the Human Research Ethics Committee of the Northern Territory Department of Health and Menzies School of Health Research and the Aboriginal Sub Ethics Committee. HREC File Reference Number 09/06.

2.1. Setting

The 2016 Australian Bureau of Statistics Census data estimated Aboriginal and Torres Strait Islander people comprised 3.3% of the Australian population (http://www.abs.gov.au/ausstats/abs@.nsf/mf/3238.0.55.001. 3238.0.55.001—Estimates of Aboriginal and Torres Strait Islander Australians, June 2016. LATEST ISSUE Released at 11:30AM (CANBERRA TIME) 31/08/2018). Darwin is the Northern Territory capital and Palmerston a nearby satellite city. Study data were collected for a period of 7 months between April 2009 and February 2010. At the time of the study population separations for Darwin and Palmerston were unavailable. Therefore, the combined total population of Darwin and Palmerston was 98,152 residents [19], with Aboriginal and Torres Strait Islander peoples comprising 7.5% of the total Palmerston population and 9.4% of the Darwin population [19]. The aim of this study was to investigate the food insecurity experiences of Aboriginal and Torres Strait Islander families in these two main centres of the Northern Territory.

2.2. Sampling

The primary author recruited potential participants through child health clinics in local health services', comprising two Aboriginal health services and two Government health services. A local Aboriginal woman was employed to assist with recruitment at one of the health service sites. Participants were also recruited from the broader community through the assistance of an Aboriginal Research Officer who had extensive networks with Aboriginal families in both Darwin and Palmerston. Convenience sampling through the local health services and known networks was used.

2.3. Participant Recruitment

The inclusion criteria were: care giver of a young Aboriginal and/or Torres Strait Islander child (aged 6 months-4 years); resided in Darwin or Palmerston for ≥12 months; and the child did not have a medical condition requiring food or nutrition supplements. A set of predetermined participant inclusion criteria were developed prior to study commencement with input from the health services during the consultation phase. During recruitment, informed consent was obtained from the eligible child's care-giver to participate in the whole study including qualitative interviews. Recruitment continued until 30 participants had completed the mUS 18-item Module, used to define the presence/absence of food insecurity. As the aim of the larger study was to test the reliability and face validity of the mUS 18-item Module among urban residing Aboriginal and Torres Strait Islander families with children 0.5 to 4 years, 30 participants were deemed a suitable number for this purpose.

2.4. Initial Discussions

Initial discussions, prompted through completion of the mUS 18-item Module, lasted from 30 min to three hours. Notes were taken (audio-recordings were not used) and read back to the participant to confirm the information and typed as a word document. Following each interview, the primary author coded text relating to food security experiences and coping strategies. These codes were explored in subsequent interviews. This iterative process continued until all initial interviews were complete. These codes informed the interview guide for the in-depth interviews (Appendix A).

2.5. In-Depth Interviews

In-depth interviews were audio recorded and notes taken. We purposively invited participants based on gender and identified age groups to reflect the overall study sample. The recordings were transcribed and the transcription read back to the participant either in person or over the telephone to verify the interview content and clarify any queries. Any adjustments or further data collected were agreed to, verified and included. The interview, transcription and analysis process continued iteratively until data saturation was reached i.e., when no new information or new themes emerged [20,21]. To achieve this, six participants were interviewed. Coding of all transcripts was undertaken firstly, by the primary author and then separately by the senior author. A set of themes identified initially by the primary author, was agreed on.

3. Results

Thirty care givers were recruited and engaged in initial discussions. Table 1 shows, the majority were female, Aboriginal and their age ranged between 17 and 58 years. Over half of the participants had partners (married or de facto relationship). The six participants were representative of the main sample in gender and age (Table 1).

Table 1. Demographic characteristics of households.

Characteristic		Initial Discussions (N = 30)	In-Depth Interviews (N = 6)
Parent gender	Female	27	4
Marital Status	Partnered	17	5
Indigenous status	Aboriginal	19	5
	Torres Strait Islander	1	0
	Aboriginal and Torres Strait Islander	6	1
	Non-Indigenous Australian	4	0
Care giver	Parent (mother/father)	27	6
	Other (grandmother/foster carer)	3	0
Parent age (yrs)	Median (range)	44.5 (17–58)	35 (25–39)
Residents in house	Median (range)	6 (3–15)	5.5 (3–10)
Number of children by age group (N = 57)	6 to 24 months	19	3
	25 to 48 months	30	5

3.1. Findings

As shown in Figure 1, themes identified from the initial interviews were grouped according to (i) factors influencing food security and (ii) coping strategies. These were explored further in the in-depth interviews with the following themes identified: *(i) Experiences of Food Insecurity; (ii) Influencing Factors; (iii) Impact on food selection; and (iv) Coping Strategies*. Themes relating to influencing factors are presented as major or minor influencing factors and determined both by the number of participants referring to these themes and whether featured prominently in their responses. (Figure 1).

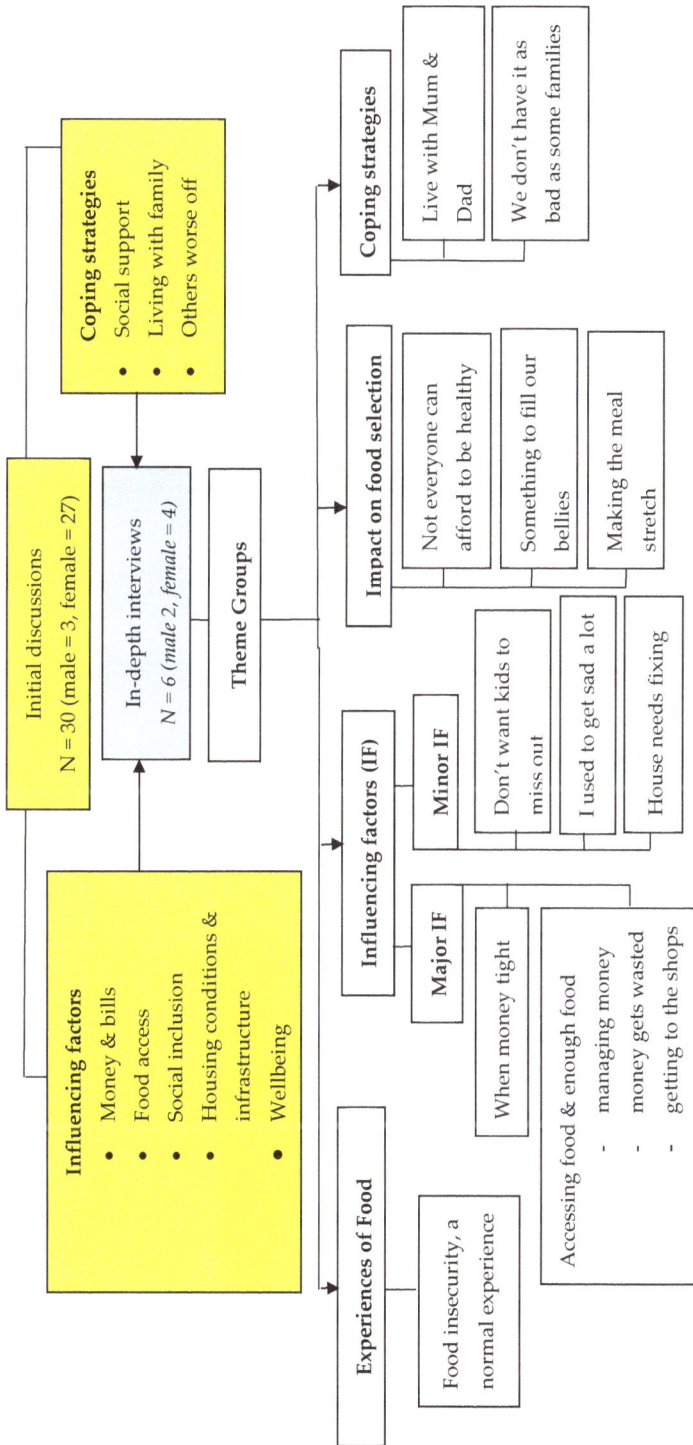

Figure 1. Overview of significant Qualitative Findings.

3.2. Experiences of Food Insecurity

Food Insecurity, a Normal Experience

Participants did not initially identify with being food insecure, although many of their experiences indicated otherwise. Whilst completing the mUS 18-item Module participants shared their own and others' experiences with not having enough food, money or both and described this situation as common among themselves and/or people close to them. The experiences of food insecurity as told by participants implied that food insecurity was seen by most as a 'normal' experience and was also considered 'the norm' within their close social interactions:

There's not enough money, full stop, to pay for food, to last from payday to payday. (Aboriginal mother with four children, aged 34 years and partnered)

Another participant shared his observations when out shopping:

. . . I've seen people put food back. Put things back because they can't get [afford] that. Or take a milk bottle back to get a smaller bottle of milk. Yes, you do see it around. (Aboriginal and Torres Strait Islander father of two children, aged 36 years and partnered).

3.3. Influencing Factors

3.3.1. Major Influencing Factors

These influencing factors were comprised of the sub-themes *"when money is tight"* and *"accessing food and enough food"*.

When Money is Tight

Many participants shared that they prioritised essentials when money was tight. Bills, such as quarterly electricity bills, were a main reason for making "money tight" and this impacted on the amount and type of food purchased. For some ($n = 9$), this situation was intermittent and occurred only when larger bills had to be paid or if there was a temporary change in household income. Whereas others ($n = 11$) described this as an everyday phenomenon. Four of these 11 participants mentioned not having enough money at all times due to an inadequate income. To ensure enough food for the family when 'money was tight' less expensive foods were chosen, such as highly processed foods of lower nutrient quality or cheaper brand options. For example, with fruit and vegetables, some participants purchased these in lesser quantity, did not buy at all, or purchased cheaper processed versions instead of fresh. Approximately half of the participants' spoke of choosing less expensive foods to ensure children had something to eat at each meal when 'money was tight'. This situation was not limited to participants who were recipients of Centrelink (The Centrelink Master Program is one of the Master Programs of the Australian Government Department of Human Services (Australia). The majority of Centrelink's services are the disbursement of social security payments (Source: Wikipedia site *en.wikipedia.org/wiki/Centrelink.*)), as some participants in paid employment, or who had partners in paid employment, also experienced this phenomenon. One Aboriginal participant shared that despite both her and her husband having paid employment, they still sometimes experienced difficulties:

Sometimes we have to be tight [with money] when the big bills (electricity, car repayments) come in and choose less expensive foods to buy. (Aboriginal mother of three children, 25 years and partnered).

This experience was echoed by an Aboriginal man, who as the sole income earner cut back on what he termed 'luxury items' such as snack foods, sweet drinks or desserts, when 'money was tight'.

Don't have real problems with food [having enough to eat] or with money. Only time may have to get tight with the budget is when the big bills come in. This just means cutting back on luxury items. (Aboriginal father of one child, 38 years and partnered).

This participant also revealed other measures used to immediately relieve a "money tight" situation and ensure adequate food, although this measure had greater cost implications:

Often the bill would come in and we would go and do a shop and then make that shop stretch to the next pay to pay the bill. I would consider putting food in people's guts (stomachs) more important than paying bills. If you don't pay the bill on time, there's a late fee $30, $40 dollars. Might as well pay it late, that's how I would look at it. (Aboriginal father of one child, 38 years, partnered).

Of the 30 participants, the sole income for nine were Centrelink payments and four of these individuals were being income managed (Income Management is an Australian Government initiative to assist individuals receiving Centrelink social security payments in managing money to meet essential household needs and expenses, and learn to better manage finances in the long term. (Source: http://www.humanservices.gov.au/customer/services/centrelink/income-management)). Three of the four participants considered these payments as inadequate in meeting their households' basic living costs. A participant told of her experience in being income managed. She viewed income management as good for families who needed help with budgeting. In her case however it was not helpful as she 'looked after her children properly' and the payment was not enough to feed her family:

I have three boys and you know, they eat a lot. One loaf of bread eaten for breakfast! I don't think we get enough money and I can't pay for all the food from my basic card Basic card (similar to a bank key card. A portion of income managed individuals' payments are deposited into a basic card to purchase food and other essential household items only. (Source: http://www.humanservices.gov.au/ customer/services/centrelink/income-management). (Aboriginal mother of four children, 34 years and partnered).

Another participant, who stated that she had money problems all the time, worked full-time and had a regular income, but her partner had been having problems with securing permanent full-time employment:

I work full-time, but don't get paid much. My partner works when he gets work and we also rely on government money [Centrelink payments]. The money that we do get seems to just cover the rent, food and basic necessities. Rent and food are expensive in Darwin. We also have a car to run and that's also expensive. (non-Indigenous mother of four children, 30 years and partnered).

Some participants shared that they experienced money problems temporarily due to a sudden change in their income, such as irregular timing in child maintenance payments:

Sometimes they [ex-partners] don't pay [child maintenance] regularly and that throws us out with budgeting for the fortnight. I don't think they [ex-partners] understand how hard it makes things sometimes. (Aboriginal and Torres Strait Islander mother of three children, 38 years, single)

Other participants spoke of full-time employment and being paid well as an enabler of food security. An Aboriginal woman who was a full-time student expressed that her husband was in secure full-time employment, earned a "good wage" that was able to meet the family's needs:

If my husband wasn't on a good wage and he didn't earn enough to cover the bills and other expenses, we would definitely be struggling. (Aboriginal mother of one child, 27 years and partnered).

Nineteen of the 30 participants identified as food secure (63.3%), raised concerns about the rising cost of living and how this would impact on their families in the future. In particular, a man of both Aboriginal and Torres Strait Islander heritage spoke of not having money issues but mentioned the rising cost of living and the impact this could have on his household:

... it's becoming very expensive. Everything has just gone up ... and not just food prices. It's electricity, phone, fuel [for car], the cost of living in general has gone up a lot. You know,

we [participant and his wife] are aware of how difficult it could be if one of us lost our job. And we don't have much in savings. And if there is an economic downturn that affects us, that's why we're trying to pay off as much of our mortgage now just to make sure that we have a buffer. (Aboriginal and Torres Strait Islander father of two children, 36 years, partnered).

Accessing Food and Enough Food

This sub-theme encompassed findings relevant to budgeting and managing money; misuse of money; and food access.

Managing Money

At least five participants spoke of how important it is to budget or "manage money" to ensure enough money for food and bills. An Aboriginal woman shared her experience:

… I've always planned a budget to include extras to make sure money for additional expenses such as car maintenance, power bills, etc. Though, power bills have gone up. Not because we're using more power, just the cost of power. Other things (essential items) are going up as well. You know, price of food, petrol, rent. So much pressure on families just to live. In our budget we always make sure the rent and bills are paid and there's money for food. You know, the kids come first. Make sure they're clothed, fed, school fees paid. Sometimes I may need new clothing, shoes, or whatever, but will go without to make sure the kids have what they need. Just make sure I have what I need budgeted for and save for it. (Aboriginal mother with three children, 25 years and partnered).

For some though, budgeting did not always prevent "money being tight":

… Sometimes things [budget] blows out and I think I mentioned it before. One month you might get your electricity bill and that. Plus, we have child care fees and that's a big chunk out of that as well. (Aboriginal and Torres Strait Islander father of two children, 36 years and partnered).

Four participants were income managed by Centrelink and had a portion of their income automatically quarantined for food and other household essentials accessed through use of a Basics card. There were mixed experiences with this system and two mentioned post-introduction of income management that money problems still occurred, whilst another two experienced improvements:

It's ok. I don't get much humbug (Humbug is a term predominantly used by Indigenous Australians in a way that means 'to pester', as in being pestered (humbugged) by someone for money) now [since introduction of basics card] for money and have enough money for food. (Aboriginal grandmother, carer of 10 grandchildren, 44 years, widowed).

Money Gets Wasted

Although participants referred to their own struggles with managing money to meet family needs, many participants expressed that there were families in worse situations than themselves, particularly when anti-social behaviour such as gambling, excessive alcohol and illicit drug use were involved. Participants defined anti-social behaviour as that of 'social problems' and associated these with food and money problems:

… there are also problems with drinking [alcohol] and gambling. It makes me wonder sometimes, when people say they have no money to pay bills or buy food. They smoke [cigarettes], drink [alcohol] and gamble and don't seem to understand this causes problems. When you have limited money, need to be smart about how to use it. (Aboriginal and Torres Strait Islander mother of three, 38 years and single).

"Other families find it hard too [money problems]. That's why some people sell drugs. Need more money. … Some problems with gambling and drinking [alcohol]. Maybe drugs. A lot of money gets

wasted. Make me sorry for the kids". (Aboriginal and Torres Strait Islander mother of five, 29 years, partnered).

Food security for some participants' households were directly affected by others' social problems:

My brother is bad. All he wants to do is drink grog [alcohol]. Then he gets hungry and comes here. Eats all my kids' tucker [food]. He takes money from me and Nanna. Other people after him cos' he steal grog [alcohol] from them. (Aboriginal mother of two, 25 years and partnered).

Getting to the Shops

This sub-theme covered the ability to access food (shops) and reliable transport. Eleven participants mentioned their experience with accessing shops and how this impacted on food purchasing as well as seeking out food specials and bargains. Having access to supermarkets was considered by most participants as important to obtain affordable food items. Supermarkets were considered as cheaper and offering a wider variety of goods when compared to the smaller convenience type stores. During the study period a major supermarket chain outlet accessed by a quarter of the participants closed. The only other food outlet option locally available to these participants and within walking distance was the service station (a service station is a motor vehicle fuel outlet and often provides a small range of grocery items, including bread, milk, juice and a few dry goods lines.) which had only a small range of goods and was expensive. The impact of the supermarket closure on food security was expressed by an Aboriginal and Torres Strait Islander woman:

[I] find it hard with shopping since local supermarket closed. Shopping Centre not within walking distance but was a short drive from my house and [I] relied on a lift or taxi that didn't cost very much. Now [I] have to pay more for taxis, as [I] travel further to go shopping. (Aboriginal and Torres Strait Islander mother of four children, 33 years and single)

Different modes of transport were used for food shopping by participants. Access to a reliable car, particularly a privately-owned car, was said to help the most and enabled access to larger supermarkets for food specials and buying food in bulk:

We didn't have a car before but have one now. Made it easier to get around and do the shopping. (Aboriginal and Torres Strait Islander mother of five children, 29 years and partnered).

I don't have transport problems and can go to the places I want to shop. Usually follow the bargains and try to buy in bulk. (Aboriginal and Torres Strait Islander mother of three, 38 years and single).

Participants who accessed public transport, particularly buses, found it difficult when travelling with small children. Using taxis was another option, though this was expensive particularly when funds were limited:

Hard to take the bus with a baby and a two year old to go shop or clinic. (Aboriginal mother of two children, 25 years and partnered).

3.3.2. Minor Influencing Factors

Social pressures, emotional wellbeing and housing featured in discussions of food security with at least one-third of the participants.

Don't Want the Kids to Miss out

Four participants spoke in detail about their school-aged children needing money for entertainment and social occasions, of which put a strain on family income. They did not want their children "to go without" or miss out on social experiences that their children's peers were perceived to have:

We have problems sometimes with having enough money . . . only when we have visitors or things the kids want to go to, like the [Darwin] Show. All the other kids going to the Show and our kids don't want to miss out. It's only fair for them, they only kids and should enjoy themselves. (Aboriginal Grandmother of 10 grandchildren, 44 years and widowed).

Kid's like to buy from the school shop [tuckshop] like the other kids. Sometimes I really don't have enough money but, give them anyway. I don't want other kids at school to think my kids are poor. (Aboriginal mother of seven children, 26 years and single).

I Used to Get Sad a Lot

At least two thirds of participants openly discussed their feelings of how they felt emotionally in relation to food insecurity. Eleven participants expressed feelings of being stressed, down, sad, lonely and of frustration or feeling inadequate in being a good provider for their children. Two of the four participants receiving Centrelink payments referred to the stigma of shopping with a Basics Card and the feeling of frustration and 'shame' (shame is a term used by Aboriginal and Torres Strait Islander peoples as feeling embarrassed either about themselves or others. I.e. feeling shame because no money on the card to purchase groceries and others looking on. Or, feeling shame for someone else in a similar situation.) in having little control over managing their finances. These two participants also believed they did not need to be income managed and described feelings of public humiliation when not having enough money on the Basic card for groceries:

Real shame job [embarrassed] for me to go shop and find out don't have enough money on the card [Basic card] to pay for groceries. Have to leave everything—trolley and all—with everyone watching. Make me real shame. (Aboriginal mother of two children, 25 years and partnered).

Other participants raised and spoke about wellbeing related issues with relevance to food and money. In particular these were emotions of feeling down or sad due to relationship breakdowns and family stresses:

I used to get sad a lot and not able to look after the kids properly. (Aboriginal mother of three children, 34 years and single).

The House Needs Fixing

Of the 30 participants, four were owner-occupiers with seven renting privately and nineteen renting through public housing. One-third of the participants in rental properties discussed problems with general home maintenance, specifically with kitchen maintenance including problems with window fly screens, kitchen benches, kitchen cupboards and stoves:

. . . There are no flyscreens on some of the windows and in others there are holes. The rats get in at night and sometimes [we] can see and hear them running in the house. Sometimes they run over us in our sleep! (Aboriginal mother of four children, 34 years and partnered).

A number of participants expressed frustration in home maintenance:

. . . We've told him [owner] about the kitchen cupboards falling apart and other problems in the house. Just doesn't seem to want to do anything about it . . . . (Aboriginal mother of two children, 29 years and partnered).

We can't use the benches properly 'cause the tiles are broken and dirty (bench top is tiled). The stove doesn't work either". We told housing [public housing authority] we have problems months ago, but they still haven't come to fix them. All we do is wait and see what happens. (Aboriginal mother of four children, 34 years and partnered).

One participant who owned their home, indicated that having adequate food storage space helped with always having food on hand!

. . . we buy frozen vegies as well, because they last longer and we have them on hand to put in our food [cooking]. Well that helps with us. So, having a freezer helps as well [with food storage]. (Aboriginal and Torres Strait Islander father of two children, 36 years and partnered).

Whereas a participant who did not have adequate cold food storage had to shop more frequently:

I have what I need in the house. [I] Need a freezer. That way can buy more meat and put away, instead of going to the shop every day to buy meat for dinner. (Aboriginal mother of seven children, 26 years and single).

3.4. Impact on Food Selection

Within this theme are sub themes that encompass participants' views regarding food affordability; relationship between food and health; and food behaviour in association with food insecurity.

3.4.1. Not Everyone Can Afford to be Healthy

Many references to food and health were made by participants. In particular, the benefits of consuming home prepared meals rather than take-away meals perceived as high in fat and sugar. Four of the 30 participants spoke in-depth about fresh fruit and vegetables being 'healthy' foods and important in the prevention of illnesses such as type 2 diabetes. These foods though were considered by these participants as expensive and not always affordable when compared with other less healthy food options. At least half of the participants referred to the high cost of food influencing food choice.

An Aboriginal woman for example understood the relationship with food and good health, yet felt she was unable to put this knowledge into practice due to limited money and high food costs:

[I] Find it hard sometimes to eat healthy like have fruit and vegetables every day. Sometimes [it's a] bit tight with money and [I] buy food that fills you up. Fruit doesn't [fill you up] and it's expensive. . . . . Always hear about why important to eat healthy to stop diseases like diabetes, but when you try to, it's very expensive. (Aboriginal mother of three children, 29 years and partnered).

We're told to eat right, exercise and be healthy, but it's hard when everything costs so much to be healthy. Not everyone can afford to be healthy. (Torres Strait Islander mother of four children, 30 years and partnered).

One participant, where money for food was not considered an issue, spoke of not wanting her children to eat too much processed foods and have more natural foods in their diets:

I like my children to eat fresh food and foods that are not over processed. Also, processed foods tend to have a lot of sugar and that's no good. (Aboriginal mother of two children, 29 years and partnered).

3.4.2. Something to Fill Our Bellies

Participants referred to compromising food quality for quantity to ensure that there was enough to eat at each meal. Most participants spoke of the importance of eating healthy food at meal times. However, for some this was not always feasible and most important to these participants was ensuring enough food to eat "to fill bellies":

I make sure my kids are fed and don't go without. Some of our meals are not that healthy, but at least we have something to fill our bellies. (Aboriginal and Torres Strait Islander mother of three, 38 years and single).

We can afford food, but not always healthy food. Sometimes, have hamper [tinned corned beef] and rice with bread for dinner. It's filling and the kids are not hungry. (non-Indigenous mother of four children, 30 years and partnered).

Some participants referred to strategies used to ensure the family did not go without a meal:

. . . Usually try to buy in bulk and cook meals in bulk to freeze and use later. Therefore, make sure my daughter never goes without food. (non-Indigenous mother of one, 28 years and single).

3.4.3. Making the Meal Stretch

Most participants mentioned the use of low cost starchy foods, such as rice, pasta and bread to 'fill children up between meals' or add quantity to 'bulk up' meals when unexpected visitors joined in a meal or to use up leftover foods:

. . . If not enough food for each meal, cook more rice or have bread. This fills you up. Only time this happens is when we have unexpected visitors at dinnertime [evening meal] and we have to stretch the food so everyone has something". (Aboriginal mother of three children, 34 years and single).

I make sure kids always eat weet-bix [wheat biscuits breakfast cereal] in the morning before go to school. Have something at school from the shop [school tuckshop] and when they get home usually have bread with something on it. Boys eat a lot and bread is cheap and fills them up. (Aboriginal mother of seven children, 26 years and single).

A male participant spoke of his family's experience with using up left over food and filler foods to bulk up meals:

It's sort of a standard way (having rice) of making the meal stretch. Not that having enough food is an issue. But when we have leftovers, it's a, way of making sure we have enough. (Aboriginal and Torres Strait Islander father of two, 36 years and partnered).

3.5. Coping Strategies

As a coping strategy, social support in the form of accessing extended family was the most prominent form of assistance sought by participants to prevent or help alleviate food insecurity.

3.5.1. Live with Mum and Dad, They Help Out a Lot

Extended family provided the most common form of support and the types of support sought were mainly for money and food, but for some families it was assistance with looking after children. For four participants, assistance was sought regularly where others sought assistance only when there were additional demands placed on the household income. Running out of money and/or food were the most common reasons for accessing social support which usually occurred during 'money tight' times when the 'big bills' were due for payment. An Aboriginal woman with a family who lived with her parents, spoke of how this living arrangement assisted with expenses and provided support with looking after her children:

Sometimes have problems with money. Especially when the bills come in at once and don't always have enough to buy food. My three kids and me live at home with my mum and dad. This makes it easier for when I run out of money. Mum and dad have money for food. (Aboriginal mother of three children, 34 years and single).

Other participants shared their experiences with accessing family for assistance when experiencing difficulties and this support being reciprocated:

My partner has family here and if we don't have food, or money for food, we go over to family's place for dinner [evening meal]. Or if someone has money, we'll lend money. Our home is open to family if we have food and someone wants something to eat or money. But I always make sure we have enough for ourselves first. (non-Indigenous mother of four, 30 years and partnered).

We do have problems with food sometimes. Especially when we get big bills and there's not enough money for food. Usually, go to my mum and dad to ask for money or food. Glad I have them. Don't know where I would go otherwise for help. (Aboriginal and Torres Strait Islander mother of five children, 29 years and partnered).

There were instances where participants who had limited or no social support found it difficult:

I am not from Darwin and don't really have family here. My mother is visiting and I know some people from the community where I come from. Bit lonely sometimes. (Aboriginal mother of seven children, 26 years and single).

For one participant however, a falling out with a family member led to this young mother of two to seek support elsewhere which was limited and resulted in food and money problems.

Four participants received support from family with household chores and looking after children:

We haven't relied on family to help us out with feeding us, only with looking after the baby and other household chores when my wife was sick. (Aboriginal father of one child, 38 years and partnered).

Most participants mentioned that living with immediate family members (parents or siblings) reduced the financial burden of expenses and assisted with raising of children. Almost one third of the participants lived with extended family and seemed to be in this arrangement for similar reasons. A participant shared her situation where she and her family had recently moved in with her parents:

We used to be in government housing, but now me and my partner earn too much and had to give up our house and find a private house to rent. But we can't afford to pay private rent. Too much and won't have much money left for food and other things we need. Me, my partner and the kids moved in with my mum and dad. That way we can save money to buy our own house. (Aboriginal mother of three children, 29 years and partnered).

A mother of one, recently separated from her partner spoke of having to move in with her family to cope with expenses:

My ex [partner] moved out about 2 months ago and it was hard paying the rent and bills, so [I] decided to move out to Palmerston and be with my family. Too expensive living in Darwin. [I] Don't know how other people like me can live there. (non-Indigenous mother of one child, 28 years and single).

3.5.2. We Don't Have It as Bad as other Families

Most participants experiencing food insecurity expressed that others were in a worse situation than their own:

We don't have it bad as some families. At least we always have something to eat, bills are paid and [have] petrol for the car". (Non-Indigenous mother of four children, 30 years and partnered).

"We are doing better than some other families. I know some have to ask for food vouchers [from Centrelink] to buy groceries. (Aboriginal and Torres Strait Islander mother of three children, 38 years and single).

It makes you feel a bit easier to know that your situation is bad, but that someone else is worse off to make yourself feel better or make light of your current situation. I don't know, but I think that it's across the board [whole population]. (Aboriginal father of one child, 38 years and partnered).

4. Discussion

This study examined issues relating to food insecurity within a cohort of urban-based care-givers of Aboriginal and Torres Strait Islander children and found common features that contributed to household food security issues and mechanisms of coping. The most striking finding was that participants did not initially identify with being food insecure, although many participants' experiences indicated otherwise. In general, participants accepted the situation of running out of money, food or both, and having to seek assistance from relatives as a normal experience. This finding has also been described in a study involving six Inuit communities of Nunavut, Canada which described an incongruence between perceived food security status and experiences in obtaining enough food to eat [7]. In contrast, another study undertaken within an Inuit population from Nunavut, found participants who reported food insecurity also reported regular use of community food programs to assist with alleviating hunger [2]. Unlike Chan et al.'s (2006) study, Ford et.al. (2012) recruited participants who were registered with food assistance programs and these participants may have shared characteristics with those considered by this study's participants as "worse off" [2,7].

A second finding was that for most, food insecurity was experienced occasionally and usually when larger bills were due for payment. Food insecurity for some however was a chronic problem and seemed to be often due to an inadequate or irregular income. Two Australian studies have found that the Commonwealth Government New Start Allowance does not provide an adequate income for families, or anyone, to meet healthy living standards [22,23]. The authors did raise whether introducing an independent mechanism, similar to that of the Minimum Wage Panel that assesses its adequacy, to review and set the New Start Allowance level [23]. Participants that reported to have enough money to meet their needs, tended to be in paid employment. Secure employment and stable housing have been shown in other studies to be strongly associated with food security [2,4,5]. In contrast seasonal employment [5,8], unemployment and underemployment (the underemployment classification includes those workers that are highly skilled but work in low paid jobs; workers that are highly skilled but work in low skill jobs and part-time workers that would prefer to be full-time. This is different from unemployment in that the individual is working but isn't working at their full capability. (Source: http://www.investopedia.com/terms/u/underemployment.asp)) [2–4,7,10,11] have been reported as problematic in ensuring a regular income to afford food and other expenses among those experiencing food insecurity. Noted in the findings, a small proportion of participants were income managed and shared mixed views of their experiences. These were, not having enough money to meet the family's groceries requirements; feeling anxious wondering if there was enough money on the card for food; and finally, that it stopped the 'humbugging' from others wanting a loan. A study undertaken by Brimblecombe et al. (2010) in ten remote communities of the Northern Territory where income management had been introduced, investigated the impact of income management on store sales [24]. Stores sale data were reviewed over a 35-month period and included 18-months of data prior to the introduction of income management. Focusing on fruit and vegetable sales and turnover, Brimblecombe et al. (2010) found income management did not have an effect on store sales over the study period [24]. However, the Government stimulus payment between November 2008 to January 2009 did have a positive effect on fruit and vegetable sales [24].

In our study, participants with and without employment, referred to the cost of living as contributing to their food insecurity experiences. In some instances, participants purposely lived with extended family to mitigate potential food insecurity with the rising cost of living, even though they reported to earn an adequate income. Chan et al. also found the cost of living and cash flow among the 'working poor' to negatively impact food security in Nunavut communities [7]. A study undertaken in a United States urban centre found the cost of home rental was the single biggest factor identified among a group of young mothers as contributing to food insecurity [4]. In the current study, not only were high rent and large bills contributing factors to the high cost of living and food insecurity experiences, but issues with housing maintenance and inadequate kitchen facilities were also associated with experiences of food insecurity.

The experience amongst this study population of "money tight" due to the payment of large bills and general cost of living has also been reported by other researchers investigating food security experiences and influencing factors [4,5,8]. Participants in these studies were either low income earners or recipients of welfare (government payments) and received support through government and non-government food and nutrition assistance programs. Food insecurity occurred when money 'ran out' before the next pay period and food and nutrition assistance was accessed at these times to alleviate food insecurity over the short term. This contrasts to the findings of this study, where participants did not report to access food assistance programs.

Whilst participants dealt with intermittent food insecurity through various coping strategies, they did not appear to seek assistance from relevant agencies to alleviate food insecurity. Instead, strategies participants put in place during the "money tight" times were to delay payment of bills or undertake part payment of larger bills through staggered payments, or to cut back "luxury foods", such as sweets, soft drinks and desserts. Similar coping strategies were reported by a study among a group of 90 food pantry users in Washington, USA, where coping strategies included putting off paying bills and using up leftover food, preparing food in bulk and freezing food for later use [11]. A study among Latino immigrant families in North Carolina, USA, also reported participants coped with times of food insecurity by reducing purchase of foods considered expensive, such as meats and fruits and unnecessary foods, such as 'soft drinks, snacks and eating out' [8].

The strategies employed to cope with "money tight" times in this study were seen to be both positive (such as limiting purchase of sweets and soft drinks) and negative (compromising quality for quantity) in respect to food behaviour and health. In other studies, shopping for specials, bulk-buying, cooking in bulk and freezing food portions are examples of other pragmatic responses [4,5,8,11] to food insecurity which were also employed by participants within this study. Negative responses to food insecurity, similar to that reported by this study, have also been reported by others including forgoing healthier food options and choosing cheaper less healthier foods, reducing meal size or going without to ensure children eat [4–6,8,11].

There is debate to whether the behavioural purchase of unhealthy foods in preference to healthy foods is driven by need, due to healthy food not being affordable [2,6,7,25] or by poor dietary habits, established food preferences and poor food purchasing knowledge [7,9]. Poor eating habits among high and low-income earners have been considered as being due to laziness [25] and time constraints [11,26]. In the current study, as similar to other studies, participants perceived healthier food to be more expensive to less healthy food and expressed frustrations at not always being able to afford healthier food options and bewilderment as to why unhealthier foods appeared cheaper. Other studies have reported the cost of healthy food options as a barrier to healthy eating and have commented that low income gave participants little option but to buy highly refined, energy dense foods that provide calories at less cost than low-calorie nutrient rich foods [4,7,15]. Similarly, a study undertaken within a low income urban Australian Aboriginal population, found participants understood what were healthy foods, but were not always able to afford these foods [13]. The same was reported for a study undertaken in an Aboriginal population in remote Australia where participants perceived healthy food to be unaffordable [17].

A fourth finding is participants' concerns for their children's needs often characterised their food behaviour responses to food insecurity. Hamelin and others (2002) also noted experiences of anxiety by some participants in ensuring enough food for the children and the accompanying feelings of despair [10]. Upon similar lines, within this study several participants expressed concerns for the acceptance and social inclusion of their children by peers and how this exacerbated the risk of food insecurity due to allocation of limited food money to non-food items or entertainment. Participants also spoke of the experiences of others' they knew, specifically with drug and alcohol use and how this impacted on families' food security situation. Temple's (2018) study looking at the association between stressful events and food insecurity in Australia, found between the food secure and food insecure respondents there was a prevalence greater than 10% that included among other stressors, drug or alcohol related problems [27].

Use of a private vehicle, as reported within the current study to access food outlets, enabled people to seek out food bargains and specials. Specifically, access to a private vehicle was advantageous in accessing larger supermarkets where food was often cheaper and of more variety. This was also noted by other studies where public transport (buses and taxis) were considered by participants as unreliable, inconvenient or expensive and therefore, found to negatively impact on food security [4,5,9,28,29].

Finally, unlike the variety of social support systems accessed by other populations experiencing food insecurity, including food assistance programs, food charity organisations, faith communities, neighbours and friends [2–11,26], this study is unique in that family support was the only resource reported to be accessed for assistance. Other studies have also identified the extended family as a social support system [2–4,8,9,11] and identified support from friends and neighbours as a main coping strategy in response to food insecurity [5]. Only one study however, mentioned living with family as a temporary measure [2]. Residing with family members, particularly parents, was mentioned within the current study as a way for families to cope with living expenses. For some, this arrangement also provided support with child care. However, we did not the food security of all family members and it is possible that other members have influence perceptions of food security e.g., food insecure members moving in with food secure persons may heighten the odds of the later experiencing food insecurity.

Central to the study participants' social support system, was the action of reciprocity where families coped through inter-reliance on each other for food, money and other necessities. For instance, participants reported that when they had food, they would provide for other extended family members. Then when they would 'run out', extended family assisted in return. Reciprocity was also mentioned in a study, where young mothers would rely on family members for assistance with food and then 'return the favour' when family members experienced difficulties [4].

Within this study, as with other literature, reciprocity forms a cultural practice of sharing among Aboriginal and Torres Strait Islander peoples that is important in maintaining and reinforcing cultural social bonds with individual and group relationships [14]. As noted by Chan et al. and Ford et al., reciprocity has a place in maintaining and reinforcing family and broader community relationship obligations as well as cultural identity and practice among Inuit [2,7]. Among the Inuit these sharing networks extended to hunted traditional foods where excess was provided to the more vulnerable members of the community who cannot obtain these foods [2,7]. For those who could not hunt, money or other services were exchanged for traditional foods to keep with continuing cultural practices [2,7]. This concept of sharing traditional foods in a reciprocated environment to help each other out is also evident in this study where food and monetary assistance was sought and provided within families.

Discussions with participants within our cohort identified reciprocation as an expectation, and a given cultural practice to maintain family relationships. Such sharing support structures however are also fragile and relationship upsets can result in limited or no support as experienced by one participant in this study. In contrast, a food insecurity study undertaken in an Aboriginal and Torres Strait Islander population living in Victoria, indicated that accessing family and friends for assistance was not reported by this population [13]. External programs providing assistance in the forms of food vouchers, as well as charity organisations providing meals and food parcels, are available within the study location. However, these services were not mentioned by participants as being accessed for assistance. This finding however should be interpreted with caution as participants may have chosen not to share this information and seeking knowledge about access to such services was not the purpose of our study.

Finally, unlike studies [4,5] indicating the importance of furthering education to gain employment or improve opportunities for higher paid work as a long-term solution to overcoming food insecurity, this was not found within our cohort. A possible reason is, as identified in this cohort being food insecure is normal i.e., 'normalisation of a pathology'. When problems with food security are encountered, reciprocated arrangements with family as a coping strategy provide an immediate solution and reinforce traditional Aboriginal and Torres Strait Islander relationships. Therefore, furthering education or skill development for employment as an option to alleviate food insecurity may not be considered by participants in our cohort. This is an important issue and further understanding of what constitute food security will be useful in the future.

5. Conclusions

We found that Aboriginal and Torres Strait Islander families in our cohort had varying direct experiences with household food insecurity. A major contributor to this is their limited financial resources in conjunction with rising living costs. For the majority, this was intermittent and occurred when the larger bills were due for payment. For some, however, food insecurity is a chronic problem where expenses outweighed income. Not having enough money to buy food and take care of living expenses is a universal experience for those on limited incomes. Similarly, for the participants in this study having a limited income impacted on their circumstances and other factors also impacted on food security, including transport and concern for social image.

We also found that the extended family was the major form of support for assistance and played possibly a broader cultural role in sharing as also identified among Inuit populations [2,7]. This was also a reciprocated arrangement where families would help each other out. However, it could also be considered fragile as support was very reliant on harmonious relationships between family members and may be considered only functional when relationships are.

5.1. Strengths and Limitations

Unlike other similar published research, a strength of this study is participant sampling in that recruitment was not undertaken through food assistance programs. This study therefore, provides a broader view of food security experiences from a perspective where people are either experiencing food insecurity or not. As previously referred to, this qualitative study is one part of a larger study. Although the sample size is small, initial discussions followed by in-depth interviews consolidated themes, as a point was reached during data collection where no new information was forthcoming and data saturation was reached. The majority of participants were however, from well-established families within the two study locations. Therefore, the findings are more applicable to families who are long term residents of Darwin and Palmerston with extended family networks. Caution is required in generalising findings to all families in the Darwin and Palmerston regions and other similar populations. There are also possibilities of bias with findings reflecting the views of one gender more so than the other. Future studies may need to consider recruitment and sampling strategies that address gender balance.

The interviews were undertaken by an Aboriginal Public Health Nutritionist which was positive in communicating and establishing a trusting relationship with participants of which was captured within the interviews. The study design and methodology could be considered for future qualitative research investigating unexplored topics to generate new knowledge in learning more about Aboriginal and Torres Strait Islander peoples' understandings and experiences of food security. Finally, this qualitative research has unveiled 'new' understandings of food insecurity experiences and coping strategies from an urban Aboriginal and Torres Strait Islander population perspective that otherwise, may have remained unknown to the broader community.

5.2. Implications

A possible solution to assist with meeting payment of expenses is support to families to set up direct debit options of smaller regular payments to offset larger bills and undue financial pressure.

Transport, preferably access to a private car, was also deemed essential by some to undertake food shopping. There could be possible scope for services and other assistance programs to consider these needs. For instance, food shopping assistance for older Australians and the disabled is provided through government and non-government services [28]. Major supermarket chains in Australia such as Coles and Woolworths provide an online shopping and delivery service for a fee. This may not be available by all stores and may not appeal to all consumers. However, it could be considered by government and non-government services to provide food shopping assistance, including a subsidised or free food shopping delivery service, for low income families with young children.

There is a widely held perception that the cost of healthy foods makes a healthy diet unaffordable for families. Participants of this study referred specifically to the cost of fresh fruit and vegetables and the importance of these in prevention of chronic disease, such as type 2 diabetes. Consideration of economic access to healthy foods in public policy seems critical for improved health outcomes. A potential solution may involve food subsidies or similar. There are also opportunities for local councils to consider availability of public allotments to encourage community or family group food gardening to supplement diets though, this was not an option identified by study participants. The perception of fresh fruit and vegetables being costly is worth further research investigation, particularly in assessing the affordability of healthy foods within the study location.

In ensuring appropriate and sustainable safety nets that provide assistance to families, it is important to acknowledge the existence of support services accessed by families that are not recognised within the mainstream and are specific to Indigenous Australians. These include positive family associations. Potential scope for current services is to consider an approach in connecting with family networks for provision of support services, such as financial counselling. Such services have potential to provide peer support family counselling where members experiencing difficulties are supported by family member(s) to engage with services and work through issues.

This study has clearly identified food insecurity experiences among the study population to be related to monetary expenditure outweighing income, particularly with the payment of larger bills. Being in a situation where money is limited and expenses out way available funds, fulfilling a family's social, cultural and physical needs requires a fragile balance of continually adjusting food access and purchasing behavior at time when 'money is tight', maintaining family support structures, and upholding social status.

Author Contributions: L.M., J.B. and A.B.C. jointly conceptualized the study, prepared, reviewed, edited and authored the manuscript. L.M. conducted data collection and analysis under the supervision of J.B. and A.B.C., J.B. finalised data analysis and consolidated findings. For research articles with several authors, a short paragraph specifying their individual contributions must be provided.

Funding: This research project received no external funding. Though, L.M. was supported by The Ian Potter Foundation Indigenous Research Fellowship (Grant ID 20070455), The National Health and Medical Research Council Public Health Postgraduate Research Scholarship (App ID APP1017539) and Menzies Foundation Allied Health Scholarship; A.B.C. is supported by a NHMRC practitioner fellowship (APP1154302). J.B. was supported by a National Heart Foundation (NHF) Future Leader Fellowship (grant number 100085).

Acknowledgments: The authors acknowledge the participants, Aboriginal and Torres Strait Islander families of Darwin and Palmerston, NT; Bagot Community Health Clinic, Darwin NT; Danila Dilba Health Service child health clinic, Palmerston NT; Northern Territory Department of Health child health clinics Darwin and Palmerston; Sian Graham, Aboriginal Research Officer, Menzies School of Health Research, Darwin NT; Helen Fejo-Frith, Aboriginal Research Assistant, Bagot Community; Bagot Community Council; and Associate Jan Ritchie, School of Public Health and Community Medicine, University of New South Wales for reviewing the qualitative chapter of LM's Ph.D. thesis.

Conflicts of Interest: The authors declare no conflict of interest.

Appendix A

Table A1. Inductive development processes towards key guiding questions for the in-depth qualitative interview.

Theme	Notes	Guiding Questions
Influencing factors		
Income quarantining (Basic Card)	Limited control over own money. Anxious when going shopping, as don't know how much money available on basic card for spending. Feelings of shame/embarrassment/anger when: - can't pay for it (not enough money on card) and don't have extra cash. - On the scheme and have no say in being on it or not.	Tell me more about your experiences with the Basic Card. Why do you like/dislike being Income managed? How does this make you feel?
Housing problems (more around maintenance)	House needs fixing, takes a long time before something is done, participant has little control over the situation. Limited availability of public housing, hard to find a place to live. Sense of feeling powerless, beyond people's control	Tell me about your house. Is everything good? i.e., windows, benches, etc.? Does anything need to be fixed?
Food preparation and cooking facilities	Food storage, preparation and cooking facilities: - Need for working stove - Need for a freezer	Do you like to cook? Can you tell me about your experiences with cooking (good/ok). What stops you from cooking?
Money problems	About not having enough money to fulfil own and families' needs/wants/requirements. Impact of the cost of living in Darwin and Palmerston—everything is expensive. Limited money, prioritise what spending on Always make sure the children are fed, don't go without.	Do you have enough money for what you need? If no money problems/worries, what do you do to make sure everything is good? Can you tell me about your money problems/worries? How often do you have money problems/worries? Are money problems ongoing (all the time)? When you have money problems, how do you prioritise spending? Are there things that do you do to cope with the problem?
Social Inclusion	Not wanting money problems to impact on children's lives to point where excluded from social events, outings, what their peers have, etc.	Is it important to you and your kids that you don't miss out on what other families have? What are some of the things you do to make sure you and your kids don't miss out on having what others have?
Budgeting	Always make sure money for food, even if not healthy. An already tight budget for food and regular expenses. Additional expenses puts a strain on the budget therefore, spend less on food and tend to eat less healthy.	How do you make sure there is enough money for things you/your family need between paydays? Does this always work, or do you sometimes find it hard? What else do you do to try and make it work?

Table A1. *Cont.*

Theme	Notes	Guiding Questions
Influencing factors		
Filler Foods	Low cost, high calorie foods to stretch meals and 'fill you up'—bread and rice. E.g of filler foods for a meal—cheap tinned meats (hamper) and rice with bread.	Do you have enough food at each meal for everybody? What do you do to make sure everyone has enough food? Tell me about these foods (filler foods) and the reasons you choose them? - Cheaper, feed more people (stretch meals) and fill you up. - Comfort, familiar food
Wellbeing	2 participants talked about feeling sad. As mentioned previously, feelings of shame, embarrassment, anger, anxiety, powerless.	*If possible, find out more if these feelings are related to money worries/problems.* How do you feel when you don't have enough money? Do you think about having enough money a lot?
Other's worse off	Acknowledge other families experiences similar problems and probably more worse off. However, also put this down to possible use of drug and alcohol and this is where money is diverted to.	From what you know, do you think your family 'has it hard' compared to other families?
Transport	Few transport issues to go places to shop, particularly when relying on public transport and travelling with small children	What are your experiences with having regular transport to go shopping?
Social problems	Identify money (income) diverted to social problems such as drug, alcohol and gambling impact on having enough food.	What are your thoughts on why some families may experience problems with having enough food?
Food Shopping	Transport and the amount of shopping undertaken impacts on where people shop. Others that 'plan' where they shop according to where bargains are—buy bulk.	Do you worry about going food shopping (regularly)? Do you plan where you will shop and what you will buy before you go? Are you able to go to the shops when you want to?
Coping Strategy		
Support Networks	Families rely on extended family and friends' networks for support and 'fill the gaps'	Tell me more about the support you have when you are having difficulties? Do you think you rely on this support network? Where would you go if you didn't have this support network?

References

1. American Dietetic Association. Position of The American Dietetic Association: Domestic food and nutrition security. *J. Am. Diet. Assoc.* **1998**, 337–342. [CrossRef]
2. Ford, J.; Lardeau, M.P.; Vanderbilt, W. The characteristics and experience of community food program users in arctic Canada: A case study from Iqaluit, Nunavut. *BMC Public Health* **2012**, *12*, 464. [CrossRef] [PubMed]
3. Sim, M.S.; Glanville, T.N.; McIntyre, L. Food management behaviours in food insecure, lone mother-led families. *Can. J. Diet. Pract. Res.* **2011**, *72*, 123–129. [CrossRef] [PubMed]
4. Stevens, C.A. Exploring food insecurity among young mothers (15–24 Years). *J. Spec. Pediatr. Nurs.* **2010**, *15*, 163. [CrossRef] [PubMed]
5. De Marco, M.; Thorburn, S.; Kue, J. "In a country as affluent as America, people should be eating": Experiences with and perceptions of food insecurity among rural and urban oregonians. *Qual. Health Res.* **2009**, *19*, 1010–1024. [CrossRef] [PubMed]
6. Hamelin, A.M.; Mercier, C.; Bedard, A. Perception of needs and responses in food security: Divergence between households and stakeholders. *Public Health Nutr.* **2008**, *11*, 1389–1396. [CrossRef] [PubMed]
7. Chan, H.M.; Fediuk, K.; Hamilton, S.; Rostas, L.; Caughey, A.; Kuhnlein, H.; Egeland, G.; Loring, E. Food security in Nunavut, Canada: Barriers and recommendations. *Int. J. Circumpolar Health* **2006**, *65*, 416–431. [CrossRef] [PubMed]
8. Quandt, S.A.; Shoaf, J.I.; Tapia, J.; Hernandez-Pelletier, M.; Clark, H.M.; Arcury, T.A. Experiences of Latino immigrant families in North Carolina help explain elevated levels of food insecurity and hunger. *J. Nutr.* **2006**, *136*, 2638–2644. [CrossRef] [PubMed]
9. Kempson, K.; Palmer Keenan, D.; Sadani, P.S.; Adler, A. Maintaining food sufficiency: Coping strategies identified by limited-resource individuals versus nutrition educators. *J. Nutr. Educ. Behav.* **2003**, *35*, 179–188. [CrossRef]
10. Hamelin, A.M.; Beaudy, M.; Habicht, J.P. Characterisation of household food insecurity in Quebec: Food and feelings. *Soc. Sci. Med.* **2002**, *54*, 119–132. [CrossRef]
11. Hoisington, A.; Armstong Shultz, J.; Butkus, S. Coping strategies and nutrition education needs among food pantry users. *J. Nutr. Educ. Behav.* **2002**, *34*, 326–333. [CrossRef]
12. Temple, J.B.; Russell, J. Food insecurity among older Aboriginal and Torres Strait islanders. *Int. J. Environ. Res. Public Health.* **2018**, *15*, 1766. [CrossRef] [PubMed]
13. Adams, K.; Burns, C.; Liebzeit, A.; Ryschka, J.; Thorpe, S.; Browne, J. Use of participatory research and photo-voice to support urban Aboriginal healthy eating. *Health Soc. Care Community* **2012**, *20*, 497–505. [CrossRef] [PubMed]
14. Markwick, A.; Ansari, Z.; Sullivan, M.; McNeil, J. Social determinants and lifestyle risk factors only partially explain the higher prevalence of food insecurity among Aboriginal and Torres Strait islanders in the Australian state of Victoria: A cross-sectional study. *BMC Pubic Health* **2014**, *14*, 598. [CrossRef] [PubMed]
15. Nolan, M.; Rikard-Bell, G.; Mohsin, M.; Williams, M. Food insecurity in three socially disadvantaged localities in Sydney, Australia. *Health Promot. J. Austr.* **2006**, *17*, 247–254. [CrossRef] [PubMed]
16. Broome, R. *Aboriginal Australians: Black Responses to White Dominance 1788–1994*, 2nd ed.; Allen and Unwin: Sydney, Australia, 1994; pp. 9–21. ISBN 186373760X.
17. Brimblecombe, J. Enough for Rations and a Little Bit Extra: Challenges of Nutrition Improvements in an Aboriginal Community in North–East Arnhem Land. Ph.D. Thesis, Charles Darwin University, Darwin, Australia, 2007.
18. Braun, V.; Clarke, V. Using thematic analysis in psychology. *Qual. Res. Psychol.* **2006**, *3*, 77–101. [CrossRef]
19. Australian Bureau of Statistics. *2006 Census of Population and Housing Quickstats: Australia*; Australian Bureau of Statistics: Canberra, Australia, 2007.
20. Tuckett, A.G. Applying thematic analysis theory to practice: A researcher's experience. *Contemp. Nurse* **2005**, *19*, 75–87. [CrossRef] [PubMed]
21. Attride-Stirling, J. Thematic networks: An analytic tool for qualitative research. *Qual. Res.* **2001**, *1*, 385–401. [CrossRef]
22. Saunders, P.; Bedford, M. New minimum healthy living budget standards for low-paid and unemployed Australians. *Econ. Labour. Relat. Rev.* **2018**, *29*, 273–288. [CrossRef]

23. Saunders, P. Using a budget standards approach to assess the adequacy of newstart allowance. *Aust. J. Soc. Issues* **2018**, *53*, 4–17. [CrossRef]

24. Brimblecombe, J.K.; McDonnel, J.; Barnes, A.; Dhurrkay, J.G.; Thomas, D.P.; Bailie, R.S. Impact of income management on store sales in the Northern Territory. *MJA* **2010**, *192*, 549–554. [CrossRef] [PubMed]

25. Eikenberry, N.; Smith, C. Healthful eating: Perceptions, motivations, barriers, and promoters in low-income Minnesota communities. *J. Am. Diet. Assoc.* **2004**, *104*, 1158–1161. [CrossRef] [PubMed]

26. Inglis, V.; Ball, B.; Crawford, D. Why do women of low socioeconomic status have poorer dietary behaviours than women of higher socioeconomic status? A qualitative exploration. *Appetite* **2005**, *45*, 334–343. [CrossRef] [PubMed]

27. Temple, J.B. The association between stressful events and food insecurity: Cross-sectional evidence from Australia. *Int. J. Environ. Res. Public Health* **2018**, *15*, 2333. [CrossRef] [PubMed]

28. Coveney, J.; O'Dwyer, L.A. Effects of mobility and location on food access. *Health Place* **2009**, *15*, 45–55. [CrossRef] [PubMed]

29. Martin, K.S.; Rogers, B.L.; Cook, J.T.; Joseph, H.M. Social Capital is associated with decreased risk of hunger. *Soc. Sci. Med.* **2004**, *58*, 2645–2654. [CrossRef] [PubMed]

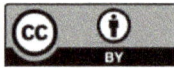

International Journal of
Environmental Research and Public Health

MDPI

Article

"A Lot of People Are Struggling Privately. They Don't Know Where to Go or They're Not Sure of What to Do": Frontline Service Provider Perspectives of the Nature of Household Food Insecurity in Scotland

Flora Douglas [1,*], Fiona MacKenzie [2], Ourega-Zoé Ejebu [3], Stephen Whybrow [4], Ada L. Garcia [5], Lynda McKenzie [3], Anne Ludbrook [3] and Elizabeth Dowler [6]

[1] School of Nursing and Midwifery, Robert Gordon University, Aberdeen AB10 7QG, Scotland
[2] Institute of Applied Health Sciences, University of Aberdeen, Aberdeen AB25 2ZD, Scotland; famackenzie68@gmail.com
[3] Health Economics Research Unit, University of Aberdeen, Aberdeen AB25 2ZD, Scotland; oejebu@abdn.ac.uk (O.-Z.E.); l.mckenzie@abdn.ac.uk (L.M.); a.ludbrook@abdn.ac.uk (A.L.)
[4] The Rowett Institute, University of Aberdeen, Aberdeen AB25 2ZD, Scotland; stephen.whybrow@abdn.ac.uk
[5] Human Nutrition, School of Medicine, Dentistry and Nursing, College of Medical, Veterinary and Life Sciences, University of Glasgow, Glasgow G31 2ER, Scotland; Ada.Garcia@glasgow.ac.uk
[6] Emeritus Professor of Food & Social Policy, Department Sociology, University of Warwick, Coventry CV4 7AL, UK; Elizabeth.Dowler@warwick.ac.uk
* Correspondence: f.douglas3@rgu.ac.uk; Tel.: +44-(0)-1224-263198

Received: 28 September 2018; Accepted: 30 November 2018; Published: 4 December 2018

Abstract: This qualitative study explored frontline service providers' perceptions of the nature of food insecurity in Scotland in 2015 to inform national policy and the provision of locally-based support for 'at risk' groups. A country-wide in-depth interview study was undertaken with informants from 25 health, social care, and third sector organisations. The study investigated informants' perspectives associated with how food insecurity was manifesting itself locally, and what was happening at the local level in response to the existence of food insecurity. Data analysis revealed three key themes. First, the *multiple faces and factors of food insecurity* involving not only increased concern for previously recognised 'at risk of food insecurity' groups, but also similar concern held about newly food insecure groups including working families, young people and women. Secondly, respondents witnessed *stoicism and struggle*, but also resistance amongst some food insecure individuals to external offers of help. The final theme identified community *participation yet pessimism* associated with addressing current and future needs of food insecure groups. These findings have important implications for the design and delivery of health and social policy in Scotland and other countries facing similar challenges.

Keywords: household food insecurity; food poverty; Scotland; low income; families; children; women; older people; qualitative

---

1. Introduction and Background

Household food insecurity has re-emerged as a subject of public health and social policy, civic and political concern in Scotland and the rest of the UK [1–8]. Household food insecurity is the experience associated with *"the inability to acquire or consume an adequate quality or sufficient quantity of food in socially acceptable ways, or the uncertainty that one will be able to do so"* [9]. Globally, household food insecurity is recognized as a problem in low income households in high income countries [10–13]. Household food insecurity prevalence data are not routinely captured and monitored in the UK [14] but it was estimated in 2014, in a one-off UN global survey, that 10.1% of the UK population were food insecure to some degree [15]. Despite the small sample size (1000 adults for the whole of the UK), this indicated the existence of a significant and real problem [16]. However, in the absence of food insecurity prevalence data, much of the current concern about this issue in the UK was triggered by the emergence of increased numbers, and greater visibility, of charitable emergency food assistance programmes (so-called food banks), which followed the UK economic crisis and reduced government spending in its aftermath [1–8]. The numbers of people seeking help from such sources has reached unprecedented levels since the mid-2000s [17], with the causes being politically disputed [7].

At the same time, within the Scottish context, a wide range of organisations and groups that had started to provide such support in their local communities expressed significant concern about the efficacy of food banks, both as a means of addressing household food insecurity and as a social justice issue [18].

Scotland is one of the four countries which makes up the United Kingdom, and operates with its own national government (within this context) which has responsibility over some devolved matters such as health care and education.

In North America, where it has been possible to compare routinely collected household food insecurity population survey data with national food bank use figures, food bank data are known to significantly underestimate population food insecurity prevalence. Twelve to fourteen percent of the Canadian population have reported some degree of food insecurity on an annual basis since 2005, yet only 20–30% of this food insecure group also reported using a food bank in the previous year [10,19]. Furthermore, it is well established that the capacity and capability of food banks to respond to growing demand for food assistance from low income communities is severely limited due to their dependence on corporate and public donations and volunteer labour [20,21]. These resources are quickly exhausted unless food is rationed or restricted and, because of the precarious and unpredictable nature of the food and volunteer labour supply, it is thought that many people who might benefit from food bank offerings do not get access to them, and therefore do not appear in food bank statistics [10,22,23]. This is of course in addition to those who might be missing from those figures through their active avoidance of this support due to shame and fear of stigma.

Scotland has a long running public health and social policy focus concerned with addressing health inequalities. This has been underpinned by an often explicit acknowledgement that life circumstances and socio-economic deprivation are primary drivers of those inequalities, and public services, including health and social care services, have been developed and delivered accordingly [24]. Population differences in self-reported dietary quality between the most and least deprived groups (as one specific domain of the experience of food insecurity) have also come under close scrutiny over some decades, related to the goal of addressing health inequalities [25]. The Scottish Diet Action Plan, (published in 1986) triggered a programme of recurring government funding over three decades, which is intended to enable low income families and neighbourhoods to gain access to affordable fruit and vegetables via local community food programmes. Typically, these include low cost food retailing outlets, budgeting and cooking skills training programmes, and in some cases, community food growing programmes [26]. It is important to note that these programmes were not set up to provide free food assistance.

Main Study Aim

These specific concerns about the lack of valid household food insecurity data and the possible under estimation of the magnitude of the problem through use of food bank data in its absence, combined with anxieties expressed about the efficacy and sustainability of community-based food assistance programmes in dealing with the issue, resulted in a national mixed methods study being commissioned to develop a better understanding of the nature and prevalence of household food in Scotland [27]. The study was commissioned by NHS Health Scotland, the national health promotion agency, and the Scottish Government's Rural Affairs and Environment Strategic Research programme with the aim of informing national policy and local practice.

This paper reports on the qualitative study component of the larger formative study [23], which set out to capture the perspectives and experiences of social, health and third sector practitioners, whose main role was concerned with supporting economically and socially vulnerable groups. These groups were considered to be key informants likely to have frontline, locally based experience and knowledge of that wider picture of household food insecurity within their respective communities, through their day-to-day engagement with people requiring their input because of food insecurity, but who may not necessarily be engaging with food assistance programmes. Some of the third sector practitioners were drawn from some of those long standing community food programmes described above. This work was commissioned to complement other research that was underway at the same time that was focused on capturing the perspectives of those with direct lived experience of food insecurity.

2. Materials and Methods

This was a qualitative research study informed by Grounded Theory (GT) principles and techniques [28]. The decision to use GT principles as the research framework within which to identify participants, generate, analyse and think about the data was largely pragmatic, i.e., it offered a conceptually congruent set of guidelines and principles to guide the research [29,30]. As discussed above, the study objectives had been developed on the basis of emergent concerns expressed by the policy, practitioner and civic society communities within Scotland. Consequently, an interview study was undertaken with community-based health, social care and third sector staff who were concerned with the care and support of so-called vulnerable groups. The sampling frame was discussed and agreed with the research commissioners as the study progressed. Older people and those who were, or were at risk of being, destitute (e.g., homeless groups, travelling people, asylum seekers) were of particular interest to the research commissioners. The rationale for participant selection was based on identifying professionals and practitioners who had primary responsibility for some aspect of health or social care at the individual and the community level, for groups considered to be economically and socially vulnerable and, importantly, had been operating in this role for some time, preferably prior to the aforementioned economic crisis. The research commissioners were also keen to capture the perspectives and experiences of those practitioners working within the community food programmes (as described above) who were perceived to have relevant local knowledge and experience of working alongside communities affected by varying degrees of economic deprivation and vulnerability, which was known to present a significant challenge in their ability to access to healthy foods.

Two interview topic guides were developed to guide the discussions and to enable the researchers to combine inductive and deductive reasoning to generate and analyse the data. The guides themselves were generated based upon the main study objectives and a series of iterative discussions between the research commissioners and the research team. Topics in the interview guides included participants' views about:

- what it means to live in household food insecurity in Scotland;
- which population groups were considered most affected by food insecurity;
- the main drivers of household food insecurity
- community responses to those trends and;
- notions of effective intervention/policy changes required to reduce the numbers of people seeking help with feeding.

Informants from community food programmes were also asked about how their organisation was alleviating food poverty at the current time, what they thought they might be doing to alleviate food insecurity in their community in the future, and their ideas or views about alternative models, or means required to address food insecurity.

The study was based on the conceptual definition of household food insecurity, which recognises the experience of food insecurity as one that negatively impacts nutritional and psycho-social domains of human existence, i.e., "*the inability to acquire or consume an adequate quality or sufficient quantity of food in socially acceptable ways, or the uncertainty that one will be able to do so*" [9].

The study protocol and associated materials were reviewed and endorsed by the University of Aberdeen's Rowett Research Institute's Human Studies Ethical Review PanelProject Review No. 2015-Douglas-01. The manuscript was written in accordance with the RATS qualitative research review guidelines [31].

A combination of purposive and maximum variation sampling was used to recruit informants to the study. As a national study, it was important to try to capture views from the different types of professional groups of interest across the whole country. Therefore we sought to engage with individuals from the different professional groups in urban, remote and rural contexts, the length and breadth of the country.

The majority of interviews took place by phone and lasted between 30 min to an hour. Two researchers (F.D. and F.McK.) undertook the interviews, and data collection stopped at the point that it became clear no new data was emerging from the interviews. All interviews were audio recorded and transcribed verbatim with informants' consent.

Data were analysed using a thematic content analysis approach. This method is commonly used for health-related research and is particularly useful for exploring questions about meaningful issues amongst a particular study group of interest [30,32]. The basis of this approach is to reduce the multiple individual responses and identify common patterns or themes in the data, as well as so-called 'deviant case' issues. At the initial stage of the analysis, a sample of interview transcripts was read and re-read independently by two researchers to identify the key concepts and themes, and a draft coding index was drawn up. The researchers met to discuss their initial analysis: areas of difference were identified and where different ideas about what particular instances of the interview discourse represented, these were discussed and agreed. The final version of the thematic index was also agreed through discussion, and all transcripts were coded manually. Memos and notes of emerging themes, issues and patterns were also recorded during this process and were referred to during the analysis. Constant comparison method was used throughout to confirm coding consistency and assignation of coded data to the emergent themes and categories, and to check that possible new themes were not being overlooked. Every attempt was made to search for disconfirming data within the data set. Data were also scrutinised for the possibility of dominant and/or marginalised viewpoints.

3. Results

Ten informants representing community food programmes and 15 informants from organisations concerned with the care and support of vulnerable groups were recruited to the study. The combined sample of informants was drawn from across Scotland and represented some of the key organisations and services that were being delivered in diverse urban, rural and remote locations. (see Appendix A for a detailed breakdown of the study participants' characteristics). The community food programme informants were people who worked in programmes that were offering multiple services, including low cost food retailing, and/or training and development programmes and/or community growing and gardening schemes. This group also contained three NHS-employed community food development staff. Although not originally set up for this purpose, six community food programmes also begun offering a take-home free food parcels (i.e., similar to a food bank service). One informant representing a recently opened food bank also took part. The 15 health, social care, and third sector participants, were drawn from a range of community-based care and support services agencies. It is important to note that those interviewed were also targeted on the basis of having been in their current post over a number of years so that they could provide insights from practice about the current position compared to their pre-recession experience.

Three major themes that emerged from this analysis are discussed in this paper, i.e., the *faces and factors of food insecurity* in Scotland associated with emergent food insecure groups, and those groups previously recognised to be at risk; *stoicism and struggle* witnessed at the individual level amongst people affected by food insecurity, and the community *participation yet pessimism* that surfaced in relation to the challenge of responding to expressed local feeding needs now and into the future.

3.1. Faces and Factors of Food Insecurity

Two fundamental issues explored at the beginning of each interview were informants' perspectives about who they believed to be, and encountered to be, most obviously affected by household food insecurity and what they believed was causing their food insecurity. The most common responses that surfaced here were not only more concern and anxiety for groups previously well known to them but also great concern for groups they had never previously considered to be affected by food insecurity.

Families with young children, young people and women were identified as emergent groups and sections of particular concern. This anxiety is illustrated by the following quotes from two different development workers based in urban locations in the north and central parts of Scotland:

> *I've got families that the parents do without, so that the child has got what they need to have, and it means that society is becoming even more uneven than it used to be before.* (Development Worker, urban),

and:

> *You've got people making choices about the kids clothing and shoes or a meal, you've got adults, women in particular I suspect, not eating properly so the kids are fed.* (Development Worker, urban).

While both quotes typify concerns for parents and children in general, the second quote illustrates the particular concern for women with children, some of whom were believed to be sacrificing their own food resources to ensure their children could eat. Some reported specific concerns about pregnant women.

The notion that families with young children were more obviously affected by food insecurity now compared to the past was linked to their having insufficient household incomes. Much of the public discourse about the rise of food banks in the UK has been linked to changes in UK government policy and related social security entitlements that were associated with unemployment (job seekers) or sickness or disability benefits. Yet many of our informants described supporting or encountering people who were working but not earning enough to cover their necessary household bills, illustrated here:

> *We have families, I have a lot of experience with people who work very hard and work long hours, to support their families, and still at the end of the week don't have enough money for basic food* (Rural, voluntary org, family worker).

Not only were people described as living on low incomes from their employment, but the issue of unpredictable levels of income was also flagged as an underlying determinant of the food insecurity. In this next illustrative quote, this welfare support worker who was based in a rural community in mid-east Scotland talks about her frustration that her clients were very keen to find work but were unable to survive on the hourly rates and number of hours on offer from local employers:

> *. . . one of the bigger employers in this area is a market gardener, who employs people through agencies, very often on short term contracts. They'll be zero hour contracts and certainly, because it's off season at the moment, a lot of people get signed off or maybe only get one shift a week, so they may be in employment, however, their income is so low that they actually can't pay their bills.* (Welfare support, rural).

Indeed, it was notable that local food production and food processing work featured in other rural participants' accounts as examples of industries which offered very low and unpredictable levels of pay for their workers.

However, picking up on the experiences of some other community-based development workers, we also found degrees of frustration expressed about recent policy changes to UK social security entitlement, which was perceived to be driving people into destitution as their benefits were reduced or removed for periods of time. These changes were viewed by many as a primary cause of household food insecurity: an argument typified in this quote:

> *He said that his benefits had changed, and he'd had to make a new claim or something, and there was a delay in getting his benefits. And this is often what we're told; that people have a delay, they've got to make a new claim, they get less money than they think they would get, they've got to wait an extra week or a fortnight to get the money. And in the meantime they often don't have anything, and they don't have any fall back.* (Social worker, island).

A few participants also talked about policy changes that were counterproductive to the aim of getting people off government support and into paid employment. These quotes from a community-based nurse located in a remote island community, and an urban-based development worker illustrate this notion of people cycling back into debt and poverty as they tried to move into paid work and off social security:

> *Younger people, who are of working age, have a much more variable source of income. If they're in employment that's fine; they might be in low employment and things are difficult. If they're moving in and out of employment, and in and out of the benefits system, it seems to me that it's very precarious* (Nurse, rural/remote).

and

> *The problem is that when they start work their first pay day may not be for four weeks. They then have got to work out how they're going to survive for that period. For many of them, the only solution is actually getting into debt of some kind. There's meant to be all kind of safety nets around that but that's just not happening in practical terms* (Development worker, urban).

These quotes also highlight the common concern expressed by our informants about younger people being amongst those new groups perceived to be most badly affected by and at risk of household food insecurity. In the next quote, the same community-based nurse, cited above, raises the issue of their existing vulnerability as an economically disadvantaged group being exacerbated by poor social support, in this case, emanating from people having to move away from the island to find work:

> *There could be any, they're working age people, and I would say that it's more typical for the younger end of working age, but it could be older people, in the working age group, who've had some other life crisis, like their family has broken up. They've had to move away from their family and from the way that they used to do things.* (Nurse, remote island).

During the time period in which the interviews took place there had also been an economic downturn in some industries in Scotland, including the oil and gas energy sector. This was linked to the experience reported by a few urban-based informants of having dealt with or being aware that previously high income earners were struggling as a consequence of losing their jobs and not being able to feed themselves, despite having a lot of expensive possessions, highlighted by this quote:

> *I've actually had people coming in with the best cars, the best fancy phones and whatever - not a lot, but I have had, coming in with all the flashiest of stuff saying that they've got a problem. The problem is they can't pay their bills. It doesn't matter that their bills are ten times higher than maybe somebody else's bills, they still come to the end of the month and they can't pay, you know? ... So it's kind of like hidden, I suppose. It's not what you expect.* (Community Food Programme Development, urban).

This quote (above) also touches on an issue that was remarked upon by many of the informants (regardless of income status) in terms of the 'hidden' nature of food insecurity; a theme that is picked up again later in the paper.

The situation for older people which was of initial, primary concern from the research commissioner's perspective, was more nuanced. Generally speaking, this study found most informants expressed less concern about older than younger people. This was often described in terms of an acknowledgement that while many older people lived on a low income, it was a predictable and relatively stable income that people had learned to live within and budget accordingly. In addition, older people were viewed as possessing all the necessary additional resources need to provide a constant, if limited, food and meal supply in the home, i.e., had the necessary food preparation, storage and cooking equipment that had been accumulated over their lifetimes. Older people were considered better able to cope with household food insecurity as illustrated here:

> ... *we very seldom have to help them [older people] out with money or with food.* (Nurse, rural/remote).

Mention was also made of older people not appearing at food banks in great numbers, which was interpreted by some to mean they were not in need of help. Interestingly, this was something that the research commissioners had noted, but had viewed as an indication of there being a problem, not a reassurance that all was well.

However, there were a minority of informants who were working directly with older people in their homes who were concerned about what they were seeing in practice (e.g., noticing that their clients' cupboards and fridges had little or no food during home visits) that led them to believe that some of their older clients were food insecure. These older people were also commonly described as denying they were having a problem with this and commonly refused offers of a referral to a food bank. Older carers were also highlighted as a group of concern.

However, even groups normally in regular contact with health and social care services were reported as being more badly affected by food poverty compared to the past, illustrated thus:

> *Definitely an increase in people who are long term sick who'd sort of settled down to a lifestyle where they understood their income so you may have had somebody who for 15 years had been in receipt of a benefit that was related to their ill-health who found themselves unchallenged around that, their rent was being paid, their council tax was being paid and they understood how much they had to live on every week.* (Development worker, urban).

This quote also illustrates a commonly cited participant observation that financial instability and unpredictability appeared to have become the norm for many people who were in receipt of social security payments due to long term ill health, and which was perceived to have occurred as a consequence of changes to government policy. Those changes to the previous pattern of timing and level of payment had made household income difficult to manage as a result.

These perceptions about the prevalence of insufficient and unpredictable income in Scottish households fit with informants' views about what it means to be food insecure in Scotland; i.e., lacking choice and being compelled to seek out cheap, nutrient poor food to survive, illustrated in this quote from an urban-based community food initiative informant:

> *I suppose the general idea is that you don't have enough food to eat but my thinking is, it's not the right food, not nutritious food that people can't afford. Or they're making choices out of necessity as to what's available rather than what they would probably like to eat. As you know, a lot of people—you see it in the supermarkets when they're reducing the food there are people queuing up just waiting for the food to be reduced.* (Community food programme informant, mixed/urban rural).

3.2. Stoicism and Struggle

It is important to stress that this study was concerned with community caregivers or support workers views' of their clients' food security status and that we were not able to explore their clients' perspectives directly during this particular study. However, this research was concerned to understand how those care givers were drawing conclusions about their clients, and what evidence they used to conclude that individuals were dealing with food insecurity. We found informants were using a wide range of different information sources, including perceptions of their clients' behaviours and attitudes, and assessments about their physical appearance, as well as their dialogue with them. It was from these data that the theme of widespread individual (and private) *struggle and stoicism* emerged.

The behaviours and attitudes participants cited ranged from actions intended to keep up appearances of being able to manage, to denial of there being a problem in the household, through to overt refusal of food bank referrals. This notion of private and long-term struggle is illustrated by this quote from a community nurse who was working in a part of the country where large numbers of long term unemployed people live:

.., a lot of people are struggling privately. They don't know where to go or they're not sure of what to do, you know, or they've been sanctioned. Can you appeal this, can you, you know, do different things about that, and they're struggling day to day. "Oh today I've got some money, tomorrow I don't have anything." They'll not worry about tomorrow, because they're managing with today; that kind of idea (Outreach community nurse, mixed urban/rural).

A few informants talked about seeing people they had been dealing with over time looking progressively unwell and noticing or being concerned about their clients' appearance, the lack of food they observed in some of their clients' homes, and noticing that basic household furniture and fittings were missing from their houses (presumably sold to raise money for food), as things that led them to believe that some people were struggling with food poverty, illustrated thus:

You know on a couple of occasions we have seen people come in who are clearly you know, look unwell and you know are struggling, (Housing Regeneration Manager, urban).

These discussions of private struggles were also underpinned by notions of underlying pride that, from the perspective of the interview participants, prevented people seeking help, highlighted here:

I think for people that are too proud to come forward . . . you know, older people who worked all their lives, who don't expect to find themselves in the kind of poverty that they find themselves in (Manager Counselling Charity, urban).

Many also talked about people they considered to be food insecure being consumed with embarrassment during conversations the informant had initiated that were intended to help, illustrated thus:

The number of people that have been referred to myself that have been working and they have described financial hardship for a number of reasons and I've offered to make these referrals to the food banks, whichever one is more accessible for them, and they really just become very embarrassed. And then when I probe just that wee bit further about how they're going to provide for their families and themselves they kind of say that they're going to rely on their families and friends to do that. (Community link worker, urban).

Perhaps another reflection of the widespread private stoicism described above was the finding that participants who were involved with the delivery or management of community food programmes had noticed increased recent uptake of, and interest in, any food and budgeting training and cooking skills development courses. It seems that this had happened 'organically' as there had been no significant increase in their promotion and marketing of those courses. Yet people were signing up to them. They also noticed increased demand for their low cost food retailing services (fruit and vegetables). Moreover, a few had noticed more people growing their own food in community gardens and allotments, and that demand for community growing spaces was increasing. This was interpreted by some to mean that people were taking active, self–initiated steps to mitigate their situation.

Conversely, a few participants reported finding some people were more willing and able to ask for help, and/or accepting of their referrals to food banks to help them acquire food, compared to their previous experience. This effect was theorised to have occurred because they believed emergency food aid centres, such as food banks, were more commonly known and talked about compared to the past. In effect, using a food bank had become more socially acceptable making it easier for some people to accept this type of help when offered.

3.3. Participation Yet Pessimism

To reiterate, we deliberately set out to engage with professionals and third sector workers who had long term experience of supporting groups who were considered to be vulnerable due to their economic or social circumstances, or had health care needs, or who had long standing and established experience of designing and running community-based food programmes intended to enable low income households to purchase, prepare and consume healthy foods. Yet we found that both groups had in-depth knowledge and experience of the role and operation of food banks within their local communities. In exploring responses to food insecurity at the community level, the overriding theme to emerge was that the community had actively *participated* in attempting to support local people in food crisis, but was *pessimistic* and sceptical about its effectiveness as a solution now or in the future.

All the community food programmes that we engaged with for this study had been operating for over a decade prior to this study, without a food bank, and all reported a very similar experience in relation to dealing with local requests for help with feeding. All had added a food bank operation to their range of programmes or services in recent months in response to those appeals. Those appeals appear to have come from two groups: health and social care professionals who had lobbied them for emergency food parcels on behalf of patients or clients they believed were in food crisis; and direct requests from local people in food crisis, who knew of their previous existence as a local, low-cost food programme.

Yet there were mixed views amongst community food programme informants about the role of food banks and the impact that they had in addressing household food insecurity in Scotland. Overriding participants' narratives about the community responses were notions of pessimism, scepticism and concern about the role and efficacy of food banks as a solution to household food insecurity. This next illustrative quote highlights the dilemma expressed by many of the deep concern they had for members of the local community who were perceived to be suffering, feeling the need to help them, but at the same time being aware that a food bank response did not address the problem:

> *I feel outrage that people have to go through this kind of terrible suffering, food poverty, in this age! And, you know, I'm sure there are many people kind of saying the same thing. You know, I'm very satisfied that I've got this kind of work, where I feel I can make a difference now and again, but I'm also overwhelmed by the fact that I know that's just almost a drop in the ocean. There are many, many people that need help and support* (Welfare support assistant, mixed urban rural).

The sense of anger expressed in this quote was also apparent in other community food informants' accounts. This anger and frustration was centred not only on the individual suffering witnessed day-to-day but was also focussed on their organisations feeling obliged to help and becoming a de facto social safety net as a consequence. This next quote highlights some resentment directed towards mainstream (government-funded) organisations and agencies about expectations that were perceived to have been placed on poorly-resourced charities to help alleviate local suffering:

Well, I think it's one of the few areas that I'm aware of that the only response is, "Go to the voluntary sector." I can't think of very many other services that are related to similar sorts of outcomes, where the response is, "Go to a food bank, go to the voluntary sector," especially food banks, who get very little money from anywhere. I think part of the problem is that it's a free service that's been offered that we may have to challenge, in the future. I can't think of anything else, in a similar situation, where people say, "Go to your local church, they'll help you out," which is what people are, in effect, saying about food banks, you know, main stream services, main stream agencies, Local Authority's and whoever else. I find that very, very worrying (Community food programme informant, mixed urban).

In addition, there was an overriding sense of pessimism amongst informants that this picture and these trends in household food insecurity were about to change in the short-term. Most believed it was likely to become worse rather than better, particularly when the additional proposed changes to the social security system were enacted in the near future. This proposed change referred to here is the introduction of new UK Government policy associated with the so-called Universal Credit system of social security payment that would see the scrapping of fortnightly payment of separate types of security payments such e.g. family tax credits, housing benefit unemployment benefit etc. in favour of a single, monthly payment system. This fear and pessimism is illustrated here:

And I don't know what would happen to the other half; I'm really frightened, and because, as I say, we have designed and promoted ourselves as a place of last resort for funders, you know, it's the only option available; the last option available. I don't know what would happen [to them]. (Community Food Program, urban).

Some informants predicted future expansion of the food bank service on the basis that there would be an ongoing need to support hungry people, highlighted in this quote:

I think food poverty in Scotland isn't something that's going to be resolved overnight. I think it's going to be a long . . . there's going to need to be looking at like longer term more sustainable solutions but I feel that until these things are achieved, food banks are now kind of part of the dialogue and will be for, maybe longer term, until adaptions are made to the welfare system and especially with regard to sanctions. But as a result of that, food banks will be . . . will have a kind of longer-term role to play (Community food programme, urban).

Almost all the community food programme informants indicated they did not believe that food banks were a positive development or an effective or sustainable solution, but could not envisage them becoming redundant soon. Some talked about wishing to develop a different 'model' of local assistance, in the future, that would enable people to buy low-cost, healthy food according to their individual dietary needs and preferences, as opposed to being handed a free food parcel. All community food programme informants talked about trying to ensure that their clients had access to as nutritious a food parcel as they were able to supply. Most also commented at some point in their interview about the limited nature (in terms of nutritional quality and dietary preference) and lack of choice their clients had in the food were given. In the context of these discussions, it was also interesting to note that a few informants also talked about the unpredictable and limited nature of the food supply available to them (sourced from public and corporate donations, and allocations from franchised food surplus distributors) and the challenge they had in meeting the needs of their local community. This next quote illustrates the limited and unhealthy nature of the food informants received from a national food surplus redistribution operation:

The council gave us money to join (food surplus distributor), but as to date since we started with (food surplus distributor), the amount of produce we've been able to use is less than 20 kg a week. Because we can't take chilled produce, we can't take frozen produce, so the ambient temperature . . . they've given us a lot more than that but the biggest item by weight we've had has been diet Irn-Bru (soft drink). I would actually use that as an example of something with no nutritional value whatsoever. The second biggest item we've had, not by weight but by quantity, has been salt and vinegar crisps (CFI mixed urban/rural).

One social care informant, working with young people at risk of homelessness, described his frustration associated with observing that the components of food bank parcels did not necessarily match the healthy eating on a budget training that his young clients were being directed towards:

Well, we've tried to work with food banks. We haven't always found that entirely easy to be honest. We've produced a range of recipes and that sort of thing aimed at healthy eating on a budget and not all of the food banks are providing a great balance of food within the food boxes and that's not in any way to throw any blame at them, they can only allocate what they get, but access to fresh food and things can be quite difficult. We've done a range of training workshops with young people primarily aimed at teaching people how to create meals that don't require cooking but it's hard to get that matched up well with the contents of the food boxes. (Homeless organisation, urban).

Moreover, it also became apparent when talking to the community food programme informants that food banks were not well placed to meet the needs of people with a long term health condition or conditions seeking help from them.

Whilst food banks were predicted to remain a response to the existence of hungry people in local communities, overall, informants believed it was action to increase the levels and predictably of people's income that would make the biggest impact on food insecurity in Scotland. Support for young people to get into employment and get access to decent housing were also high on the list of things informants mentioned here. While a few described their aspirations that locally grown food would be part of the answer, they expressed disbelief that it ever would be for those on very low incomes, as it was considered well out of reach, cost wise, for those people.

4. Discussion

While this study revealed observations and concerns about groups of people historically well known to services due to their economic and social vulnerability, or frank destitution, this study also revealed widespread perceptions and concern about groups (particularly) families with young children and young people never previously considered to have been so obviously affected by food insecurity in affluent contexts. Income insufficiency was thought to be the primary cause of this by the majority of our study participants. This was related to the nature of work i.e., low wages, and insufficient and unpredictable hours of work, as well as changes to social security entitlement changes that previously boosted the take-home pay of those in low wage employment. While concepts of food insecurity and those affected by it, described in this study, did include descriptions of destitute life circumstances and/or crisis situations involving obvious hunger, those accounts also included concern for a growing number of people living within communities who were perceived to be dealing with food insecurity but were not necessarily totally insolvent or going hungry per se. This was characterized by our study participants as something they associated with having to eat (or survive) on cheap, poor quality foods due to having insufficient household income. Concerns about groups and households not obviously experiencing destitution but who are still considered to be at risk of food insecurity, due to inadequate income, has also been highlighted elsewhere [33,34].

The UK's Joseph Rowntree Foundation, for example, has found that those living in the lowest income decile households in the UK are routinely spending 20–23% of their household income on food and non-alcoholic beverages compared to 11% allocated to this expenditure by those living in average to above average income households [35]. Our quantitative study found those living in households with below 60% average income were routinely spending between 18–23% on food and non-alcoholic beverages in Scotland between 2005 and 2012 [27]. Caraher and Furey also estimated that the lowest income decile group in the UK would have to spend 40% of their household income if they were to buy what they describe as a consensually healthy diet in the year ending 2016/2017 [16]. Furthermore, the cost of purchasing healthy food and beverages (compared to unhealthy foods) has been steadily been rising in the UK since 2002, and predictions that healthy diets will become less affordable over time suggests, as Jones et al. also argue, that there are significant implications for individual food security and population health going forward [36]. It should perhaps be no surprise therefore, that low income households in Scotland are consistently failing to achieve population healthy eating targets in Scotland [37].

In addition, while hunger due to destitution is no less a public health and social concern in its own right in the UK and elsewhere, food insecurity without hunger in high income countries (like Scotland) is increasingly understood to be the more common experience, but also as damaging to health [33,38,39]. Recent UK research indicates that the numbers of people who report skipping meals in the previous year due to economic constraints had risen from 13% in 1983 to 28% in 2012 [40]. Our participants' observations and experiences of encountering an increasing number of people and groups of people affected by food insecurity, characterized by many of them to be synonymous in the Scottish context with having to eat cheap, nutrient poor food to deal with household income insufficiency, and is also consistent with this finding.

These findings therefore have important implications for public health and social policy makers, researchers and practitioners concerned with population health improvement and promotion, who are facing growing health care costs associated with non-communicable diseases. There is growing, evidence-based recognition that chronic compromises in dietary quality (due to the experience of food insecurity), rather than periodic episodes of hunger, are not only the more common experience of food insecurity in high income countries like Scotland, but also the more likely cause of a wide range of negative physical and mental health outcomes [41]. Food insecurity is known to increase the risk of a range of chronic, non-communicable health conditions and mental health related problems such as depression [42–44]. It is also notable that Scotland ranks second behind the US (in the top 20 OECD countries) in terms of the population prevalence of overweight and obesity. The Scottish Public Health Observatory has estimated that a fifth of all cases of obesity here can be attributed to living in deprivation [45]. Living in poverty in high income countries increases the risk for overweight and obesity [46], and while the mechanisms behind this are not fully understood, it is suggested that those living in poverty consume large quantities of highly energy dense foods (and therefore excessive calories) due to their appealing combination of affordability and palatability [45,47]. Therefore it maybe that policy interventions aimed at maximizing household income, such as those currently being tested in the Scottish context associated with addressing child poverty [48] and a universal basic income [49], hold more promise in addressing the root causes and health consequences of food insecurity, compared with an emergency food-based policy response.

It is also important to remember that those living in destitution (and their food security status) remain a significant public health concern in the UK [17,50], and those interviewed for this study were acutely aware of this, regularly highlighting their observations of increased hardship and concern about the significant challenges faced by those groups they were more commonly used to dealing with in their work. This increase in adversity was frequently linked to changes to social security entitlements associated with unemployment and sickness benefits due to changes in UK government policy [48,51].

In relation to older people, the target group of concern at the outset of this research, the mixed picture that emerged here reinforces the need for vigilance and continued close monitoring of this group in relation to food insecurity. Whilst pensioner poverty has declined in Scotland in recent times [51] and some older people were perceived and observed to be living without obvious barriers to food resources, from our study participants' perspectives there was still cause for concern. That older people are not turning up at food banks in the same numbers of younger people is not an indication that all is well with this group.

Stoic struggle, and resistance to the notion of being thought of as being unable to feed oneself, was featured amongst accounts of encounters with older people, and other groups too. This study found that professional offers of referrals to food banks were being turned down by some who had given such cause for concern. This resistance to being considered or revealed as being incapable of feeding oneself should be no surprise when considering Poppendieck's and Chilton's arguments that, relying on charity (to feed oneself) not only undermines basic human dignity, but also risks drawing public attention to one's reduced capability as family providers, protectors and consumers [22,52]. In consumer societies like the UK, this defective status represents a significant challenge to an individual's self-worth and wellbeing [53]. Indeed, the experience of living in poverty is known to be accompanied by feelings of great shame and fear of stigma [54]. Moreover, the drive to 'keep up appearances' and pretence to appear 'normal' and 'respectable' is universally experienced in cultures of widely varying economic circumstances throughout the world [55]. There is certainly a growing body of experiential studies, investigating food bank users' perspectives, that has revealed that their use is the action of last resort, and is commonly accompanied by feelings of great shame and powerlessness [56–61]. This apparently human instinct, to hide individual household food insecurity from public and professional scrutiny, has significant implications for the design and delivery of policies intended to address it. For example, vigilance needs to be maintained through research and service evaluations to reduce the risk that people and households struggling to cope with food insecurity are missing out on support they are entitled or eligible to receive, by those front line service providers who interact with them.

Whilst families with young children were considered to be amongst those groups giving cause for concern amongst our participants, a few expressed specific anxiety about the food security status of mothers and pregnant women. Women with children, living in very low income households, are believed to be at particular risk in relation to coping with food insecurity and its potential impacts on their own food intake and health [62–64]. Moreover, it is not uncommon for mothers to try to optimise their children's dietary intake at the expense of their own diets [65]. Women have been found to be less likely to present at a food bank for help in the UK [7,61], but are notably more likely to report moderate or severe food insecurity in population surveys compared to men [66]. While Loopstra and Lalor (2017) reported in their recent study of UK food bank users that men were the largest group of users (39%), lone mothers with children were the next most prominent group (13%), with households with three or more children particularly prominent amongst this group and the most vulnerable to severe food insecurity [67]. Therefore, the fears expressed by our participants appear plausible.

Almost all the community food programmes we engaged with had been operating without a food bank for over a decade but reported very similar experiences in relation being compelled to add this facility to their service offerings in response to locally expressed need in recent times. Nevertheless, there were mixed views amongst study participants about the extent to which they thought their food banks were effectively addressing their clients' needs, a finding which concurs with the lived experiences of food bank users reported elsewhere [56–60]. There was also some concern expressed in this study in relation to food banks not being able to meet the needs of people with a long term health condition or conditions. This is an important issue to take note of, as people with long term conditions are disproportionately represented in UK food bank use statistics. For example, the 2017 Loopstra and Lalor survey of food banks in the UK found that 63% of food bank user respondents had a health condition, and a further 5% had someone living with a health condition in the household [67]. The experience of living with food insecurity is known to adversely affect individuals' ability to manage their health condition and achieve optimal health outcomes [68–70]. Furthermore, there is also an emerging trend in the UK to suggest that more people are relying on food bank parcels on a regular basis, as opposed to this being a one off, rarely-used food crisis support [56,71]. Therefore, there is a need to undertake research with people in Scotland and the rest of the UK, who are living with a long term condition or conditions and who are affected by chronic or periodic food insecurity, to develop a better understanding of these experiences and their impacts.

These findings raise important considerations for public health and health care policy addressing household food insecurity in Scotland. Whilst Scottish Government investment in feeding assistance programmes like food bank operations and children's holiday feeding programmes, through their Fairer Food Fund [72], might make a short term difference to those subsets of the food insecure population using them, this investment will not reach the remainder who either do not access or have no access to such support.

Almost all the study food programme informants were pessimistic about any prospect of a future reduction in demand for food banks. There is certainly evidence to indicate that those predictions have been well founded [73]. Concerns were also expressed about the sustainability of some food banks in relation to local demand outstripping supply and in relation to being unable to provide healthy nutritious food in sufficient quantity and quality to supply the needs of people seeking help from them; concerns that have been highlighted elsewhere [21,22,72,74].

This study has some important limitations that need to be borne in mind. For example, the relatively small number of participants we were able to reach within the study timeframe means that it is problematic to generalize to all possible participants throughout Scotland. However, we attempted to gain the perspectives of as varied and relevant a sample of participants as possible (as described in Section 2) and argue that the findings are theoretically generalizable for two reasons. Firstly, there is a dearth of existing studies that has explored social, health care and third sector practitioner's perspectives and experiences of these issues. Secondly, after the study was finished we found from a series of knowledge exchange events that took place throughout Scotland, that our respondents and their narratives were not atypical [75].

A further limitation is that the study was not designed to engage with people directly affected by the lived experience of food insecurity. As discussed above, some additional work was being undertaken to explore that lived experience perspective in a separate but simultaneous piece of work in Scotland. Nevertheless, there is still a significant gap in the published literature particularly with respect to those individuals and households perceived to be experiencing food insecurity and believed to be at risk of food insecurity by practitioners and professionals working in health and social care arenas, but who are choosing not to use, or are having difficulty accessing, feeding assistance programmes. This study does not purport to represent the views of people with lived experience food insecurity, but to provide important insights into the perspectives and experiences of those frontline health and social care service providers, including those third sector and community-based programmes. These individuals are more commonly and historically used to dealing with groups and individuals who are financially or socially vulnerable; for example, who are not necessarily destitute but affected by in-work poverty, and, or who have routine health care needs. To the best of our knowledge, this is the first study of its kind to represent these views, for much of the emerging, published studies focusing on household food insecurity in the UK have been directed towards the experiences and perspectives of food assistance programme providers.

Finally, it was beyond the scope of this study to measure the extent of food insecurity but the findings stress the need to monitor food insecurity. A routine population survey tool could be added to an existing survey, such as the Scottish Health Survey, as the means by which policy can be informed by a more accurate picture of the population food insecurity prevalence, particularly given the evidence presented here of there being groups and individuals thought to be in need of help with feeding, due to income insufficiency, but who are not engaging with feeding programmes that might benefit them. However, routine surveys may still fail to capture fully the experiences of hard-to-reach groups.

5. Conclusions

This study set out to understand the nature of food insecurity beyond food bank provider's experiences and it revealed widespread concern for highly vulnerable groups more commonly known to be affected or at risk of destitution; and this remains a pressing public health issue. However, it also identified concern about groups, particularly families with young children, young people, women, and some older people, who were never previously considered to have been so obviously affected by food insecurity. The notion of food insecurity underpinning this view point was frontline observations of households having to survive on cheap, poor quality foods due to insufficient income; a conclusion that may explain why low income households have been consistently failing to achieve dietary targets in Scotland over some decades. The study also revealed a sense of commonplace stoic and private struggle within some food insecure households that seemed designed to avoid revealing their condition to public view. This apparently basic human instinct to try to conceal lived experiences of food insecurity from public and professional scrutiny has significant implications for the design and delivery of policies intended to address it. Furthermore, community-created and delivered food-based responses, that have been accessed by those willing and able to use them, were understood by those setting up and operating them to be insufficient and ineffective in addressing the root causes, and for those with health conditions, not well suited to meet their needs. Therefore, these findings point to some important public health, health care, and social policy implications.

Focusing on optimizing food bank operations seems unlikely to impact on the experience of food insecurity for those people who are unable or unwilling to access a food bank. Even for those who do access food banks, their operation can be viewed as alleviating the symptoms of food insecurity rather than addressing its causes. However, in Scotland, this has recently been a primary response to addressing food insecurity at the local level, through the provision of competitive grant funding to food bank operators. Policies that focus on income maximization, on the other hand, would seem to hold more promise in enabling more people to feed themselves, according to the perspective of frontline service providers interviewed in this study. In addition, we believe it is important to capture and monitor the experience of food insecurity both quantitatively through routine population surveys, as is the case already in Canada and the US, but also qualitatively through regular engagement with people with direct, lived experience of food insecurity, both those who use and don't use food banks, through research and dialogue. Both types of data are required to develop and monitor policy interventions intended to address food insecurity and to understand the impact of any policy changes arising.

Author Contributions: Conceptualization, F.D., O.-Z.E., A.L.G., S.W., L.M., A.L. and E.D.; methodology F.D., A.L.G., E.D. and F.M.; validation F.D. and F.M.; formal analysis F.D. and F.M.; data curation F.M.; writing—original draft preparation F.D.; writing—review and editing F.D., F.M., A.L.G., A.L. and E.D.; supervision F.D.; project administration F.D.; funding acquisition F.D., O.-Z.E., L.M., S.W., A.L. and E.D.

Funding: This research was funded by NHS Health Scotland with additional funding support provided for Flora Douglas' and Stephen Whybrow's time from the Scottish Government's RESAS programme. Core support to HERU from the Chief Scientist Office Scottish Government Health and Social Care Directorates and the University of Aberdeen is gratefully acknowledged.

Acknowledgments: We would like to acknowledge Bill Gray and Dionne MacKinnon (BG NHS Health Scotland and DMcK, formerly of NHS Health Scotland) for their professional review and support during the project and our study participants for their time and expertise. We are also grateful to the anonymous reviewers of our paper for their time and extremely helpful contributions to this work.

Conflicts of Interest: The authors declare no conflict of interest. The funders had no role in the design of the study; in the collection, analyses, or interpretation of data; in the writing of the manuscript, or in the decision to publish the results.

Appendix A

Table A1. Service Provider Informant Details.

Type of Organisation	Role of Interviewee	Project or Service Description	Location	Population Group Served
Service Provider	Staff nurse, Vulnerable Populations Team	Health Service representative supporting vulnerable adults	Greater Glasgow & Clyde	Vulnerable adults of all ages (16 and over)
Service Provider	Pre School Educational Home Visitor. Provides support & education to parents regarding their children's development needs	Education & children's services	Fife	Vulnerable parents regarding their children's development needs
Service Provider	Deputy manager of advice and information service for vulnerable groups	Supports homeless or those at risk of homelessness	Grampian	Homeless & other groups at risk of homelessness
Service Provider	Family worker supporting vulnerable families via parent and toddler groups	Supports vulnerable families	Highlands	Vulnerable families with young children
Service Provider	Principal adult social worker for vulnerable groups	Supports disabled and other vulnerable adults	Orkney	Disabled and other vulnerable adults
Service Provider	Welfare Support Assistant for unemployed people	Supports unemployed people back into work	Fife	Unemployed people
Service Provider	Community Health Improvement Advisor	Promotes healthy eating and the prevention of chronic illnesses	Grampian	Vulnerable adults of all ages (16 and over)
Service Provider	Community Links Practitioner working in Primary Care—supports all patients in GP practice	Supports vulnerable patients	Greater Glasgow & Clyde	All patients in GP practice in community
Service Provider	Manager. Supports vulnerable groups in city	Supports people back into work. Counselling services	Grampian	Vulnerable adults of all ages (16 and over)
Service provider	Adult befriending Service co-Ordinator. Supports adults who are socially isolated in community	Supports vulnerable adults in community	Orkney	All adults who are socially isolated in community

Table A1. *Cont.*

Type of Organisation	Role of Interviewee	Project or Service Description	Location	Population Group Served
Service Provider	Assistant Chief Executive. Supports vulnerable young people	Supports young people at risk of homelessness back into employment	Highlands	Young people at risk of homelessness
Service Provider	Development officer. Supports vulnerable adults	Supports vulnerable adults in community	Grampian	Vulnerable adults of all ages (16 and over)
Service Provider	Re-generation manager. Supports vulnerable adults	Supports vulnerable adults in community	Greater Glasgow & Clyde	Vulnerable adults of all ages (16 and over)
Service Provider	Administrator. Supports vulnerable adults	Supports vulnerable adults in community	Grampian	Vulnerable adults of all ages (16 and over)
Service Provider	Integration Development worker. Supports asylum-seekers and refugees	Supports asylum-seekers and refugees	Greater Glasgow and Clyde	Asylum-seekers and refugees

Table A2. Community Food Programme Informant Details.

Type of Organisation	Role of Interviewee	Project or Service Description	Health Board Area	Population Group Served
Community Food Initiative: Community food programme with food bank	Manager of community food and health initiative	To improve people's health by providing them with nutritious food and cooking and nutrition classes	Greater Glasgow & Clyde	Vulnerable adults on a low income
Community Food Initiative: Food bank only	Manager of food bank	Food bank	Greater Glasgow & Clyde	Vulnerable children and adults on a low income
Community Food Initiative: Community food programme without food bank	Project Assistant at voluntary community health project	Voluntary community project which promotes healthy eating/living	Forth Valley	Vulnerable adults on a low income
Community Food Initiative: Community food programme with food bank	Chief Executive. Supports vulnerable adults	To improve health and wellbeing and to increase employability	Grampian	Vulnerable adults on a low income
Community Food Initiative: Community food programme without food bank	Community Food Development Worker for community food and health project	Supports people at risk of homelessness, offenders or those at risk of offending	Fife	Vulnerable adults on a low income

Table A2. *Cont.*

Type of Organisation	Role of Interviewee	Project or Service Description	Health Board Area	Population Group Served
Community Food Initiative: Community food programme without food bank	Manager of a healthy living centre	Tries to alleviate food poverty through their education and promotion work	Greater Glasgow & Clyde	Vulnerable adults on a low income
Community Food Initiative: Food bank only	Development worker at the foodbank	Promotes healthy eating in local schools and nurseries and runs cookery classes	Greater Glasgow & Clyde	Vulnerable children and adults living in community
Community Food Initiative: Community food programme with food bank	Foodbank coordinator at national voluntary organisation	Food bank and drop-in advice service	Dumfries and Galloway	Vulnerable children and adults on a low income
Community Food Initiative: Community garden	Volunteer coordinator at community food and health project	Promotes healthy eating via cookery classes and workshops. Sells cheap fruit and veg	Fife	All residents living in the local village
Community Food Initiative: Community food programme with food bank	Food and Health Development Worker for this Community food and health project	Supports vulnerable people living in food poverty. Promotes healthy eating via cookery classes	Lothian	Disadvantaged groups in deprived areas of city—mainly serves families with young children

References

1. Cooper, N.; Purcell, S.; Jackson, R. Below the Breadline: The Relentless Rise of Food Poverty in Britain. Available online: https://oxfamilibrary.openrepository.com/bitstream/handle/10546/317730/rr-below-breadline-food-poverty-uk-090614-en.pdf;jsessionid=2DBEBAA5229576B20714001FDF50F88C?sequence=1 (accessed on 2 December 2018).
2. UK Parliament. Hansard Report of House of Commons Food Banks Debate 18th December. Available online: http://www.publications.parliament.uk/pa/cm201314/cmhansrd/cm131218/debtext/131218-0003.htm (accessed on 20 August 2018).
3. Ashton, J.R.; Middleton, J.; Lang, T. Open letter to prime minister david cameron on food poverty in the UK. *Lancet* **2014**, *383*, 1631. [CrossRef]
4. Duggan, E. The Food Poverty Scandal that Shames Britain: Nearly 1m People Rely on Handouts to Eat–and Benefit Reforms May Be to Blame. Available online: https://www.independent.co.uk/news/uk/politics/churches-unite-to-act-on-food-poverty-600-leaders-from-all-denominations-demand-government-u-turn-on-9263035.html (accessed on 2 December 2018).
5. Sosenko, F.; Livingstone, N.; Fitzpatrick, S. *Overview of Food Aid Provision in Scotland*; Scottish Government Edinburgh: Edinburgh, UK, 2013.
6. Lambie-Mumford, H. *The Right to Food and the Rise of Charitable Emergency Food Provision in the United Kingdom*; University of Sheffield: Sheffield, UK, 2014.
7. MacLeod, M.A.; Curl, A.; Kearns, A. Understanding the prevalence and drivers of food bank use: Evidence from deprived communities in Glasgow. *Soc. Policy Soc.* **2018**, 1–20. [CrossRef]
8. All-Party Parliamentary Inquiry into Hunger. *Feeding Britain: A Strategy for Zero Hunger in England, Wales, Scotland and Northern Ireland*; Children's Society: London, UK, 2014.
9. Radimer, K.L.; Olson, C.M.; Campbell, C.C. Development of indicators to assess hunger. *J. Nutr.* **1990**, *120* (Suppl. 11), 1544–1548. [CrossRef] [PubMed]
10. Tarasuk, V.; Dachner, N.; Hamelin, A.M.; Ostry, A.; Williams, P.; Bosckei, E.; Poland, B.; Raine, K. A survey of food bank operations in five canadian cities. *BMC Public Health* **2014**, *14*, 1234. [CrossRef] [PubMed]
11. Martin-Fernandez, J.; Grillo, F.; Parizot, I.; Caillavet, F.; Chauvin, P. Prevalence and socioeconomic and geographical inequalities of household food insecurity in the paris region, France, 2010. *BMC Public Health* **2013**, *13*, 486. [CrossRef] [PubMed]
12. Pfeiffer, S.; Ritter, T.; Hirseland, A. Hunger and nutritional poverty in Germany: Quantitative and qualitative empirical insights. *Crit. Public Health* **2011**, *21*, 417–428. [CrossRef]
13. Reeves, A.; Loopstra, R.; Stuckler, D. The growing disconnect between food prices and wages in Europe: Cross-national analysis of food deprivation and welfare regimes in twenty-one EU countries, 2004–2012. *Public Health Nutr.* **2017**, *20*, 1414–1422. [CrossRef]
14. Food Foundation. Household Food Insecurity: The Missing Data. 2016. Available online: https://foodfoundation.org.uk/wp-content/uploads/2016/11/FF-Food-insecurity-4pp-V3.pdf (accessed on 1st September 2018).
15. Taylor, A.; Loopstra, R. *Too Poor to Eat: Food Insecurity in the UK*; Food Foundation: London, UK, 2016; Available online: http://foodfoundation.org.uk/wp-content/uploads/2016/07/FoodInsecurityBriefing-May-2016-FINAL.pdf (accessed on 2 December 2018).
16. Caraher, M.; Furey, S. The cultural and economic dimensions of food poverty. In *The Economics of Emergency Food Aid Provision*; Palgrave Pivot: Cham, Switzerland, 2018; pp. 1–24.
17. Loopstra, R. Rising food bank use in the UK: Sign of a new public health emergency? *Nutr. Bull.* **2018**, *43*, 53–60. [CrossRef]
18. Faith in Community Scotland. Beyond Foodbanks? Growing a Food Justice Movement. Available online: https://www.faithincommunityscotland.org/beyond-foodbanks-2015-conference-outputs/ (accessed on 1 September 2018).
19. Loopstra, R.; Tarasuk, V. The relationship between food banks and household food insecurity among low-income Toronto families. *Can. Public Policy* **2012**, *38*, 497–514. [CrossRef]
20. Bazerghi, C.; McKay, F.H.; Dunn, M. The role of food banks in addressing food insecurity: A systematic review. *J. Community Health* **2016**, *41*, 732–740. [CrossRef]

21. Iafrati, S. We're not a bottomless pit: Food banks' capacity to sustainably meet increasing demand. *Volunt. Sect. Rev.* **2018**, *9*, 39–53. [CrossRef]

22. Poppendieck, J. *Sweet Charity?: Emergency Food and the End of Entitlement*; Penguin: New York, NY, USA, 1999.

23. Thompson, C.; Smith, D.; Cummins, S. Understanding the health and wellbeing challenges of the food banking system: A qualitative study of food bank users, providers and referrers in London. *Soc. Sci. Med.* **2018**. [CrossRef] [PubMed]

24. The Scottish Government. Equally Well—The Report of the Ministerial Task Force on Health Inequalities. Available online: https://www2.gov.scot/Resource/Doc/229649/0062206.pdf (accessed on 5 November 2018).

25. Fraser, P.L.F.B.; Douglas-Hamilton, J. Eating for Health: A Diet Action Plan for Scotland; Scottish Executive 1996. Available online: https://www2.gov.scot/Resource/0040/00400745.pdf (accessed on 5 November 2018).

26. Lang, T.; Dowler, E.; Hunter, D.J. *Review of the Scottish Diet Action Plan: Progress and Impacts 1996–2005*; NHS Scotland Edinburgh: Edinburgh, UK, 2006.

27. Douglas, F.; Ejebu, O.Z.; Garcia, A.; MacKenzie, F.; Whybrow, S.; McKenzie, L.; Ludbrook, A.; Dowler, E. *The Nature and Extent of Food Poverty in Scotland*; NHS Health Scotland: Glasgow, UK, 2015.

28. Strauss, A. *Basics of Qualitative Research: Techniques and Proceduare for Developing Grounded Theory*; Sage: Thousand Oaks, CA, USA, 1998.

29. Hussein, M.E.; Hirst, S.; Salyers, V.; Osuji, J. Using grounded theory as a method of inquiry: Advantages and disadvantages. *Qual. Rep.* **2014**, *19*, 1–15.

30. Green, J.; Thorogood, N. *Qualitative Methods for Health Research*; Sage: London, UK, 2010.

31. Clark, J. How to peer review a qualitative manuscript. *Peer Rev. Health Sci.* **2003**, *2*, 219–235.

32. Ritchie, R.; Lewis, J.; Nicholls, C.M.; Ormston, R. *Qualiative Research Practice: A Guide for Social Science Students and Researchers*; Sage: London, UK, 2013.

33. Tarasuk, V. Discussion Paper on Household and Individual Food Insecurity. Available online: https://www.researchgate.net/profile/Valerie_Tarasuk/publication/245946029_Discussion_Paper_on_Household_and_Individual_Food_Insecurity/links/566eefd508ae4bef40611e55.pdf (accessed on 1 September 2018).

34. Patil, S.P.; Craven, K.; Kolasa, K.M. Food insecurity: It is more common than you think, recognizing it can improve the care you give. *Nutr. Today* **2017**, *52*, 248–257. [CrossRef]

35. Joseph Rowntree Foundation. *UK Poverty 2017: A Comprehensive Analysis of Poverty Trends and Figures*; Joseph Rowntree Foundation: York, UK, 2017.

36. Jones, N.R.; Conklin, A.I.; Suhrcke, M.; Monsivais, P. The growing price gap between more and less healthy foods: Analysis of a novel longitudinal uk dataset. *PLoS ONE* **2014**, *9*, e109343. [CrossRef] [PubMed]

37. Food Standards Scotland. *The Scottish Diet Needs to Change: Situation Report Update*; Food Standards Scotland: Aberdeen, UK, 2018.

38. Butcher, L.; Ryan, M.; O'Sullivan, T.; Lo, J.; Devine, A. What drives food insecurity in Western Australia? How the perceptions of people at risk differ to those of stakeholders. *Nutrients* **2018**, *10*, 1059. [CrossRef] [PubMed]

39. Ward, P.R.; Verity, F.; Carter, P.; Tsourtos, G.; Coveney, J.; Wong, K.C. Food stress in Adelaide: The relationship between low income and the affordability of healthy food. *J. Environ. Public Health* **2013**, *2013*, 968078. [CrossRef]

40. Lansley, S.; Mack, J. *Breadline Britain: The Rise of Mass Poverty*; Oneworld Publications: London, UK, 2015.

41. Gundersen, C.; Ziliak, J.P. Food insecurity and health outcomes. *Health Aff. (Millwood)* **2015**, *34*, 1830–1839. [CrossRef]

42. Tarasuk, V.; Mitchell, A.; McLaren, L.; McIntyre, L. Chronic physical and mental health conditions among adults may increase vulnerability to household food insecurity-3. *J. Nutr.* **2013**, *143*, 1785–1793. [CrossRef]

43. Maynard, M.; Andrade, L.; Packull-McCormick, S.; Perlman, C.; Leos-Toro, C.; Kirkpatrick, S. Food insecurity and mental health among females in high-income countries. *Int. J. Environ. Res. Public Health* **2018**, *15*, 1424. [CrossRef] [PubMed]

44. Martin, M.S.; Maddocks, E.; Chen, Y.; Gilman, S.E.; Colman, I. Food insecurity and mental illness: Disproportionate impacts in the context of perceived stress and social isolation. *Public Health* **2016**, *132*, 86–91. [CrossRef] [PubMed]

45. Grant, I.; Fischbacher, C.; Whyte, B. *Obesity in Scotland: An Epidemiology Briefing*; Scottish Public Health Observatory: Edinburgh, UK, 2007.

46. Butland, B.; Jebb, S.; Kopelman, P.; McPherson, K.; Thomas, S.; Mardell, J.; Parry, V. Foresight. Tackling Obesities: Future Choices. Available online: https://assets.publishing.service.gov.uk/government/uploads/system/uploads/attachment_data/file/287937/07-1184x-tackling-obesities-future-choices-report.pdf (accessed on I1 September 2018).

47. Drewnowski, A. Obesity, diets, and social inequalities. *Nutr. Rev.* **2009**, *67*, S36–S39. [CrossRef] [PubMed]

48. Scottish Government. *Child Poverty (Scotland) Act 2017*; Scottish Government: Scotland, UK, 2017.

49. Scottish Government, Citizen's Income. Available online: http://www.parliament.scot/parliamentarybusiness/CurrentCommittees/103211.aspx (accessed on 5 November 2018).

50. Fitzpatrick, S.; Bramley, G.; Sosenko, F.; Blenkinsopp, J. *Destitution in the UK 2018*; The Joseph Rowntree Foundation: York, UK, 2018; Available online: https://www.jrf.org.uk/report/destitution-uk-2018?gclid=EAIaIQobChMI96jcnoaE3wIVGeR3Ch2wBA3iEAAYASAAEgJuhPD_BwE (accessed on 5 November 2018).

51. Joseph Rowntree Foundation. Poverty in Scotland: Briefing Paper. Available online: https://www.jrf.org.uk/report/poverty-scotland-2018 (accessed on 30 July 2018).

52. Chilton, M.; Rose, D. A rights-based approach to food insecurity in the United States. *Am. J. Public Health* **2009**, *99*, 1203–1211. [CrossRef] [PubMed]

53. Bauman, Z. *Consuming Life*; John Wiley & Sons: Hoboken, NJ, USA, 2013.

54. Shildrick, T. *Poverty Propaganda: Exploring the Myths*; Policy Press: Bristol, UK, 2018.

55. Walker, R.; Kyomuhendo, G.B.; Chase, E.; Choudhry, S.; Gubrium, E.K.; Nicola, J.Y.; Lødemel, I.; Mathew, L.; Mwiine, A.; Pellissery, S. Poverty in global perspective: Is shame a common denominator? *J. Soc. Policy* **2013**, *42*, 215–233. [CrossRef]

56. Holmes, E.; Black, J.L.; Heckelman, A.; Lear, S.A.; Seto, D.; Fowokan, A.; Wittman, H. "Nothing is going to change three months from now": A mixed methods characterization of food bank use in greater vancouver. *Soc. Sci. Med.* **2018**, *200*, 129–136. [CrossRef]

57. Middleton, G.; Mehta, K.; McNaughton, D.; Booth, S. The experiences and perceptions of food banks amongst users in high-income countries: An international scoping review. *Appetite* **2018**, *120*, 698–708. [CrossRef]

58. Garthwaite, K.A.; Collins, P.J.; Bambra, C. Food for thought: An ethnographic study of negotiating ill health and food insecurity in a uk foodbank. *Soc. Sci. Med.* **2015**, *132*, 38–44. [CrossRef]

59. Purdam, K.; Garratt, E.A.; Esmail, A. Hungry? Food insecurity, social stigma and embarrassment in the UK. *Sociology* **2016**, *50*, 1072–1088. [CrossRef]

60. Van der Horst, H.; Pascucci, S.; Bol, W. The "dark side" of food banks? Exploring emotional responses of food bank receivers in the netherlands. *Br. Food J.* **2014**, *116*, 1506–1520. [CrossRef]

61. Douglas, F.; Sapko, J.; Kiezebrink, K.; Kyle, J. Resourcefulness, desperation, shame, gratitude and powerlessness: Common themes emerging from a study of food bank use in Northeast Scotland. *AIMS Public Health* **2015**, *2*, 297. [CrossRef] [PubMed]

62. Tarasuk, V.S. Household food insecurity with hunger is associated with women's food intakes, health and household circumstances. *J. Nutr.* **2001**, *131*, 2670–2676. [CrossRef] [PubMed]

63. Ivers, L.C.; Cullen, K.A. Food insecurity: Special considerations for women. *Am. J. Clin. Nutr.* **2011**, *94*, 1740S–1744S. [CrossRef] [PubMed]

64. Pederson, A.; Haworth-Brockman, M.; Clow, B.; Isfeld, H.; Liwander, A. *Rethinking Women and Healthy Living in Canada*; Centre of Excellence for Women's Health: Vancouver, BC, Canada, 2013.

65. Hall, S.; Knibbs, S.; Medien, K.; Davies, G. *Child Hunger in London: Understanding Food Poverty in the Capital*; Greater London Authority: London, UK, 2013.

66. Jung, N.M.; de Bairros, F.S.; Pattussi, M.P.; Pauli, S.; Neutzling, M.B. Gender differences in the prevalence of household food insecurity: A systematic review and meta-analysis. *Public Health Nutr.* **2017**, *20*, 902–916. [CrossRef] [PubMed]

67. Loopstra, R.; Lalor, D. *Financial Insecurity, Food Insecurity, and Disability: The Profile of People Receiving Emergency Food Assistance from the Trussell Trust Foodbank Network in Britain*; Trussell Trust: Oxford, UK, 2017.

68.	Galesloot, S.; McIntyre, L.; Fenton, T.; Tyminski, S. Food insecurity in Canadian adults: Receiving diabetes care. *Can. J. Diet. Pract. Res.* **2012**, *73*, e261–e266. [CrossRef] [PubMed]

69.	Seligman, H.K.; Davis, T.C.; Schillinger, D.; Wolf, M.S. Food insecurity is associated with hypoglycemia and poor diabetes self-management in a low-income sample with diabetes. *J. Health Care Poor Underserved* **2010**, *21*, 1227. [PubMed]

70.	Gucciardi, E.; Vahabi, M.; Norris, N.; Del Monte, J.P.; Farnum, C. The intersection between food insecurity and diabetes: A review. *Curr. Nutr. Rep.* **2014**, *3*, 324–332. [CrossRef] [PubMed]

71.	Garratt, E. Please sir, I want some more: An exploration of repeat foodbank use. *BMC Public Health* **2017**, *17*, 828. [CrossRef] [PubMed]

72.	The Scottish Government. Tackling Food Poverty. Available online: https://news.gov.scot/news/tackling-food-poverty-1 (accessed on 5 November 2018).

73.	Trussell Trust. UK Food Bank Use Continues to Rise. Available online: https://www.trusselltrust.org/2017/04/25/uk-foodbank-use-continues-rise/ (accessed on 6 August 2018).

74.	Loopstra, R.; Tarasuk, V. Food bank usage is a poor indicator of food insecurity: Insights from Canada. *Soc. Policy Soc.* **2015**, *14*, 443–455. [CrossRef]

75.	Mason, J. Making convincing arguements with qualitative data. In *Qualitative Resaerching*; Sage: London, UK, 2002.

International Journal of
Environmental Research and Public Health

MDPI

Article

What can Secondary Data Tell Us about Household Food Insecurity in a High-Income Country Context?

Ourega-Zoé Ejebu [1], Stephen Whybrow [2], Lynda Mckenzie [1], Elizabeth Dowler [3], Ada L Garcia [4], Anne Ludbrook [1], Karen Louise Barton [5], Wendy Louise Wrieden [6] and Flora Douglas [2,*]

[1] Health Economics Research Unit, University of Aberdeen, Aberdeen AB25 2ZD, UK;
   oejebu@abdn.ac.uk (O.E.); l.mckenzie@abdn.ac.uk (L.M.); a.ludbrook@abdn.ac.uk (A.L.)
[2] Rowett Institute, University of Aberdeen, Aberdeen AB25 2ZD, UK; stephen.whybrow@abdn.ac.uk
[3] Department of Sociology, University of Warwick, Coventry CV4 7AL, UK; Elizabeth.Dowler@warwick.ac.uk
[4] Human Nutrition, University of Glasgow, Glasgow G31 2ER, UK; Ada.Garcia@glasgow.ac.uk
[5] Division of Food and Drink, Abertay University, Dundee DD1 1HG, UK; K.Barton@abertay.ac.uk
[6] Human Nutrition Research Centre and Institute of Health & Society, Newcastle University,
   Newcastle upon Tyne NE2 4HH, UK; Wendy.Wrieden@newcastle.ac.uk
* Correspondence: f.douglas3@rgu.ac.uk

Received: 29 November 2018; Accepted: 27 December 2018; Published: 29 December 2018

Abstract: In the absence of routinely collected household food insecurity data, this study investigated what could be determined about the nature and prevalence of household food insecurity in Scotland from secondary data. Secondary analysis of the Living Costs and Food Survey (2007–2012) was conducted to calculate weekly food expenditure and its ratio to equivalised income for households below average income (HBAI) and above average income (non-HBAI). Diet Quality Index (DQI) scores were calculated for this survey and the Scottish Health Survey (SHeS, 2008 and 2012). Secondary data provided a partial picture of food insecurity prevalence in Scotland, and a limited picture of differences in diet quality. In 2012, HBAI spent significantly less in absolute terms per week on food and non-alcoholic drinks (£53.85) compared to non-HBAI (£86.73), but proportionately more of their income (29% and 15% respectively). Poorer households were less likely to achieve recommended fruit and vegetable intakes than were more affluent households. The mean DQI score (SHeS data) of HBAI fell between 2008 and 2012, and was significantly lower than the mean score for non-HBAI in 2012. Secondary data are insufficient to generate the robust and comprehensive picture needed to monitor the incidence and prevalence of food insecurity in Scotland.

Keywords: food insecurity; food poverty; prevalence; household; food surveys; secondary data; Scotland

1. Introduction

Household food insecurity (HFI) is a common problem for low-income households in high-income countries [1–4]. HFI exists when a household experiences the inability "to acquire or consume an adequate quality or sufficient quantity of food in socially acceptable ways, or the uncertainty that one will be able to do so" [5]. It has been empirically established to manifest itself involuntarily across four dimensions: (i) quantity and (ii) quality of food; (iii) psychological impacts; and (iv) socially unacceptable food and ways of obtaining food [6–8]. In high-income countries, food insecurity is more commonly characterised by chronic compromises in dietary quality and anxiety associated with accessing food. In contrast, low and middle income countries most generally experience acute and chronic episodes of food deprivation, hunger, and starvation [8]. Critically, for health and social care policy makers in high-income countries, the experience of food insecurity featuring poor diet quality leads to negative health outcomes i.e., cancer, stroke, cardiovascular disease, diabetes and obesity, and depression [8–15]. Much of the epidemiological evidence highlighting these associations has been generated in the North American context where routine capture of HFI data has taken place for some decades [16]. Nationally representative food security monitoring was established in the U.S. in 1995 with the highest recorded HFI prevalence observed during the global recession of 2008–2009 (14.5% of the population) [17]. While there has been an observed decline in those figures, they remain in the region of 12% of the population (15 million households) [18]. Canadian HFI prevalence runs roughly in line with the U.S. at 11–12% of the population found to have been food insecure since food security monitoring was established there in 1994 [19]. HFI prevalence is also higher in specific population subgroups including households with children, single-parent households and indigenous, black and Hispanic households [18,20], a pattern also observed in Australia and New Zealand [21,22]. It is also widely argued that HFI is an outcome of income insufficiency in relation to necessary household expenditures [20,22–26] and the decisions of policy makers [27]. In the late-2000s, HFI had re-emerged as a subject of public health, social policy, civic and political concern in Scotland and the rest of the UK. This is attributed to an increase in the numbers of people turning to emergency food supply centres (so-called food banks) for help with feeding themselves and their families [28–32]. Food bank use data became a de facto measure of food insecurity across the UK, largely through the high profile reporting of the Trussell Trust, which is one of the best known charitable organizations providing emergency food aid in the UK [33]. Yet the ability of emergency food supply centres to address HFI, or provide an insight into the nature and scale of food insecurity at the local and national level is problematic [6,17,18,34]. In similar international contexts, where it is possible to make comparisons with routinely collected food insecurity data, food bank use data tend to significantly underestimate the prevalence of food insecurity [35,36]. This presents challenges for policy makers tasked with the development, implementation, and evaluation of policy measures aimed at addressing the problem [37]. It is particularly problematic for governments and policy makers given that food banks, as a de facto public policy response to the problem, are unable to meet local demand for food assistance for a variety of inherent resource constraints, unless food is rationed by restricting access for those who want and are able to access them [34,38,39].

It was in this context, and in the absence of any purposively collected and experiential household food insecurity population survey data, that research was undertaken in Scotland, in 2014, to explore the nature and prevalence of HFI. This paper reports on the study component that screened and analysed relevant existing secondary data, with the specific aim of finding out what could be determined about the nature and prevalence of HFI in Scotland, as defined above [5]. The study was also guided by a particular focus on the years preceding the UK economic recession (2008 to 2009) [40] and the period of rapid increase in food prices (2007 to 2012) [41]. Additionally, the analysis included a comparison of the diets of households at risk of food insecurity compared to those at less risk. The paper discusses what analysis of existing data sources is able to reveal (or not) about two of the four defined dimensions of the experience of food insecurity in the Scottish context, i.e., dietary quantity and quality, and reflects on the absence of data on psychological and social experiences, and the implications of this research for future policy making in this area.

2. Materials and Methods

The secondary data analysis proceeded in three stages.

2.1. First stage—Scoping and Data Source Selection

The first stage involved a scoping, consultation and decision making process to identify suitable Scottish data sources to explore food insecurity patterns covering the 2008 UK recession. It was at this stage also that consideration and agreement was reached about the 'at risk' household income threshold that would be used during the analysis, to take account of the lack of a UK food insecurity measure [37].

The threshold level agreed for identifying those at risk of food poverty was equivalised net household income of less than 60% of the median value [42,43], which is the commonly used measure of poverty in the UK. Household income is equivalised to take account of household size and composition (including numbers of adults and children, and their ages [44]). Households below the threshold are referred to as households below average income (HBAI). Households with income above this threshold are referred as non-HBAI. Income was measured before housing costs were deducted [43].

Using the aforementioned HFI definition [5], datasets were identified where relevant variables for analysing HFI trends and prevalence in Scotland were available. Six potentially suitable datasets were identified, with four being rejected. These were, (i) the General Lifestyle Survey [45] (excluded due to difficulties gaining timely data access); (ii) the European Union Statistics on Income and Living Conditions [46] (Scotland is not identified as a separate UK region); the Family Resources Survey [47] (insufficient information on food purchase data); and Kantar Worldpanel [48] (which includes very few low income households and insufficient information to calculate equivalised income). The two remaining datasets, the Living Costs and Food Survey (LCFS) [49] and the Scottish Health Survey (SHeS) [50], were used for this analysis.

The LCFS is an annual stratified random sample survey conducted by the Office for National Statistics. It includes approximately 500 households in Scotland. The survey collects information on household spending patterns from diaries of daily expenditure recorded over a 2-week period. LCFS data from 2007 and 2012 were used for the present study. Variables include weekly household expenditure on food and non-alcoholic drinks brought home, eaten away from home (e.g., at a restaurant or hotel) and take-away items. Weekly food expenditures were adjusted to 2013 prices using the food and non-alcoholic drinks Consumer Price Index (CPI). Food expenditure-to-income ratios were calculated by dividing weekly household food expenditure by weekly equivalised household income using the McClement equivalence scale [44]. Household income was adjusted for inflation using the overall 2013 CPI.

From 2008, the SHeS was conducted annually. It contains information on the prevalence of different health conditions and health-related behaviours, including dietary intake collected on alternate years. Data are collected at an individual (both adults and children) and a household level. It includes around 6500 individual observations in 2008 and 4800 in 2012. Information on usual daily food eating patterns (type of food and frequency of consumption) are provided. SHeS also collects data on annual household income and converts this value to equivalised income using the McClement equivalence scale.

Both datasets were weighted using available sampling weights, which adjust for non-response and to match the population distribution [49,51].

2.2. Second Stage—Prevalence Estimation and Sub Group Analysis

Using both LCFS and SHeS, the second stage involved estimating the numbers of households at risk of being in food poverty, and investigating how prevalence had changed over time, and comparing these changes with data from the Family Resources Survey. Information on household income and prevalence of HBAI from the Family Resources Survey [47] was included to place the Scottish data in the context of data for the whole of the UK. The FRS (Family Resources Survey) is the most comprehensive survey of household financial circumstances using a large sample of UK households, and is the government source for poverty level analyses.

Using LCFS, this stage also included analysis of food expenditure (£) and food-to-income shares (%) between lower and higher income households. Mean weekly expenditure on food and non-alcoholic drinks, and their corresponding values in terms of percentage by food group based on the Eatwell Plate [52] were also calculated. Two-tailed independent t-tests were used to compare mean food expenditure (overall and by food group) and food-to-income shares between HBAI and non-HBAI, and to compare percentage DQI score (see below) between HBAI and non-HBAI and over time.

2.3. Third Stage—Dietary Quality Assessment and Analysis

The third stage involved assessing differences in overall diet quality between those considered at risk, and those not at risk, of being in food poverty. Dietary recommendations are based on the amounts of foods consumed, whereas food and drink are recorded in the LCFS "as purchased". These were adjusted to "as consumed" values per person by accounting for food waste, and food preparation and cooking weight changes [53–55]. Nutrient intakes were calculated using the LCFS food composition database [56].

Within the SHeS, an Eating Habits Module (EHM) assesses consumption of a simple list of foods that are relevant to the Scottish Dietary Goals [57]. The EHM focuses on frequency of consumption of specific foods and was not designed to quantify amounts of foods or nutrients consumed, or meal patterns. It is not possible to assess nutrient intake, household food practices, meal patterns or experiences of the stability of the household food supply from the EHM. The EHM consists of two sections, the first being a series of questions on the consumption of food and drink items to gather information on general eating habits using a food frequency questionnaire methodology. The second assesses fruit and vegetable intake by a 24 h recall method using "everyday" food portion terms (such as tablespoons, cereal bowls and slices). Information on the number and type of fruit and vegetables eaten by respondents the day prior to the interview was used to compare the percentage of individuals in HBAI and non-HBAI reaching the 5-a-day goal for portions of fruit and vegetables.

A more comprehensive measure of diet quality, using the Diet Quality Index (DQI) devised by Barton and colleagues [58,59], was also used to calculate scores for SHeS and LCFS. Diet quality indexes are frequently used to summarise how well an individual's diet compares to a collection of dietary recommendations, based on foods and nutrients considered to be important to health [60]. For example, adherence to the Dietary Guidelines for Americans can be assessed using the Healthy Eating Index, which has been shown to be a valid and reliable index of diet quality [61].

Diet Quality Index scores were calculated for the LCFS (2007 and 2012) and SHeS (2008 and 2012). For the LCFS data, DQI scores were calculated for a combination of foods (fruit and vegetables, fish, and red meat) and nutrients (percentage energy from fat and saturated fat, sugar and complex carbohydrates, and fibre) [58]. For the SHeS data, DQI scores were calculated from seven food components: oil-rich fish; red meat and processed meat; starchy foods; fibre in foods; sugary foods; fatty foods; and fruit and vegetables. The difference in food items used to calculate the DQI is because of the variations in dietary information available from the LCFS and SHeS. Absolute values for the DQI from the two surveys are therefore not directly comparable and have been expressed in the results as a percentage of the maximum possible score for each survey. Higher scores indicate greater adherence to dietary guidelines.

The proportions of food groups contributing to each diet were estimated using the Eatwell Plate recommendations. In the UK, the Eatwell Plate [52] (now updated and renamed the Eatwell Guide) was developed for representing nutrient intake information in a picture format to make dietary recommendations easier for consumers to understand. The Eatwell Plate is a pie-chart diagram consisting of five food group segments, the recommended proportions of which are based on the dietary reference values for the population. The five groups being: 1. bread, rice, potatoes, pasta and other starchy foods (starchy, which should make up around 33% of the diet), 2. fruit and vegetables (F&V, 33%), 3. milk and dairy foods (dairy, 15%), 4. meat, fish, eggs, beans and other non-dairy sources of protein (protein, 12%) and 5. foods and drinks that are high in fat or sugar, or both (HFHS, 8%).

Statistical analyses were carried out using STATA Version 13 (StataCorp LP, College Station, Texas, TX, USA) and SPSS Version 22 (SPSS/IBM Corp, Armonk, New York, NY, USA).

3. Results

3.1. Households at Risk of Food Insecurity—Prevalence Estimates

Table 1 shows the number and proportion of HBAI estimated in the LCFS, SHeS, and from the FRS.

Table 1. Prevalence of households below 60% median income in Living Costs and Food Survey (LCFS), Scottish Health Survey (SHeS) and the Family Resources Survey (FRS), along with mean weekly expenditure and measures of diet quality.

Year of Survey	LCFS		SHeS		FRS	
	2007	2012	2008	2012	2007/8	2012/13
Scottish observations (households)	501	483	3567	2697	NA	NA
Monthly equivalised median household income (£)	£2079	£2039	£1842	£1954	£1699	£1907
Poverty threshold * (£)	£1247	£1223	£1105	£1172	£1019	£1144
Percentage of HBAI (Number)	23.4% (117)	18.9% (92)	26.3% (940)	23.4% (632)	17%	16%
Percentage of non-HBAI (Number)	76.7% (384)	81.1% (391)	73.6% (2627)	76.6% (2065)	NA	NA
Weekly expenditure on food and drinks (£)—HBAI $$	£54.08 [48.30–59.86]	£53.85 [45.11–62.6]	NA	NA	NA	NA
Weekly expenditure on food and drinks (£)—non-HBAI $$	£102.14 [95.41–108.87]	£86.73 [81.43–92.02]	NA	NA	NA	NA
p-values of mean food expenditure between HBAI and non-HBAI	$p < 0.001$	$p < 0.001$				
Weekly expenditure on food and drinks (% income)—HBAI $$	30.7% [22.36–39.04]	29.4% [23.19–35.53]	NA	NA	NA	NA
Weekly expenditure on food and drinks (% income)—Non-HBAI $$	14.1% [13.14–15.06]	15.5% [14.38–16.59]	NA	NA	NA	NA
p-values of food-to-income ratios between HBAI and non-HBAI	$p < 0.001$	$p < 0.001$				
DQI score (%)—HBAI	35.1% [31.9–38.3]	36.2% [31.8–40.5]	50.4%	48.5%	NA	NA
DQI score (%)—non-HBAI	36.5% [34.7–38.4]	34.7% [33.0–36.5]	51.6%	51.6%	NA	NA
p-values of DQI scores between HBAI and non-HBAI	$p = 0.327$	$p = 0.506$				

* 60% of monthly equivalised median household income (£). $$ weekly food includes grocery shopping, non-alcoholic drinks, food eaten away from home (e.g., at a restaurant or hotel) and take-away food. Confidence interval into [brackets]. HBAI: households below average income.

Prevalence estimates from the LCFS and SHeS are similar. In contrast, the results using LCFS data are weighted to adjust for non-response and to match population distributions, and give higher levels than those in the FRS. However, all estimates show an apparent decline in the prevalence of HBAI between 2007 and 2012.

Table 1 also shows the mean weekly expenditure on food (including food eaten away from home and take away food) and non-alcoholic drinks using LCFS. Results are displayed for HBAI and non-HBAI for 2007 and 2012, respectively. HBAI spent less actual money per week on food than non-HBAI (Table 1) ($p < 0.001$ in both years), but the proportion (%) of equivalised household income spent on food was approximately twice the proportion spent by non-HBAI ($p < 0.001$ in both years). There is a slight decrease in both food expenditure and the share of food expenditure to income from 2007 to 2012 for HBAI. However, there is a bigger drop in food expenditure by non-HBAI combined with an increasing share of income being spent on food. This suggests that non-HBAI had more discretion to reduce food spending in the face of declining real incomes during the period of recession.

3.2. Dietary Analysis and Assessment

Table 2 reports the (mean) weekly expenditure of HBAI and non-HBAI, by Eatwell Plate food group, as well as the corresponding percentage share of income (%). In contrast to the results in Table 1, any other food expenditure (e.g., food eaten away from home and take-away food) are excluded from this calculation.

For each food group, while HBAI spend significantly less of their weekly income in pounds (£), they spend proportionately (%) more in comparison to non-HBAI ($p < 0.001$ for each food group in both years). There is no statistically difference of expenditure between HBAI and non-HBAI for Non-alcoholic drinks in year 2012 and 'Other' food (for both years).

Non-HBAI households spend more on both 'healthy' food (fruit and vegetables) and 'unhealthy food' (foods high in fat and sugar (HFHS)), suggesting that poor dietary choices are not necessarily determined solely by spending power. Meat and other sources of proteins, and HFHS represent the largest share of food expenditure in both HBAI and non-HBAI alike. Noticeably, fruit and vegetables constitute the third largest food expenditure in both household types.

Figure 1 shows the percentage of SHeS individuals from HBAI and non-HBAI by number of portions of fruits and vegetables consumed on the day prior to the interview. In both years, there is a marked difference in the proportion of individuals reaching the 5-a-day target between those in HBAI and non-HBAI (14% and 32%, $p < 0.001$ in 2008 and 12% and 21%, $p < 0.001$ in 2012). Respondents in HBAI were more likely to report consuming no, or only one portion of, fruit or vegetables the previous day compared to their non-HBAI counterparts.

The proportion of individuals in HBAI who reported eating no fruit and vegetables the day prior to the interview was higher in 2012 (18%) than in 2008 (11%). Nevertheless, 14% of individuals from HBAI reported eating five or more portions of fruits and vegetables in 2008; this proportion fell to 11% by 2012. However, there was little change in the proportion of individuals from non-HBAI eating five or more portions of fruits and vegetables over time (22% and 21% respectively).

Examination of the DQI scores calculated from the LCFS revealed no significant differences between HBAI and non-HBAI households for percentage DQI score (35.1% and 36.5%, $p = 0.327$ in 2007, and 36.2% and 34.7%, $p = 0.506$ for 2012) (Table 1). Examination of the DQI score based on the SHeS data showed the overall mean percentage DQI scores were similar in 2008 for HBAI and non HBAI (50.4% and 51.6% respectively, $p = 0.196$). However, by 2012, the overall percentage DQI score was significantly lower for HBAI than non-HBAI (48.5% and 51.6% respectively, $p = 0.001$).

Table 2. Mean weekly expenditure * (£ and % of income) of HBAI (households below average income.) and non-HBAI, by food group.

Food type	2007 HBAI	2007 non-HBAI	2012 HBAI	2012 non-HBAI
Starchy food	£5.91 [5.16–6.67] 2.49% [1.80–3.17]	£8.06 [7.45–8.66] 0.87% [0.79–0.94]	£5.28 [4.24–6.31] 3.01% [2.06–3.95]	£6.93 [6.42–7.43] 1.25% [1.13–1.37]
p-values		_p_ < 0.001 _p_ < 0.001		_p_ = 0.005 _p_ < 0.001
Fruits and vegetables	£6.85 [5.73–7.97] 2.54% [2.00–3.09]	£12.83 [11.82–13.85] 1.31% [1.20–1.41]	£7.22 [5.59–8.86] 3.70% [2.81–4.59]	£10.83 [9.98–11.69] 1.86% [1.69–2.03]
p-values		_p_ < 0.001 _p_ < 0.001		_p_ < 0.001 _p_ < 0.001
Milk and dairy	£5.16 [4.47–5.85] 2.09% [1.64–2.53]	£7.75 [7.02–8.46] 0.83% [0.75–0.90]	£5.10 [4.26–5.94] 2.71% [2.13–3.28]	£6.28 [5.84–6.73] 1.09% [1.01–1.1]
p-values		_p_ < 0.001 _p_ < 0.001		_p_ = 0.015 _p_ < 0.001
Meat and protein	£12.22 [10.53–13.92] 4.20% [3.53–4.87]	£19.87 [18.35–21.38] 2.09% [1.92–2.25]	£12.08 [9.67–14.48] 6.52% [4.82–8.23]	£18.2 [16.70–19.71] 3.15% [2.86–3.44]
p-values		_p_ < 0.001 _p_ < 0.001		_p_ < 0.001 _p_ < 0.001
HFHS	£10.72 [9.26–12.19] 4.71% [3.07–6.36]	£19.39 [17.69–21.10] 2.07% [1.88–2.27]	£11.78 [9.80–13.76] 5.95% [4.91–6.99]	£17.12 [15.81–18.44] 3.05% [2.75–3.35]
p-values		_p_ < 0.001 _p_ = 0.0018		_p_ < 0.001 _p_ < 0.001
Non-alcoholic drinks	£1.07 [0.84–1.30] 0.37% [0.28–0.45]	£1.72 [1.46–1.98] 0.18% [0.15–0.21]	£1.11 [0.78–1.44] 0.71% [0.25–1.17]	£1.46 [1.22–1.71] 0.25% [0.21–0.30]
p-values		_p_ < 0.001 _p_ < 0.001		_p_ =0.095 _p_ = 0.053
Other food	£0.08 [0.01–0.14] 0.03% [0.004–0.05]	£0.13 [0.003–0.23] 0.02% [0.00–0.03]	£0.05 [0.01–0.09] 0.02% [0.006–0.04]	£0.14 [0.08–0.20] 0.03% [0.02–0.04]
p-values		_p_ = 0.3756 _p_ = 0.4632		_p_ = 0.014 _p_ = 0.856
Total *	£42.01 [37.40–46.65] 16.42% [13.26–19.60]	£69.73 [65.06–74.41] 7.37% [6.82–7.90]	£42.62 [35.77–49.47] 22.62% [18.05–27.18]	£60.96 [57.24–64.70] 10.68% [9.99–11.37]
p-values		_p_ < 0.001 _p_ < 0.001		_p_ < 0.001 _p_ < 0.001
Observations	117	384	92	391

* Excludes spending on food eaten away from home and takeaway food. Confidence interval into [brackets]. _p_-values represent the statistical differences between HBAI and non-HBAI for (i) mean weekly expenditure and (ii) food-to-income ratios respectively. Source: computed by the authors based on LCFS 2007 and 2012. Weighted and adjusted for inflation.

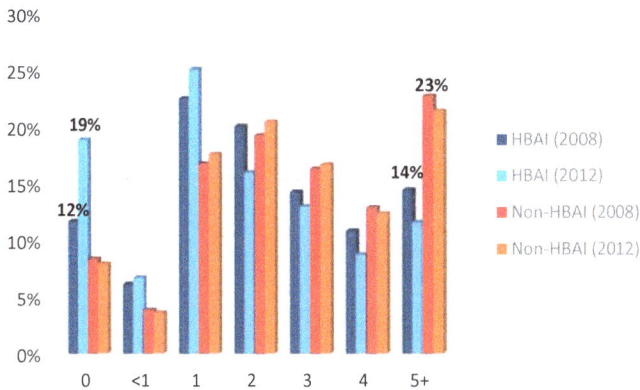

Figure 1. Percentage of individuals from HBAI (households below average income.) and non-HBAI by fruit and vegetables consumption (number of portions on the day prior to the interview). Source: computed by the authors based on SHeS (2008 and 2012)—weighted data.

4. Discussion

This study aimed to establish what could be determined about the nature and prevalence of household food insecurity in Scotland from secondary data. The scoping study established that it was possible to gain only a partial picture of HFI in the Scottish context, allowing a focus on quantity and quality of diets. Therefore, the subsequent analyses centered on an exploration of food expenditure-to-income shares and levels of food expenditure, and a dietary quality analysis of foods purchased and reported as consumed. The analysis focused on HBAI and non-HBAI households, over the period following the recent economic recession. Consequently, this discussion proceeds in two parts, focusing firstly on the findings of the 'partial picture' data able to be accessed and analysed, and secondly, reflecting on the policy and practice implications arising from the lack of routine capture of psychosocial domain data of the experience of household food insecurity in the population.

4.1. Household Expenditure and Food and Nutrition Security

This analysis revealed that low income households in Scotland have continued to allocate a greater income share (%) to food over the period following the recession, with food expenditure a particularly prominent component of all household expenditure, compared to wealthier households. This is consistent with the expenditure patterns reported for the whole of the UK [62]. Findings from the current study suggest that the HBAI group had less margin to reduce food expenditure than their wealthier counterparts. For, at the same time that there was a reduction in food spending for this group, the income share devoted to it increased, as it did for non-HBAI. These findings also align with the current position, as more recent UK figures suggest that increases in food prices have continued to exacerbate the situation of low-income households due to the larger income share they devote to food expenditure, compared with higher income households [63]. Given the relative stasis of, and in many cases decline in, household incomes in low income households in the UK [64], the net effect on those lower income households is that they probably have less available income to spend on other essential household items.

Indeed, although there appear to be few differences in the diets of HBAI and non-HBAI when the frequencies of consumption of all key food groups were compared using the DQI, in both the LCFS and SHeS data, the consistent exception is in fruit and vegetable consumption. Fruit and vegetable consumption is commonly used as proxy indicator of diet quality. Lower income households have lower expenditure on fruit and vegetables than do higher income households (LCFS); and their self-reported consumption was lower compared with non-HBAI (SHeS). These results from the SHeS partially support previous research indicating that the quality of dietary intake is poor across all income groups in Scotland, but tends to be worse in the poorer households [65], and that these effects have worsened over time. Overall, the indicators of HFI and the subsequent analysis used in this study are innovative and could be adapted in other studies to bridge the gap in the literature.

As this research was designed to examine the usefulness of existing relevant data sources in enabling the characterization of HFI in Scotland, it is important to note that the SHeS is designed to estimate frequency of consumption rather than provide estimates of the amounts of foods consumed. This makes interpretation of dietary quality difficult, since the Scottish Dietary Targets are based on amounts of food groups consumed. It is conceivable that those on the lowest incomes have already made all possible adjustments to expenditure and cannot further reduce spending, as argued above [62]. This finding might also be explained by the relatively short shelf life of fresh fruit and vegetables, which often makes such items relatively unattractive to purchase compared to other less perishable items for those whose room for financial manoeuver is more limited.

Consequently, when considering and interpreting these findings, it is important to note that virtually no attention had been paid to people's lived experience of food insecurity in Scotland until very recently. No study has focused on the experience of food (in)security in the context of other necessary household expenditures [66], that might explain these patterns of difference in diet quality and, for example, expenditure on fruit and vegetables. Why these patterns persist, despite longstanding educational campaigns exhorting the benefits of healthy eating, has also not been investigated. Where empirical research (in high income country contexts) has been conducted to investigate the direct perspectives and motivations of different socioeconomic households regarding "healthy" food provisioning and meal preparation (as opposed to drawing inferences from dietary pattern data), low income/food insecure households are no less likely than their wealthy counterparts to express a desire to consume healthy food [67]. Indeed, there is some evidence to suggest that very low-income households possess significant food knowledge and skills, and employ multiple strategies with the aim of feeding the family nutritious foods [68–72]. The evidence presented above regarding income shares devoted to food in Scotland in recent years suggests that the capacity for very low income households to be able to take action according to their aspirations and preferences could be constrained; which is consistent with the views of health, social care and third sector practitioners supporting economically and social vulnerable groups in Scotland [73].

The analysis also revealed an apparent decrease in the proportion of households whose household income fell below 60% of the median income value between 2007 and 2012, which some may construe to mean a subsequent decline in the numbers of households affected by food insecurity. The poverty threshold used in this study was based on the median income of each sample survey, and not the UK or Scottish median income; this might partially explain disparities in the percentage of HBAI within the FRS. In addition, since the "HBAI at risk marker" is based on a single threshold each year, any change in the overall nature of the distribution of equivalised household income between survey years could affect the position of the median relative to the mean equivalised income. This could influence the proportion of households above and below the poverty threshold level. Median income was likely to be falling in real terms due to the recession. Existing Scottish Government surveys and reports provide a more thorough and complete view of the prevalence of poverty per se [74,75].

In addition, the food poverty threshold used in this study (<60% of the median equivalised household income) masks the experiences of households with considerably lower incomes, which are also likely to be underrepresented in the datasets used in this analysis. Individuals whose household income is below 50% or 40% of the UK median income are considered as living in severe or extreme poverty, respectively [74]. Moreover, those just above or below this threshold may be quite similar, and experience similar financial difficulties from increased household costs.

Furthermore, households living on remote Scottish islands are not included in the LCFS, for data collection cost reasons. This is an important omission, given that incomes are known to be lower in rural areas, and that those living in remote and rural areas in Scotland need to spend "10–40% more on everyday requirements than elsewhere in the UK" [76]. In the LCFS, sampling variability was also affected by a higher non-response rate of households whose head had no post-school qualification or was in a manual social class group [56]. In the SHeS, deprived areas were over-sampled however [56]. In both LCFS and SHeS, weights were used to reduce the effect of non-response bias so that the sample distribution matches the population distribution in terms of region, age group and sex [49,77].

However, international evidence derived from jurisdictions where food insecurity is routinely monitored shows that while household income is an important determinant, it does not fully explain the circumstances of all those who are food insecure. Housing costs (i.e., mortgage, rent, fuel and insurances), and other necessary household expenditures (such as travel and debt) have been shown to significantly contribute to the observed prevalence of food insecurity [78,79].

4.2. Study Implications

While the current analysis revealed some important and worrying patterns of population dietary deterioration in HBAI households at the same time as they are apportioning more and more of their income to food expenditure in Scotland, it also revealed some crucial gaps in the available data. For example, it was not possible to show which groups of people were most at risk from food insecurity. As highlighted previously, in other high income jurisdictions it has been possible to identify specific household types that are more at risk of severe and enduring HFI, and with it, the theoretical possibility of targeted policy interventions [18,20]. The need for this data has been brought into sharp relief in recent times in the UK as a recently published report by the UN Rapporteur for Extreme Poverty and Human Rights expressed great concern for the working poor, female-headed households, children and those living with disabilities, pensioners, asylum seekers and refugees and those living in rural poverty as most at risk of extreme poverty in the UK at the present time [80].

An analysis of children living in households at risk of HFI was not possible either. Such analysis would be very informative considering the latest finding of a UNICEF report [81]. It revealed that in 2014, 19.7% children aged 0–17 were living in HBAI in the UK. Whilst this stands below the average of developed countries (21.0%), it is an indication of the extent to which HFI affects vulnerable groups.

Another important gap revealed was the lack of data that could provide a picture of the people and groups who were affected by uncertainty/anxiety associated with being able to afford to feed oneself or the family. Nor was it possible to determine the duration and frequency of these types of experiences at the household level. Based on U.S. observational studies [6], markers of food deprivation are regarded as more sensitive than income-based measures alone, in capturing not only the material aspects of deprivation (largely caused by income poverty), but also its combined biological and psychosocial effects on health and well-being. A number of international studies have also concluded that the experience of HFI is likely to be impacting human health as much through 'non-nutritional' mechanisms, such as worry, anxiety, feelings of deprivation, and social isolation, as through nutritional routes [6,82–84].

Indirect measures of HFI, such as food availability, purchasing power, consumption patterns and anthropometric measures were deemed to be insufficient for HFI monitoring and the evaluation of interventions intended to address it as far back as the late 1970's [85]. Within other high-income country contexts, where routine HFI monitoring takes place, a now significant body of research has linked HFI with negative physical and psychological health consequences [16,68,86,87]. It is also known to impair chronic condition management [88,89] and is independently associated with increased health care use and costs [90].

Therefore, it has been encouraging to witness the discussion and policy shifts in recent years highlighting the need for routine monitoring of HFI across the UK. However, there is still no agreement about the means and measures by which this should be done, with policy differences emerging within the different nations of the UK regarding these [91,92]. For example, the Scottish Government have recently accepted the main recommendations of the Independent Working Group on Food Poverty in Scotland [93] and have introduced a HFI measure (a derivative of the UN Food Insecurity Experience Scale) [94] into the SHeS. The SHeS operates on a continuous annual reporting basis, and provides sufficient data for each individual health board area in Scotland to understand their population health dynamics over time, and has the potential for data linkage with other population data sets including disease registers [95]. The SHeS is specifically funded to monitor population health outcomes and trends. Therefore, the inclusion of a HFI measure in this survey should make it possible to determine the effectiveness of policy interventions intended to address HFI, as well as understanding the role of HFI in the poor health outcomes of the Scottish population. The benefits of placing this measure here, and with it the potential routine capture the more multi-dimensional HFI experience, are manifold. Firstly, it provides the facility to assess and monitor food insecurity experience for different subgroups (e.g., geographic location, age, ethnicity, household type, occupational status and health status). Secondly, embedded HFI monitoring in such a survey enables data linkage with other population data sets including disease registers, and therefore enables better scrutiny of the impact of food insecurity experience on population health outcomes [95]. Thirdly, the inclusion of a such HFI measure also provides the facility to monitor prevalence and severity (if not chronicity), and with it the potential to develop better understanding of the role different HFI experiences (in terms of nature and severity) has in relation to health outcomes within the Scottish population, something that was beyond the scope of this study. Fourthly, it should also provide a robust means to determine the effectiveness of policy interventions intended to address HFI. Indeed, it is important to stress the benefits of introducing and retaining such a measure compared to the HFI indicator used in Europe, which uses a more unidimensional indicator that is based primarily on the prevalence of the household's inability to afford meat/fish/poultry (or a vegetarian equivalent) every second day [25]. Fifthly as the SHeS survey routinely also captures household income data, it should be possible to monitor and model changes in HFI prevalence in the context of changing national and household economic circumstances and social policy changes, something one-off cross-sectional studies cannot undertake. There have been calls for a similar type of measure to be introduced in England and Wales [96].

In 2003, the UK Food Standards Agency used a piloted questionnaire based on the USDA (United States Department of Agriculture) experience to investigate household food security in a UK-wide survey of diet and nutrition in low-income households [97]. A similar questionnaire was used in the Food Standard Agency's 'Food and You' consumer survey in England in 2016 [98]. However, this seems unlikely to offer the same depth and functionality as the data collected by the SHeS going forward. In addition, none of the measures mentioned above include questions about children's food security status. This is a serious omission given the reported levels of child poverty and so-called 'holiday hunger' in the UK, relating to the important role that is played by provision of free school meals to low income families during term time [99], and the associated poor child health and educational outcomes that have been observed in international contexts where children's HFI status is captured and recorded [100].

It is important also to acknowledge that, while routine food insecurity measurement offers the potential to characterise and monitor HFI prevalence more comprehensively, and provides a means to evaluate policy and programmatic interventions aimed at addressing it, challenges will remain in capturing the experiences of homeless and destitute individuals and families, and representing them in secondary data. Routine HFI monitoring and evaluation endeavors must therefore also include direct qualitative engagement with those highly vulnerable groups and the services and/or agencies responsible for their care and support, to inform and evaluate social, economic and health policy changes intended to address HFI [73]. In addition, whilst periodic episodes of absolute food deprivation are a public health and ethical concern of any country, it is also the case that the less severe experience of food insecurity resulting in chronic dietary quality compromises over time, is likely to be the more prevalent experience in high income countries like Scotland. This is an important distinction to be able to capture as accurately as possible as chronic food insecurity experience is considered to be as damaging to health and well-being over the long term as periodic deprivation experiences [68] and this phenomenon needs more research attention in HFI monitoring work in the UK and elsewhere than it currently receives. Related to this is the need in the UK to develop a better understanding to the impact of food insecurity on chronic or long-term health condition management in the UK [73]. Having a clearer picture of the severity and chronicity of people's HFI experience as well as national and subnational prevalence would assist researchers and policy makers to develop more insight into this overlooked health care issue, and create better informed policy responses to address HFI in the Scotland and elsewhere in the UK.

5. Conclusions

This study provided a partial picture of the prevalence of HFI in Scotland. It revealed that low income households have been consuming a diet that has further deteriorated in nutritional quality over the period following the recession and have been spending a significantly higher proportion of their household incomes compared to wealthier households. Other important dimensions of HFI are unavailable for scrutiny for monitoring and evaluation purposes. Additional or alternative measures to identify at-risk households are required to inform the development and evaluation of policy and programmatic interventions intended to address the problem. Routine and systematic monitoring would not only enable HFI incidence and prevalence to be better characterised, but would enable the relationship between household-level problems of food insecurity and changing social and economic conditions to be monitored and understood. In order to develop, implement and evaluate social and public health policy interventions intended to reduce the numbers of households affected by food insecurity, the routine capture of household food insecurity data suitable for Scottish and UK population health monitoring is urgently needed.

Author Contributions: Conceptualisation, F.D., A.L.G., S.W., L.M., A.L., E.D.; methodology, O.E., S.W., L.M., A.G., A.L., K.L.B., W.L.W., F.D.; validation formal analysis O.E., S.W., L.M., K.L.B., A.L.G.; data curation O.E., S.W., L.M.; writing—original draft preparation O.E.; F.D.; writing—review and editing F.D., O.E., S.W., L.M., K.L.B., A.L., A.L.G., E.D.; supervision A.L., L.M.; project administration F.D.; funding acquisition F.D., L.M., S.W., A.L., E.D.

Funding: This research was funded by NHS Health Scotland with additional funding support provided for Flora Douglas' and Stephen Whybrow's time from the Scottish Government's RESAS programme. Core support to HERU from the Chief Scientist Office Scottish Government Health and Social Care Directorates and the University of Aberdeen is gratefully acknowledged.

Acknowledgments: This study was also like to acknowledge Bill Gray NHS Health Scotland and Dionne MacKison formerly of NHS Health Scotland for their professional review and support during the project. The authors would also like to acknowledge the anonymous reviewers of this manuscript, whose observations and suggestions improved this paper.

Conflicts of Interest: The authors declare no conflict of interest. The funders had no role in the design of the study; in the collection, analyses, or interpretation of data; in the writing of the manuscript, or in the decision to publish the results.

References

1. Tarasuk, V.; Dachner, N.; Hamelin, A.M.; Ostry, A.; Williams, P.; Bosckei, E.; Poland, B.; Raine, K. A survey of food bank operations in five Canadian cities. *BMC Public Health* **2014**, *14*, 1234. [CrossRef] [PubMed]
2. Martin-Fernandez, J.; Grillo, F.; Parizot, I.; Caillavet, F.; Chauvin, P. Prevalence and socioeconomic and geographical inequalities of household food insecurity in the Paris region, France, 2010. *BMC Public Health* **2013**, *13*, 486. [CrossRef] [PubMed]
3. Pfeiffer, S.; Ritter, T.; Hirseland, A. Hunger and nutritional poverty in Germany: Quantitative and qualitative empirical insights. *Crit. Public Health* **2011**, *21*, 417–428. [CrossRef]
4. Reeves, A.; Loopstra, R.; Stuckler, D. The growing disconnect between food prices and wages in Europe: Cross-national analysis of food deprivation and welfare regimes in twenty-one EU countries, 2004–2012. *Public Health Nutr.* **2017**, *20*, 1414–1422. [CrossRef] [PubMed]

5. Radimer, K.L.; Olson, C.M.; Campbell, C.C. Development of indicators to assess hunger. *J. Nutr.* **1990**, *120*, 1544–1548. [CrossRef] [PubMed]

6. Habicht, J.-P.; Pelto, G.; Frongillo, E.; Rose, D. Conceptualization and instrumentation of food insecurity. In Proceedings of the Workshop on the Measurement of Food Insecurity and Hunger, Washington, DC, USA, 15 July 2004.

7. Fram, M.S.; Bernal, J.; Frongillo, E.A. *The Measurement of Food Insecurity Among Children: Review of Literature and Concept Note*; Innocenti Working Paper No. 2015-08; UNICEF Office of Research: Florence, Italy, 2015.

8. Tarasuk, V. *Discussion Paper on Household and Individual Food Insecurity*; Health Canada: Ottawa, ON, Canada, 2001; Volume 13.

9. Patil, S.P.; Craven, K.; Kolasa, K.M. Food insecurity: It is more common than you think, recognizing it can improve the care you give. *Nutr. Today* **2017**, *52*, 248–257. [CrossRef]

10. Butcher, L.; Ryan, M.; O'Sullivan, T.; Lo, J.; Devine, A. What drives food insecurity in Western Australia? How the perceptions of people at risk differ to those of stakeholders. *Nutrients* **2018**, *10*, 1059. [CrossRef]

11. Ward, P.R.; Verity, F.; Carter, P.; Tsourtos, G.; Coveney, J.; Wong, K.C. Food stress in Adelaide: The relationship between low income and the affordability of healthy food. *J. Environ. Public Health* **2013**, *2013*, 968078. [CrossRef]

12. Gundersen, C.; Ziliak, J.P. Food Insecurity And Health Outcomes. *Health Aff. (Millwood)* **2015**, *34*, 1830–1839. [CrossRef]

13. Maynard, M.; Andrade, L.; Packull-McCormick, S.; Perlman, C.; Leos-Toro, C.; Kirkpatrick, S. Food Insecurity and Mental Health among Females in High-Income Countries. *Int. J. Environ. Res. Public Health* **2018**, *15*, 1424. [CrossRef] [PubMed]

14. Martin, M.S.; Maddocks, E.; Chen, Y.; Gilman, S.E.; Colman, I. Food insecurity and mental illness: Disproportionate impacts in the context of perceived stress and social isolation. *Public Health* **2016**, *132*, 86–91. [CrossRef] [PubMed]

15. Butland, B.; Jebb, S.; Kopelman, P.; McPherson, K.; Thomas, S.; Mardell, J.; Parry, V. *Foresight, Tackling Obesities: Future Choices*; UK Government Office for Science: London, UK, 2007.

16. Nord, M. What have we learned from two decades of research on household food security? *Public Health Nutr.* **2014**, *17*, 2–4. [CrossRef]

17. Riches, G.; Silvasti, T. Hunger in the rich world: Food aid and right to food perspectives. In *First World Hunger Revisited*; Springer: Berlin, Germany, 2014; pp. 1–14.

18. Coleman-Jensen, A.; Rabbitt, M.; Gregory, C.; Singh, A. *Household Food Security in the United States in 2015*; ERR-215; U.S. Department of Agriculture, Economic Research Service: Washington, DC, USA, September 2016.

19. Riches, G.; Tarasuk, V. Canada: Thirty years of food charity and public policy neglect. In *First World Hunger Revisited*; Springer: Berlin, Germany, 2014; pp. 42–56.

20. Tarasuk, V.; Mitchell, A.; Dachner, N. *Household Food Insecurity in Canada, 2014: Research to Identify Policy Options to Reduce Food Insecurity*; Research to Identify Policy Options to Reduce Food Insecurity (PROOF): Toronto, ON, Canada, 2016.

21. Rosier, K. *Food Insecurity in Australia: What Is It, Who Experiences It and How Can Child and Family Services Support Families Experiencing It?* Australian Commonwealth Government: Melbourne, Australia, 2011.

22. Carter, K.N.; Lanumata, T.; Kruse, K.; Gorton, D. What are the determinants of food insecurity in New Zealand and does this differ for males and females? *Aust. N. Z. J. Public Health* **2010**, *34*, 602–608. [CrossRef]

23. Riches, G. Food banks and food security: Welfare reform, human rights and social policy. Lessons from Canada? *Soc. Policy Adm.* **2002**, *36*, 648–663. [CrossRef]

24. Loopstra, R.; Reeves, A.; Taylor-Robinson, D.; Barr, B.; McKee, M.; Stuckler, D. Austerity, sanctions, and the rise of food banks in the UK. *BMJ* **2015**, *350*, h1775. [CrossRef] [PubMed]

25. Davis, O.; Geiger, B.B. Did Food Insecurity rise across Europe after the 2008 Crisis? An analysis across welfare regimes. *Soc. Policy Soc.* **2017**, *16*, 343–360. [CrossRef]

26. Dowler, E. Food banks and food justice in 'Austerity Britain'. In *First World Hunger Revisited*; Springer: Berlin, Germany, 2014; pp. 160–175.

27. McIntyre, L.; Patterson, P.B.; Mah, C.L. The application of 'valence' to the idea of household food insecurity in Canada. *Soc. Sci. Med.* **2019**, *220*, 176–183. [CrossRef]

28. Cooper, N.; Purcell, S.; Jackson, R. Below the Breadline: The Relentless Rise of Food Poverty in Britain. Available online: https://policy-practice.oxfam.org.uk/publications/below-the-breadline-the-relentless-rise-of-food-poverty-in-britain-317730 (accessed on 27 December 2018).

29. Government, H.U. Hansard Report of House of Commons Food Banks Debate 18th December. 2013. Available online: http://www.publications.parliament.uk/pa/cm201314/cmhansrd/cm131218/debtext/131218-0003.htm (accessed on 20 August 2018).

30. Ashton, J.R.; Middleton, J.; Lang, T. Open letter to Prime Minister David Cameron on food poverty in the UK. *Lancet* **2014**, *383*, 1631. [CrossRef]

31. Duggan, E. The Food Poverty Scandal that Shames Britain: Nearly 1m People Rely on Handouts to Eat—And Benefit Reforms May Be to Blame. Available online: https://www.independent.co.uk/news/uk/politics/churches-unite-to-act-on-food-poverty-600-leaders-from-all-denominations-demand-government-u-turn-on-9263035.html (accessed on 27 December 2018).

32. Sosenko, F.; Livingstone, N.; Fitzpatrick, S. *Overview of Food Aid Provision in Scotland*; Scottish Government: Edinburgh, UK, 2013.

33. Trust, T. UK Food Bank Use Continues to Rise. 2017. Available online: https://www.trusselltrust.org/2017/04/25/uk-foodbank-use-continues-rise/ (accessed on 6 August 2018).

34. Bazerghi, C.; McKay, F.H.; Dunn, M. The role of food banks in addressing food insecurity: A systematic review. *J. Community Health* **2016**, *41*, 732–740. [CrossRef]

35. Loopstra, R.; Tarasuk, V. The relationship between food banks and household food insecurity among low-income Toronto families. *Can. Public Policy* **2012**, *38*, 497–514. [CrossRef]

36. Loopstra, R.; Tarasuk, V. Food bank usage is a poor indicator of food insecurity: Insights from Canada. *Soc. Policy Soc.* **2015**, *14*, 443–455. [CrossRef]

37. Food Foundation. *Household Food Insecurity: The Missing Data*; The Food Foundation: London, UK, 2016.

38. Iafrati, S. "We're not a bottomless pit": Food banks' capacity to sustainably meet increasing demand. *Volunt. Sect. Rev.* **2018**, *9*, 39–53. [CrossRef]

39. Poppendieck, J. *Sweet Charity?: Emergency Food and the End of Entitlement*; Penguin: London, UK, 1999.

40. Crossley, T.F.; Low, H.; O'Dea, C. Household consumption through recent recessions. *Fisc. Stud.* **2013**, *34*, 203–229. [CrossRef]

41. Griffith, R.; O'Connell, M.; Smith, K. *Food Expenditure and Nutritional Quality over the Great Recession*; IFS Briefing Note BN143; Institute of Fiscal Studies: London, UK, 2013.

42. Adams, N.; Carr, J.; Collins, J. *Households Below average Income: An Analysis of the Income Distribtution, 1994/95 to 2010/11*; Department for Work and Pensions: London, UK, 2012.

43. McGuinness, F. *Poverty in the UK: Statistics*; House of Commons Library: London, UK, 2018.

44. McClements, L.D. Equivalence scales for children. *J. Public Econ.* **1977**, *8*, 191–210. [CrossRef]

45. UK Data Service. General Lifestyle Survey. 2017. Available online: https://discover.ukdataservice.ac.uk/series/?sn=200019 (accessed on 5 April 2017).

46. Eurostat. European Union Statistics on Income and Living Conditions EU-SILC. 2017. Available online: http://ec.europa.eu/eurostat/web/microdata/european-union-statistics-on-income-and-living-conditions (accessed on 5 April 2017).

47. Service, U.D. Family Resources Survey. 2017. Available online: https://discover.ukdataservice.ac.uk/series/?sn=200017 (accessed on 5 April 2017).

48. Kantar. Kantar World Panel. 2017. Available online: https://www.kantarworldpanel.com/global/Consumer-Panels (accessed on 5 April 2017).

49. Department for Environment, Food and Rural Affairs. Living Costs and Food Survey. 2015. Available online: https://www.ons.gov.uk/file?uri=/peoplepopulationandcommunity/personalandhouseholdfinances/incomeandwealth/methodologies/livingcostsandfoodsurvey/livingcostsfoodtechnicalreport2015.pdf (accessed on 5 November 2017).

50. Scottish Health Survey. 2015. Available online: http://discover.ukdataservice.ac.uk/series/?sn=2000047 (accessed on 27 December 2018).

51. Scottish Government. Scottish Household Survey—Survey Details. 2009. Available online: http://www.gov.scot/Topics/Statistics/16002/Methodology (accessed on 27 December 2018).

52. Food Standards Agency. The Eatwell Plate. Available online: https://www.gov.uk/government/publications/the-eatwell-guide (accessed on 25 March 2014).

53. Barton, K.L.; Wrieden, W.L.; Sherriff, A.; Armstrong, J.; Anderson, A.S. Trends in socio-economic inequalities in the Scottish diet: 2001–2009. *Public Health Nutr.* **2015**, *18*, 2970–2980. [CrossRef] [PubMed]

54. Wrieden, W.; Armstrong, J.; Anderson, A.; Sherriff, A.; Barton, K. Choosing the best method to estimate the energy density of a population using food purchase data. *J. Hum. Nutr. Diet.* **2015**, *28*, 126–134. [CrossRef] [PubMed]

55. Wrieden, W.L.; Armstrong, J.; Sherriff, A.; Anderson, A.S.; Barton, K.L. Slow pace of dietary change in Scotland: 2001–2009. *Br. J. Nutr.* **2013**, *109*, 1892–1902. [CrossRef] [PubMed]

56. Office for National Statistics. *Living Costs and Food Survey. User Guide Volume A—Introduction*; Office for National Statistics: Newport, UK, 2013.

57. Scottish Government. *Revised Dietary Goals*; Scottish Government: Edinburgh, UK, 2013.

58. Barton, K.L. An Exploratory Analysis of the Scottish Diet 2001–2009 Using Household Purchase Data. Ph.D. Thesis, Universtiy of Dundee, Dundee, UK, 2014.

59. Armstrong, J.; Sherriff, A.; Wrieden, W.L.; Brogan, Y.; Barton, K.L. *Deriving and Interpreting Dietary Patterns in the Scottish Diet: Further Analysis of the Scottish Health Survey and Expenditure and Food Survey*; Food Standards scotland: Aberdeen, UK, 2009.

60. Waijers, P.M.; Feskens, E.J.; Ocké, M.C. A critical review of predefined diet quality scores. *Bri. J. Nutr.* **2007**, *97*, 219–231. [CrossRef]

61. Guenther, P.M.; Kirkpatrick, S.I.; Reedy, J.; Krebs-Smith, S.M.; Buckman, D.W.; Dodd, K.W.; Casavale, K.O.; Carroll, R.J. The Healthy Eating Index-2010 Is a Valid and Reliable Measure of Diet Quality According to the 2010 Dietary Guidelines for Americans1–3. *J. Nutr.* **2013**, *144*, 399–407. [CrossRef]

62. Department for Environment, Food & Rural Affairs. *Family Food*; Department for Environment, Food & Rural Affairs: London, UK, 2012.

63. Department for Environment, Food & Rural Affairs. *Food Statistics in Your Pocket 2017: Prices and Expenditure*; Department for Environment, Food & Rural Affairs: London, UK, 2018.

64. Thompson, S. *The Low-Pay, No-Pay Cycle*; Joseph Rowntree Foundation: York, UK, 2015.

65. Food Standards Scotland. *The Scottish Diet Needs to Change: Situation Report Update*; Food Standards Scotland: Aberdeen, UK, 2018.

66. Douglas, F.; Ejebu, O.Z.; Garcia, A.; MacKenzie, F.; Whybrow, S.; McKenzie, L.; Ludbrook, A.; Dowler, E. *The Nature and Extent of Food Poverty in Scotland*; NHS Health Scotland: Glasgow, UK, 2015.

67. Nevarez, L.; Tobin, K.; Waltermaurer, E. Food Acquisition in Poughkeepsie, NY: Exploring the Stratification of "Healthy Food" Consciousness in a Food-Insecure City. *Food Cult. Soc.* **2016**, *19*, 19–44. [CrossRef]

68. Tarasuk, V. A critical examination of community-based responses to household food insecurity in Canada. *Health Educ. Behav.* **2001**, *28*, 487–499. [CrossRef] [PubMed]

69. Hamelin, A.-M.; Mercier, C.; Bédard, A. Discrepancies in households and other stakeholders viewpoints on the food security experience: A gap to address. *Health Educ. Res.* **2009**, *25*, 401–412. [CrossRef] [PubMed]

70. Hamelin, A.M.; Mercier, C.; Bédard, A. Needs for food security from the standpoint of Canadian households participating and not participating in community food programmes. *Int. J. Consum. Stud.* **2011**, *35*, 58–68. [CrossRef]

71. Harden, J.; Dickson, A. Low-income mothers' food practices with young children: A qualitative longitudinal study. *Health Educ. J.* **2015**, *74*, 381–391. [CrossRef]

72. Douglas, F.; Sapko, J.; Kiezebrink, K.; Kyle, J. Resourcefulness, desperation, shame, gratitude and powerlessness: Common themes emerging from a study of food bank use in northeast Scotland. *AIMS Public Health* **2015**, *2*, 297–317. [CrossRef] [PubMed]

73. Douglas, F.; MacKenzie, F.; Ejebu, O.-Z.; Whybrow, S.; Garcia, A.L.; McKenzie, L.; Ludbrook, A.; Dowler, E. "A Lot of People Are Struggling Privately. They Don't Know Where to Go or They're Not Sure of What to Do": Frontline Service Provider Perspectives of the Nature of Household Food Insecurity in Scotland. *Int. J. Environ. Res. Public Health* **2018**, *15*, 2738. [CrossRef]

74. Scottish Government. *Severe Poverty in Scotland*; Scottish Government: Edinburgh, UK, 2015.

75. Scottish Government. *Poverty and Income Inequality in Scotland 2009–10*; Scottish Government: Edinburgh, UK, 2015.

76. Hirsch, D.; Bryan, A.; Davis, A.; Smith, N. *A Minimum Income Standard for Remote and Rural Scotland*; Highlands and Islands Enterprise: Inverness, UK, 2013.

77. ScotCen Social Research. *Scottish Health Survey, 2012: User Guide*; Scottish Government: Edinburgh, UK, 2013.

78. Fafard, A.-A.; Tarasuk, V. Shelter Expenditures Increase Vulnerability to Household Food Insecurity. *FASEB J.* **2015**, *29*, 261.6.

79. Sriram, U.; Tarasuk, V. Economic predictors of household food insecurity in Canadian metropolitan areas. *J. Hunger Environ. Nutr.* **2016**, *11*, 1–13. [CrossRef]

80. Alston, P. Statement on Visit to the United Kingdom, by Professor Philip Alston, United Nations Special Rapporteur on Extreme Poverty and Human Rights. 2018. Available online: https://www.ohchr.org/EN/NewsEvents/Pages/DisplayNews.aspx?NewsID=23881&LangID=E (accessed on 14 December 2018).

81. UNICEF. *Building the Future: Children and the Sustainable Development Goals in Rich Countries*; UNICEF: New York, NY, USA, 2017.

82. Kirkpatrick, S.I.; McIntyre, L.; Potestio, M.L. Child hunger and long-term adverse consequences for health. *Arch. Pediatr. Adolesc. Med.* **2010**, *164*, 754–762. [CrossRef]

83. Seligman, H.K.; Laraia, B.A.; Kushel, M.B. Food insecurity is associated with chronic disease among low-income NHANES participants. *J. Nutr.* **2009**, *140*, 304–310. [CrossRef]

84. Gowda, C.; Hadley, C.; Aiello, A.E. The association between food insecurity and inflammation in the US adult population. *Am. J. Public Health* **2012**, *102*, 1579–1586. [CrossRef] [PubMed]

85. Marques, E.S.; Reichenheim, M.E.; de Moraes, C.L.; Antunes, M.M.; Salles-Costa, R. Household food insecurity: A systematic review of the measuring instruments used in epidemiological studies. *Public Health Nutr.* **2015**, *18*, 877–892. [CrossRef]

86. Muldoon, K.A.; Duff, P.K.; Fielden, S.; Anema, A. Food insufficiency is associated with psychiatric morbidity in a nationally representative study of mental illness among food insecure Canadians. *Soc. Psychiatry Psychiatr. Epidemiol.* **2013**, *48*, 795–803. [CrossRef] [PubMed]

87. Fitzpatrick, T.; Rosella, L.C.; Calzavara, A.; Petch, J.; Pinto, A.D.; Manson, H.; Goel, V.; Wodchis, W.P. Looking beyond income and education: Socioeconomic status gradients among future high-cost users of health care. *Am. J. Prev. Med.* **2015**, *49*, 161–171. [CrossRef]

88. Seligman, H.K.; Davis, T.C.; Schillinger, D.; Wolf, M.S. Food insecurity is associated with hypoglycemia and poor diabetes self-management in a low-income sample with diabetes. *J. Health Care Poor Underserved* **2010**, *21*, 1227–1233. [PubMed]

89. Chan, J.; DeMelo, M.; Gingras, J.; Gucciardi, E. Challenges of diabetes self-management in adults affected by food insecurity in a large urban centre of Ontario, Canada. *Int. J. Endocrinol.* **2015**, *2015*, 903468. [CrossRef] [PubMed]

90. Tarasuk, V.; Cheng, J.; de Oliveira, C.; Dachner, N.; Gundersen, C.; Kurdyak, P. Association between household food insecurity and annual health care costs. *Can. Med. Assoc. J.* **2015**, *187*, 429–436. [CrossRef] [PubMed]

91. All-Party Parliamentary Inquiry into Hunger in the United Kingdom. *Feeding Britain: A Strategy for Zero Hunger in England, Wales, Scotland and Northern Ireland*; Children's Society: London, UK, 2014.

92. Scottish Food Comission. *Scottish Food Commission Interim Report*; Scottish Food Comission: Edinburgh, UK, 2016.

93. Scottish Government. *Dignity: Ending Hunger Together in Scotland—The Report of the Independent Working Group on Food Poverty*; Scottish Government: Edinburgh, UK, 2016.

94. Cafiero, C.; Nord, M.; Viviani, S. *Methods for Estimating Comparable Prevalence Rates of Food Insecurity Experienced by Adults throughout the World*; IOP Publishing: Bristol, UK, 2016.

95. Observatory, S.P.H. Scottish Health Survey. 2016. Available online: http://www.scotpho.org.uk/publications/overview-of-key-data-sources/surveys-cross-sectional/scottish-health-survey (accessed on 17 July 2017).

96. Tait, C. *Hungry for Change: The Final Report of the Fabian Commission on Food and Poverty*; Fabian Society: London, UK, 2015.

97. Nelson, M.; Erens, B.; Bates, B.; Church, S.; Boshier, T. *Low Income Diet and Nutrition Survey*; TSO: London, UK, 2007; Volume 3.

98. Agency, F.S. 'Food and You' Survey Wave 4. 2017. Available online: https://www.food.gov.uk/science/research-reports/ssresearch/foodandyou (accessed on 28 March 2017).

99. Machin, R.J. Understanding holiday hunger. *J. Poverty Soc. Justice* **2016**, *24*, 311–319. [CrossRef]

100. Cook, J.T.; Frank, D.A. Food security, poverty, and human development in the United States. *Ann. N. Y. Acad. Sci.* **2008**, *1136*, 193–209. [CrossRef]

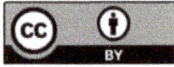

International Journal of
*Environmental Research
and Public Health*

MDPI

Article

Food Reference Budgets as a Potential Policy Tool to Address Food Insecurity: Lessons Learned from a Pilot Study in 26 European Countries

Elena Carrillo-Álvarez [1,*], Tess Penne [2], Hilde Boeckx [3], Bérénice Storms [4] and Tim Goedemé [5]

[1] Blanquerna School of Health Sciences—Universitat Ramon Llull-Global Research on Wellbeing—GRoW Research group, Padilla, 08025 Barcelona, Spain

[2] Research Foundation—Flanders, Herman Deleeck Centre for Social Policy—University of Antwerp, 2000 Antwerp, Belgium; tess.penne@uantwerpen.be

[3] Thomas More Kempen, 2440 Malle, Belgium; hilde.boeckx@thomasmore.be

[4] Herman Deleeck Centre for Social Policy—University of Antwerp, 2000 Antwerp, Belgium; bereniceML.storms@uantwerpen.be

[5] Institute for New Economic Thinking at the Oxford Martin School and Department of Social Policy and Intervention, University of Oxford, Oxford OX2 6ED, UK; tim.goedeme@uantwerp.be

[*] Correspondence: elenaca@blanquerna.url.edu; Tel.: +34-93-325-32-56

Received: 31 October 2018; Accepted: 14 December 2018; Published: 24 December 2018

Abstract: The aim of this article is to present the development of cross-country comparable food reference budgets in 26 European countries, and to discuss their usefulness as an addition to food-based dietary guidelines (FBDG) for tackling food insecurity in low-income groups. Reference budgets are illustrative priced baskets containing the minimum goods and services necessary for well-described types of families to have an adequate social participation. This study was conducted starting from national FBDG, which were translated into monthly food baskets. Next, these baskets were validated in terms of their acceptability and feasibility through focus group discussions, and finally they were priced. Along the paper, we show how that food reference budgets hold interesting contributions to the promotion of healthy eating and prevention of food insecurity in low-income contexts in at least four ways: (1) they show how a healthy diet can be achieved with limited economic resources, (2) they bring closer to the citizen a detailed example of how to put FBDG recommendations into practice, (3) they ensure that food security is achieved in an integral way, by comprising the biological but also psychological and social functions of food, and (4) providing routes for further (comparative) research into food insecurity.

Keywords: reference budgets; food insecurity; cost of a healthy diet; Food-based dietary guidelines

1. Introduction

In a moment in which 18.8% of the global burden of disease has been attributed to unhealthy eating [1], and in the context of growing inequalities in many countries [2–6], policy-makers face the challenge of developing strategies that are sufficiently powerful to revert long-standing patterns of unhealthy eating.

While ecologic approaches and upstream actions have been argued to be indispensable to effectively tackle the situation, actions addressed to the individual are still timely [7–9]. Food-Based Dietary Guidelines (FBDG) constitute the closest set of nutritional standards for the population and are primarily intended for consumer information and education. Starting from the available evidence on the most relevant diet-disease relationships for the targeted population, FBDG are science-based policy recommendations in the form of guidelines that describe dietary patterns that can facilitate the adherence to eating habits that maintain and promote health [10,11].

Since there exists a strong link between diet and the most prevalent diseases in developed societies, the development and implementation of FBDG has the potential to substantially influence the burden of disease within its citizenship, to the extent that the quality of such tools may accentuate or blur diet-related health inequalities between and within countries [10,12–14]. As the EFSA explains in its 'Scientific Opinion on establishing Food-Based Dietary Guidelines' [10], the development of pan-European detailed and effective FBDG is not possible due to wide cross-country variations in nutritional priorities, which are the result of differences in terms of nutrient intake [15], eating habits and traditions [16] and diet-related health situation [14].

In 1996, the FAO and WHO published a set of recommendations on the development of FBDG that remains a point of reference for policy makers on the field [11]. In Europe, additionally, this work was taken further by the EURODIET project, which proposed an updated framework for the development of FBDG in the European Union [17]. Their main recommendations can be summarized in five points: (1) FBDG must start from recognized public health problems; (2) FBDG are prepared for a particular socio-economic context and must reflect the particularities of the territory with regard to food availability and consumption patterns; (3) FBDG should be updated systematically, ideally every 5 years, to adapt to the evolution of consumption patterns and food availability; (4) FBDG must reflect patterns of consumption, rather than numerical goals in terms of nutrients; and (5) they must be relatively consistent with prevailing patterns of consumption (otherwise they will hardly be accepted). A sixth point was added by Roth and Knai in a report issued in 2003 by the WHO Regional Office for Europe, concerning the need for government endorsement of FBDG to further articulate health policies coherent with dietary recommendations [13]. At that moment, only 25 of the 48 countries participating in the study reported having national, government-endorsed food-based dietary guidelines.

Fifteen years later, we conducted a similar research to the EURODIET project, in which the FBDG available in 26 EU Member States were analysed in the light of the previously mentioned guidelines (Carrillo et al., submitted for publication). Our findings were consistent with the conclusions of previous studies [18–20], indicating little advancement on the topic in the last two decades. Among the different findings, we highlight the fact that none of the FBDG includes any specific recommendation for low-income groups, for which regular FBDG have been described as insufficient, as they do not address one of the main factors conditioning food decisions in this population: the cost of a diet [21,22].

In this paper, we present food reference budgets (RBs) for 26 EU Member States, as a tool that can complement regular FBDG to better orientate the dietary intake of low-income groups. RBs are defined as illustrative priced baskets of goods and services that represent the minimum necessary resources for well-described types of families that allow for an adequate diet. In this context, not only the biological function of food is taken into account, but also the social, hedonistic and gastronomic role that food has in current societies [23]. While food reference budgets have been published for individual countries [24,25], to the best of our knowledge, this is the first attempt to document and illustrate in a comparative perspective the cost of a healthy diet in the European Union.

The aim of this article is to discuss the development of cross-country comparable food reference budgets in 26 European countries, as well as their added-value for FBDG for tackling food insecurity in low-income groups.

2. Materials and Methods

The research that we describe here is part of the pilot project for the development of a common methodology on Reference Budgets in Europe. The pilot project was funded by the European Commission's DG Employment, Social Affairs and Inclusion to develop a common methodology to construct high-quality comparable reference budgets in all EU Member States [26] (participating countries: AT, Austria; BE, Belgium; BG, Bulgaria; CY, Cyprus; CZ, Czech Republic; DE, Germany; DK, Denmark; EE, Estonia; EL, Greece; ES, Spain; FI, Finland; FR, France; HR, Croatia; HU, Hungary; IT, Italy; LT, Lithuania; LU, Luxembourg; LV, Latvia; MT, Malta; NL, Netherlands; PL, Poland; PT, Portugal; RO, Romania; SE, Sweden; SK, Slovakia; SI, Slovenia). For the purpose of this project, a common method was developed, along with food baskets for 26 EU Member States that illustrate what families need to access a diet that allows for adequate social participation. Being able to participate adequately means that people would have the essentials to play their various social roles in a particular society [26]. This is why, in the concrete context of food, we started from a broader perspective on the functions of food, beyond the necessities of a healthy diet, strictly speaking. The research was carried out by 26 country teams and coordinated by the Herman Deleeck Centre for Social Policy at the University of Antwerp together with three domain coordinators. The geographical coverage is the European Union, except for Ireland and the United Kingdom. Each country team collaborated with a nutritionist and started from the existing national FBDG. The choice to start from FBDG rather than, for instance, common nutritional guidelines from the WHO, was motivated by the fact that FBDG represent the country-specific recommendations on what people need to eat to achieve and/or maintain a good health, while at the same time respecting the cross-national differences in food habits and health priorities. The underlying assumption is that the overall objective of FBDG is the same across countries: facilitating a healthy diet, based on relevant insights from the scientific literature, while respecting local conditions. Finally, each country team organised three focus group discussions in order to test the completeness and acceptability of the food baskets. The items in the food basket were priced in accessible and affordable shops in the capital city.

For the construction of the food baskets we focused primarily on the required budget that should enable people to consume a healthy diet. Although we also considered the other functions of food (e.g., psychological and social) and the necessities for a minimum level physical activity, as recommended in many FBDG, in this paper we report only on the part related to having access to a healthy diet. The main reason is that the nature of collecting robust budgets for the other functions of food and physical activity required more time and resources than were available in our project. As a result, the budgets for the other functions of food and physical activity are not sufficiently robust and comparable. Obviously, in order to be able to afford a healthy diet, one should also have access to kitchen equipment, clean water, and energy to cook. However, due to the specific requirements to estimate their cost, also these are not considered here (see [26] for a discussion of kitchen equipment and energy costs).

Given the large variation in needs between individuals and households, and our objective to construct cross-country comparable baskets that represent what is needed at the minimum, in all countries the food baskets were developed for household types with the same specific characteristics:

(1)   a single man [35–45-years-old]
(2)   a single woman [35–45-years-old]
(3)   a couple [man, woman; 35–45-years-old]
(4)   a single woman [35–45-years-old] + 2 children [primary school boy, 10-years-old + secondary school girl, 14-years-old].
(5)   a couple [35–45-years-old] + 2 children [primary school boy, 10-years-old + secondary school girl, 14-years-old].

Furthermore, for assessing and pricing the concrete lists of items, the following assumptions were made:

-   The household types are assumed to live in the capital city of each participant country. This point is particularly relevant in terms of the pricing of the items and the frequency in which people rely on the production of food for own consumption.
-   All meals are prepared and eaten at home. All food is acquired, prepared and consumed in the most economical way possible. This means families are well-informed about prices and are able to shop in the most economic retailers that are accessible with public transport. However, we do not assume that people can always buy all their ingredients in the cheapest available supermarket. Hence, we allowed for a certain freedom of choice to shop within a range of cheap retailers.

-    All household members are in good health and do not have specific dietary requirements. The reason for this assumption is not so much that this is the most common health condition, but rather that the cost of a diet varies depending on the kind and severity of health problems, each having different implications for the needs of the person affected.
-    The ingredients should give families access to healthy, tasty and well varied meals. The food basket should be acceptable for citizens with different background characteristics provided that the healthy aspect is not compromised.
-    Finally, we assume that the budget for food is allocated to each household member in accordance with her/his needs.

By making these assumptions, we focus on the minimum below which a healthy diet in accordance with the FBDG is not possible. In real-life situations, though, more resources will usually be needed because resources are not always spent in the most economical way, people could be confronted with diseases or special needs, people might lack the necessary capacities or information to buy and prepare healthy food at economical prices, and some household members may consume a share of the food budget that is not in proportion to their needs. The procedure that the various country teams followed was structured in five standardized steps or milestones.

(1)   For the first milestone, the national experts provided a clear description of the scientific basis (DRVs) of the national FBDG, the results of the last food consumption survey and the model of health education in their country.
(2)   In the following step, in cooperation with a nutritionist, country teams translated the FBDG into a concrete list of food items, including the necessary amounts for each hypothetical household.
(3)   For the third milestone, three different focus groups were organized in the capital city. Several focus group trainings were organized and instructions were developed by the coordinating team to make sure that the focus groups were conducted and analysed in a standardized way (cf. Annex 1 in [26]). The national partners recruited for each focus group 5–11 participants of active age (30–50), through a questionnaire for recruitment ensuring a mix of different family situations, and a variety of socio-economic backgrounds. Involving people with different backgrounds increases the variation of opinions, the quality of discussions (in terms of argumentation) and validity of the outcome [27–29]. The recruitment of different socio-economic backgrounds was measured based on three variables: activity status, level of education and burden of housing costs as a proxy for income. Because of the limited number of focus groups, it was difficult to make sure ethnic minorities were equally involved. Therefore, this pilot project aimed in the first place at capturing the dominant cultural patterns through FG discussions, acknowledging that more research is necessary to reveal the cultural variety within cities. Each focus group followed a predefined topic list, with an estimated time of three hours. The first half of the discussion was devoted to evaluating the broader theoretical framework (the assessment of needs and essential social roles) and the underlying assumptions we made (characteristics of the reference family), and the second half was used to discuss the acceptability, feasibility and completeness of the food basket, the kitchen equipment and the other non-physical functions of food—as well as the related purchasing patterns. For the purpose of this article, we only make use of the second part of the focus group discussions, which had an average duration of approximately 90 min. To facilitate the discussion, an illustrative weekly menu was developed by the nutritionist, in accordance with the proposed food basket. The results were analysed by the country teams in accordance with a common template of analysis. Each focus group was recorded, and, during the discussion, an assistant wrote down the various arguments in a structured template. For each topic a final column was completed with the overall conclusions and general remarks on interaction processes, proxemics and paralinguistic information. In literature they call this a micro-interlocutor analysis [30], which allows to focus on the group as well as on the individual data while taking into account group dynamics. The purpose of the focus

groups was not to decide on specific quantities but rather to assess the nature, the origin and the construction of the arguments regarding why items are needed or not and what is acceptable and feasible within a given socio-cultural context.

(4) Next, the food baskets had to be adapted in function of feasibility and acceptability, based on the arguments put forward during focus group discussions. This was done in accordance with a common decision procedure that country teams had to follow to ensure that the healthy character of the diet was respected and to facilitate the consistency and robustness of the results across countries (cf. Annex 2 in [26]).

(5) The last milestone consisted of estimating the minimum feasible cost of the food basket. Again, several common assumptions were made. First of all, the food budget should represent the minimum resources that people need to get access to all essential food items. Further, people should have a minimum acceptable degree of freedom in the choice of shops and products. Thirdly, market prices are used, unless other purchasing patterns are common practice, but no sales prices are used. Another important guideline was that economies of scale in buying and preparing food should be taken into account. For the choice of shops to buy food, the national teams had to choose a few retailers or markets which were suggested by the participants in the focus groups. The retailers had to meet the following criteria: (1) they offer a wide variety of food items of acceptable quality at low prices, (2) the shops are well spread over the city, (3) the shops are well accessible by public transport. Being well spread over the country was another criterion that could be considered, as this could facilitate the future pricing of reference budgets developed for other regions. All countries priced the food baskets between March and April 2015 (exceptions are the food baskets for Luxembourg, Denmark and Slovakia which were priced in December 2014, July 2015 and October 2015, respectively). Prices were collected on the basis of a small-scale survey, carried out by researchers from each country team, making use of a standardised excel sheet (with the exception of Luxembourg, where the country team had access to the official price survey). To price pre-packaged food, the lowest price of suitable products had to be chosen. With regard to fresh food and food categories which contain a large variety of products, country teams had to follow a specific predefined pricing procedure, such that a weighted price could be estimated which takes into account the available range of relevant products. The food categories for which a weighted price procedure had to be used are the following: fresh fruit, canned fruit, fruit puree, frozen fruit, dried fruit, fresh vegetables, frozen prepared & unprepared vegetables, canned vegetables, fresh fish, frozen fish, canned fish, lean meat, fat meat, charcuterie and cheese. For instance, the cost of fresh fruit is based on a weighted average of all fresh fruit available in the shop, taking from each type of fruit the cheapest alternative of sufficient quality (e.g., the cheapest apple, the cheapest pear, etc.). The cheapest products are weighted 5/7, whereas the average weight of the more expensive items is given a weight of 2/7, while discarding the 10% most expensive fruits. This procedure aims to meet the dual objective of identifying the minimum cost to prepare healthy menus that still offer sufficient variation (see Annex 3 in [26] for the detailed instructions for assessing the cost of the food basket).

The applied pricing procedure was explicitly designed to balance standardisation, sensitivity to the local context, cross-national variations in purchasing patterns and considerations of acceptability. At the same time, it is clear that the procedure is open for improvement. More in particular, the number of shops frequented was generally low and the price survey typically shows a snapshot of the prices at one particular moment in time, collected by a single observer. A much more extensive price survey would be very useful and facilitate representativeness and reliability. In this context, building on the official price survey, especially for assessing the cost of food, could result in a significant improvement of the quality of the pricing procedure.

3. Results

3.1. The Contents of the Food Basket

What Constitutes a Healthy Diet?

Although there is little difference in the main food groups included in the country-specific FBDG, the type of foods and the recommended amounts within these main food groups differ substantially across countries [10]. These differences follow a clear geographical pattern which may be understood to be mainly a reflection of cultural background and food availability. For instance, in Eastern and Southern European countries the recommended quantities for protein-based foods such as meat or fish are higher compared to Western Europe. Nonetheless, the cross-national variation in FBDG can not only be explained by the differences in cultural habits. Also other factors play a role, including variations in health priorities and the availability of food products between EU member states, as well as the fact that the FBDGs have been updated at different points in time, by different institutions and aimed at different kind of age groups. Furthermore, the interpretation of international recommendations differs across EU Member States, which is reflected in differences in concrete guidelines. Figure 1 shows the content of the national healthy food baskets for a single woman expressed in daily food amounts (mg, and mL for liquids).

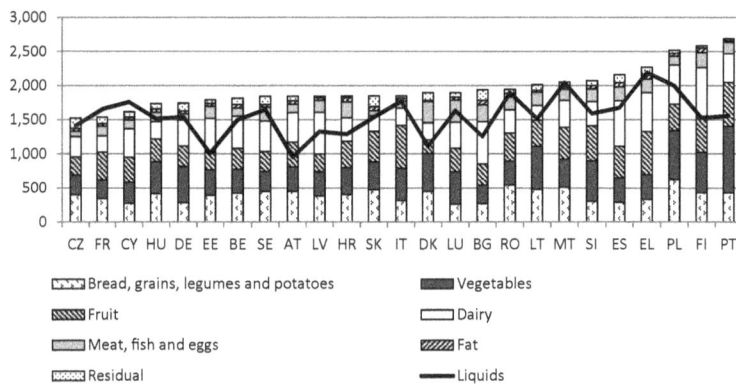

Figure 1. Daily food (mg/mL) amounts for a single woman, healthy food basket, 2015. Country abbreviations: AT, Austria; BE, Belgium; BG, Bulgaria; CY, Cyprus; CZ, Czech Republic; DE, Germany; DK, Denmark; EE, Estonia; EL, Greece; ES, Spain; FI, Finland; FR, France; HR, Croatia; HU, Hungary; IT, Italy; LT, Lithuania; LU, Luxembourg, LV, Latvia; MT, Malta; NL, Netherlands; PL, Poland; PT, Portugal; RO, Romania; SE, Sweden; SK, Slovakia; SI, Slovenia.

The amounts included in the graph refer to the quantity of food in the healthy food baskets that were developed by the country teams, taking account of the edible portions and typical wastes. Net amounts of fresh fruits, vegetables, potatoes, fish, fatter meat and eggs as recommended in the FBDG were increased with a waste percentage of respectively 22%, 28%, 10%, 30%, 20% and 12%. All countries have used the same edible portions, following guidelines that have originally been developed for Belgium [31]. An exception is Portugal, where –slightly different- national criteria were applied.

With regard to the amount of *vegetables* and *fruits*, country teams included on average between 300–400 g per day for each group. As explained above, the source of variation in the amounts relates to various factors, such as cultural differences (e.g., inclusion of vegetarian meals) or to differences in FBDG, e.g., some countries differentiate between fruit and vegetables while others formulate a joint recommendation. The amount of *dairy products* varies more across countries, ranging from 215 g in Latvia to 710 g in Finland. Also, for the group of meat, fish and eggs, variations fluctuate between long than 100 g per day (CZ, DE) to 339 g per day (LU). These variations reflect not only differences in guidelines but also, for instance, cultural differences in the composition of the meals. Countries with higher amounts usually include a portion of these foods in two of their meals per day, while others only include them for one daily meal. For the *liquids* group, the large variation is partly due to whether or not countries included wine and beer, and by the varying amounts of coffee and tea across countries. Water was the basic beverage in all countries and products like fruit juices or sodas were not included in this group, as they are not recommended on a regular basis. Milk was placed in the dairy group.

For some food groups, the variation can also be explained by the differences in the type of foods. For example, the food group *grains* includes foods such as bread, rice, pasta, pulses and potatoes. Nutritionally these items are considered as exchangeable, but the size of the portion in a daily meal varies considerably (e.g., for an adult: 70–100 g rice compared to 150–250 g potatoes). The *fat* group mainly includes cooking oil/fat. The Mediterranean countries nuts were also included in this group following some national guidelines. The type of fat included varies across countries. In Mediterranean countries the main source of recommended fat is olive oil and nuts, while in most of the other countries, butter and other spreadable fats are the most common type of fat. Hence, it is important to bear in mind that comparing food group amounts among the different countries does not necessarily provide information about the nutritional value of the baskets, since food items belonging to the same food group may have a different nutritional composition and/or different portion size.

The *residual* group is the food group with the highest variations, with amounts ranging from 25 g to 155 g. These differences are likely to be a consequence of the lack of guidelines with regard to these kind of products. All the countries include some salt, sugar and spices, but also sauces (such as mayonnaise and ketchup), dressings and sweets, especially for children, albeit with large variations.

3.2. The Cost of the Food Baskets

In this section, we present the results of the food baskets, priced in the capital cities in March-April 2015. Figure 2 shows the total food baskets for a single woman in EUR/month. The baskets represent the budget a single person needs to have a healthy diet.

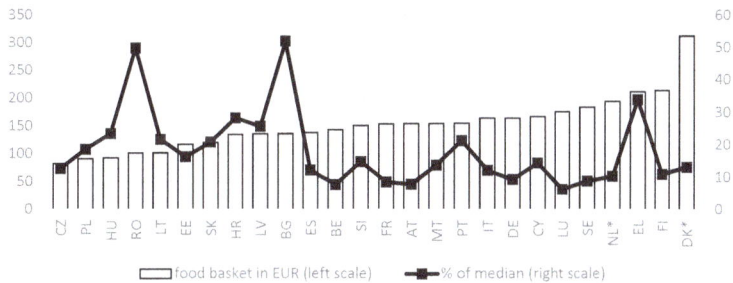

Figure 2. Total food baskets for a single woman in EUR / month (left axis) and as a percentage of the national median equivalent disposable household income (right axis). Results refer to the capital city of each country. Prices 2015. * Pricing procedure for DK and NL is not fully comparable. Source: [26] and Eurostat online database (median income).

When we compare the total food baskets, we observe large variations between EU Member States. The highest price can be found in Denmark, while the lowest cost can be observed for the Czech Republic. In Denmark a single woman needs about three times as much (312 EUR) for eating healthily as compared to a single woman in the Czech Republic (82 EUR). Even if we leave out Denmark (in which the pricing procedure was somewhat different), the difference between the most expensive food basket (Finland) and the cheapest one remains quite large. This substantial variation between countries is mainly a combination of differences in dietary guidelines on the one hand and price differences on the other hand.

At the same time, it is well known that the level of average household incomes varies a lot between EU Member States. In the context of food security, it is therefore relevant to consider the cost of a healthy diet also in relation to the level of incomes. Therefore, Figure 2 also depicts the food basket for a single person as a percentage of the median equivalent disposable household income in each country, as measured in the EU survey on Income and Living Conditions (EU-SILC) of 2016 (the source of the data on disposable household incomes is the Eurostat online database, last accessed 7 December 2018). This representative household survey collects on a yearly basis information on household incomes (including taxes, social contributions and benefits) in the previous calendar year [32]. We express the budgets as a percentage of the median disposable income (after taxes and transfers), adjusted for household size. This reveals a very different pattern of the relative cost of the food basket: it is lowest in Luxembourg (about 6% of the median income) and the highest in Romania (50%) and Bulgaria (52%), implying that in the latter countries, at the median income, households in the capital city would have to spend half of their income on food in order to have a diet in accordance with their national FBDG. Also, in Greece the relative cost of the food basket is remarkably high. Obviously, the implications for variations in food security require a much more in-depth analysis, with a focus on households with the lowest incomes, but this falls outside the scope of the present paper. In any case, this preliminary analysis shows that the cost of a healthy diet is a non-negligent factor to better understand patterns of food insecurity across the European Union.

4. Discussion

In the text above, we have described the process of development and the content of the Food Reference Budgets for 26 European countries, as constructed in the framework of the European Commission's DG Employment, Social Affairs and Inclusion funded *Pilot Project for the development of a common methodology on Reference Budgets in Europe.* We follow a normative perspective [33], and use guidelines and expert opinions to establish what is needed for an adequate diet. However, such an exercise is only helpful for health promotion if the resulting food baskets are sufficiently acceptable and feasible. Therefore, focus group discussions played a central role for assessing the acceptability and feasibility baskets.

The process of building food reference budgets is confronted with several limitations. First, there are a number of unavoidable arbitrary choices that condition the final budgets, such as the decision of not including promotions or discounts, the assumption that people are sufficiently informed and skilled to follow a healthy diet, or have enough time to do so. While we are aware that skills and capability to shop and cook healthily as well as time availability are important constraints towards a healthy eating [34,35], and that some studies describe that these aspects are even more critical in vulnerable groups [36–38], the decision to develop RBs for these types of family was consistent with the need of having a common and clear family type to facilitate the robustness of the results and the focus on the minimum required resources for an adequate diet. It would be worthwhile to expend the results of this pilot project to household types based on other assumptions regarding time constraints and competences, to reveal the importance of these personal factors in having access to a healthy diet. At the same time, we are convinced that the current food budgets, with their specific assumptions, can already be used in tailored nutrition education programs, as has been done in some countries [39,40]. Second, although the Supplementary materials (Table S1) contain the budgets for additional household types, the budgets have been developed for a limited number of types only and cannot be extrapolated to the entire population. Moreover, since food RBs start from FBDG, in their current form they only represent the *official* healthy way of eating, while they leave out a myriad of other possible ways of following a healthy diet. In this sense, future research should be able to take into account a greater variation of reference situations in terms of age, cultural background, personal choices and health conditions. Fourth, the pricing procedure that was applied could be further improved to increase representativeness and reliability by working with a larger, random sample of food products. Fifth, due to their detailed character, the budgets risk to be used in a prescriptive way. Given previously mentioned limitations, food reference budgets do not pretend to *define* what people should eat, but to illustrate a way in which an adequate diet can be achieved, and how much that would cost at the minimum. Finally, when using the food budgets for comparative research, researchers should be aware of the limits to their comparability that we have highlighted above. In particular, it should be clear that is the healthy food basket is comparable only in the sense that it reflects everywhere the state of affairs of FBDG in 2015. We are well aware that the extent to which the FBDG are an adequate cultural and scientific reflection of what a healthy diet should be in different national contexts can be criticised [41].

Notwithstanding these limitations, we are convinced that food reference budgets hold interesting contributions to the promotion of healthy eating and prevention of food insecurity in low-income contexts in at least four ways: First, because they show how a healthy diet can be achieved with limited economic resources, they constitute not only a guideline in terms of budgeting, but also offer policy-makers more insight into the cost of a healthy diet and how this may be a hurdle to achieve a healthy eating pattern.

Second, food reference budgets also bring closer to the citizen a detailed example of how to put general recommendations (as the ones contained in FBDG) into practice. Several studies show that the main motivators in the choice of food differ depending on the socioeconomic and educational level. We know that even though the price is a great determinant of the intake, culinary skills and food knowledge is also a determining factor among low-income people [36,37]. FBDG are designed to be easy to interpret and to translate into physical dishes and food preparations. However, in a moment in which most population is losing culinary referents and less and less familiar with cooking [42], much people do not have the necessary knowledge to translate dietary recommendations into daily eating practices (this is what the nutritionist on each country team did). Hence, a guide that shows how to cook a healthy diet with very few resources is most useful.

Third, if, when ensuring food security, we really aim at promoting a bio-psycho-social understanding of the person, healthy eating promotion must compulsorily include foods to share, foods to enjoy and foods to celebrate. This is something the focus groups laid bare. In all countries, FG participants stressed how food is not only about being in a good health, but it is an essential part of cultural and social life. Eating and drinking is playing a crucial role for social activities and gatherings with family, friends and colleagues in all different cultural contexts. The people in FGs emphasize the importance of cooking and dining together but also of eating out in order to maintain social relations and to socialize. Food can be a means to show care and respect, to create hospitality and to create a feeling of belonging. Further, the FG participants often mentioned the role of food in the preservation of traditions and in the expression of a certain cultural, religious or personal identity. These foods and activities are not essential for a healthy diet, nevertheless, they are seen as important to participate adequately in society. As mentioned above, in this project, the inclusion of these items was not done in a very standardized and cross-nationally comparable way, which is why we did not report their estimated levels. Nevertheless, we should acknowledge the importance of these functions in order to create more acceptable and complete food baskets that allow for adequate social participation in the different EU countries. Ultimately this is the only pathway to work toward narrowing diet-related health inequalities in a comprehensive and empowering manner. Therefore, it would be worthwhile to spend more time and resources on collecting high quality information on this aspect of an adequate diet.

Finally, it is worthwhile pointing out that although there is quite some variation between countries in the cost of a healthy diet, this variation is much smaller than the variation in median disposable household incomes we find in the EU. For instance, while the cost of a healthy diet is about 214 EUR/month in Finland as compared to just 102 EUR per month in Romania, its median equivalent disposable household income in EUR is about ten times higher [43]. As a result, it is clear that people living in countries with a relatively low median disposable will have a much harder time spending sufficient income to ensure a healthy diet. Furthermore, the ranking in the cost of a healthy diet differs from the ranking of countries in terms of their median disposable household income. For instance, even though Romania clearly is the EU country with the lowest median household incomes, the cost of a healthy diet in Bucarest is clearly higher than the cost of a healthy diet in, for instance, the Czech Republic, which in terms of household incomes is considerably less poor. This has clear implications for policies, especially at the EU level, but it also shows the potential of the food reference budgets for further research into better understanding patterns of food insecurity across the EU.

5. Conclusions

In this paper, food reference budgets are presented and their potential utility as a complement for FBDG in low-income contexts is discussed. These reference budgets are built upon cross-nationally comparable food baskets which reflect the minimum cost for a healthy diet, taking national food patterns and recommendations into account by starting from national FBDG. Food baskets were constructed for the capital city in 26 countries, including all EU Member States except Ireland and the United Kingdom. In Denmark and the Netherlands, the procedure that was applied was not fully comparable. The figures show that even though cross-national differences in the minimum cost of a healthy diet are large, they vary much less than net disposable median incomes. We are convinced that the part of the food baskets which relates to having a healthy diet is comparable across countries in the sense that it reflects dominant institutionalized expectations regarding what constitutes a healthy diet, as embedded in national FBDG, and so will be useful for further comparative research.

The procedure we set up for developing and pricing the cost of a healthy diet has been conceived to optimise the balance between the following objectives: (1) It should allow for a healthy diet in line with recommendations in the applicable food-based dietary guidelines; (2) It should be the most economical option possible, while allowing some room for choice; and (3) It should be acceptable, tasty and feasible for the wider public, that is, it should be in line with local food habits. This setup seemed to work well and led to reasonable outcomes. However, further efforts should be undertaken to develop strategies to also collect comparable information on the cost of other functions of food, kitchen equipment and national recommendations regarding physical activity.

We are strongly convinced that the food reference budgets offer a useful tool for the promotion of healthy eating and prevention of food insecurity in low-income contexts in at least four ways: (1) help with budgeting for a healthy diet and making the financial hurdles for realising a healthy diet visible to policy makers; (2) educational illustration of how to cook in accordance with national food recommendations as embedded in the FBDGs; (3) showing that also other functions of food matter, apart from having access to a healthy diet; (4) providing routes for further (comparative) research into food insecurity.

While the results of this pilot project have proven to be very useful, we have also pointed to several limitations that indicate the potential for further improvement. Overcoming these limitations is strongly dependent on having access to better data, including price data and comparable food consumption surveys in all EU Member States. Also, to make the food baskets more comparable in the sense of the minimum necessary for an adequate diet, it would be welcome to have up-to-date high quality FBDGs everywhere.

Supplementary Materials: The following are available online at http://www.mdpi.com/1660-4601/16/1/32/s1, Table S1: The complete food baskets for each country.

Author Contributions: All authors contributed equally to this paper.

Funding: This research was funded by DG Employment and Social Affairs of the European Commission (contract no. VC/2013/0554).

Acknowledgments: We are very grateful to two anonymous reviewers for very constructive comments and suggestions and to all national experts who contributed to the development of the national food baskets. A complete list of the research teams involved in the Pilot Project can be found in ref. 26.

Conflicts of Interest: The authors declare no conflict of interest. The funders had no role in the design of the study; in the collection, analyses, or interpretation of data; in the writing of the manuscript, and in the decision to publish the results.

References

1. GBD 2016 Risk Factors Collaborators. Global, regional, and national comparative risk assessment of 84 behavioural, environmental and occupational, and metabolic risks or clusters of risks, 1990–2016: A systematic analysis for the global burden of disease study 2016. *Lancet* **2017**. [CrossRef]
2. Thomson, K.; Hillier-Brown, F.; Todd, A.; McNamara, C.; Huijts, T.; Bambra, C. The effects of public health policies on health inequalities in high-income countries: An umbrella review. *BMC Public Health* **2018**, *18*, 869. [CrossRef] [PubMed]
3. World Health Organization. *World Health Statistics 2017. Monitoring Health for the SDGs*; World Health Organization: Geneva, Switzerland, 2017.
4. OECD. *It Together: Why Less Inequality Benefits All*; OECD Publishing: Paris, France, 2015.
5. Brian, N. *Inequality and Inclusive Growth in Rich Countries: Shared Challenges and Contrasting Fortunes*; Oxford University Press: Oxford, UK, 2018.
6. Milanovic, B. *Global Inequality. A New Approach for the Age of Globalization*; Harvard University Press: Cambridge, MA, USA, 2016.
7. Roberto, C.A.; Swinburn, B.; Hawkes, C.; Huang, T.T.-K.; Costa, S.A.; Ashe, M.; Zwicker, L.; Cawley, J.H.; Brownell, K.D. Patchy progress on obesity prevention: Emerging examples, entrenched barriers, and new thinking. *Lancet* **2015**, *385*, 2400–2409. [CrossRef]
8. Carrillo-Álvarez, E.; Riera-Romaní, J. Childhood obesity prevention: Does policy meet research? Evidence-based reflections upon the Spanish case. *MOJ Public Heal.* **2017**, *6*, 1–14. [CrossRef]
9. Kumanyika, S.; Libman, K.; Garcia, A. Strategic Action to Combat the Obesity Epidemic. Available online: http://www.wish.org.qa/wp-content/uploads/2018/02/27425_WISH_Obesity_Report_web14.pdf (accessed on 14 December 2018).
10. EFSA Panel on Dietetic Products, Nutrition, and Allergies (NDA). Scientific opinion on establishing food-based dietary guidelines. *EFSA J.* **2010**, *8*, 1–42. [CrossRef]
11. FAO/WHO. *Preparation and Use of Food-Based Dietary Guidelines*; WHO: Nicosia, Cyprus, 1996.
12. Stockley, L. Toward public health nutrition strategies in the European Union to implement food based dietary guidelines and to enhance healthier lifestyles. *Public Health Nutr.* **2001**, *4*, 307–324. [CrossRef] [PubMed]
13. Roth, N.; Knai, C. *Food Based Dietary Guidelines in the Who European Region*; WHO: Geneva, Switzerland, 2003.
14. WHO. *Global Status Report on Noncommunicable Diseases 2014*; WHO: Geneva, Switzerland, 2014.
15. Pomerleau, J.; McKee, M.; Lobstein, T.; Knai, C. The burden of disease attributable to nutrition in Europe. *Public Health Nutr.* **2003**, *6*, 453–461. [CrossRef]
16. Naska, A.; Fouskakis, D.; Oikonomou, E.; Almeida, M.; Berg, M.; Gedrich, K.; Moreiras, O.; Nelson, M.; Trygg, K.; Turrini, A.; et al. Dietary patterns and their socio-demographic determinants in 10 European countries: Data from the DAFNE databank. *Eur. J. Clin. Nutr.* **2006**, *60*, 181–190. [CrossRef]
17. Gibney, M.; Sandstrom, B. A framework for food-based dietary guidelines in the European Union. *Public Health Nutr.* **2000**, *4*, 293–305. [CrossRef]
18. European Food Information Council Food Based Dietary Guidelines in Europe. Available online: www.eufic.org/en/healthy-living/article/food-based-dietary-guidelines-in-europe (accessed on 14 December 2018).
19. Montagnese, C.; Santarpia, L.; Buonifacio, M.; Nardelli, A.; Caldara, A.R.; Silvestri, E.; Contaldo, F.; Pasanisi, F. European food-based dietary guidelines: A comparison and update. *Nutrition* **2015**, *31*, 908–915. [CrossRef]
20. Brown, K.A.; Timotijevic, L.; Barnett, J.; Shepherd, R.; Lähteenmäki, L.; Raats, M.M. A review of consumer awareness, understanding and use of food-based dietary guidelines. *Br. J. Nutr.* **2011**, *106*, 15–26. [CrossRef] [PubMed]
21. Drewnowski, A.; Eichelsdoerfer, P. Can low-income Americans afford a healthy diet? *Nutr. Today* **2010**, *44*, 246–249. [CrossRef] [PubMed]
22. Schönfeldt, H.C.; Hall, N.; Bester, M. Relevance of food-based dietary guidelines to food and nutrition security: A South African perspective. *Nutr. Bull.* **2013**, *38*, 226–235. [CrossRef]
23. Poulain, J.-P. *The Sociology of Food: Eating and the Place of Food in Society*; Bloomsbury: New York, NY, USA; ISBN 9781472586209.
24. Chrysostomou, S.; Andreou, S.N.; Polycarpou, A. Developing a food basket for fulfilling physical and non-physical needs in Cyprus. Is it affordable? *Eur. J. Public Health* **2017**, *27*, 553–558. [CrossRef] [PubMed]

25. Carrillo Álvarez, E.; Cussó-Parcerisas, I.; Riera-Romaní, J. Development of the Spanish Healthy Food Reference Budget for an adequate social participation at the minimum. *Public Health Nutr.* **2016**, *19*. [CrossRef] [PubMed]

26. Goedemé, T.; Storms, B.; Penne, T.; Van den Bosch, K. *Pilot Project for the Development of a Common Methodology on Reference Budgets in Europe. Final Report*; European Commission: Antwerp, Belgium, 2015; ISBN 9789279540912.

27. Deeming, C. The historical development of family budget standards in britafrom the 17th century to the present. *Soc. Policy Adm.* **2010**. [CrossRef]

28. Vranken, J. Using Reference Budgets for Drawing up the Requirements of a Minimum Income Scheme and Assessing Adequacy. Available online: https://ec.europa.eu/social/main.jsp?catId=1024&langId=en&newsId=1392&moreDocuments=yes&tableName=news (accessed on 14 December 2018).

29. Devuyst, K.; Storms, B.; Penne, T. *Methodologische Keuzes Bij De Ontwikkeling Van Referentiebudgetten: Welke Rol Voor Focusgroepen?* Aromede: Antwerp, Belgium, 2014.

30. Onwuegbuzie, A.J.; Dickinson, W.B.; Leech, N.L.; Zoran, A.G. A Qualitative Framework for Collecting and Analyzing Data in Focus Group Research. *Int. J. Qual. Methods* **2009**. [CrossRef]

31. Gezondheidsraad, H. *Maten en Gewichten: Handleiding Voor Een Gestandaardiseerde Kwantificering Van Voedingsmiddelen [Measures and Weights: Manual for Standardized Quantification of Foods]*; Belgische Hoge Gezondheidsraad: Brussels, Belgium, 2005.

32. Atkinson, T.; Guio, A.C.; Marlier, E. Monitoring Social Inclusion in Europe. Available online: https://ec.europa.eu/eurostat/web/income-and-living-conditions/publications/-/asset_publisher/zdEOYZhr9af3/content/KS-05-14-075/3217494?inheritRedirect=false (accessed on 14 December 2018).

33. Storms, B.; Goedemé, T.; Van den Bosch, K.; Penne, T.; Schuerman, N.; Stockman, S. Pilot Project for a Development of a Common Methodology on Reference Budgets in Europe. Review of Current State of Play on Reference Budget Practices at National, Regional and Local Level. Available online: http://www.referencebudgets.eu/ (accessed on 25 July 2014).

34. Sobal, J.; Bisogni, C.A. Constructing food choice decisions. *Ann. Behav. Med.* **2009**, *38*, 37–46. [CrossRef]

35. Leng, G.; Adan, R.A.H.; Belot, M.; Brunstrom, J.M.; de Graaf, K.; Dickson, S.L.; Hare, T.; Maier, S.; Menzies, J.; Preissl, H.; et al. The determinants of food choice. *Proc. Nutr. Soc.* **2017**, *76*, 316–327. [CrossRef]

36. Antentas, J.M.; Vivas, E. Impacto de la crisis en el derecho a una alimentación sana y saludable. *Informe SESPAS 2014. Gac. Sanit.* **2014**, *28*, 58–61. [CrossRef]

37. Darmon, N.; Drewnowski, A. Does social class predict diet quality? *Am. J. Clin. Nutr.* **2008**, *87*, 1107–1117. [CrossRef] [PubMed]

38. Tiwari, A.; Aggarwal, A.; Tang, W.; Drewnowski, A. Cooking at home: A strategy to comply with U.S. Dietary guidelines at no extra cost. *Am. J. Prev. Med.* **2017**, *52*, 616–624. [CrossRef] [PubMed]

39. Cornellis, I.; Vandervoort, B. *Een Hele Dag Lekker en Gezond Eten Voor 5 Euros*; Borgerhoff & Lamberigst: Ghent, Belgium, 2013.

40. Muro, P.; Carrillo-Álvarez, E.; Marzo, T. Empoderar en hábitos saludables a familias vulnerables. In *REPS 2018: Políticas sociales ante horizontes de incertidumbre y desigualdad*; Red Española de Política Social: Zaragoza, Spain, 2018.

41. Carrillo-Álvarez, E.; Boeckx, H.; Penne, T.; Palma, I.; Goedemé, T.; Storms, B. Promoting healthy eating in Europe: A comparison of European countries FBDG. 2019. In press.

42. Sainz García, P.; Carmen Ferrer Svoboda, M.; Sánchez Ruiz, E.; Pedro Sainz García, C. Competencias culinarias y consumo de alimentos procesados o preparados en estudiantes universitarios de barcelona. *Rev. Esp. Salud. Pública* **2016**, *90*, 1–13.

43. Eurostat Eurostat Online Database. Available online: https://ec.europa.eu/eurostat/data/database (accessed on 14 December 2018).

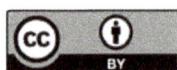

International Journal of
*Environmental Research
and Public Health*

MDPI

Protocol

Protocol for the Development of a Food Stress Index to Identify Households Most at Risk of Food Insecurity in Western Australia

Timothy J. Landrigan *[ID], Deborah A. Kerr[ID], Satvinder S. Dhaliwal and Christina M. Pollard[ID]

School of Public Health, Curtin University, Kent Street, GPO Box U1987, Perth 6845, Australia;
D.Kerr@curtin.edu.au (D.A.K.); S.Dhaliwal@curtin.edu.au (S.S.D.); C.Pollard@curtin.edu.au (C.M.P.)
* Correspondence: timothy.landrigan@postgrad.curtin.edu.au

Received: 7 November 2018; Accepted: 26 December 2018; Published: 29 December 2018

Abstract: Food stress, a similar concept to housing stress, occurs when a household needs to spend more than 25% of their disposable income on food. Households at risk of food stress are vulnerable to food insecurity as a result of inadequate income. A Food Stress Index (FSI) identifies at-risk households, in a particular geographic area, using a range of variables to create a single indicator. Candidate variables were identified using a multi-dimensional framework consisting of household demographics, household income, household expenses, financial stress indicators, food security, food affordability and food availability. The candidate variables were expressed as proportions, of either persons or households, in a geographic area. Principal Component Analysis was used to determine the final variables which resulted in a final set of weighted raw scores. These scores were then scaled to produce the index scores for the Food Stress Index for Western Australia. The results were compared with the Australian Bureau of Statistics' Socio-Economic Indexes for Areas to determine suitability. The Food Stress Index was found to be a suitable indicator of the relative risk of food stress in Western Australian households. The FSI adds specificity to indices of relative disadvantage specifically related to food insecurity and provides a useful tool for prioritising policy and other responses to this important public health issue.

Keywords: food insecurity; food stress; food affordability

1. Introduction

The different Socio-Economic Indexes for Areas (SEIFA) developed by the Australian Bureau of Statistics (ABS) measure various aspects of socio-economic status. The four different indexes measure relative socio-economic disadvantage (IRSD), relative socio-economic advantage or disadvantage (IRSAD), education and occupation (IEO), and economic resources (IER) [1], however, none of those indexes provide a suitable measure of food insecurity or food stress. The variables used in constructing these indexes are wider socio-economic measures and don't relate specifically to food insecurity. In order to measure food insecurity, these indexes need to be used in conjunction with other data such as food costs to provide an indication of the impact of socio-economic status and food costs on health [2–6].

The concept of a Food Stress Index (FSI) is to provide a simple indication of the potential for food stress of households in a particular geographic location which may be postcode, Statistical Area, Local Government Area or another region. It is a single index that encompasses all aspects of food insecurity to provide information about the likelihood households in a geographic area are suffering food stress.

Housing stress is usually defined as occurring for those households who spend more than 30% of their income on housing costs, whether that is rent or mortgage [7]. This is particularly critical for those households whose income is in the 1st or 2nd quintile. Housing affordability relates to a household's or a person's ability to pay for their housing. The impacts of housing stress are widespread as this impacts a household's spending patterns and has wider effects on the economy as a whole.

Food stress is a similar concept to housing stress and occurs when a household needs to spend more than 25% of their disposable income on food [8]. Australian research has shown that welfare-dependent and low-income households are suffering food stress [9–11]. Between 2008 and 2012, this food inequality has risen in Australia [12].

Households at risk of food stress are vulnerable to food insecurity as a result of inadequate income. Food security is "when all people, at all times, have physical and economic access to sufficient, safe and nutritious food to meet their dietary needs and food preferences for an active and healthy life." [13]. The 2011–2012 Australian Health Survey (AHS) found that four per cent of all Australian households 'ran out of food in the last 12 months and couldn't afford to buy more', increasing to seven per cent of households in the most disadvantaged areas, compared to only one per cent in the least disadvantaged areas. The prevalence was higher among Aboriginal and Torres Strait Islander households with 22% overall and 31% of those households in remote areas running out of food in the previous year [14]. Research looking at the relationship between food security status and multiple socio-demographic variables found that 36% of survey participants had low or very low food security [15].

The United States Department of Agriculture has a Food Security Survey Module (FSSM) [16,17] that is run every two years to measure levels of food security in the United States. In Australia the only routine food security measure is the single-item question on the AHS which does not effectively measure levels of food insecurity [18]. There is no measure, equivalent to the USDA FSSM, that allows routine monitoring of the prevalence of food insecurity at a population level in Australia with the only research to date being undertaken in small geographic areas using small samples [15,18].

Food affordability is defined as the amount of money a household spends on food, relative to income of that household. It is of greater concern for lower income households as they spend a greater proportion of their income on food [19]. Food affordability impacts not only the wider economy through the impacts on spending patterns, but also on health by affecting the ability to purchase healthy and nutritious food [20,21]. While some household expenses are fixed (e.g., rent or utility expenses), the food budget is changeable and can be cut back if needed with nutrition consequences [22]. If one household expense increases (e.g., an increase in rent) then this will impact on that household's food affordability leading to additional stress on the food budget; i.e., food stress. As a household becomes food stressed, they become vulnerable to food insecurity as they have less available income to meet their dietary needs.

The Food Stress Index is designed as a single measure, using currently available data without the need for additional and expensive surveillance, that ranks geographic areas based on the likelihood that households in those areas are food stressed. The FSI is not a measure of food insecurity as not every household in geographic areas at high risk of food stress would be food insecure; the FSI shows particular geographic areas where households would be more vulnerable to food insecurity. A FSI could be used to measure the impact food affordability has on chronic disease such as diabetes and cardiovascular disease. It could also be used to highlight areas or households in need of food relief.

2. Materials and Methods

2.1. Developing a Food Stress Index

The methodology used to create the Food Stress Index is similar methodology to that used to develop the Australian Bureau of Statistics' SEIFA [1] index. The FSI is a weighted combination of select variables that results in a score that can be used to rank areas according to the likelihood of food stress in each area. The index is assigned to areas and reflects the characteristics of the households of people living in an area.

Starting with a broad list of potential or candidate variables covering all aspects of food stress and socio-economic indicators, Principal Component Analysis [23] was used to reduce these variables to a single index which indicates the likelihood households in the selected geographic area are suffering food stress. Low index scores indicate less likelihood of food stress while high index scores indicate more likelihood of food stress. The methodology is discussed in detail below.

2.2. The List of Candidate Variables

In order to encapsulate various aspects of food affordability and food stress a wide range of candidate variables were considered when constructing the Food Stress Index. This resulted in an initial set of over 50 candidate variables from eight different datasets from existing surveys. The framework for the selection of variables was based around the following dimensions:

- Household demographics
- Household income
- Household expenses
- Financial stress
- Food affordability
- Geographic information.

Table 1 outlines the dimensions and candidate variables that were considered when developing the index. At this stage, no consideration was made to the availability of the data, only what variables ideally would be suitable when constructing a Food Stress Index. Final decisions on the availability and suitability of the candidate variables were made in the next step.

Table 1. Candidate variables for a Food Stress Index.

Dimensions	Description of Measure	Description of Candidate Variables	Data Source
Household demographics	Proportion households by family composition	Couple families with children under 15 Single parent families with children under 15 Couple families with no children under 15 Single parent families with no children under 15	ABS: 2016 Census, Datapacks, General Community Profile, Western Australia [24]
Aboriginal and Torres Strait Islander Peoples	Proportion of Aboriginal and Torres Strait Islander households	Indigenous status	ABS: 2016 Census, Datapacks, General Community Profile, Western Australia [24]
Household income	Income quintiles of household	Proportion of households in the lowest income quintile Proportion of households in the highest income quintile	ABS: 2016 Census, Tablebuilder, Counting Persons, Place of Enumeration, Equivalised Total Household Income (weekly) [24]
Household expenses	Proportion of income used for household expenses (excluding food)	Housing costs (rent/mortgage) Transport Utilities Education	ABS: Household Expenditure Survey [25]
Financial stress indicators	A measure of whether households may be experiencing economic hardship, based on how many of the financial stress indicators a household experiences.	Financial stress experiences (e.g., unable to raise funds for an emergency, unable to pay bills on time) Missing out experiences (e.g., could not afford a holiday for at least a week, could not afford a special meal once a week)	ABS: Household Expenditure Survey [25]
Food affordability and access	Food affordability for the household. Access to food for the household.	Proportion of income required to purchase a healthy meal plan. Number of supermarkets within geographic area as an indication of access to affordable food.	2013 Food Access and Cost Survey [26]

The initial set of candidate variables was reduced before constructing the final index. When reducing the variables to a more manageable set, consideration was made of the suitability of each variable, and the potential to match variables by the selected geography, in this case the ABS' geographic classification of Statistical Area 2. This meant that variables that were not available on the same geographic basis for the respective households were not considered further. It is anticipated that the index will be regularly updated, and it was important that data was available from within the last five years to maintain relevance. Census data met both of these considerations and was the preferred source of data. In the case of the Food Access and Cost Survey (FACS) [26], the most recent data was from 2013 and the 2016 Census of Population and Housing [24] was used for all other variables.

From the list of variables in Table 1, household expense variables and financial stress indicators weren't available within the five-year period, or at the desired geography for this work. The sources for these variables are irregular surveys run by the ABS; as a result these variables were excluded from the Food Stress Index.

2.3. Description of Variables Used

The variables relate to persons, families or households and were expressed as a proportion of units in an area with the specified characteristic. Each of the dimensions is discussed below.

2.3.1. Household Demographics

Household composition, including family size, the number of parents and the age of any children provides a good indicator of household size, income and expenses. A single parent household with children under the age of 15 will have more difficulty earning income and meeting weekly expenses as they are generally able to only work on a part-time or casual basis due to child care commitments [27]. Single parent households also have to spend a greater proportion of their income to purchase a healthy meal plan [19].

The 2016 Australian Census shows that 45% of families were families with two parents and children while 38% of families were couples without children, and 16% were single parent families [24]. Using this information, the variables selected to demonstrate most, and least likelihood of food stress are the proportions of single parent or two parent households, with or without children under 15, within the selected geographic area.

2.3.2. Indigenous Status

The Indigenous status of a household provides a strong indicator of whether or not that household is likely to suffer from food stress. There are high unemployment rates and low income among Aboriginal and Torres Strait Islander peoples as well as significant disparities in health status between Aboriginal and Torres Strait Islander peoples and other Australians [28]. The proportion of Indigenous households from the 2016 Census was used.

2.3.3. Household Income

Income is an important indicator of the likelihood of food stress with households in the lowest income quintiles needing to spend a higher proportion of the income on food than those households in the highest income quintiles [19]. The income variable used was the Equivalised Total Household Income variable from the 2016 Census. Equivalised household income is household income which has been adjusted by an 'equivalence scale' based on the number of adults and children in the household [1].

Low income was defined as the proportion of households in the first quintile of the equivalised household income distribution; i.e., those households earning between $1 and $25,999 per year. These households represent those most likely to suffer food stress. The households least likely to suffer food stress were defined as those in the top income quintile, earning more than $78,000 per year.

2.3.4. Food Affordability

Food costs, as measured by the proportion of income required to purchase a healthy meal plan for a household, vary depending on the income of the household. Households that need to spend more than 25% of their income on food are suffering food stress [8] and the proportion of income required provides the strongest indicator of food stress.

Data from the 2013 FACS [26] was used to estimate food affordability; i.e., the proportion of income required to purchase a healthy meal plan for households of different compositions and incomes.

2.3.5. Geographic Information

Most of the data was taken from ABS datasets so each of the variables was available on ABS geography and Statistical Area 2 (SA2) was used as the base geography. Data from the FACS was also available by SA2s. Various SA2s were excluded from the list of SA2s because of the type of area (e.g., national parks, airports and industrial areas) or there was insufficient data (i.e., two or more variables unavailable). When the invalid areas were removed, 228 SA2s remained of the 253 SA2s in Western Australia. Data from the 2013 FACS was only available for 76 SA2s so the Food Stress Index was created for these SA2s.

2.4. Reduced Set of Variables

The final set of 13 variables selected is shown in Table 2.

Table 2. Reduced set of variables used to construct the Food Stress Index.

Dimensions	Description
Household demographics	Proportion of couple families with no children under 15 Proportion of couple families with children under 15 Proportion of one parent families with no children under 15 Proportion of one parent families with children under 15
Aboriginal and Torres Strait Islander Peoples	Proportion of Aboriginal and Torres Strait Islander households
Household income	Proportion of households in the lowest equivalised household income quintile (i.e., less than $500 per week) Proportion of households in the highest equivalised household income quintile (i.e., more than $1499 per week)
Food affordability	Proportion of income required to buy healthy food–couple family on welfare income Proportion of income required to buy healthy food–couple family on low income Proportion of income required to buy healthy food–couple family on average income Proportion of income required to buy healthy food–one parent family on welfare income Proportion of income required to buy healthy food–one parent family on low income Proportion of income required to buy healthy food–one parent family on average income

Once the initial variables were identified, Principal Component Analysis (PCA) [23] was used to create the Food Stress Index. The PCA technique summarises a number of correlated variables into a set of new uncorrelated components to allow for easier analysis. By removing correlated variables, the technique reduces the number of variables to a set that summarises the information and enables easier analysis. The PCA process results in a set of weighted raw scores that can then be scaled to produce the index scores for the Food Stress Index.

2.4.1. Create Proportions for the List of Initial Variables

Each variable was created as a proportion of units within the selected geography. For household composition, this was the proportion of families within the area. For the household income and Indigenous status variables, the proportion of households was used. For the food affordability variables, the proportion of income was used.

Each variable was then standardised to a mean of 0 and a standard deviation of 1 using R [29].

2.4.2. Create Correlation Matrix

The correlation matrix was calculated, and highly correlated variables were removed to avoid over-representation of food stress. When two variables measuring conceptually similar aspects of food affordability or food stress had a correlation coefficient of 0.8 in absolute value, one of them was removed.

2.4.3. Conduct Initial PCA

Next, Principal Component Analysis was conducted on the reduced set of variables to obtain the loadings for each variable on the first principal component. Any variables with resulting loadings less than 0.3 were removed on the grounds they were not strong enough to indicate food stress. The PCA step was then repeated until there were no variables with loadings less than 0.3 in absolute value. This resulted in a reduced set of variables, with at least one variable in each of the dimensions covering the food stress and food affordability measures.

2.5. Calculate and Scale the Index

Once there was a reduced set of variables, the final step was to calculate the final index. For each SA2, each standardised variable was multiplied by its weight, then summed across all variables. The weight was obtained by dividing the loading for each variable by the square root of the eigenvalue. In order to ensure that low scores indicate least likely to suffer food stress, and high scores indicate most likely to suffer food stress, the sign (positive or negative) for each indicator was set accordingly. That is, indicators of high food stress were given positive signs and indicators of low food stress were given negative signs.

This resulted in scores for each SA2. See the formula below.

$$Z_{SA2} = \sum_{j=1}^{p} \frac{L_j}{\sqrt{\lambda}} \times v_{j,SA2}$$

where

Z_{SA2} = raw score for the SA2
$v_{j,SA2}$ = standardised variable of the j-th variable for the SA2
L_j = loading for the j-th variable
λ = eigenvalue of the principal component
p = total number of variables in the index

To create a meaningful index, the scores were scaled with a mean of 1000 and standard deviation of 100 to create a new set of scores ranking the SA2s in order from least likely to suffer food stress to most likely to suffer food stress.

3. Results

The Food Stress Index was created for 76 SA2s in Western Australia. The scores ranged from 873.5 for North Perth (which is in the most advantaged SEIFA quintile), to 1400.4 for Halls Creek (in the most disadvantaged SEIFA quintile). This meant that households in the inner Perth suburb of North Perth are the least likely to suffer food stress in Western Australia and households in the remote north-west town of Halls Creek are most likely to suffer food stress. Table 3 shows the SA2s in each quintile of the Food Stress Index.

Table 3. Food Stress Index for Statistical Areas in Western Australia by quintile, ranging from 1 (least likelihood of food stress) to 5 (most likelihood of food stress).

Food Stress Index Quintile	Western Australia Statistical Areas
1	Applecross—Ardross, Ashburton, Baldivis, Booragoon, Greenwood—Warwick, Innaloo—Doubleview, Karratha, Mount Hawthorn—Leederville, Murdoch—Kardinya, Newman, North Perth, Ocean Reef, Subiaco—Shenton Park, Success—Hammond Park, Wembley—West Leederville—Glendalough, Wembley Downs—Churchlands—Woodlands
2	Australind—Leschenault, Belmont—Ascot—Redcliffe, Bentley—Wilson—St James, Byford, Carramar, Coolbellup, Craigie—Beldon, Eaton—Pelican Point, Esperance Region, Kalgoorlie, Margaret River, Murray, Rivervale—Kewdale—Cloverdale, South Bunbury—Bunbury, Thornlie
3	Albany, Augusta, Busselton, Capel, Denmark, East Bunbury—Glen Iris, Esperance, Geraldton—North, Gingin—Dandaragan, Gnowangerup, Harvey, Maddington—Orange Grove—Martin, Manjimup, Pinjarra, Rockingham
4	Alexander Heights—Koondoola, Beckenham—Kenwick—Langford, Bridgetown—Boyup Brook, Broome, Dowerin, Exmouth, Kambalda—Coolgardie—Norseman, Kulin, Merredin, Moora, Mukinbudin, Narrogin, Northam, Pemberton, Roebourne
5	Armadale—Wungong—Brookdale, Calista, Carnarvon, Cooloongup, Derby—West Kimberley, East Pilbara, Geraldton, Girrawheen, Gosnells, Halls Creek, Kununurra, Leinster—Leonora, Meekatharra, Parmelia—Orelia, Plantagenet, Roebuck

The Food Stress Index scores were compared with SEIFA Index of Relative Socio-economic Advantage and Disadvantage (IRSAD) for consistency. For example, the IRSAD for Mt Hawthorn/Leederville falls in the tenth decile, meaning persons living there are most advantaged. This aligns well with the Food Stress Index for Mt Hawthorn/Leederville which falls in the first decile, meaning persons living there have the least likelihood of food stress. To test the suitability of the FSI, a Spearman's correlation was run to determine the relationship between the Food Stress Index and the IRSAD index. There was a strong, negative correlation with the IRSAD index ($r = -0.89$, $p < 0.001$).

4. Discussion

The Food Stress Index provides a measure of the likelihood that households in a geographic area are vulnerable to food stress. When applied to Statistical Area 2 (SA2), households in the more remote areas of Western Australia are most likely to suffer food stress (e.g., East Pilbara, Halls Creek, Kununurra). Households in Perth metropolitan areas are least likely to suffer from food stress (e.g., North Perth, Mount Hawthorn and Ocean Reef). The FSI provides more information on food security than the widely used SEIFA which measures socioeconomic status. For example, although Ashburton is in a remote part of Western Australia and is in the third quintile for SEIFA, the FSI takes into account the high proportion of households in Ashburton that are in the highest income quintile and the low proportion of single parent families, resulting in a low Food Stress Index. Similarly, within the Perth metropolitan area, households in Girrawheen, are more likely to suffer food stress due the high proportion of households in the lowest income quintile and the high proportion of Indigenous households.

One of the limitations of this research was that some of the candidate variables (i.e., household expense and financial stress data) were not available at the required level of detail when the analysis was undertaken. Although this data wasn't included it was still possible to construct a suitable index with the available data. Further research is planned to determine the implications of including this data if it becomes available.

5. Conclusions

The Food Stress Index, the first of its kind in Australia, is a suitable indicator of the risk of food stress in Western Australian households. It incorporates a range of variables to measure food stress including food costs, household composition and household incomes. Further research is needed to develop the FSI methodology for smaller geographic areas such as Statistical Area 1 (SA1) to be more representative of households. Population weighted averages of the SA1s would be used to construct indexes for larger geographies. The FSI could be applied to all Australian households, providing a useful tool for national food security. The FSI can be used for to highlight areas where households are more likely to be food stressed and more vulnerable to food insecurity. Policy and intervention planning can then better target services to where they are needed.

Author Contributions: T.J.L. conceived the study and undertook the analysis. T.J.L. and C.M.P. authored the original manuscript. All authors read and approved the final manuscript. T.J.L. undertook this work as part of his Doctor of Philosophy.

Funding: This research received no external funding.

Acknowledgments: T.J.L. is supported through an Australian Government Research Training Program Scholarship.

Conflicts of Interest: The authors declare no conflict of interest.

References

1. ABS. Census of Population and Housing: Socio-Economic Indexes for Areas (SEIFA). Available online: http://www.abs.gov.au/websitedbs/censushome.nsf/home/seifa (accessed on 18 June 2018).
2. Backholer, K.; Spencer, E.; Gearon, E.; Magliano, D.J.; McNaughton, S.A.; Shaw, J.E.; Peeters, A. The association between socio-economic position and diet quality in Australian adults. *Public Health Nutr.* **2016**, *19*, 477–485. [CrossRef] [PubMed]
3. Barosh, L.; Friel, S.; Engelhardt, K.; Chan, L. The cost of a healthy and sustainable diet—Who can afford it? *Aust. N. Z. J. Public Health* **2014**, *38*, 7–12. [CrossRef] [PubMed]
4. Brimblecombe, J.; Ferguson, M.; Liberato, S.C.; Ball, K.; Moodie, M.L.; Magnus, A.; Miles, E.; Leach, A.J.; Chatfield, M.D.; Ni Mhurchu, C.; et al. Stores Healthy Options Project in Remote Indigenous Communities (SHOP@RIC): A protocol of a randomised trial promoting healthy food and beverage purchases through price discounts and in-store nutrition education. *BMC Public Health* **2013**, *13*, 744. [CrossRef] [PubMed]
5. Godrich, S.; Lo, J.; Davies, C.; Darby, J.; Devine, A. Prevalence and socio-demographic predictors of food insecurity among regional and remote Western Australian children. *Aust. N. Z. J. Public Health* **2017**, *41*, 585–590. [CrossRef] [PubMed]
6. Palermo, C.; McCartan, J.; Kleve, S.; Sinha, K.; Shiell, A. A longitudinal study of the cost of food in Victoria influenced by geography and nutritional quality. *Aust. N. Z. J. Public Health* **2016**, *40*, 270–273. [CrossRef] [PubMed]
7. Yates, J.; Gabriel, M. *Housing Affordability in Australia*; Australian Housing and Urban Research Institute: Melbourne, Australia, 2006.
8. Ward, P.R.; Coveney, J.; Verity, F.; Carter, P.; Schilling, M. Cost and affordability of healthy food in rural South Australia. *Rural Remote Health* **2012**, *12*, 1938. [PubMed]
9. Ward, P.R.; Verity, F.; Carter, P.; Tsourtos, G.; Coveney, J.; Wong, K.C. Food stress in Adelaide: The relationship between low income and the affordability of healthy food. *J. Environ. Public Health* **2013**, *2013*, 968078. [CrossRef] [PubMed]
10. Williams, P.; Hull, A.; Kontos, M. Trends in affordability of the Illawarra healthy food basket 2000–2007. *Nutr. Diet.* **2009**, *66*, 27–32. [CrossRef]
11. Wong, K.C.; Coveney, J.; Ward, P.; Muller, R.; Carter, P.; Verity, F.; Tsourtos, G. Availability, affordability and quality of a healthy food basket in Adelaide, South Australia. *Nutr. Diet.* **2011**, *68*, 8–14. [CrossRef]
12. Pollard, C.; Begley, A.; Landrigan, T. The Rise of Food Inequality in Australia. In *Food Poverty and Insecurity: International Food Inequalities*; Caraher, M., Coveney, J., Eds.; Springer International Publishing: Cham, Switzerland, 2016; pp. 89–103.
13. FAO. Rome Declaration on World Food Security. 1996. Available online: http://www.fao.org/docrep/003/w3613e/w3613e00.htm (accessed on 13 September 2018).
14. ABS. Australian Aboriginal and Torres Strait Islander Health Survey: Nutrition Results—Food and Nutrients. Available online: http://www.abs.gov.au/AUSSTATS/abs@.nsf/Lookup/4727.0.55.005Main+Features12012-13?OpenDocument (accessed on 14 March 2018).

15. Butcher, L.M.; O'Sullivan, T.A.; Ryan, M.M.; Lo, J.; Devine, A. Utilising a multi-item questionnaire to assess household food security in Australia. *Health Promot. J. Austr.* **2018**. [CrossRef] [PubMed]

16. Bickel, G.; Nord, M.; Price, C.; Hamilton, W.; Cook, J. *Guide to Measuring Household Food Security, Revised 2000*; U.S. Department of Agriculture, Food and Nutrition Service: Alexandria, VA, USA, 2000.

17. Coleman-Jensen, A.; Rabbitt, M.P.; Gregory, C.A.; Singh, A. *Household Food Security in the United States, 2017*; ERR-256; U.S. Department of Agriculture, Economic Research Service: Alexandria, VA, USA, 2018.

18. McKechnie, R.; Turrell, G.; Giskes, K.; Gallegos, D. Single-item measure of food insecurity used in the National Health Survey may underestimate prevalence in Australia. *Aust. N. Z. J. Public Health* **2018**, *42*, 389–395. [CrossRef] [PubMed]

19. Landrigan, T.J.; Kerr, D.A.; Dhaliwal, S.S.; Savage, V.; Pollard, C.M. Removing the Australian tax exemption on healthy food adds food stress to families vulnerable to poor nutrition. *Aust. N. Z. J. Public Health* **2017**, *41*, 591–597. [CrossRef] [PubMed]

20. Booth, S.; Smith, A. Food security and poverty in Australia-challenges for dietitians. *Aust. J. Nutr. Diet.* **2001**, *58*, 150–156.

21. Lee, A.; Mhurchu, C.N.; Sacks, G.; Swinburn, B.; Snowdon, W.; Vandevijvere, S.; Hawkes, C.; L'Abbé, M.; Rayner, M.; Sanders, D.; et al. Monitoring the price and affordability of foods and diets globally. *Obes. Rev.* **2013**, *14*, 82–95. [CrossRef] [PubMed]

22. Lloyd, S.; Lawton, J.; Caraher, M.; Singh, G.; Horsley, K.; Mussa, F. A tale of two localities. *Health Educ. J.* **2010**, *70*, 48–56. [CrossRef]

23. Joliffe, I.T. *Principal Component Analysis*, 2nd ed.; Springer: New York, NY, USA, 2002.

24. ABS. Census of Population and Housing. Available online: http://www.abs.gov.au/websitedbs/censushome.nsf/home/data?opendocument#from-banner=LN (accessed on 31 May 2018).

25. ABS. Household Expenditure Survey, Australia. Available online: http://www.abs.gov.au/AUSSTATS/abs@.nsf/mf/6530.0 (accessed on 22 May 2018).

26. Pollard, C.; Savage, V.; Landrigan, T.J.; Hanbury, A.; Kerr, D.A. Food Access and Cost Survey Western Australia. 2013. Available online: https://ww2.health.wa.gov.au/~{}/media/Files/Corporate/Reports%20and%20publications/Chronic%20Disease/Food-Access-and-Cost-Survey-Report-2013-Report.pdf (accessed on 13 September 2018).

27. Western Australian Council of Social Service Inc. *2017 Cost of Living Report*; Western Australian Council of Social Service Inc.: West Perth, Australia, 2017.

28. AHMAC. *Aboriginal and Torres Strait Islander Health Performance Framework Report 2006*; AHMAC: Canberra, Australia, 2006.

29. R Core Team. *R: A Language and Environment for Statistical Computing*; R Foundation for Statistical Computing: Vienna, Austria, 2014.

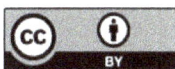

International Journal of
*Environmental Research
and Public Health*

MDPI

Article

Testing the Price of Healthy and Current Diets in Remote Aboriginal Communities to Improve Food Security: Development of the Aboriginal and Torres Strait Islander Healthy Diets ASAP (Australian Standardised Affordability and Pricing) Methods

Amanda Lee [1,2,*] and Meron Lewis [1]

[1] School of Public Health, Faculty of Medicine, The University of Queensland, Herston, Queensland 4006, Australia; m.lewis@uq.edu.au
[2] The Australian Prevention Partnership Centre, The Sax Institute, Ultimo 2007, New South Wales, Australia
*   Correspondence: amanda.lee@uq.edu.au; Tel.: +61-0-412-975-197

Received: 8 November 2018; Accepted: 18 December 2018; Published: 19 December 2018

Abstract: Aboriginal and Torres Strait Islander peoples suffer higher rates of food insecurity and diet-related disease than other Australians. However, assessment of food insecurity in specific population groups is sub-optimal, as in many developed countries. This study tailors the Healthy Diets ASAP (Australian Standardised Affordability and Pricing) methods protocol to be more relevant to Indigenous groups in assessing one important component of food security. The resultant Aboriginal and Torres Strait Islander Healthy Diets ASAP methods were used to assess the price, price differential, and affordability of healthy (recommended) and current (unhealthy) diets in five remote Aboriginal communities. The results show that the tailored approach is more sensitive than the original protocol in revealing the high degree of food insecurity in these communities, where the current diet costs nearly 50% of disposable household income compared to the international benchmark of 30%. Sixty-two percent of the current food budget appears to be spent on discretionary foods and drinks. Aided by community store pricing policies, healthy (recommended) diets are around 20% more affordable than current diets in these communities, but at 38.7% of disposable household income still unaffordable for most households. Further studies in urban communities, and on other socioeconomic, political and commercial determinants of food security in Aboriginal and Torres Strait Islander communities appear warranted. The development of the tailored method provides an example of how national tools can be adapted to better inform policy actions to improve food security and help reduce rates of diet-related chronic disease more equitably in developed countries.

Keywords: food security; diet price; food price; affordability; food policy; nutrition policy; fiscal policy; obesity prevention; non-communicable disease; monitoring and surveillance; INFORMAS

1. Introduction

1.1. Background

Poor diet is now the major preventable risk factor contributing to the burden of disease globally [1]. In Australia, Aboriginal and Torres Strait Islander peoples suffer the poorest health of all population groups and have a lower life expectancy [2]. At least 75% of the mortality gap between Aboriginal and Torres Strait Islanders and other Australians is attributed to diet-related chronic diseases such as cardiovascular disease, chronic kidney disease, and type 2 diabetes [3]. Malnutrition is a major problem in Aboriginal and Torres Strait Islander communities. This includes both over-nutrition, particularly the consumption of too many 'discretionary' food and drinks (those not necessary for health, that are high in saturated fat, added sugar, salt and/or alcohol), and under-nutrition, particularly dietary deficiencies related to inadequate intake of healthy foods in the five food groups and unsaturated spreads and oils allowance, as recommended by the Australian Dietary Guidelines [3,4]. Forty-one percent of the energy intake reported by Aboriginal and Torres Strait Islanders in the Australian Health Survey (AHS) 2011–2013 was derived from 'discretionary' food and drinks [5]. This was higher than reported by non-Indigenous Australians, for whom 35% of the energy intake of adults and 39% of the energy intake of children was derived from discretionary choices [6].

Few Australians (<4%) consume diets consistent with the Australian Dietary Guidelines (ADGs) [4,7]. The contribution of poor diets to the rising rates of overweight and obesity associated with chronic disease is of particular concern. Twenty-five percent of all Australian children aged two to 17 years and 63% of Australian adults aged 18 years and over are overweight or obese [8]. These proportions are even higher for Aboriginal and Torres Strait Islander groups, with 30% of children aged two to 17 years and 66% of adults being overweight or obese [3]. Nutrition policy actions are needed urgently to improve the current diet of the whole Australian population and particularly of Aboriginal and Torres Strait Islander groups.

Good nutrition is underscored by food security. This is when "all people, at all times, have physical, social and economic access to sufficient, safe and nutritious food that meets their dietary needs and food preferences for an active and healthy life" [9]. Food security has been deemed to be a fundamental human right [10]. The Universal Declaration of Human Rights affirms that "everyone has the right to a standard of living adequate for the health and well-being of himself and of his family, including food" [11]. The right to adequate food has been seen as "a right of people to be given a fair opportunity to feed themselves, now and in the future" [12] rather than a right to be fed. In this way, food security is impacted by the availability, accessibility, affordability and acceptability (appropriateness) of the food supply. The experience of these determinants of food security can vary greatly amongst different groups of the population in developed economies like Australia [3,4].

One specific barrier to food security in Australia is believed to be the relative expense of healthy foods. This is particularly the case, among low socioeconomic groups [13–17] in which Aboriginal and Torres Strait Islanders are over-represented. More than one in five Aboriginal and Torres Strait Islanders reported living in a household that had run out of food in the past year and had not been able to afford to buy more in 2011–2013 [18]. This proportion was much higher than in the non-Indigenous population (3.7%) [6]. The affordability of healthy food is believed to be a key aspect of the inequitable distribution of household food security in developed economies such as Australia [13] and a major challenge to food security in remote Aboriginal and Torres Strait Islander communities particularly [3,19]. For over twenty years food prices have been shown consistently to be around 30% higher in remote Aboriginal and Torres Strait Islander communities than in urban centres [20], yet median household incomes are lower in remote areas than in urban areas [3].

However, past food price surveys in Australia have applied a wide variety of 'food basket' costing tools and methods [20] and results are not comparable across different locations or times due to dissimilarity of metrics in the different approaches [20]. These include: number and type of foods surveyed; application of availability and/or quality measures; definition of reference households; estimated household income calculation methods; food store sampling frameworks; data collection methods; and analysis [20]. Until recently, standardised methods to assess and compare the price and affordability of healthy diets with currently consumed, unhealthy diets were lacking in Australia [20] and globally [21]. Such methods are essential to provide robust, meaningful data to inform health and fiscal policy actions, for example, decisions around exemption of basic, healthy foods from Goods and Services Tax (GST) and introduction of health levies on sugary drinks [17,22].

The Healthy Diets ASAP methods protocol was developed to assess, compare and monitor the price and affordability of healthy and current diets among the general population in Australia [22,23]. The method was based on the 'optimal' approach to monitor food price and affordability globally proposed by the International Network for Food and Obesity/non-communicable Diseases Research, Monitoring and Action Support (INFORMAS) [21]. Surprisingly, testing of the Healthy Diets ASAP methods protocol demonstrated that the price of healthy diets recommended by the Australian Dietary Guidelines were 12–15% less expensive than reported current (unhealthy) diets in Australia [22,24]. The results also suggested that Australians were spending 49–64% of their household food budget on discretionary foods and drinks [22,24].

In addition to application at international and national levels, the 'optimal' approach of the INFORMAS diet price and affordability framework [21] has the potential to be modified for use in specific populations and localities. This allows for comparison of diet price and affordability in specific population groups and locations with that of the general population, to inform the development of targeted health and fiscal policies. For example, in Australia, the Healthy Diets ASAP approach has been applied in country Victoria, as reported elsewhere in this special edition [25]. As another example, the INFORMAS 'optimal' approach to assessing diet price and affordability has been tailored to different population groups in New Zealand [26]; results showed that a healthy diet would be more affordable than the current diet for both the total New Zealand population (3.5% difference) and Pacific households (4.5% difference) but the cost of both diets would be similar for Māori households (0.57% difference). However, while previous surveys have used market baskets to estimate the price of 'healthy' basic foods in remote Aboriginal and Torres Strait Island communities [3,20,27], the 'optimal' approach in the INFORMAS step-wise framework to monitor food price data [20] had not been adapted for use in Aboriginal and Torres Strait Islander groups in Australia to enable generation of policy-relevant data.

1.2. The Healthy Diets ASAP Methods Protocol

The Healthy Diets ASAP methods protocol for application with the Australian population as a whole has been reported in detail elsewhere [23]. The protocol consists of five parts; (i) construction of the healthy (recommended) and current (unhealthy) diet pricing tools, (ii) calculation of both median and low-income household incomes; (iii) store location and sampling, (iv) price data collection, and (v) analysis and reporting. To modify the protocol for Aboriginal and Torres Strait Islander groups only the first and second parts of the protocol required adjustment. The remaining three parts of the protocol were retained exactly to optimise comparability of results.

Part one of the Healthy Diets ASAP methods protocol covers the development of two diet pricing survey tools. These are the current (unhealthy) diet pricing tool and the healthy (recommended) diet pricing tool. The current (unhealthy) diet pricing tool comprises the mean fortnightly intake of specific foods and drinks reported in the AHS 2011–2013, expressed in grams or millilitres, by each age/gender group corresponding to the four individuals comprising a reference household (an adult male 31–50 years old, an adult female 31–50 years old, a 14-year-old boy and an eight-year-old girl) in the AHS 2011–2013 [28]. The amounts of foods and drinks consumed per day were derived from the AHS 2011–2013 Confidentialised Unit Record Files (CURFs) of reported dietary intake at 5-digit code level [28]. The mean reported daily dietary intakes for the four individuals were multiplied by 14 to produce the quantities consumed per household per fortnight. The healthy (recommended) diet pricing tool reflects the types and amounts of corresponding foods and drinks for the reference household for a fortnight consistent with the ADGs [4]. In both diet pricing tools, an allowance for edible portion foods/as cooked, as specified in AUSNUT 2011-13 [28], was included; however, post-plate wastage was not estimated or included.

In the second part of the Healthy Diets ASAP methods protocol pertaining to household income, median household income is sourced from national Australian census data which provide a total (gross) amount per household per week (i.e. before taxation). To estimate household income at time points between the five-yearly census, national wage price indexes (published quarterly) are applied [29].

The indicative low (minimum) income for the household is calculated from minimum wage and welfare payments provided by the Department of Human Services [30,31]. A set of assumptions relating to employment, housing type, education attendance, disability status, savings and investments and children's immunisation status are used to determine the appropriate welfare payments and taxation payable. As taxation payable is included, the indicative low (minimum) income is considered disposable income.

Affordability of the healthy and current diets for the reference household is determined by comparing the cost of each diet with the median (gross) household income and with the indicative low (minimum) disposable income of low income households per fortnight. Internationally, a benchmark of 30% of income has been used as a cut-off point to indicate affordability of a diet [16,21].

1.3. Aim

The aim of this study was to modify and test the Healthy Diets ASAP methods protocol to be more relevant to the Aboriginal and Torres Strait Islander population. It developed methods and tools to assist others to apply the approach in order to compare the price, price differential and affordability of healthy (recommended) and current (unhealthy) diets of Aboriginal and Torres Strait Islanders living in different locations with other population groups in Australia.

2. Methods

2.1. Development of the Aboriginal and Torres Strait Islander Healthy Diets ASAP Methods

It was not necessary to amend the Healthy Diets ASAP healthy (recommended) diet pricing tool to adapt the Healthy Diets ASAP methods protocol for application with Aboriginal and Torres Strait Islander groups as the Australian Dietary Guidelines already include culturally-appropriate and commonly available food and drink options and are similar at broad food group level for both Aboriginal and Torres Strait Islanders and non-Indigenous people [4].

However, the Healthy Diets ASAP current (unhealthy) diet pricing tool required modification to reflect the mean intake of each relevant Aboriginal and Torres Strait Islander age and gender group in the National Aboriginal and Torres Strait Islander Nutrition and Physical Activity Survey component of the AHS 2011–2013 [5]. This was compared with the mean dietary intake of each relevant age and gender group of the whole Australian population reported in the AHS 2011–2013 [5,6] to calculate a reported consumption ratio for each food group or, where data were available, for component food and drinks in each food group. This ratio was applied to derive estimates of the current dietary intake of all foods and drinks included in the current diet pricing tool in Aboriginal and Torres Strait Islander groups.

In relation to assessment of household income, it was not necessary to adapt the Healthy Diets ASAP methods protocol to determine the median (gross) household income in Aboriginal and Torres Strait Islander communities in remote areas as census data is reported for relevant Statistical Areas (SA2).

However, assumptions regarding characteristics of the household members were reviewed in relation to any welfare and taxation policies specific to Aboriginal and Torres Strait Islander people and/or to those people living in remote locations in order to better reflect Aboriginal and Torres Strait Islander households living in remote areas for the calculation of indicative low (minimum) disposable income [30,32]. The current quantums of relevant welfare and taxation payments were applied to calculate the indicative low (minimum) disposable household income.

2.2. Testing of the Aboriginal and Torres Strait Islander Healthy Diets ASAP Methods

Prices of food and drinks were collected in five community stores on the Anangu Pitjantjatjara Yankunytjatjara (APY) Lands of South Australia (Figure 1) using the Healthy Diets ASAP food price data collection sheet as per the Healthy Diets ASAP methods protocol [23] by AL in June 2017 as part of ongoing Nganampa Health Council service delivery. In each location, a single store is the main source of food in the community. Further information about the communities is available elsewhere [27].

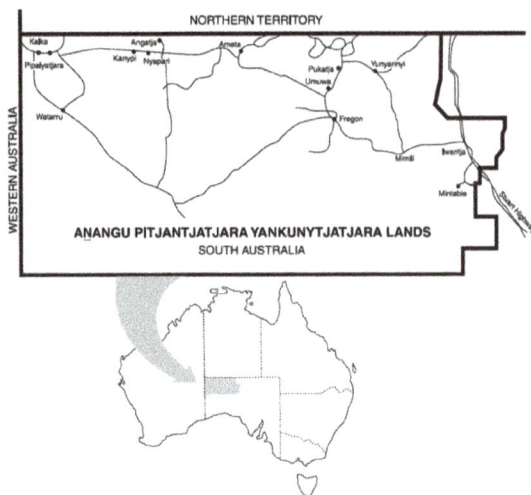

Figure 1. Map showing the Anangu Pitjantjatjara Yankunytjatjara (APY) Lands of South Australia.

Under the Healthy Diets ASAP pricing collection methods protocol, several discretionary food prices are collected from commercial premises outside of a supermarket, including for pizza, hamburger, beef pie and hot chips. As such premises were not available in the remote communities, relevant prices were collected from the store's hot takeaway section, or if not available, for frozen pizza, frozen hamburger and frozen pies, as these items were commonly heated by the purchaser in a microwave at the store for immediate consumption. Frozen potato chip prices were not collected however, due to the large price differential between a single serve of hot chips and the significantly larger bag of frozen chips, and the requirement for more complex cooking methods than microwaving. Alcohol prices were not collected as the communities are 'dry' and alcohol was not available for sale.

Price data were double entered by ML into data entry and analysis Excel© spreadsheets developed for the Healthy Diets ASAP methods protocol [23,33]. If the price of a specific food item was unavailable, the average price for that item in the other four stores was used. If an item was out of stock, the shelf price was collected. The mean prices for each diet and component food groups were calculated. The data were analysed according to both the Healthy Diets ASAP methods protocol and the Aboriginal and Torres Strait Islander Healthy Diets ASAP methods, and results were compared.

Median (gross) household income data from the Community Profile for the APY Lands SA2 [34] was transcribed directly and adjusted by the Wage Price Index percentage increase from June 2016 (at census data collection) to June 2017 (when the food price data were collected) [29].

2.3. Ethical Standards Disclosure

The QUT University Human Research Ethics Committee assessed this study as meeting the conditions for exemption from Human Research Ethics Committee review and approval in accordance with section 5.1.22 of the National Statement on Ethical Conduct in Human Research (2007); the exemption numbers are 1500000161 and 1800000151. All data were obtained from publicly available sources and did not involve human participants.

3. Results

3.1. Developing the Aboriginal and Torres Strait Healthy Diets ASAP Methods Part One: Construct of the Diet Pricing Tools

3.1.1. The Aboriginal and Torres Strait Islander Healthy Diets ASAP Current (Unhealthy) Diet Pricing Tool

The reported consumption ratio calculated by comparing the reported dietary intakes of each food group, and relevant components, by Aboriginal and Torres Strait Islanders [5] with the whole Australian population [7] in the AHS 2011–2013 is presented in Table 1.

Table 1. Reported consumption ratios of each food group and food group component for Aboriginal and Torres Strait Islanders [5] compared with the broader Australian population [7].

Food Group and Food Group Component	Reported Consumption Ratio
Vegetables & legumes	0.67
Fruit	0.8
Grain (cereal) foods—wholegrains	0.74
Grain (cereal) foods—others	1
Meat, poultry, fish & alternatives—red meat & poultry	1.14
Meat, poultry, fish & alternatives—others	0.94
Milk, yoghurt, cheese & alternatives	0.8
Unsaturated oils & spreads	0.7
Discretionary foods—sugar-sweetened drinks	1.8
Discretionary foods—others	1.1
Water	1
Alcohol	1

The reported consumption ratios were applied to calculate the amounts of foods and drinks comprising the Aboriginal and Torres Strait Islander Healthy Diets ASAP current (unhealthy) diet pricing tool as presented in Table 2. The composition of the original Healthy Diets ASAP current (unhealthy) diet pricing tool for the whole population is also presented in Table 2.

Table 2. Composition of the Healthy Diets ASAP and Aboriginal and Torres Strait Islander Healthy Diets ASAP current (unhealthy) diet and healthy (recommended) diet pricing tools (pertaining to the diet of a reference household per fortnight [1]).

Current (Unhealthy) Diet Pricing Tool			Healthy (Recommended) Diet Pricing Tool	
Food or Drink	Healthy Diets ASAP Quantity	Aboriginal and Torres Strait Islander Healthy Diets ASAP Quantity	Food or Drink	Healthy Diets ASAP and Aboriginal and Torres Strait Islander Healthy Diets ASAP Quantity
Bottled water, still (mL)	5296	5296	Bottled water, still (mL)	5296
Artificially sweetened 'diet' soft drink (mL)	2391	2630		
Fruit			*Fruit*	
Apples, red, loose (g)	3497	2797	Apples, red, loose (g)	5460
Bananas, Cavendish, loose (g)	899	719	Bananas, Cavendish, loose (g)	5460
Oranges, loose (g)	1664	1331	Oranges, loose (g)	5460
Fruit salad, canned in juice (g)	2046	1637		
Fruit juice	3026	3329		
Vegetables			*Vegetables*	
Potato, white, loose (g)	1460	978	Potato, white, loose (g)	2320
Sweetcorn, canned, no added salt (g)	206	138	Sweetcorn, canned, no added salt (g)	1160
Broccoli, loose (g)	422	282	Broccoli, loose (g)	1470
White cabbage, loose (g)	235	157	White cabbage, loose (g)	1470
Iceberg lettuce, whole (g)	795	533	Iceberg lettuce, whole (g)	1470
Carrot, loose (g)	753	505	Carrot, loose (g)	2205
Pumpkin (g)	240	161	Pumpkin (g)	2205
Four bean mix, canned (g)	74	50	Four bean mix, canned (g)	1005
Diced tomatoes, canned, in tomato juice (g)	234	157	Diced tomatoes, canned, in tomato juice (g)	1638
Onion, brown, loose (g)	84	57	Onion, brown, loose (g)	1638
Tomatoes, loose (g)	488	327	Tomatoes, loose (g)	1638

Table 2. *Cont.*

Current (Unhealthy) Diet Pricing Tool			Healthy (Recommended) Diet Pricing Tool	
Food or Drink	Healthy Diets ASAP Quantity	Aboriginal and Torres Strait Islander Healthy Diets ASAP Quantity	Food or Drink	Healthy Diets ASAP and Aboriginal and Torres Strait Islander Healthy Diets ASAP Quantity
Frozen mixed vegetables, pre-packaged (g)	1184	793	Frozen mixed vegetables, pre-packaged (g)	1638
Frozen peas, pre-packaged (g)	273	183	Frozen peas, pre-packaged (g)	1638
Baked beans, canned (g)	369	247	Baked beans, canned (g)	1005
Salad vegs in sandwich	120	120	Salad vegs in sandwich	120
Veg in tinned meat and vegetable casserole (g)	646	736		
Grain (cereal) foods			*Grain (cereal) foods*	
Wholegrain cereal biscuits Weet-bix™ (g)	430	319	Wholegrain cereal biscuits Weet-bix™ (g)	2216
Wholemeal bread, pre-packaged (g)	1054	780	Wholemeal bread, pre-packaged (g)	4272
Rolled oats, whole (g)	870	870	Rolled oats, whole (g)	6648
White bread, pre-packaged (g)	3033	3033	White bread, pre-packaged (g)	893
Cornflakes (g)	680	680	Cornflakes (g)	670
White pasta, spaghetti (g)	1326	1326	White pasta, spaghetti (g)	2042
White rice, medium grain (g)	1622	1622	White rice, medium grain (g)	2042
Dry water cracker biscuit (g)	258	258	Dry water cracker biscuit (g)	781
Bread in sandwich	120	120	Bread in sandwich	120
Meats, poultry, fish, eggs, nuts and seeds			*Meats, poultry, fish, eggs, nuts and seeds*	
Beef mince, lean (g)	267	305	Beef mince, lean (g)	1168
Lamb loin chops (g)	257	293	Lamb loin chops (g)	1169
Beef rump steak (g)	1056	1204	Beef rump steak (g)	1172
Tuna, canned in vegetable oil (g)	1052	989	Tuna, canned in vegetable oil (g)	1841
Whole barbeque chicken, cooked (g)	1661	1893	Whole barbeque chicken, cooked (g)	1471
Eggs (g)	872	820	Eggs (g)	2208
Meat in tinned meat and vegetable casserole (g)	646	736	Peanuts, roasted, unsalted (g)	780
Chicken in sandwiches	120	120	Chicken in sandwiches	120
Milk, yoghurt, cheese and alternatives			*Milk, yoghurt, cheese and alternatives*	
Cheddar cheese, full fat (g)	624	499	Cheddar cheese, full fat (g)	704
Cheddar cheese, reduced fat (g)	44	35	Cheddar cheese, reduced fat (g)	516
Milk, full fat (mL)	5961	4769	Milk, full cream (mL)	6438
Milk, reduced fat (mL)	2929	2344	Milk, reduced fat (mL)	12000
Yoghurt, full fat plain (g)	204	163	Yoghurt, full fat plain (g)	2576
Yoghurt, reduced fat, flavoured (vanilla) (g)	676	541	Yoghurt, reduced fat, flavoured (vanilla) (g)	5100
Flavoured milk (mL)	2416	2658		
Unsaturated oils				
Canola margarine (g)	170	119	Canola margarine (g)	412
Sunflower oil (mL)	7	5	Sunflower oil (mL)	291
Olive oil (mL)	7	5	Olive oil (mL)	291
Discretionary choices				
Beer, full strength (mL)	4661	4661		
White wine, sparkling (mL)	863	863		
Whisky (mL)	266	266		
Red wine (mL)	1078	1078		
Butter (g)	280	308		
Muffin, commercial (g)	1455	1601		
Cream-filled sweet biscuit, pre-packaged (g)	496	546		
Muesli bar, pre-packaged (g)	373	410		
Mixed nuts, salted (g)	255	281		
Pizza, commercial (g)	1182	1300		
Savoury flavoured biscuits (g)	222	244		
Confectionary (g)	418	460		
Chocolate (g)	441	485		
Sugar-sweetened beverages (Coca Cola) (mL)	12012	21621		
Meat pie, commercial (g)	1638	1802		
Frozen lasagne, pre-packaged (g)	4322	4754		
Hamburger, commercial (g)	2413	2654		
Beef sausages (g)	1048	1152		
Ham (g)	189	208		
Potato crisps, pre-packaged (g)	518	570		
Potato chips, hot, commercial (g)	670	737		
Ice cream (g)	1830	2013		
White sugar (g)	564	621		
Salad dressing (mL)	277	305		
Tomato sauce (mL)	569	626		
Chicken soup, canned (g)	1340	1474		
Orange juice (mL)	3027	3330		
Fish fillet crumbed, pre-packaged (g)	302	332		
Instant noodles, wheat-based (g)	381	419		

[1] The reference household comprises four people: adult male 19–50 years old; adult female 19–50 years old; boy 14 years old; girl 8 years old.

3.1.2. The Aboriginal and Torres Strait Islander Healthy Diets ASAP Healthy (Recommended) Diet Pricing Tool

The amounts of foods and drinks comprising the Aboriginal and Torres Strait Islander Healthy Diets ASAP healthy (recommended) diet pricing tool (unchanged from the original protocol [23]) are presented in Table 2.

3.2. *Developing the Aboriginal and Torres Strait Healthy Diets ASAP Methods Part Two: Determination of Median and Low-Income Household Income*

The Community Profile for the APY Lands SA2 states that the median weekly household income in 2016 was $AUD1150 and the average household contained 3.8 people [34]. The Australian Wage Price Index [29] increased from June 2016 (at census data collection) to June 2017 (when the food price data was collected) by 1.9%. Applying this index gave an estimated median weekly household income on the APY Lands in June 2017 of $AUD1171. Thus, the fortnightly median (gross) household income for the reference household in the APY Lands in June 2017 was $AUD2342.

The method to determine the indicative low (minimum) disposable household income was modified to include in the underlying assumptions (Table 3) that the reference family is comprised of people identifying as Aboriginal and/or Torres Strait Islanders and that they live in a remote location as determined by the Australian Tax Office [32]. Compared with the Healthy Diets ASAP methods protocol, the assumptions included an AbStudy school term allowance for the 14-year-old boy [30] and a remote area tax offset amount applied in assessment of taxation for the adult male, as shown in Table 4. All other assumptions were the same as those for non-Indigenous households and those living in non-remote areas [30].

Table 3. Assumptions used to determine the indicative low (minimum) disposable household income of the reference household.

Assumptions for the Reference Household Consisting of an Adult Male, an Adult Female, a 14-Year-Old Boy and an 8-Year-Old Girl
• The family is privately renting a house at $AUD75/week [34]
• The adult male works on a permanent basis at the national minimum wage ($AUD17.29 per hour [31]) for 38 h a week
• The adult female works on a part-time basis at the national minimum wage ($AUD17.29 per hour) for 6 h a week
• Both children attend school and are fully immunised
• None of the family are disabled
• The family has some emergency savings that earn negligible interest
• The family are Aboriginal and/or Torres Strait Islanders
• The family live in a remote location

Table 4. Calculation of the indicative low (minimum) disposable household income of the reference Aboriginal and Torres Strait Islander household.

Income Type	Amount Per Fortnight ($AUD)
Paid employment–adult male	1345.20
Paid employment–adult female	212.40
Family Tax Benefit A	420.70
Family Tax Benefit A Supplement	55.87
Family Tax Benefit B	108.64
Family Tax Benefit B Supplement	13.62
Clean Energy Supplement (across all payments)	9.94
Rent Assistance	nil
AbStudy School term allowance–14 yr old boy	20.80
Income tax paid (tax owing on employment income of adult male, less low income tax offset, less remote area tax offset)	−48.09
Total Fortnightly Income	**2139.08**

3.3. Testing the Aboriginal and Torres Strait Islander Healthy Diets ASAP Methods: The Cost of The Diets and Component Food Groups

The mean (± standard deviation) cost of the healthy diet was $AUD827.63 (± $42.24) in the five remote Aboriginal communities surveyed.

The cost of the current diet in the five remote Aboriginal communities using the Healthy Diets ASAP methods protocol and Aboriginal and Torres Strait Islander Healthy Diets ASAP methods, and the difference between the two, are presented in Table 5. Application of the Aboriginal and Torres Strait Islander Healthy Diets ASAP methods assessed the cost of the current diet at $AUD1023.16 (± $40.90) which was 7% higher than the cost of $AUD956.18 (± $39.60) assessed by application of the original Healthy Diets ASAP methods protocol.

Table 5. Mean cost of the current (unhealthy) diet in five remote Aboriginal communities using the Healthy Diets Australian Standardised Affordability and Pricing (ASAP) methods protocol and Aboriginal and Torres Strait Islander Healthy Diets ASAP methods.

Diet Component	Healthy Diets ASAP (Whole Population) Methods Protocol		Aboriginal and Torres Strait Islander Healthy Diets ASAP Methods		Cost Difference between Using Aboriginal and Torres Strait Islander Healthy Diets ASAP Methods and Healthy Diets ASAP Methods Protocol
	Mean Cost ($AUD)	Std Dev ($AUD)	Mean Cost ($AUD)	Std Dev ($AUD)	Difference $AUD (% Change)
Water	8.83	—	8.83	—	—
Fruit	80.66	8.70	68.13	6.93	−12.54 (−15%)
Vegetables & Legumes	56.31	3.21	43.48	2.15	−12.83 (−23%)
Grains & Cereals	66.42	2.35	63.37	2.29	−3.05 (−5%)
Meats, nuts, seeds, eggs	110.65	3.33	119.95	3.16	9.30 (+8%)
Milk, yoghurt, cheese	80.66	13.72	71.93	14.08	−8.73 (−11%)
Unsaturated oils & spreads	2.03	0.01	1.42	0.01	−0.61 (−30%)
Artificially sweetened soft drink	10.52	—	11.57	—	1.05 (+10%)
Take-away foods	181.32	17.53	199.45	19.28	18.13 (+10%)
Sugar-sweetened drinks	68.18	—	115.35	—	47.18 (+69%)
Discretionary choices-other	290.62	13.36	319.68	14.70	29.06 (+10%)
Total cost	**956.18**	**39.60**	**1023.16**	**40.90**	**66.97 (+7%)**

[1] The current diet for a fortnight for the reference household comprising four people: adult male 19–50 years old; adult female 19–50 years old; boy 14 years old; girl 8 years old.

Using the Aboriginal and Torres Strait Islander Healthy Diets ASAP methods, the cost of a healthy diet was 24% less than the cost of the current diet. If the original Healthy Diets ASAP methods protocol was used, the cost of the healthy diet was 16% less than the current diet.

Using the Healthy Diets ASAP methods protocol, the proportion of the total cost of the current diet derived from discretionary foods and drinks was 56.5%. This figure was 62.0% when the Aboriginal and Torres Strait Islander Healthy Diets ASAP methods were used.

The total cost of the current (unhealthy) diet was $AUD66.97 per fortnight (7%) more expensive when the Aboriginal and Torres Strait Islander specific methods were used rather than the original Healthy Diets ASAP methods protocol for the whole population (Table 5). The main source of difference for healthy foods was that the cost of all fruit and vegetables included in the current diet was $AUD25.37 per fortnight (19%) less when assessed by the Aboriginal and Torres Strait Islander Healthy Diets ASAP methods than by the Healthy Diet ASAP methods protocol. The healthy unsaturated oils and spreads were cost 30% less using the Aboriginal and Torres Strait Islander specific methods; however, this was a difference of only $AUD0.61 per fortnight, given the low quantities of these foods consumed. Conversely, the cost of all unhealthy discretionary foods and drinks included in the current diet was $AUD94.37 (17%) more expensive per fortnight when assessed by the Aboriginal and Torres Strait Islander Healthy Diets ASAP methods than by the Healthy Diets ASAP methods protocol. The major source of this variance was the cost of sugar-sweetened drinks which were $AUD47.18 per fortnight (69%) more expensive when assessed by the Aboriginal and Torres Strait Islander specific methods.

3.4. Testing of the Aboriginal and Torres Strait Islander Healthy Diets ASAP Methods: Affordability of Healthy Diets

The affordability of healthy diet and the current diets determined by both the Healthy Diets ASAP methods protocol and the Aboriginal and Torres Strait Islander Healthy Diets ASAP methods in five remote Aboriginal communities are shown in Table 6. When determined by the Aboriginal and Torres Strait Islander Healthy Diets ASAP methods, the affordability of the current diet was around 7% poorer than when assessed by the original Healthy Diets ASAP methods protocol. When assessed by the Aboriginal and Torres Strait Islander Healthy Diets ASAP methods, the affordability of the current diet as a proportion of both the median (gross) household income (35.3%) and indicative low (minimum) disposable household income (38.7%) respectively was above the internationally acceptable benchmark of 30% [16,21]. As assessed by the Aboriginal and Torres Strait Islander Healthy Diets ASAP methods, the healthy diet would be around 20% more affordable than the current diet, but at 35.3% of the median (gross) household income and 38.7% of the indicative low (minimum) disposable household income, would still be unaffordable compared to the internally acceptable benchmark of 30% [16,21].

Table 6. Affordability of current diets and healthy diets in remote Aboriginal communities on the APY Lands.

Diet	Mean Diet Cost (±Std Dev) ($AUD)	Affordability with Median (Gross) Household Income ($AUD2342)	Affordability with Indicative Low (Minimum) Disposable Household Income ($AUD2139.08)
Healthy (recommended) diet	827.63 (42.24)	35.3%	38.7%
Current (unhealthy) diet determined by the Healthy Diets ASAP methods protocol	956.18 (39.60)	40.8%	44.7%
Current (unhealthy) diet determined by the Aboriginal and Torres Strait Islander Healthy Diets ASAP methods	1023.16 (40.90)	43.7%	47.8%

4. Discussion

4.1. Discussion of Approach

Food insecurity is a key factor contributing to the high double-burden of malnutrition experienced by Indigenous Australians [3]. However, as in many developed nations, food security is poorly assessed in Australia, where, for over twenty years irregular national dietary surveys have included a single question on individual food security around running out of food and not being able to afford to buy more [3]. This measure, while a useful indicator, is likely to underestimate the full extent of the problem. There is a pressing need to better understand food insecurity from an Aboriginal and Torres Strait Islander perspective in order to develop Indigenous-specific tools for assessment of availability, affordability, accessibility and acceptability of healthy food and drinks and other determinants of food security, particularly at household and community level [3,35]. This paper attempted to do this in the area of food price and affordability, in order to provide relevant data to inform the development of tailored fiscal and nutrition policy actions with Aboriginal and Torres Strait Islander communities.

Adjustment of the whole-of-population Healthy Diets ASAP current (unhealthy) diet pricing tool by the reported consumption ratio method, proved to be a simple, expedient method to customise the tool for application in remote Aboriginal and Torres Strait Islander communities, particularly as it did not require redevelopment of the original data collection tools. However, this method does rely on the availability of quality dietary (food and drink) intake survey data for both the whole population at the national level and for specific population groups, which may not always be available, even in developed countries [21].

The total cost of the current diet was 7% more expensive when the Aboriginal and Torres Strait Islander specific methods were used rather than the original Healthy Diets ASAP methods protocol for the whole population. This was due to differences in the reported intakes of foods and drinks that contributed substantially to the current diet in Aboriginal and Torres Strait Islander groups compared with the broader Australian population. Major differences were seen for sugar-sweetened drinks (with reported intakes nearly double that of broader Australia) contributing most (69%) of the additional expense, and reported intakes of fruit and vegetables (which were 30% less than the broader population) reducing the current diet costs by 19%, when determined by the Aboriginal and Torres Strait Islander Healthy Diets ASAP methods.

While data on median (gross) household income of Aboriginal and Torres Strait Islanders specifically are not readily available, the use of median (gross) household income from the relevant 2016 Census data Community Profiles [34] did provide meaningful information once updated with the wage price index [29], and at $AUD2342 per household per fortnight (gross), was consistent with expectations given the low (minimum) disposable household income of $AUD2139 estimated in the test communities using different methods. This study demonstrated that determination of the indicative low (minimum) disposable household income for Aboriginal and Torres Strait Islander households living in remote areas was feasible. This figure for Aboriginal and Torre Strait Islander households living in non-remote areas would be slightly less, due to the non-applicability of the remote area tax offset.

Testing demonstrated that it is feasible to apply the Aboriginal and Torres Strait Islander Healthy Diets ASAP methods stores in remote communities. However, further studies would be required to test utility of the approach in urban centres. Among other differences, remote community stores, stock a much smaller range of items than supermarkets in urban areas. In this study there were four instances where the listed food item in the pricing tool was unavailable in any size or brand. Each store outlet surveyed in the five remote communities operates as a general store selling fresh fruit, vegetables, meat, bread, frozen foods, pantry items, and other goods. Four of the stores also sold a range of hot takeaway food items. Some food items were available only in sizes much smaller than stated on the price collection data sheet; for example, plain yoghurt is listed as 1kg on the Healthy Diets ASAP food price data collection sheet, but was only available in 200g tubs in three of the five stores. This contributed to the high standard deviation in the cost of the food groups observed where larger items were missing, particularly the milk, yoghurt and cheese food group. Conversely, as part of the nutrition policy in place in the five stores surveyed, the price of 600mL bottled water is mandated at $AUD1.00, so that for this item the standard deviation of prices across the five stores was zero.

Testing of the Aboriginal and Torres Strait Islander Healthy Diets ASAP methods supported the notion that the approach has acceptable face validity in providing assessment of the price, price differential and affordability of current (unhealthy) and healthy (recommended) diets of Aboriginal and Torres Strait Islander groups living in remote communities. The results were consistent with expectations arising from consideration of the reported dietary intake data of the two different populations [5,7] and the relative prices of foods in the remote Aboriginal community stores [27].

Consistent with similar surveys, particularly in Australia where the GST of 10% is not applied to basic, healthy foods [22–25], application of the Aboriginal and Torres Strait Islander Healthy Diets ASAP methods in remote Aboriginal communities showed that a healthy diet ($AUD827.63) was less expensive than the current diet ($AUD1,023.16) per household per fortnight. However, at 76% of the cost of the current diet, a healthy diet was potentially more affordable in the remote Aboriginal communities studied than in other places, where the cost of the healthy diet ranges between 80–85% [22–25]. Surprisingly, this price differential between the current and healthy diets was larger than in other studies even though alcohol was not included in the current diet, as the communities are 'dry' and alcohol is not available for sale. One likely reason for this is that the five community stores surveyed on the APY Lands have in place a prescribed nutrition policy which mandates, among other potential benefits, that fruit and vegetables are sold at cost price, that 600mL bottled water is priced at $AUD1.00, and that low mark ups on the wholesale price of other healthy foods, such as lean meat and wholemeal bread, are standard. Previous studies have found that this nutrition policy contributes to relative affordability of healthy foods, particularly fruit and vegetables, compared to unhealthy, discretionary choices [27].

Despite these promising findings, further scrutiny showed that healthy diets would be unaffordable due to the low household incomes in the communities surveyed. When assessed by the Aboriginal and Torres Strait Islander Healthy Diets ASAP methods, healthy diets would cost over 35% of median (gross) household income and nearly 39% of indicative low (minimum) disposable household incomes in these communities, compared to the international affordability benchmark of 30% of disposable household income [16,21].

The high level of food insecurity and food stress in these communities was confirmed, as the current diet cost over 43% of median (gross) household income and nearly 48% of indicative low (minimum) disposable household incomes when assessed by the Aboriginal and Torres Strait Islander Healthy Diets ASAP methods.

The tailored Aboriginal and Torres Strait Islander Healthy Diets ASAP methods were more sensitive than the original Healthy Diets ASAP methods protocol in revealing the current degree of food security in the communities surveyed. If the tailored methods developed and tested in this study had not been used, the severity of food security issues in the remote Aboriginal communities surveyed would have been partially masked, and valuable data relevant to potential policy actions would have remained undetected.

Worryingly, while 41% of the energy intake of the diet was derived from discretionary choices [5], application of the Aboriginal and Torres Strait Islander Healthy Diets ASAP methods showed that 62% of the current food budget in the remote communities surveyed was spent on discretionary food and drinks; of this over 18% was spent on sugary drinks and over 30% on take-away foods. This high reliance on discretionary food and drinks has been described previously and appears to be driven by the increasing availability, range and variety of unhealthy discretionary foods and drinks in community stores over the last three decades [27]. Such changes in the food supply reflect those seen more broadly in Australia, and globally [27].

These results highlight that, given the high proportion of food insecurity and diet-related disease in Aboriginal and Torres Strait Islander groups, nothing should be done to risk increasing the price differential of healthy to discretionary food and drinks in remote Aboriginal communities, as this could act as a further barrier to healthy diets. While better understanding of price elasticities and access to income entitlements in remote communities would be useful, the findings also suggest that investigation into the nature and effect of drivers of food choice other than price, such as housing, access to educational and employment opportunities, availability and functionality of food preparation/cooking facilities, transport, convenience, product placement in stores, promotion, advertising and food preferences appears warranted.

4.2. Limitations

Similar to the original Healthy Diets ASAP methods protocol, there are several inherent limitations in the Aboriginal and Torres Strait Islander Healthy Diets ASAP methods. Given that the approach is based on the reported mean dietary intakes of select age and gender groups of Aboriginal and Torres Strait Islanders at the national level, the diet pricing tools should be considered as reference instruments and the cost of the current diet is unlikely to be the same as actual expenditure on food and drinks by all Aboriginal and Torres Strait Islander people or households currently [36].

All diet pricing tools should ideally include foods that are culturally acceptable, commonly consumed and widely available. Whilst the amounts of the foods included in the diet survey pricing tools are reflective of the respective food and food group consumption of Aboriginal and Torres Strait Islander groups reported in the AHS 2011-13 [5] at the three digit-level, the Healthy Diet ASAP methods protocol includes foods and drinks reported in the AHS 2011-13 [6] at the five-digit level. Therefore, a very small number of the specific foods and drinks included tend to reflect reported consumption of the Australian population as a whole, rather than Aboriginal and Torres Strait Islander peoples specifically. While all foods in the pricing tools were generally available and accessible in the remote community stores surveyed, formal assessment of their cultural acceptability has not been undertaken as yet. Subsequent modifications may be required to accommodate specific food preferences; for example, further reduction of the quantities of plain yoghurt included as this item was frequently out of stock and was considered by store managers to be a low demand item.

No adjustments were made to account for the marked under-reporting in the AHS 2011-13 [5,6]. Nor were adjustments made for the greater proportion of 'convenience' items in the current (unhealthy) diet pricing tool compared with the healthy (recommended) diet pricing tool. Given the high rates of overweight/obesity in Aboriginal and Torres Strait Islander groups, and that the Foundation Diets of the modelling used to inform the Australian Guide to Healthy Eating component of the Australian Dietary Guidelines were prescribed for the shortest and least active in each age group [37], the healthy (recommended) diet tool under-estimates the requirements of taller, more active and healthy weight individuals.

5. Conclusions

The Aboriginal and Torres Strait Islander Healthy Diets ASAP methods tailor nationally-standardised diet price and affordability method protocols to improve applicability to Indigenous Australians. The method incorporates relevant household income data and reported dietary intakes of Aboriginal and Torres Strait Islander groups to more appropriately assess, compare, monitor and benchmark the price, price differential and affordability of current (unhealthy) and healthy (recommended) diets in different communities.

The development of the tailored Aboriginal and Torres Strait Islander Healthy Diets ASAP methods provides an example of how standardised national tools can be adapted at sub-population and regional levels to provide better data to inform policy actions to improve food security and help reduce rates of diet-related disease more equitably in developed countries.

Author Contributions: Conceptualisation, A.L.; Methodology, A.L.; Formal Analysis, M.L.; Investigation, A.L.; Writing—Original Draft Preparation, M.L. and A.L.; Writing—Review & Editing, A.L.; Project Administration, A.L.

Funding: Data collection was funded by Nganampa Health Council as part of ongoing service delivery. Funding for data analysis and preparation of the manuscript has been provided from the Australian Government's Medical Research Future Fund (MRFF). The MRFF provides funding to support health and medical research an innovation, with the objective of improving the health and wellbeing of Australians. MRFF funding has been provided to The Australian Prevention Partnership Centre under the Boosting Preventative Health Research Program. Further information on the MRFF is available at www.health.gov.au/mrffwere funded by The Australian Prevention Partnership Centre.

Acknowledgments: We acknowledge the support and assistance of the Nganampa Health Council, the Ngaanyatjarra Pitjantjatjara Yankunytjatjara Women's Council (NPYWC), and the Mai Wiru Regional Stores Council Aboriginal Corporation.

Conflicts of Interest: The authors declare no conflict of interest.

References

1. Institute for Health Metrics and Evaluation. Global Burden of Disease Country Profile Australia. Available online: http://www.healthdata.org/sites/default/files/files/country_profiles/GBD/ihme_gbd_country_report_australia.pdf (accessed on 12 November 2017).
2. Australian Institute of Health and Welfare. *Australian Burden of Disease Study: Impact and Causes of Illness and Death in Aboriginal and Torres Strait Islander People 2011*; Series No. 6; Australian Burden of Disease Stufy: Canberra, Australia, 2015.
3. Lee, A.; Ride, K. *Review of Nutrition among Aboriginal and Torres Strait Islander People*; Australian Indigenous HealthInfoNet: Perth, Australia, 2018.
4. National Health and Medical Research Council. *Australian Dietary Guidelines—Providing the Scientific Evidence for Healthier Australian Diets*; National Health and Medical Research Council: Australia, Canberra, 2013. Available online: https://www.eatforhealth.gov.au/sites/default/files/content/n55_australian_dietary_guidelines.pdf (accessed on 9 February 2016).

5. Australian Bureau of Statistics. 4727.0.55.008—Australian Aboriginal and Torres Strait Islander Health Survey: Consumption of Food Groups from the Australian Dietary Guidelines, 2012–2013. Available online: http://www.abs.gov.au/ausstats/abs@.nsf/PrimaryMainFeatures/4727.0.55.008?OpenDocument (accessed on 20 September 2018).

6. Australian Bureau of Statistics. 4364.0.55.007—Australian Health Survey: Nutrition First Results—Foods and Nutrients, 2011–2012. Available online: http://www.abs.gov.au/AUSSTATS/abs@.nsf/DetailsPage/4364.0.55.0072011-12?OpenDocument (accessed on 12 November 2017).

7. Australian Bureau of Statistics. 4364.0.55.012—Australian Health Survey: Consumption of Food Groups from the Australian Dietary Guidelines, 2011–2012. Available online: http://www.abs.gov.au/ausstats/abs@.nsf/mf/4364.0.55.012 (accessed on 12 November 2017).

8. Australian Bureau of Statistics. 4364.0.55.003—Australian Health Survey: Updated Results, 2011–2012—Overweight and Obesity. Available online: http://www.abs.gov.au/ausstats/abs@.nsf/lookup/33C64022ABB5ECD5CA257B8200179437?opendocument (accessed on 12 November 2017).

9. FAO. *The State of Food Insecurity in the World 2001*; Food and Agriculture Organization of the United Nations: Rome, Italy, 2002.

10. Davy, D. Australian's efforts to improve food security for Aboriginal and Torres Strait Islander peoples. *Health Hum. Rights* **2016**, *18*, 209. [PubMed]

11. United Nations. *Universal Declaration of Human Rights*; Unated Nations: Geneva, Switzerland, 1948.

12. Eide, W.B.; Kracht, U. Towards a definition of the right to food and nutrition: Reflections on General Comment No. 12. *SCN News* **1999**, *18*, 39–40.

13. Kettings, C.; Sinclair, A.J.; Voevodin, M. A healthy diet consistent with Australian health recommendations is too expensive for welfare-dependent families. *Aust. N. Z. J. Public Health* **2009**, *33*, 566–572. [CrossRef] [PubMed]

14. Williams, P.G. Can the poor in Australia afford healthy food? *Nutr. Diet.* **2011**, *68*, 6–7. [CrossRef]

15. Ward, P.R.; Verty, F.; Cartrer, P.; Tsurtos, G.; Conveney, J.; Wong, C.K. Food Stress in Adelaide: The Relationship between Low Income and the Affordability of Healthy Food. *J. Environ. Public Health* **2013**, *2013*, 10. [CrossRef] [PubMed]

16. Barosh, L.; Friel, S.; Engelhardt, K.; Chan, L. The cost of a healthy and sustainable diet—Who can afford it? *Aust. N. Z. J. Public Health* **2014**, *38*, 7–12. [CrossRef] [PubMed]

17. Landrigan, T.J.; Kerr, D.A.; Dhaliwal, S.S.; Pollard, C.M. Removing the Australian tax exemption on healthy food adds food stress to families vulnerable to poor nutrition. *Aust. N. Z. J. Public Health* **2017**, *41*. [CrossRef] [PubMed]

18. Australian Bureau of Statistics. 4727.0.55.005—Australian Aboriginal and Torres Strait Islander Health Survey: Nutrition Results—Food and Nutrients, 2012–2013. Available online: http://www.abs.gov.au/ausstats/abs@.nsf/PrimaryMainFeatures/4727.0.55.005?OpenDocument (accessed on 20 September 2018).

19. Queensland Health. 2014 Healthy Food Access Basket Survey. Available online: https://www.health.qld.gov.au/research-reports/reports/public-health/food-nutrition/access/overview (accessed on 8 February 2016).

20. Lewis, M.; Lee, A. Costing 'healthy' food baskets in Australia—A systematic review of food price and affordability monitoring tools, protocols and methods. *Public Health Nutr.* **2016**, *19*, 2872–2886. [CrossRef] [PubMed]

21. Lee, A.; Murchu, C.N.; Sacks, G.; Swinburn, B.A.; Snowdon, W.; Vandevijvre, S.; Hawkes, C.; L Abbe, M.; Rayner, M.; Sandres, D. Monitoring the price and affordability of foods and diets globally. *Obes. Rev.* **2013**, *14* (Suppl. S1), 82–95. [CrossRef] [PubMed]

22. Lee, A.J.; Kane, S.; Ramsey, R.; Good, E.; Dick, M. Testing the price and affordability of healthy and current (unhealthy) diets and the potential impacts of policy change in Australia. *BMC Public Health* **2016**, *16*, 315. [CrossRef] [PubMed]

23. Lee, A.J.; Kane, S.; Lewis, M.; Good, E.; Pollard, C.M.; Landrigan, J.T.; Dick, M. Healthy diets ASAP—Australian Standardised Affordability and Pricing methods protocol. *Nutr. J.* **2018**, *17*, 88. [CrossRef] [PubMed]

24. Lee, A.; Lewis, M.; Kane, S. Are Healthy Diets really More Expensive? Findings Brief. The Australian Prevention Partnership Centre. Available online: https://preventioncentre.org.au/our-work/research-projects/are-healthy-diets-really-more-expensive/ (accessed on 18 November 2018).

25. Love, P.; Wheland, J.; Bell, C.; Garinger, F.; Russell, C.; Lewis, M.; Lee, M. Healthy diets in rural Victoria—Cheaper than unhealthy alternative, yet affordable. *Int. J. Environ. Res. Public Health* **2018**, *15*, 2469. [CrossRef] [PubMed]

26. Mackay, S.; Buch, T.; Vandevijvere, S.; Goodwin, R.; Korohina, E.; Tahifote, M.F.; Lee, A.J.; Swinburn, B.A. Cost and Affordability of Diets Modelled on Current Eating Patterns and on Dietary Guidelines, for New Zealand Total Population, Māori and Pacific Households. *Int. J. Environ. Res. Public Health* **2018**, *15*, 1255. [CrossRef] [PubMed]

27. Lee, A.; Rainow, S.; Tregenza, J.; Tregenza, L. Nutrition in remote Aboriginal communities: Lessons from Mai Wiru and the Anangu Pitjantjatjara Yankunytjatjara Lands. *Aust. N. Z. J. Public Health* **2016**, *40*, S81–S88. [CrossRef] [PubMed]

28. Australian Bureau of Statistics. 4324.0.55.002 Microdata: Australian Health Survey: Nutrition and Physical Activity, 2011–2012. Available online: http://www.abs.gov.au/ausstats/abs@.nsf/PrimaryMainFeatures/4324.0.55.002?OpenDocument (accessed on 12 November 2017).

29. Australian Bureau of Statistics. 6345.0—Wage Price Index, Australia, June 2017. Available online: http://www.abs.gov.au/AUSSTATS/abs@.nsf/allprimarymainfeatures/A52F591B2454B045CA2581D8000E926D?opendocument (accessed on 29 September 2018).

30. Department of Human Services. Online Estimators. Available online: http://www.humanservices.gov.au/customer/enablers/online-estimators (accessed on 22 October 2015).

31. Fair Work Ombudsman. Minimum Wages. Available online: https://www.fairwork.gov.au/how-we-will-help/templates-and-guides/fact-sheets/minimum-workplace-entitlements/minimum-wages (accessed on 22 October 2015).

32. Australian Taxation Office. Individual Offsets and Rebates: Zone and Overseas Forces. Available online: https://www.ato.gov.au/Individuals/Income-and-deductions/Offsets-and-rebates/Zones-and-overseas-forces/ (accessed on 27 January 2018).

33. Microsoft Corporation. *Microsoft Office*, Version 2007; Microsoft Corporation: Washington, WA, USA, 2007.

34. Australian Bureau of Statistics. QuickStats. 2016. Available online: http://quickstats.censusdata.abs.gov.au/census_services/getproduct/census/2016/quickstat/406021138 (accessed on 29 September 2018).

35. Lee, A.; Ride, K. *Review of Programs and Services to Improve Aboriginal and Torres Strait Islander Nutrition and Food Security*; Australian Indigenous HealthInfoNet: Perth, Australia, 2018.

36. Mhurchu, C.N.; Eyles, H.; Schilling, C.; Yang, Q.; Kaye-Blake, W.; Genc, M.; Blakely, T. Food prices and consumer demand: Differences across income levels and ethnic groups. *PLoS ONE* **2013**, *8*, e75934. [CrossRef] [PubMed]

37. National Health and Medical Research Council. *A Modelling System to Inform the Revision of the Australian Guide to Healthy Eating*; National Health and Medical Research Council: Canberra, Australia, 2011. Available online: https://www.eatforhealth.gov.au/sites/default/files/files/the_guidelines/n55c_australian_dietary_guidelines_food_modelling_140121.pdf (accessed on 11 February 2016).

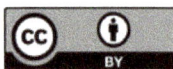

International Journal of
*Environmental Research
and Public Health*

MDPI

Article

Healthy Diets in Rural Victoria—Cheaper than Unhealthy Alternatives, Yet Unaffordable

Penelope Love [1,2,*], Jillian Whelan [3], Colin Bell [3], Felicity Grainger [2], Cherie Russell [1,2], Meron Lewis [4] and Amanda Lee [4,5]

[1] Institute for Physical Activity and Nutrition (IPAN), Deakin University, Geelong 3220, Australia; caru@deakin.edu.au
[2] School of Exercise and Nutrition Sciences, Deakin University, Geelong 3220, Australia; fgrainge@deakin.edu.au
[3] School of Medicine, Global Obesity Centre, Deakin University, Geelong 3220, Australia; jill.whelan@deakin.edu.au (J.W.); colin.bell@deakin.edu.au (C.B.)
[4] The Australian Prevention Partnership Centre (TAPPC), Sax Institute, Sydney 2007, Australia; meron.lewis@saxinstitute.org.au (M.L.); amanda.lee@saxinstitute.org.au (A.L.)
[5] School of Public Health, University of Queensland, Herston QLD 4006, Australia
* Correspondence: penny.love@deakin.edu.au

Received: 15 September 2018; Accepted: 1 November 2018; Published: 5 November 2018

Abstract: Rural communities experience higher rates of obesity and reduced food security compared with urban communities. The perception that healthy foods are expensive contributes to poor dietary choices. Providing an accessible, available, affordable healthy food supply is an equitable way to improve the nutritional quality of the diet for a community, however, local food supply data are rarely available for small rural towns. This study used the Healthy Diets ASAP tool to assess price, price differential and affordability of recommended (healthy) and current diets in a rural Local Government Area (LGA) (pop ≈ 7000; 10 towns) in Victoria, Australia. All retail food outlets were surveyed ($n = 40$). The four most populous towns had supermarkets; remaining towns had one general store each. Seven towns had café/take-away outlets, and all towns had at least one hotel/pub. For all towns the current unhealthy diet was more expensive than the recommended healthy diet, with 59.5% of the current food budget spent on discretionary items. Affordability of the healthy diet accounted for 30–32% of disposable income. This study confirms that while a healthy diet is less expensive than the current unhealthier diet, affordability is a challenge for rural communities. Food security is reduced further with restricted geographical access, a limited healthy food supply, and higher food prices.

Keywords: Healthy Diets ASAP tool; food security; food prices; diet affordability; rural communities; INFORMAS

1. Introduction

'If it's not available or you cannot afford it, then you cannot eat it even if you wanted to!'. [1] (p. 363)

The cost of food and the financial resources to procure it are key economic determinants of food choice [1]. Food security is defined as the physical, social and economic access to a stable and safe food supply, in sufficient quantity and quality to meet dietary needs and food preferences, within an environment that supports a healthy and active lifestyle [2]. In high income countries, like Australia, people identified as being most at risk for food insecurity have typically been those on low incomes, experiencing homelessness, refugees and migrants, and Aboriginal and Torres Strait Islander communities [3]. More recently, however, households on middle incomes, experiencing financial stress, have been identified as food insecure [3]. The national food insecurity prevalence of 4% [4] for Australia is therefore considered an underestimation, with predictions of 10–25% of households in some areas being food insecure [3].

The link between food insecurity and overweight/obesity [5] is of particular concern given the global prevalence of this complex public health problem [6]. In Australia, 25% of children and 63% of adults are overweight/obese [4], with rural Australian communities generally experiencing higher rates of obesity and decreased food security than their urban counterparts [7]. Despite having a higher disease burden, rural communities in Australia are frequently overlooked and under-researched regarding prevention, and therefore less informed about appropriate solutions. Providing an accessible, available and affordable healthy food supply is a well-established [8,9] and equitable way to improve the nutritional quality of food consumed by a community or population [10].

Unhealthy diets, and associated overweight/obesity, are now the major preventable risk factor contributing to the burden of disease [11], yet adherence to the Australian Dietary Guidelines is poor [12]. Unhealthy diets are caused by a range of complex and inter-related determinants including 'obesogenic' food environments, defined as an environment that promotes weight gain and hinders weight loss, affecting food promotion, availability, accessibility and affordability [9]. A key determinant is the perception that healthy diets are expensive and a barrier to the purchase of healthier foods [13]. Increased food prices, poorer quality produce and a limited variety of healthier options are primary contributors to food insecurity for Australian households [14]. The price and affordability of a healthy diet is of particular concern for rural communities where geographic location and low population density pose significant challenges for the food supply chain, resulting in an infrequent supply of healthy food to at risk communities [15], often of poorer quality [16] and less varied in terms of product brand, size and type [17,18]. A lack of infrastructure in these areas with low-density transport networks and high car dependency also make access to food outlets more difficult than in larger towns and cities [15].

Food pricing information in Australia has most commonly been collected using "healthy food basket" (HFB) methodology, using a predefined list of indicator food items representative of the total diet for different reference households [13]. Different HFB methodology exists across Australian States and Territories, with Victoria using the Victorian Healthy Food Basket (VHFB) comprising 44 listed food items. The VHFB approach poses limitations for small rural towns with food stores that often do not meet the inclusion criterion to stock at least 90% of the listed food items [19] as well as not including generic food product brands which are becoming increasingly prominent in Australian food stores [20].

The recent development of the Healthy Diets Australian Standardised Affordability and Price (ASAP) tool, through the global INFORMAS (International Network for Food and Obesity/non-communicable diseases Research, Monitoring and Action Support) network, may overcome these challenges. The Healthy Diets ASAP tool seeks to provide a standardised method to assess and compare the price and affordability of the recommended Australian diet with the current Australian diet [21–23], to enable informed community specific food supply decisions. The Healthy Diets ASAP tool comprises 76 food items [23] indicative of the recommended Australian diet (based on the quantitative modelled Foundation Diets within the Australian Dietary Guidelines) [24] and the current Australian diet (based on reported dietary intakes within the Australian Health Survey 2011–2012) [25]. Food item prices (n = 43), adjusted for edible proportion, representative of the recommended Australian diet encompass the five food groups (fruit; vegetables and legumes; grain/cereal foods; meats, poultry, fish and alternatives; milk, yoghurt, cheese and alternatives); and unsaturated oils and spreads. Additional food item prices (n = 33) representative of the current Australian diet include discretionary high in saturated fats, sugars, salt and/or alcohol (described as energy dense) and considered not necessary as part of a healthy diet. Discretionary items include cakes, biscuits, pastries, pies; chocolate, confectionery, ice confections; butter, cream, spreads which contain predominantly saturated fats; potato chips, crisps and other fatty or salty snack foods; sugar-sweetened soft drinks and cordials; sports and energy drinks; and alcoholic drinks) [24] (p. 144).

This study assessed and compared the price, price differential (relative price) and affordability of the recommended Australian diet (as defined by the Australian Dietary Guidelines) and the current Australian diet (as described by the Australian Health Survey) for a small rural Local Government Area in Victoria, Australia. Ethical approval for this study was obtained through Deakin University (HEAG-H 80_2016).

2. Materials and Methods

2.1. Study Context and Selection of Study Site

The LGA selected for this study was determined by its rurality, modifiable chronic disease risk factor profile, and limited exposure to State-funded health promotion/obesity prevention initiatives.

The study LGA is predominately a rural area, growing mainly wheat, barley, oilseeds and legumes, and grazing sheep [26]. Geographically classified as remote (population size 5000–10,000), the LGA is described as having moderate accessibility based on minimum road distance from populated localities to nearest service centres [27]. At the time of this study, the LGA had a total population of 6674 residents across 7158 km^2, comprising one main town (≈2300 residents), eight small towns (≈130 to 800 residents) and eight smaller localities (<100 residents) [26]. The LGA is subdivided into three wards (north, central, south) defined by electoral boundaries, influencing the provision of services and creating three distinct community hubs within the LGA. The LGA scores below the regional State average on the Index of Relative Disadvantage, with up to 59% of families in some towns on low incomes; a high proportion of people aged over 65 and people with a disability; and high levels of social isolation [28,29]. Compared with State averages, the LGA experiences a high prevalence of overweight (38.3% vs. Victorian average 31.2%) and obesity (38.3% vs. Victorian average 18.8%); low fruit and vegetable consumption (4.5% vs. Victorian average 5.2%); high sugar sweetened beverage consumption (30.3% vs. Victorian average 15.9%); high take-away meal consumption (80.9% eating takeaway once per week vs. Victorian average 71.2%); and similar levels of food insecurity (4.6%) [30].

2.2. Selection of Data Collection Tool

The Healthy Diets ASAP tool was used to collect food pricing information (Supplementary File S1) [21,23] for the recommended Australian diet, defined by the Australian Dietary Guidelines (ADG) [24], and the current Australian diet, described by the Australian Health Survey (AHS) [25] (Table 1). The current Australian diet is comparable with that reported for the study LGA [30]; namely; low daily fruit consumption (LGA 1.3 serves vs. AHS 1.2 serves vs. ADG 2 serves); low daily vegetable consumption (LGA 2.5 serves vs. AHS 2.7 serves vs. ADG 5 serves).

Table 1. Comparison of the recommended and current Australian diets for males and females (19–50 years) [12].

Food Groupings (Recommended Serves/Day)	Australian Dietary Guidelines—Recommended Dietary Intakes		Australian Health Survey—Current Dietary Intakes	
	Males	Females	Males	Females
Bread and Cereals	6	6	5.2	3.7
Fruit	2	2	1.2	1.1
Vegetables	6	5	2.8	2.7
Dairy	2.5	2.5	1.6	1.3
Meat and alternatives	3	2.5	2.2	1.6
Discretionary items	0	0	6.4	4.2

2.3. Selection of Retail Food Outlets

Thirty-nine retail food outlets (supermarkets, general stores, bakeries, take-away outlets, cafes, hotels/pubs and service stations) were identified across the LGA using the community directory available on the LGA website. Validation of these business listings, using 'ground truthing' (physically viewing and recording of outlets) [31], identified that three outlets had closed and four new outlets had opened. All outlets operating at the time of the study were surveyed (*n* = 40). These outlets were located across ten towns within the LGA.

2.4. Data Collection

Assistance was provided by AL and ML regarding the use of the Healthy Diets ASAP tool protocols [23] and data were collected by four researchers, working in pairs (PL, JW, FG, CR), within one week in June 2017. As per protocol, within each town, all supermarkets and general stores were surveyed first, followed by bakeries, take-away outlets, cafes, hotels/pubs, and service stations. Permission to participate was obtained verbally from each outlet manager immediately prior to data collection, with all outlets agreeing to participate. Data collected included usual price for specified brands and sizes; sale/special promotion price if usual price was unavailable; price of cheapest brand if specified brand was unavailable; price of nearest larger size (or nearest smaller size) if specified size was unavailable; and cheapest usual price for loose fresh produce. Alternate product brand names and sizes were recorded. Unavailable items were cross checked with outlet managers to determine if out of stock or never stocked. Information for out of stock items was provided by outlet managers, and never stocked items were recorded as missing.

2.5. Data Entry

Eleven data sheets were compiled representing the main town with two supermarkets, and the nine smaller towns each with one supermarket or general store. Data entry was done by F.G. and C.R. with all entries cross-checked by PL and JW. As per protocol, missing items within an outlet were allocated the mean price for that item from all other outlets across the LGA.; and price conversions were calculated for alternate product sizes. The Healthy Diets ASAP tool uses the reference household of two parents (one full-time employed; one part-time employed) and two children (boy aged 14 years; girl aged 8 years). Median disposable family income for this reference household was derived from recent census data for the LGA, calculated at $AUD2358/fortnight [26]. Using the Healthy Diets ASAP tool protocol, indicative minimum disposable income for this reference household was calculated based on minimum wage rates, family tax benefits and relevant welfare payments derived from the Australian Government Department of Human Services [32], calculated at $AUD2167.24/fortnight as detailed in Table 2. The LGA scores below the regional State average on the Index of Relative Disadvantage [28] with only 7.3% of households on high incomes [26].

2.6. Data Analysis

Data were analysed to explore price differential and affordability of the recommended diet and current diet for the reference household for the whole LGA; by ward (south, central and north); and each town within the LGA. Mean food prices were used for whole of LGA and by ward analyses. Price differentials were compared using the following metrics: total diet; each of the five food groups (fruit; vegetables/legumes; grains/cereals; meats/nuts/seeds/eggs; and milk/yoghurt/cheese); unsaturated oils/spreads; discretionary items (take-away foods, soft drinks, alcoholic beverages). Data were also entered into SPSS version 25 and Wilcoxon-signed ranks test were used to compare total diet costs between towns, and between the northern, central and southern areas of the LGA. Affordability of the recommended diet and current diet was calculated as a proportion of household income using median and indicative minimum disposable incomes for an average and low income household, respectively.

Table 2. Low income household calculations ($AUD) for reference household of two parents with two children within the Local Government Area (adult male; adult female; boy 14 years; girl 8 years).

Assumptions [a]	Fortnightly Income	
The family is privately renting a 3 bedroom house at $130/week	Paid employment—adult male	$1390.04
The adult male works on a permanent basis at national minimum wage * ($18.29/h) for 38 h/week	Paid employment—adult female	$219.00
The adult female works on a part-time basis at national minimum wage * ($18.29/h) for 6 h/week	Family Tax Benefit A ^	$420.70
Both children attend school and are fully immunised	Family Tax Benefit A supplement	$55.87
None of the family are disabled	Family Tax Benefit B ^^	$108.64
The family have some emergency savings that earn negligible interest	Family Tax Benefit B Supplement	$13.62
The family has negligible tax deductions	Clean Energy Supplement	$9.94
	Rent Assistance **	$132.61
	INCOME TAX PAID #	−$185.66
	TOTAL FORTNIGHTLY INCOME	**$2167.24**

[a] Verification of assumptions: https://profile.id.com.au/; * Minimum Wage: https://www.fairwork.gov.au/how-we-will-help/templates-and-guides/fact-sheets/minimum-workplace-entitlements/minimum-wages. # current-national-minimum-wage; ^ Family Tax A: https://www.humanservices.gov.au/customer/enablers/payment-rates-family-tax-benefit-part; ^^ Family Tax B: https://www.humanservices.gov.au/customer/enablers/payment-rates-family-tax-benefit-part-b; ** Rent Assistance: Full amount of rent assistance paid to couple with 1 or 2 children if rent is >$436.19 per fortnight, minimum rent is $229.8/fortnight. Full amount is $155.26/fortnight. Rent assistance is paid at the rate of 75 cents for every dollar of rent paid in excess of that threshold up to the maximum rate applicable to the person. Rental at $260/fortnight; rent assistance = 155.26 − [260 − 229.80 × 0.75] = $132.61 https://www.humanservices.gov.au/individuals/enablers/how-much-rent-assistance-you-can-get; # Income tax paid: (income tax due + income tax offset + remote area tax offset) => −5147.45 + 372.29 + 0 = $4775.16; Annual income tax due: tax bracket >$37,000 − $87,000 => $3572 plus 32.5c for each $1 over $37,000; Annual income at $41,847.52; Tax paid = 3572 + [(41,847.52 − 37,000.00) × 0.325] = $5147.45; Annual income tax offset: available if taxable income is <$66,667. Maximum tax offset of $445 applies if taxable income is $37,000 or less. This amount is reduced by 1.5 cents for each dollar over $37,000. Annual income at $41847.52; Tax offset = 445 − [(41,847.52 − 37,000.00) × 0.015] = $372.29 https://www.ato.gov.au/individuals/income-and-deductions/offsets-and-rebates/low-income-earners/.

3. Results

Forty retail food outlets were included in the study, located across 10 towns, and categorized as supermarkets (*n* = 5), general stores (*n* = 6), bakeries (*n* = 2), take-away outlets (*n* = 6), cafés (*n* = 7), hotels/pubs (*n* = 12) and service stations (*n* = 2) (Table 3). The majority of outlets (*n* = 14) were in the main town, with a range of 2–5 outlets in the smaller towns. Supermarkets were located in four towns; two in the main town and one each in the three next most populated towns. General stores were located in the six remaining towns. All towns had at least one hotel/pub, and the majority of towns had a café and/or take-away outlet. Three towns, all with populations less than 150, had no cafés or take-away outlets (Figure 1).

Pricing for the recommended and current diets, using the reference household, are presented for the whole LGA, and the southern, central and northern communities of the LGA in Figure 2 and Appendix A. Figure 2 also illustrates the contribution of the cost of component food groups to total diet costs. Data for each town is available in Supplementary File S2.

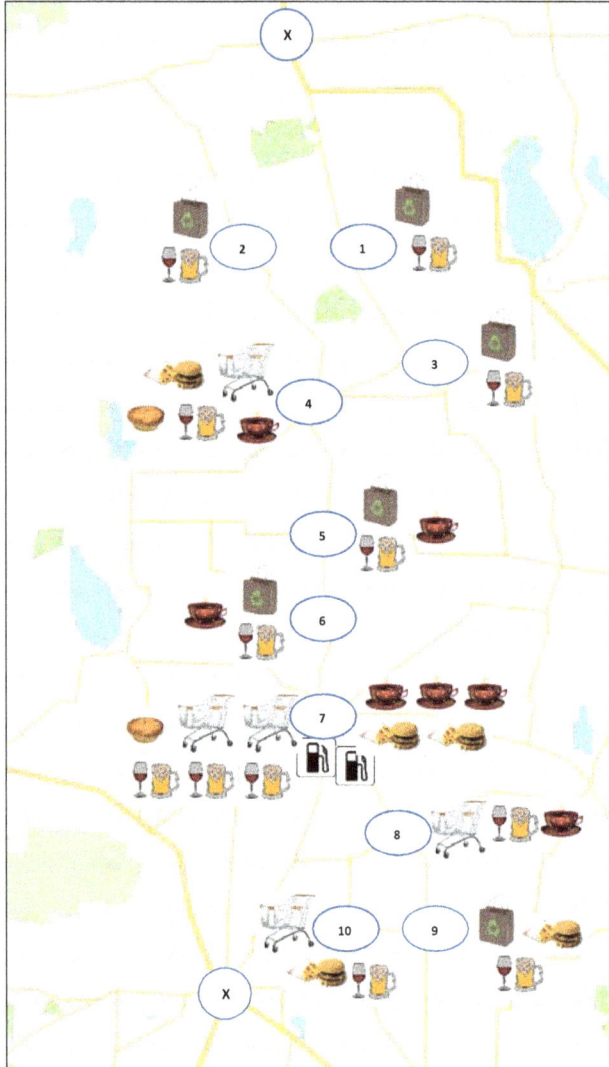

X - nearest next town
(153.9km from main town)
(pop≈1190)

①115km from main town
(pop≈<150)

② 112km from main town
(pop≈<150)

③ 93km from main town
(pop≈<150)

④ 63km from main town
(pop≈525)

⑤ 37km from main town
(pop≈175)

NORTH-------------------------

⑥26km from main town
(pop≈175)

⑦ **MAIN TOWN**
(pop≈2300)

SOUTH-------------------------

⑧ 31km from main town
(pop≈420)

⑨ 49km from main town
(pop≈345)

⑩ 55km from main town
(pop≈785)

X - nearest next town
(59km from main town)
(pop≈16800)

LEGEND:
Supermarket   General Store   Service Station   Bakery

Take-away   Hotel/Pub   Café   pop = population of town

(x)   **Nearest town outside LGA boundary**   (#)   **Town in LGA (km from main town in LGA)**

Figure 1. Distribution of food retail outlets across ten towns within the Local Government Area indicating type of outlet and distance (km) of towns from the main town (https://www.google.com/maps).

Table 3. Number and type of retail food outlet surveyed across the Local Government Area (LGA).

Retail Food Outlet by Town		Super-Market [a]	General Store [b]	Bakery	Take-Away	Café	Hotel/Pub	Service Station	Total Outlets by Town
North of LGA	Town 1		1				1		2
	Town 2		1				1		2
	Town 3		1				1		2
	Town 4	1		1	1	1	1		5
	Town 5		1				1	1	3
Centre of LGA	Town 6		1			1	1		3
	Town 7	2		1	3	3	3	2	14
South of LGA	Town 8	1				1	1		3
	Town 9		1		1		1		3
	Town 10	1			1		1		3
Total Outlets by Type		5	6	2	6	7	12	2	40

[a] Supermarket—chain store, selling food products predominantly, open for extended hours on most day; [b] General stores—privately owned, selling food products and other items, open for limited hours.

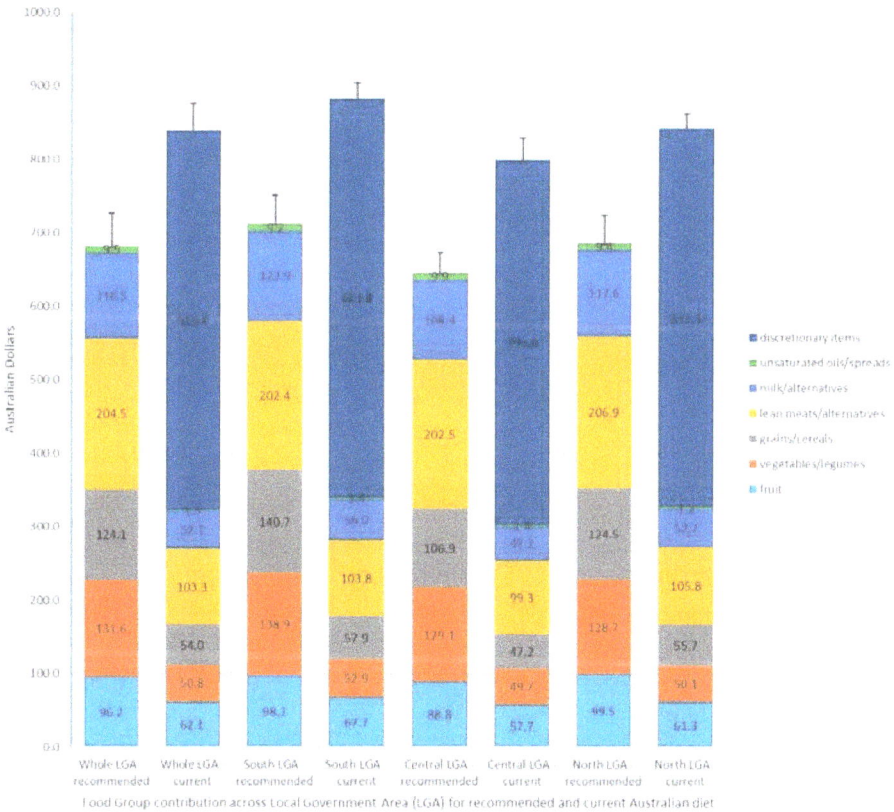

Figure 2. Food group contribution and total diet costs for recommended and current diets for the Local Government Area ($AUDmean ± SD per fortnight).

Across the LGA, the recommended diet was cheaper than the current diet ($AUD702.41 ± 44.80 vs. $AUD866.19 ± 37.54 per fortnight/reference household), costing an average 81.1% of the current diet budget. Within the current diet, expenditure for all five food groups was less than half what would be required to achieve recommended intakes of these foods; namely, fruit and vegetables (13% current vs. 32% required); grains/cereal-based foods (6.2% current vs. 17.7% required); lean meats, poultry, fish, eggs (11.9% current vs. 29.1% required); and milk, cheese, yoghurt (6.0% vs. 16.6%). The majority of the current diet budget was spent on discretionary items (59.5%), particularly take-away foods/beverages (18.1%) and alcoholic beverages (11.2%).

For each of the three LGA wards, the recommended diet was cheaper than the current diet, costing an average 81.3% of the current diet budget for southern and northern wards, and an average of 80.4% for central towns (Supplementary File S2). Food item prices were higher in the southern (8.7%) and northern (5.5%) towns than the central towns in the LGA. Food item prices in the southern towns were highest for four of the five food groups (especially fruits, grains, and milk, cheese and yoghurt); take-away food items were the most expensive (approximately 12–13%); and sugar-sweetened beverages were the cheapest. For towns in the centre of the LGA, take-away food items were the cheapest and sugar-sweetened beverages the most expensive (approximately 19–23%). For both the southern and northern towns, price differences were greatest for grains (approximately 15–19%) and milk, cheese and yoghurt (approximately 10–16%) than the other five food groups.

Across the LGA the cost of the current diet was statistically significantly higher than the recommended diet at $p < 0.05$. There were no significant differences between the three LGA wards.

Affordability of the recommended and current diets was calculated using median and indicative minimum disposable incomes for an average and low income household, respectively (Table 4). Across the LGA, the recommended diet ($AUD702.41 ± 44.80/fortnight/reference household) would expend 30–32% of a median and low income household, respectively; and the current diet ($AUD866.19 ± 37.54/fortnight/reference household) would expend 37–40% of a median and low income household. Affordability of the recommended diet as a proportion of household income was similar for the southern and northern towns, approximately 2% higher than towns in the centre of the LGA.

Availability of food items listed on the Healthy Diets ASAP tool protocol ($n = 76$) varied across the ten towns within the LGA. All items were available within the main town, which had two supermarkets and twelve other food retail outlets. Towns with supermarkets appeared to have fewer missing food items (3–12 missing items) compared to towns with only a general store (18–38 missing items). Most commonly missing food items were low fat yoghurt and low fat cheese (available only in the main town); cooked whole chicken (available in two towns); canned sweetcorn (no added salt) and extra virgin olive oil (both available in three towns); and unsalted peanuts (available in four towns). Yoghurt (full or reduced fat) was unavailable in five towns. Specific product brands and product sizes were unavailable for 36 (47%) and 43 (75%) of the listed food items, respectively, requiring substitution with price of cheapest brand and price of nearest larger (or nearest smaller) size. As per protocol, missing items within an outlet were allocated the mean price for that item from all other outlets across the LGA, thereby minimizing effects to food budget calculations.

Table 4. Affordability (% household income) of the recommended diet and current diet across the Local Government Area (LGA) for the reference household by median and low income ($AUD).

LGA Area and Town	Median Household Income ($2358)		Low Household Income ($2167)	
	Recommended Diet (%)	Current Diet (%)	Recommended Diet (%)	Current Diet (%)
Whole of LGA	30	37	32	40
Town 1	28	36	30	39
Town 2	28	37	31	40
Town 3	32	37	35	41
Town 4	30	32	33	34
Town 5	32	38	34	42
North of the LGA	30	37	33	40
Town 6	27	35	30	38
Town 7	27–30	33–36	30–32	36–40
Centre of the LGA	28	35	31	38
Town 8	31	37	33	40
Town 9	33	39	36	42
Town 10	29	39	32	42
South of the LGA	30	37	32	40

4. Discussion

This study assessed the price, price differential (relative price) and affordability of the recommended and current diets in a small rural LGA in Victoria, Australia. Study findings confirm the paradoxical co-existence of food insecurity, low income and obesity, linked to limited geographical access to a healthy, fresh food supply; limited variety of healthy food options; the ubiquitous availability of highly palatable energy-dense foods, drinks and discretionary items; higher overall food prices; and low incomes reducing affordability of a healthy diet.

Findings suggest that a healthy diet, consistent with national dietary guidelines, is less expensive than the current diet consumed by Australians. For some rural towns, this differential may be as much as 18.9%. The Healthy Diets ASAP tool has only recently been used within Australia, with available studies of the pilot approach limited to urban areas reporting a finding of 16.3% for a low income household [21]. These findings challenge the perception that a healthy diet is more expensive, as described in a systematic review of food pricing studies across 10 countries (excluding Australia) [33] which found little difference between the cost of healthier and unhealthy dietary patterns. As explained by Lewis and Lee [13], studies included in this review did not consider the contribution of alcoholic beverages or most other discretionary items[1] to the cost of the diet nor the application of a goods and sales tax (GST) exemption to certain food items. The inclusion of discretionary items is important in the Australian context, as over a third (35%) of the total daily intake of Australians comprises discretionary items in the form of biscuits, cakes, confectionary, sugar-sweetened beverages and alcoholic beverages [12]. Additionally Australia applies a 10% GST exemption to basic, healthy foods in the five food groups such as fruit, vegetables, bread, fresh meat, eggs and milk [34], increasing the affordability of these food items.

On average the income of Australian families in rural and remote areas is 15–20% lower than in metropolitan areas, which together with higher food prices in these areas, makes it difficult to afford a healthy diet [15]. While purchasing a recommended diet may be less expensive than the current diet, findings from this study highlight that it would account for almost a third of the budget for median (30%) and low (32%) income households in the LGA. These levels of affordability align with those reported by the Healthy Diets ASAP pilot tool, where a recommended diet accounted for 20–29% of a low income household budget in an urban area [21]. Study findings are similar however to research using 'healthy food basket' methodologies which found the recommended diet accounted for between 26–32% of a low income household budget across urban and rural towns of South Australia [17], Victoria [16,35] and Queensland [36]. While there is no accepted benchmark for affordability of a healthy diet [22], relative unaffordability is commonly associated with food costs accounting for 30% or more of the household budget [1,35]. Recently, Ward et al. [17] have proposed that 'food stress' occurs when food costs account for 25% or more of the household income.

Australian studies consistently show significant increases in food pricing as one moves from inner city to suburban to regional and rural areas [16,17,35,36]. "Out-shopping", purchasing food outside of one's local area from a larger centre, is therefore a common practice in rural areas [37] to benefit from lower prices and greater variety. In this study, differences in food prices were observed across the LGA, with prices 8–10% higher in the south. Furthermore, a comparison of the cost of a 'Victorian Healthy Food Basket' for the LGA ($AUD528.41), with neighbouring regional towns ($AUD438.30—town population ≈ 17,000; $AUD453.34—town population ≈ 30,000) reveals that food prices are lower in regional towns outside the LGA boundary [38,39]. In addition to higher food pricing and out-shopping, rural communities often experience low density transport networks, leading to an increased reliance on motor vehicles, with associated time, fuel and vehicle maintenance costs, when purchasing food [15].

This study also found that the majority of the food budget was spent on discretionary items (59.5%), of which take-away foods comprised 18%. The Australian Dietary Guidelines food price indexes report [40] estimates that 58.2% of the 2014 household food budget was spent on discretionary items; and Lee et al. [21] report a similar figure of 58% for households in an urban area. While study findings on discretionary item expenditure are higher than reported by others, they do align with the Victorian Population Health Survey [30], with the LGA having high sugar sweetened beverage consumption (30.3% vs. Victorian average 15.9%), low fruit and vegetable consumption (4.5% vs. Victorian average 5.2%) [30]; and high take-away meal consumption (80.9% eating takeaway once per week vs. Victorian average 71.2%).

While a recommended diet may cost less than the current diet, it would appear that price is not the main driver of food choice for this community. In addition to the cost of foods, LGA residents have reported poor quality, limited variety (especially culturally appropriate foods), and inadequate or unreliable public transport as other reasons limiting their food choices [28]. The abundant supply of 'convenience' outlets (bakeries, take-away outlets, cafes, hotels/pubs, service stations) also appears to meet consumer demand for convenience [32] and taste [14], overcoming the challenges of limited geographic access, busy lifestyles and limited cooking skills, while also contributing to the local economy.

The rising cost of foods [16] combined with a limited number of food retail outlets, stocking a reduced variety of food items, lowers the likelihood of rural communities adhering to a healthier diet [41]. Rural areas with few supermarkets and several 'convenience' outlets have been found to have higher food prices, and limited availability of fresh produce and healthier food choices, particularly skim/low fat milk, whole wheat bread, fruits and vegetables [42]. Of the 40 food retail outlets included in this study, 11 (27.5%) were supermarkets and general stores selling predominantly healthy five food group items; and 29 (72.5%) were 'convenience' outlets selling predominately discretionary and take-away food items. Rural towns in Victoria have consistently been excluded from 'Victorian Healthy Food Basket' studies as they do not meet the inclusion criterion of stocking at least 90% (40 of 44) of listed food items [16,19]. Similarly, this study found that healthier food items were frequently unavailable in smaller general stores compared with supermarkets.

There is potential for supermarkets to increase variety and quality of fresh and healthy food options; provide competitive, lower pricing for healthy foods; and improve geographic access in areas described as 'food deserts' [41]. However, studies in the United States show that while supermarkets improve the perceptions of healthy food access amongst residents, improvements in net availability of healthy foods may be minimal, with residents continuing to shop outside their local area; more food stores stocking a wider variety of all food products; and greater market segmentation with 'convenience' outlets reducing stocks of healthy foods [41]. Positive impacts on food pricing however may be experienced with healthy foods offered at lower prices and discretionary item prices increasing as 'convenience' outlets attempt to compensate for reduced stocks of healthy foods [41]. In Australia, supermarkets are described by Pulker et al. [43] (p. 1) as having *"a powerful position in the Australian food system . . . . . . acting as gate-keepers between food producers and consumers"*, thereby influencing the range and price of food choices available, and shaping consumer preferences and social norms. While Australian supermarkets demonstrate some commitment to nutrition promotion and the prevention of obesity, Sacks et al. [44] argue that more is needed across this sector, especially to address the availability, affordability and promotion of healthy food choices.

In contrast to the establishment of new supermarkets, improvements to existing stores is suggested as a less time consuming and less expensive strategy to improve the variety and relative price of healthy food options in underserved areas with 'food deserts' [41]. In-store activities found to be feasible and acceptable to food retailers in rural communities, with modest levels of effectiveness, appear to focus predominately on health promotional practices, such as the provision of recipes and shopping lists for healthy meals, in-store displays with healthy samples, promotional signage within the store, and point-of-purchase signage for fruits and vegetables [45]. In a recent systematic review of 30 studies across nine countries regarding the effectiveness of food pricing strategies, Gittelsohn et al. [46] found that nearly all studies (*n* = 27) used in-store pricing strategies to promote healthy foods, most commonly fruits and vegetables (usually through price discounts, coupons and vouchers). Few studies (*n* = 6) used pricing strategies to specifically discourage unhealthy foods such as sugar-sweetened beverages and foods high in fat and/or sugar (using a price increase). It was noted that using pricing strategies that target only fruits and vegetables may be difficult for small retail outlets to implement, especially in low income communities, as fresh produce is often hard to source and highly perishable; and therefore any price incentives should cover a broad range of healthy food items [46].

In one of few studies exploring the perspectives of retailers, Kim et al. [47] found that small store owners in a low income community, regardless of their ethnic background, regarded customer preferences and wholesaler availability of food products as critical barriers to the provision of healthy options. The stocking of 'low customer demand' items was perceived to be a high-risk investment resulting in possible sales loss. When queried about pricing strategies, concerns were raised about offering discounts on multiple items given the small range of products the stores usually stocked. Retailers felt that discounts created price fluctuations and customer dissatisfaction when prices returned to normal. They also described the availability and pricing/discounting of items as being highly dependent on what wholesalers can offer [47].

Rural communities in Australia are serviced by long food supply chains which are not flexible to sudden changes or able to keep inventories to a minimum; instead they encourage the delivery of set quotas of items with a long shelf life [15]. Small stores not aligned to major supermarket chains are therefore at a disadvantage in acquiring fresh produce regularly and at competitive prices. Strategies to improve and/or subsidise the freighting of food to remote Australian communities have been suggested for communities who face similar challenges of vast distances, extreme temperatures and variable road conditions [48,49]. For example, 'group freight buying' where a group of stores combines their volumes to fill transport units on a geographically logical freight route that are not at full capacity, resulting in increased service frequency and/or lower freight costs per unit transported [49]. Such strategies will require leadership across all levels of government, and a strong commitment to the development and implementation of a National Nutrition Policy [50] and a National Food Plan that considers health [51].

At a policy level, food pricing options exist in the form of taxation, subsidisation, or a combination of these [22,52]. The taxing of unhealthy foods is considered of benefit for raising revenue as well as an effective strategy to improve dietary behaviours [53]; and subsidising healthy food is considered of benefit in making these foods more affordable and also, though to a smaller effect, appear to improve dietary behaviours [21,52]. For Australia, the exemption of 'healthy' foods from goods and sales tax (GST) is a means of reducing 'food stress' for low income families. Without this safeguard, Lee et al. [21] estimate that the cost of a healthy (recommended) diet would increase by approximately 10%, with the likelihood of a greater proportion of the food budget being spent on discretionary items.

5. Strengths and Limitations

To our knowledge, this is the first study in rural Australia to utilize the Healthy Diets ASAP tool to explore the price, price differential and affordability of the recommended and current diet. This study was also able to survey all supermarkets and general stores given the relative low number of outlets available, thereby providing a true representation for this LGA. While an advantage to data collection, a small sample size of retail outlets poses limitations for statistically analysis.

As a cross sectional study, data collection reflects a single time point, occurring on random days of the week during Winter, and therefore pricing information is indicative of seasonal and wholesaler availability at that time. 'Ground truthing' was used to identify and verify the presence of operational food stores, however food environments are constantly subject to change, and food stores included in this study may have since closed and/or new businesses opened.

No data was collected regarding consumer shopping venue preferences, especially the phenomena of 'out-shopping' which is known to occur anecdotally; nor other means through which food items may be obtained such as the community garden, food swaps, the food pantry or food bank. It was also out of scope for this study to conduct in-depth interviews with food store owners which may have elicited information regarding food pricing strategies.

The Healthy Diets ASAP tool was a practical and time efficient survey to conduct across the LGA. While some product brands/sizes were different to those specified on the protocol, the tool allowed for alternate brands/sizes to be included. The use of average prices for missing/unavailable items may have led to an underestimation of the cost of the diet for these towns as residents would have travelled to purchase this item elsewhere. Information on unavailable items will be used to update the tool for greater utility. The tool has been developed for different reference households, with the default being two adults and two children. It may be necessary to enable a wider application to other reference households to better reflect the demographics of rural, remote communities with higher numbers of elderly couples with no children and single-parent families.

6. Conclusions

This study confirms that while a healthy diet is less expensive than the current unhealthy diet, affordability is a challenge for Australians living in rural Victoria, especially for families on median or low incomes. For these communities, food security is compromised by limited geographical access to food retail outlets, with most outlets, especially in smaller towns, offering a reduced variety of healthy food choices at higher prices.

Implications for research: Research shows that rural, remote communities have poor adherence to recommended dietary guidelines, experience higher rates of overweight/obesity and associated chronic disease, and are disproportionately affected by the influence of their food environment compared with their urban counterparts. There appears to be a gap, however, in research regarding the influence of food environments among rural communities. Continued research in this area is therefore warranted to improve our understanding and identification of important determinants of diet for these Australian communities.

Implications for practice and policy: It would appear that price is not the main driver of food choice for rural, remote Australian communities. A preference for unhealthier foods, that meet the needs of convenience and taste, undermines the establishment of a reliable demand-supply cycle that would be economically viable for small food retailers. The challenge of food distribution across vast distances to provide affordable, quality produce also serves as a barrier within rural communities affecting accessibility and availability of supply. Understanding the associations between these factors will help to shape appropriate interventions needed at the individual, organizational, community and policy level. It is evident that a combination of strategies is required, including public health campaigns and programs targeting the individual to improve food literacy knowledge and skills; interventions in food retail outlets to improve affordability and promotion of healthier foods/drinks; establishing alternative community-led food supply options such as food cooperatives, farmers' markets and community gardens; safeguarding agricultural land use and monitoring the zoning of fast food retail outlets through local, regional and state government planning mechanisms; developing a flexible, responsive food supply chain; and retaining a General Sales Tax (GST) exemption for basic healthy foods.

Supplementary Materials: The following are available online at http://www.mdpi.com/1660-4601/15/11/2469/s1, File S1: Healthy Diets ASAP tool collection sheet; File S2: Food pricing data for LGA and towns.

Author Contributions: P.L. and J.W. conceived and designed the study with input from C.B.; A.L. and M.L. provided expertise on the Healthy Diets ASAP tool methodology; P.L., J.W., F.G. and C.R. undertook data collection and analysis; M.L. cross-checked data analysis; P.L. led the writing of the manuscript with input from all authors. All authors approved the manuscript for submission.

Funding: This research received no external funding. J.W. was funded through the Royal Flying Doctors Services, Victoria.

Acknowledgments: The authors thank all retail outlet owners within the study area for their willingness and time to participate in this study.

Conflicts of Interest: The authors declare no conflict of interest.

Appendix

Table A1. Price of recommended and current diets for the Local Government Area (using a reference household of two parents and two children).

Northern LGA = towns 1,2,3,4,5; Central LGA = towns 6,7; Southern LGA = towns 8,9,10	Whole LGA—Recommended Diet	Whole LGA—Current Diet	Southern LGA—Recommended Diet	Southern LGA—Current Diet	Central LGA—Recommended Diet	Central LGA—Current Diet	Northern LGA—Recommended Diet	Northern LGA—Current Diet
TOTAL DIET $mean ±sd	702.41 ± 44.89	866.19 ± 37.54	733.31 ± 39.70	901.38 ± 20.87	661.96 ± 27.66	823.23 ± 29.55	708.14 ± 37.96	870.86 ± 21.02
CORE 5 FOOD GROUP FOODS $mean +sd (%total diet cost)	702.41 ± 44.89 (100.0%)	343.47 ± 26.93 (39.65%)	733.31 ± 39.70 (100%)	360.24 ± 23.33 (39.97%)	661.96 ± 27.66 (100%)	318.79 ± 19.23 (38.72%)	708.14 ± 37.96 (100%)	348.20 ± 22.15 (39.98%)
FRUIT $mean ±sd (%total diet cost)	96.20 ± 13.89 (13.70%)	62.06 ± 11.45 (7.16%)	98.14 ± 15.29 (13.38%)	67.73 ± 12.11 (7.51%)	88.77 ± 2.48 (13.41%)	57.65 ± 2.35 (7.00%)	99.49 ± 15.30 (14.05%)	61.31 ± 12.87 (7.04%)
VEGETABLES/LEGUMES $mean ±sd (%total diet cost)	131.61 ± 8.71 (18.74%)	50.77 ± 4.39 (5.86%)	138.87 ± 1.15 (18.94%)	52.90 ± 2.75 (5.87%)	129.14 ± 10.15 (19.51%)	49.74 ± 5.13 (6.04%)	128.74 ± 7.80 (18.18%)	50.10 ± 4.26 (5.75%)
FRUIT & VEG/LEGUMES $mean ±sd (%total diet cost)	227.81 ± 18.81 (32.43%)	112.83 ± 13.00 (13.03%)	237.01 ± 15.77 (32.32%)	120.64 ± 12.67 (13.38%)	217.90 ± 11.33 (32.92%)	107.39 ± 7.33 (13.04%)	228.23 ± 21.02 (32.23%)	111.41 ± 13.66 (12.79%)
GRAINS/CEREALS $mean ±sd (%total diet cost)	124.11 ± 17.69 (17.67%)	53.98 ± 5.13 (6.23%)	140.70 ± 13.93 (19.19%)	57.93 ± 3.86 (6.43%)	106.86 ± 8.71 (16.14%)	47.22 ± 2.06 (5.74%)	124.50 ± 13.52(17.58%)	55.68 ± 2.63 (6.39%)
LEAN MEATS & ALT $mean ±sd (%total diet cost)	204.48 ± 9.05 (29.11%)	103.27 ± 6.56 (11.92%)	202.41 ± 11.03 (27.60%)	103.80 ± 6.06 (11.44%)	202.54 ± 10.10 (30.60%)	99.32 ± 7.22 (12.06%)	206.88 ± 5.94 (29.22%)	105.76 ± 5.08 (12.14%)
MILK & ALT $mean ±sd (%total diet cost)	116.54 ± 6.64 (16.59%)	52.08 ± 4.82 (6.01%)	122.86 ± 3.30 (16.75%)	55.99 ± 4.79 (6.21%)	108.40 ± 5.41 (16.38%)	47.17 ± 2.80 (5.73%)	117.64 ± 2.83 (16.61%)	52.67 ± 2.94 (6.05%)
UNSATURATED OILS/SPREADS $mean ±sd (%total diet cost)	9.47 ± 0.86 (1.35%)	1.30 ± 0.19 (1.15%)	9.16 ± 1.25 (1.25%)	1.43 ± 0.19 (0.16%)	9.92 ± 0.22 (1.50%)	1.36 ± 0.07 (0.17%)	9.39 ± 0.69 (1.33%)	1.19 ± 0.17 (0.14%)
WATER $mean +sd (%total diet cost)	20.00 ± 5.90 (2.85%)	20.00 ± 5.90 (2.31%)	21.18 ± 8.31 (2.89%)	21.18 ± 8.31 (2.35%)	16.33 ± 5.55 (2.47%)	16.33 ± 5.55 (1.98%)	21.50 ± 2.32 (3.04%)	21.50 ± 2.32 (2.47%)
ALL DISCRETIONARY FOODS $mean +sd (%total diet cost)		515.42 ± 22.77 (59.50%)		534.77 ± 28.41 (59.33%)		496.63 ± 17.77 (60.33%)		515.08 ± 5.49 (59.15%)
TAKE-AWAY FOODS $mean +sd (%total diet cost)		156.67 ± 15.29 (18.09%)		172.48 ± 19.10 (19.13%)		149.97 ± 3.06 (18.22%)		151.20 ± 9.14 (17.36%)
ARTIFICIALLY SWEETENED BEVERAGES $mean +sd (%total diet cost)		7.31 ± 1.10 (0.84%)		6.37 ± 0.93 (0.71%)		7.81 ± 0.91 (0.95%)		7.58 ± 0.96 (0.87%)
SUGAR SWEETENED BEVERAGES $mean +sd (%total diet cost)		44.03 ± 6.66 (5.08%)		38.37 ± 5.63 (4.26%)		47.05 ± 5.46(5.72%)		45.61 ± 5.79 (5.24%)
ALCOHOLIC BEVERAGES $mean +sd (%total diet cost)		97.33 ± 9.74 (11.24%)		102.63 ± 12.40 (11.39%)		88.45 ± 6.96 (10.74%)		99.47 ± 4.30 (11.42%)

References

1. Burns, C.; Friel, S. It's time to determine the cost of a healthy diet in Australia. *ANZJPH* **2007**, *31*, 363–365. [CrossRef]
2. HLPE. *Food Security and Climate Change*; Committee on World Food Security: Rome, Italy, 2012.
3. McKechnie, R.; Turrell, G.; Giskes, K.; Gallegos, D. Single-item measure of food insecurity used in the national health survey may underestimate prevalence in Australia. *ANZJPH* **2018**, *42*, 389–395. [CrossRef] [PubMed]
4. ABS. *Australian National Health Survey—First Results 2014–2015*; Australian Bureau of Statistics: Canberra, Australia, 2015.
5. Franklin, B.; Jones, A.; Love, D.; Puckett, S.; Macklin, J.; White-Means, S. Exploring mediators of food insecurity and obesity: A review of recent literature. *J. Community Health* **2012**, *37*, 253–264. [CrossRef] [PubMed]
6. Abarca-Gómez, L.; Abdeen, Z.A.; Hamid, Z.A.; Abu-Rmeileh, N.M.; Acosta-Cazares, B.; Acuin, C.; Adams, R.J.; Aekplakorn, W.; Afsana, K.; Aguilar-Salinas, C.A.; et al. Worldwide trends in body-mass index, underweight, overweight, and obesity from 1975 to 2016: A pooled analysis of 2416 population based measurement studies in 128·9 million children, adolescents, and adults. *Lancet* **2017**, *390*, 2627–2642. [CrossRef]
7. AIHW. *Australian Burden of Disease: Impact of Overweight and Obesity as a Risk Factor for Chronic Conditions*; Australian Institute of Health and Welfare: Canberra, Australia, 2017.
8. Glanz, K.; Johnson, L.; Yaroch, A.L.; Phillips, M.; Ayala, G.X.; Davis, E.L. Measures of retail food store environments and sales: Review and implications for healthy eating initiatives. *J. Nutr. Educ. Behav.* **2016**, *48*, 280.e1–288.e1. [CrossRef] [PubMed]
9. Swinburn, B.A.; Sacks, G.; Hall, K.D.; McPherson, K.; Finegood, D.T.; Moodie, M.L.; Gortmaker, S.L. The global obesity pandemic: Shaped by global drivers and local environments. *Lancet* **2011**, *378*, 804–814. [CrossRef]
10. Backholer, K.; Spencer, E.; Gearon, E.; Magliano, D.J.; McNaughton, S.A.; Shaw, J.E.; Peeters, A. The association between socio-economic position and diet quality in Australian adults. *Public Health Nutr.* **2016**, *19*, 477–485. [CrossRef] [PubMed]
11. AIHW. *Australian Burden of Disease Study: Impact and Causes of Illness and Deaths in Australia 2011*; Australian Institute of Health and Welfare: Canberra, Australia, 2016.
12. ABS. *Australian Health Survey—Consumption of Food Groups from the Australian Dietary Guidelines 2011–2012*; Australian Bureau of Statistics: Canberra, Australia, 2016.
13. Lewis, M.; Lee, A. Costing 'healthy' food baskets in Australia—A systematic review of food price and affordability monitoring tools, protocols and methods. *Public Health Nutr.* **2016**, *19*, 2872–2886. [CrossRef] [PubMed]
14. State Government of Victoria. *Victorian Population Health Survey 2012*; Department of Health and Human Services: Melbourne, Australia, 2016.
15. National Rural Health Alliance. *Food Security and Health in Rural and Remote AUSTRALIA*; Rural Industries Research and Development Corporation, Australian Government: Deakin West, ACT, Australia, 2016.
16. Palermo, C.; McCartan, J.; Kleve, S.; Sinha, K.; Shiell, A. A longitudinal study of the cost of food in victoria influenced by geography and nutritional quality. *ANZJPH* **2016**, *40*, 270–273. [CrossRef] [PubMed]
17. Ward, P.R.; Coveney, J.; Verity, F.; Carter, P.; Schilling, M. Cost and affordability of healthy food in rural South Australia. *Rural Remote Health* **2012**, *12*, 1938. [PubMed]
18. Innes-Hughes, C.; Boylan, S.; King, L.; Lobb, E. Measuring the food environment in three rural towns in New South Wales, Australia. *Health Promot. J. Aust.* **2012**, *23*, 129–133. [CrossRef]
19. Palermo, C.E.; Walker, K.Z.; Hill, P.; McDonald, J. The cost of healthy food in rural Victoria. *Rural Remote Health* **2008**, *8*, 1074. [PubMed]
20. Chapman, K.; Innes-Hughes, C.; Goldsbury, D.; Kelly, B.; Bauman, A.; Allman-Farinelli, M. A comparison of the cost of generic and branded food products in Australian supermarkets. *Public Health Nutr.* **2013**, *16*, 894–900. [CrossRef] [PubMed]

21. Lee, A.J.; Kane, S.; Ramsey, R.; Good, E.; Dick, M. Testing the price and affordability of healthy and current (unhealthy) diets and the potential impacts of policy change in Australia. *BMC Public Health* **2016**, *16*, 315. [CrossRef] [PubMed]

22. Lee, A.; Mhurchu, C.N.; Sacks, G.; Swinburn, B.; Snowdon, W.; Vandevijvere, S.; Hawkes, C.; L'Abbe, M.; Rayner, M.; Sanders, D.; et al. Monitoring the price and affordability of foods and diets globally. *Obes. Rev.* **2013**, *14* (Suppl. 1), 82–95. [CrossRef]

23. Lee, A.; Kane, S.; Lewis, M.; Good, E.; Pollard, C.M.; Landrigan, T.J.; Dick, M. Healthy Diets ASAP—Australian Standardised Affordability and Pricing methods protocol. *BMC Nutr. J.* **2018**, *17*, 88. [CrossRef] [PubMed]

24. NHMRC. *Australian Dietary Guidelines*; National Health and Medical Research Council: Canberra, Australia, 2013. Available online: http://www.eatforhealth.gov.au (accessed on 26 August 2018).

25. ABS. *Australian Health Survey—First Results 2011–2012*; Australian Bureau of Statistics: Canberra, Australia, 2012.

26. ABS. Census of Population and Housing—Quickstats, Community Profiles and Datapacks User Guide. Available online: http://quickstats.censusdata.abs.gov.au/census_services/getproduct/census/2016/quickstat/LGA27630 (accessed on 28 August 2017).

27. AIHW. *Rural, Regional and Remote Health: A Guide to Remoteness Classifications*; Australian Institute of Health and Welfare: Canberra, Australia, 2004.

28. Wimmera Primary Care Partnership. *Wimmera Population Health and Wellbeing Profile 2016*; Wimmera Primary Care Partnership: Horsham, Victoria, Australia, 2016.

29. State Government of Victoria. *Change and Disadvantage in the Grampians Region, Vvictoria*; Department of Planning and Community Development: Melbourne, Australia, 2011.

30. State Government of Victoria. *Victorian Population Health Survey 2014: Modifiable Risk Factors Contributing to Chronic Disease in Victoria*; Department of Health and Human Services: Melbourne, Australia, 2016.

31. Caspi, C.E.; Friebur, R. Modified ground-truthing: An accurate and cost-effective food environment validation method for town and rural areas. *IJBNPA* **2016**, *13*, 37. [CrossRef] [PubMed]

32. Australian Government Department of Human Services. Social and Health Payments and Services. Available online: https://www.humanservices.gov.au/ (accessed on 28 August 2017).

33. Rao, M.; Afshin, A.; Singh, G.; Mozaffarian, D. Do healthier foods and diet patterns cost more than less healthy options? A systematic review and meta-analysis. *BMJ Open* **2013**, *3*, e004277. [CrossRef] [PubMed]

34. Australian Taxation Office, A.G. GST-Free Food. Available online: https://www.ato.gov.au/Business/GST/In-detail/Your-industry/Food/GST-and-food/?anchor=GSTfreefood (accessed on 3 July 2018).

35. Rossimel, A.; Han, S.S.; Larsen, K.; Palermo, C. Access and affordability of nutritious food in metropolitan Melbourne. *Nutr. Diet.* **2016**, *73*, 13–18. [CrossRef]

36. Harrison, M.; Lee, A.; Findlay, M.; Nicholls, R.; Leonard, D.; Martin, C. The increasing cost of healthy food. *ANZJPH* **2010**, *34*, 179–186. [CrossRef] [PubMed]

37. Bardenhagen, C.J.; Pinard, C.A.; Pirog, R.; Yaroch, A.L. Characterizing rural food access in remote areas. *J. Community Health* **2017**, *42*, 1008–1019. [CrossRef] [PubMed]

38. State Government of Victoria. *VLGA Food Scan Report: Mildura Rural City Council*; Healthy Together Victoria: Mildura, Australia, 2013.

39. Wimmera Food Security Group. *Victorian Healthy Food Basket Survey—Summer 2016–2017*; Wimmera Primary Care Partnership: Horsham, Victoria, Australia, 2017.

40. ABS. Australian Dietary Guideline Food Price Indexes Series 6401.1. Available online: http://www.abs.gov.au/AUSSTATS/abs@.nsf/Previousproducts/6401.0Feature%20Article1Dec%202015?opendocument&tabname=Summary&prodno=6401.0&issue=Dec%202015&num=&view= (accessed on 12 November 2017).

41. Ghosh-Dastidar, M.; Hunter, G.; Collins, R.L.; Zenk, S.N.; Cummins, S.; Beckman, R.; Nugroho, A.K.; Sloan, J.C.; Wagner, L.; Dubowitz, T. Does opening a supermarket in a food desert change the food environment? *Health Place* **2017**, *46*, 249–256. [CrossRef] [PubMed]

42. Vilaro, M.; Barnett, T. The rural food environment: A survey of food price, availability, and quality in a rural Florida community. *Food Public Health* **2013**, *3*. [CrossRef]

43. Pulker, C.E.; Trapp, G.S.A.; Scott, J.A.; Pollard, C.M. What are the position and power of supermarkets in the Australian food system, and the implications for public health? A systematic scoping review. *Obes. Rev.* **2018**, *19*, 198–218. [CrossRef] [PubMed]

44. Sacks, G.; Robinson, E.; Cameron, A.; INFORMAS. *Inside Our Supermarkets—Assessment of Company Policies and Committments Related to Obesity Prevention and Nutrition*; Deakin University: Melbourne, Australia, 2018.

45. Martinez-Donate, A.P.; Riggall, A.J.; Meinen, A.M.; Malecki, K.; Escaron, A.L.; Hall, B.; Menzies, A.; Garske, G.; Nieto, F.J.; Nitzke, S. Evaluation of a pilot healthy eating intervention in restaurants and food stores of a rural community: A randomized community trial. *BMC Public Health* **2015**, *15*, 136. [CrossRef] [PubMed]

46. Gittelsohn, J.; Trude, A.C.B.; Kim, H. Pricing strategies to encourage availability, purchase, and consumption of healthy foods and beverages: A systematic review. *Prev. Chronic Dis.* **2017**, *14*, E107. [CrossRef] [PubMed]

47. Kim, M.; Budd, N.; Batorsky, B.; Krubiner, C.; Manchikanti, S.; Waldrop, G.; Trude, A.; Gittelsohn, J. Barriers to and facilitators of stocking healthy food options: Viewpoints of Baltimore city small storeowners. *Ecol. Food Nutr.* **2017**, *56*, 17–30. [CrossRef] [PubMed]

48. *Freight Improvement Toolkit*; National Rural Health Alliance: Canberra, ACT, Australia, 2007.

49. Queensland Health. *Vegetable and Fruit Supply to South West Queensland: An Information Paper*; Queensland Government: Brisbane, Australia, 2006.

50. Lee, A.; Baker, P.; Stanton, R.; Friel, S.; O'Dea, K.; Weightman, A. *Scoping Study to Inform the Development of the New National Nutrition Policy*; (rft 028/1213); Released under FOI, March 2016; QUT, Australian Department of Health and Ageing: Queensland, Brisbane, Australia, 2013.

51. *The People's Food Plan*; Australian Food Sovereignty Alliance: Canberra, ACT, Australia, 2013.

52. Kern, D.M.; Auchincloss, A.H.; Stehr, M.F.; Roux, A.V.D.; Moore, L.V.; Kanter, G.P.; Robinson, L.F. Neighborhood prices of healthier and unhealthier foods and associations with diet quality: Evidence from the multi-ethnic study of atherosclerosis. *Int. J. Environ. Res. Public Health* **2017**, *14*, 1394. [CrossRef] [PubMed]

53. Powell, L.M.; Maciejewski, M.L. Taxes and sugar-sweetened beverages. *JAMA* **2018**, *319*, 229–230. [CrossRef] [PubMed]

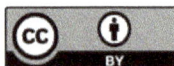

International Journal of
Environmental Research and Public Health

MDPI

Article

Cost and Affordability of Diets Modelled on Current Eating Patterns and on Dietary Guidelines, for New Zealand Total Population, Māori and Pacific Households

Sally Mackay [1,*], Tina Buch [2], Stefanie Vandevijvere [1], Rawinia Goodwin [1], Erina Korohina [3], Mafi Funaki-Tahifote [2], Amanda Lee [4] and Boyd Swinburn [1]

[1] School of Population Health, University of Auckland, Auckland 1142, New Zealand;
    s.vandevijvere@auckland.ac.nz (S.V.); rawiniagoodwin@icloud.com (R.G.);
    boyd.swinburn@auckland.ac.nz (B.S.)
[2] The Heart Foundation of New Zealand, Auckland 1051, New Zealand; TinaB@heartfoundation.org.nz (T.B.);
    mafift@heartfoundation.org.nz (M.F.-T.)
[3] Toi Tangata, Auckland 1010, New Zealand; erina@toitangata.co.nz
[4] The Australian Prevention Partnership Centre, The Sax Institute, Sydney 1240, Australia;
    amanda.lee@saxinstitute.org.au
*   Correspondence: sally.mackay@auckland.ac.nz; Tel.: +64-9-923-8733

Received: 11 April 2018; Accepted: 12 June 2018; Published: 13 June 2018

Abstract: The affordability of diets modelled on the current (less healthy) diet compared to a healthy diet based on Dietary Guidelines was calculated for population groups in New Zealand. Diets using common foods were developed for a household of four for the total population, Māori and Pacific groups. Māori and Pacific nutrition expert panels ensured the diets were appropriate. Each current (less healthy) diet was based on eating patterns identified from national nutrition surveys. Food prices were collected from retail outlets. Only the current diets contained alcohol, takeaways and discretionary foods. The modelled healthy diet was cheaper than the current diet for the total population (3.5% difference) and Pacific households (4.5% difference) and similar in cost for Māori households (0.57% difference). When the diets were equivalent in energy, the healthy diet was more expensive than the current diet for all population groups (by 8.5% to 15.6%). For households on the minimum wage, the diets required 27% to 34% of household income, and if receiving income support, required 41–52% of household income. Expert panels were invaluable in guiding the process for specific populations. Both the modelled healthy and current diets are unaffordable for some households as a considerable portion of income was required to purchase either diet. Policies are required to improve food security by lowering the cost of healthy food or improving household income.

Keywords: INFORMAS; diet prices; food affordability; Pacific diets; Māori diets; food security

1. Introduction

Dietary risks and a high body mass index are major risk factors contributing to health loss globally and in New Zealand (NZ) with dietary risk factors contributing to the highest proportion of total disability-adjusted life years in 2015 compared to other risk factors [1]. New Zealanders consume too much saturated fat, sodium and sugar and not enough dietary fibre, fruit and vegetables [2]. NZ has high rates of obesity with 32.2% of all adults, 50.2% of Māori adults and 68.7% of Pacific adults, obese [3]. For children (aged 2 to 14), 11% of the total population, 18.1% of Māori and 29.1% of Pacific children are obese [3]. Māori and Pacific people are more likely than non-Māori and non-Pacific to experience food insecurity [2].

An 'obesogenic' environment is 'the sum of influences that the surroundings, opportunities, or conditions of life have on promoting obesity in individuals or populations' [4]. A focus on creating healthy food environments is required to move populations towards diets that meet food-based dietary guidelines [5]. It is fundamental to consider cultural factors when discussing environmental influences on obesity [6].

Non-Māori are more advantaged than Māori across socioeconomic indictors related to education, employment, income and household crowding [7]. Inequities in health outcomes for Māori are influenced by the negative experiences of colonisation, institutional racism, alienation of land and thus identity and historical trauma [8]. In NZ, the Pacific Island community is a large and diverse ethnic group. Pacific communities, while being an integral part of New Zealand's society, continue to face challenges with lower levels of education and qualifications, lower incomes and a higher unemployment rate than the total population [9].

The International Network for Food and Obesity/NCDs Research, Monitoring and Action Support (INFORMAS) aims to monitor key aspects of food environments related to obesity and non-communicable diseases (NCDs) [10]. The INFORMAS food price module provides a framework to examine the price differential of healthy and unhealthy foods, meals and diets with this research focusing on the diet component.

Food prices are a major influence on household food purchases [11]. When the household budget is limited, fixed costs are prioritized so the money allocated for food reduces, which often results in food insecurity with potential health consequences [12].

Researchers have successfully used expert or focus panels to develop diets and select pricing outlets to ensure the costing of diets reflects intakes [13,14]. This is important in this research as eating patterns of Māori and Pacific households in NZ are influenced by traditional foods and eating patterns.

The relative difference in the affordability of a diet modelled to meet dietary guidelines compared with a modelled current (less healthy) diet has not been measured before in NZ, and there are few international studies. A systematic review by Rao et. al. (2013) concluded that healthier diets cost more than less healthy diets, though this depended on whether the cost of the total diet or cost per 2000 kcal was compared [15].

The affordability of a healthy diet compared to the current diet can be used to estimate the affordability component of food security for households on different income levels, for social planning and to advocate for fiscal policies and examine the influence on diet cost of taxes and subsidies on foods [16,17].

This study aims to assess the affordability of diets modelled on current eating patterns (current diet) and on dietary guidelines (healthy diet), for the total population, Māori and Pacific households, and to explore the feasibility of using expert panels to guide the process.

2. Materials and Methods

The methodology follows the guidelines set out in the INFORMAS food prices foundation paper [10] and the INFORMAS food prices module (www.INFORMAS.org). Māori and Pacific expert panels provided guidance for the selection of common foods, menus and price collection methods appropriate to the population group. Figure 1 illustrates the phases in assessing the cost of a modelled healthy versus the current diet. The diets for the total population were developed by a Registered Nutritionist (SM) rather than an expert panel.

The research was approved by the University of Auckland Human Participant Ethics Committee on 22 June 2016 for the Pacific diets (reference 017579) and on 26 September 2016 for the Māori diets (reference 018028). All expert panel participants provided written informed consent prior to participation.

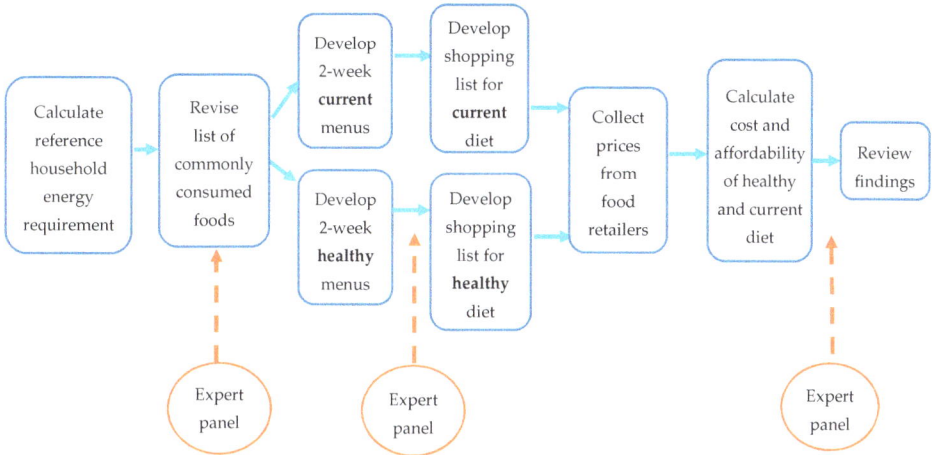

Figure 1. Phases in assessing the cost of a healthy and the current diet.

2.1. Expert Panels

The members of the Māori (four members) and Pacific (six members) expert panels were health professionals knowledgeable about foods and dietary patterns of their communities. The members were selected on the advice of Māori and Pacific non-governmental health organisations.

Phase 1: The expert panel reviewed a list of commonly consumed foods for Māori or Pacific people, provided feedback on menus for the diets and suggested the type and location of retailers for price collection. The initial discussion was face-to-face. The revised commonly consumed foods list and menu plans were emailed to the experts for review.

Phase 2: The results were presented to each expert panel who provided input into the interpretations and implications of the findings.

2.2. Common Foods

Commonly consumed foods were identified from the micro-data of the 2008/09 Adult Nutrition Survey [18] for the total population and for Māori and Pacific separately. Within each of the major food groups (33), the minor groups (395) with the most people consuming the item, or the most grams consumed were identified. Foods consumed by at least 5% of people were considered frequent. The amount consumed of a minor group depended on the food, for example, bread was consumed in higher amounts than butter.

A list of 109/107 common foods was presented to the Māori and the Pacific expert panels respectively. Items were then added or excluded based on the consensus of the expert panel on whether the foods were frequently consumed by the respective population group [Table S1]. The revised Māori common food list included traditional foods such as watercress and mussels. The revised Pacific common food list included taro, green bananas, cabin bread, canned corned beef, mutton flaps, panipopo (sweet coconut buns) and coconut cream.

The number of foods included on the list needed to be manageable for price collection, while ensuring sufficient variety for a two-week menu. The initial revised lists were too extensive so were refined by expert consensus, with some foods acting as proxies for similar foods e.g., jam represented all sweet spreads. The final selection contained 106 foods for the total population, 120 foods for Māori and 127 foods for Pacific populations.

2.3. Household Energy Requirements

The reference household used was that recommended in the INFORMAS food prices module: 45-year old man, 45-year old woman, 14-year old boy, 7-year old girl. The energy requirement for the adults for the healthy diet was calculated using the Body Weight Planner [19] based on a weight derived from a Body Mass Index (BMI) of 23 kg/m^2 calculated from mean population height [20] for moderate physical activity [Table S2]. The energy requirement for children for the healthy diet was based on the recommended energy requirements per KJ/kg per day by FAO/WHO/UNU [21] for moderate physical activity. The target weight was calculated from the 50th percentile BMI from the Centres for Disease Control and Prevention growth charts [22] using mean height [20].

The energy requirement for the current diet for adults was based on the current BMI [Table S2]. The average physical activity level (PAL) was unknown for the population, but approximately half of NZ adults met the physical activity guidelines [20] so a moderate physical activity level was selected. The energy requirement for the current diet for children was based on actual weight [20] and moderate physical activity as most children met the NZ physical activity guidelines [23]. The additional energy required for the actual weight was calculated using a validated equation for the excess energy intake per unit excess weight in childhood [24].

2.4. Diet Constraints

The current diets were modelled to reflect the median intake of the macronutrients (percentage of energy), fibre and total sugar, serves of fruits, vegetables, grains, meat and alternatives and dairy products reported in the 2008/09 Adult Nutrition Survey [2] and the Children's Nutrition Survey 2002 [25] [Tables S3 and S4]. The estimated intakes of sodium were from a later survey using a 24-h urine collection [26]. The current diets met Recommended Dietary Intakes (RDIs) and Adequate Intakes (AIs) for micronutrients except for iodine for all household members, and calcium, iron or Vitamin A for some household members.

The healthy diets were modelled to meet the NZ Eating and Activity Guidelines food group recommendations for number of servings [27] [Table S3] and the acceptable macronutrient distribution range, adequate intake for fibre and the upper limit for sodium (2.3 g per day) from the Nutrient Reference Values and the RDIs and AIs for micronutrients [28] [Table S4]. The intake of iodine could not be assessed due to incomplete food composition data on this micronutrient. The RDI for iron was not met by the adult female of each population group. Foods recommended by the Eating and Activity Guidelines (for example, whole-grain bread, lean meat, reduced-fat milk) were selected. There were no discretionary foods (high in added salt, sugar, saturated fat) in the standard healthy diets. An additional scenario was modelled which replaced 6% of energy from a wide range of foods with discretionary foods and alcohol (adult's diets) to compare a realistic healthy diet rather than an aspirational diet with the current diet.

Additional healthy foods were added to the list of common foods to enable the NZ Eating and Activity Guidelines recommendations for whole-grains, low-fat dairy and legumes to be met; for example, unsalted peanuts, reduced fat corned beef, brown rice, hummus, canned beans. The additional foods were selected based on frequency of consumption in the nutrition surveys and advice from the expert panels.

2.5. Gifting and Gathering of Food

The Māori expert panel identified the gifting and gathering of kai (food) as an important part of accessing food. Foods commonly gifted and/or gathered were seasonal fruit and vegetables and seafood. An additional scenario was analysed where the foods commonly gifted or gathered were priced in the original diet at $0 (mandarins, fresh fish, mussels, puha and watercress).

2.6. Menu Development

A fortnightly menu was developed for the current and healthy diets for each household member separately using the commonly consumed foods for breakfast, lunch, dinner, snacks and beverages. The expert panels advised on the menu structure. For example, the Pacific expert panel highlighted that on Sunday there is a large shared church feast so people only have a cup of tea and cabin bread for breakfast. The Māori expert panel considered it important to include sauces and spreads in the healthy diet to ensure the diet was realistic. The nutrient content of the menus was analysed using FoodWorks [29] with the NZ Food Composition Database. The nutrient composition of some Pacific foods were entered as additional foods, sourced from the Pacific Island Food Composition Tables [30]. Modifications were made to ensure diets met the constraints.

2.7. Price Collection

The amount to purchase for the household, allowing for inedible portion, yield and retention factors, [31] was calculated [Tables S5 and S6]. The expert groups advised that households would select the cheapest brand. Therefore, the brand with the cheapest price was collected from each store, including discount prices and generic brands. For items sold per unit, for example head of broccoli or a donut, three units were weighed and averaged to calculate the price per 100 g.

For the total population, prices were collected from a convenience sample of twelve supermarkets representing the three major supermarket chains and twelve neighbouring fresh produce stores in greater Auckland in November 2016 over two weeks. The prices for takeaway items were sourced from the INFORMAS meals cost study [32]. All items were available.

The Māori expert panel advised to collect prices from urban and rural grocery stores because price and access may be a barrier in rural areas. Prices were collected from three supermarkets (two large, one small) in an urban area and from three supermarkets (one large, two small) in rural areas and takeaway outlets in the Waikato region. Price collection was for one week in July 2017. Six items were not available in some of the smaller grocery stores, mainly fresh fish and meat.

The Pacific expert panel advised that prices should be collected in South Auckland to ensure specific Pacific foods were available. Prices were collected from three supermarkets (each major chain), three neighbouring fruit and vegetable shops, three bakeries and takeaway outlets. Price collection was for two weeks in September 2016. Not all items were available in stores such as mutton flaps, wholemeal pasta, light coconut cream and taro leaves.

2.8. Analysis

The cost of the household diet was calculated for the healthy and current diet (Table 1) for the three populations. A scenario was calculated with the 15% Goods and Services Tax (GST) removed from core foods (fruits, vegetables, less processed meat, seafood, poultry, legumes, nuts, dairy, healthy oils, grains).

To assess affordability of the diets, the percentage of household income required to purchase each diet was calculated for three scenarios:

Scenario 1: Median disposable income [33]

Scenario 2: Household receiving income support

- Jobseeker Support [34]
- Accommodation Supplement (area 2) [34]
- Family tax credit [35]

Scenario 3: Minimum wage [36]

- 60 h per week = one adult 40 h + one adult 20 h Jobseeker Support [34]
- Family tax credit calculated online using gross wages [35]

3. Results

3.1. Energy Requirements

The household energy requirement for the modelled healthy diet is 39.9 MJ and for the current diet is 43.6 MJ for the total population, 46 MJ for Māori and 47.3 MJ for Pacific. The current diet has 8.5% more energy than the healthy diet for the total population household, 13.3% for Māori and 15.6% for Pacific households.

3.2. Cost of Diets

The cost of the diets, and composite food groups, for each population group is outlined in Table 1. For the total population and Pacific Island households, the cost of a modelled healthy diet per fortnight is slightly less than the current diet by 3.5% and 4.5%, with a cost differential over one year of $588 and $575 respectively. For the Māori household, the cost of a healthy and current diet is similar (0.57% difference). When the diets are equivalent in energy, the healthy diet is more expensive than the current diet for all population groups (by 8.5% for the total population, 13.3% for Māori, and 15.6% for Pacific). When 6% of energy in the healthy diet is replaced by discretionary foods and alcohol, the healthy diet reduces in cost by 0.5% ($3.23 per fortnight).

Discretionary foods, beverages and takeaways comprise 36%, 46% and 41% respectively of the current diet costs for the total population, Māori and Pacific Islander populations. The healthy diets have more protein foods, vegetables, grains, fruit and dairy foods than the current diets, and no takeaways, discretionary foods, alcohol, or sugary beverages.

Table 1. Percentage of diet cost of each food group.

Food Group	Healthy Diet	Current Diet	Healthy Diet	Current Diet	Healthy Diet	Current Diet
	All	All	Māori	Māori	Pacific	Pacific
Fruits	18.1%	9.4%	13.6%	8.0%	14.1%	7.0%
Vegetables	17.6%	11.8%	20.8%	10.4%	25.2%	12.9%
Grains	13.8%	6.9%	14.0%	5.5%	15.4%	6.8%
Dairy	11.0%	5.5%	11.2%	6.8%	12.4%	5.2%
Protein	37.9%	31.4%	37.9%	22.0%	30.1%	26.6%
Fats and Oils	1.5%	1.3%	0.7%	1.4%	1.50%	0.9%
Sauces and Spreads	0	2.0%	1.6%	2.3%	0	3.0%
Snacks, sweets	0	6.9%	0	11.5%	0	8.0%
Processed meats	0	4.4%	0	5.3%	0	5.2%
Beverages	0	3.3%	0	5.2%	0	3.8%
Takeaway	0	10.8%	0	15.9%	0	14.9%
Alcohol	0	6.4%	0	5.7%	0	5.8%
Proportion less healthy food	0	35.5%	1.6%	45.9%	0	40.7%
Total cost	$649.06	$671.69	$558.50	$561.68	$526.92	$550.52

3.3. Affordability of Diets

The percentage of income required to purchase either diet is outlined in Table 2. When the 15% Goods and Services Tax (GST) is removed from core foods, affordability for a household improves more for the healthy diet than the current diet.

Table 2. Percentage of household income required to purchase diets.

	Standard Diet		GST off Core Foods	
	Healthy Diet % Income	Current Diet % Income	Healthy Diet % Income	Current Diet % Income
Median Household income ($1733 per week)				
Total population	18.7%	19.4%	16.3%	17.7%
Māori	16.1%	16.2%	14.0%	15.1%
Pacific	15.2%	15.9%	13.2%	15.2%
Minimum Wage ($1115 per week)				
Total population	32.8%	33.9%	28.5%	31.0%
Māori	28.2%	28.3%	24.5%	26.3%
Pacific	26.6%	27.8%	23.1%	26.6%
Income support ($636 per week)				
Total population	51.0%	52.8%	44.4%	48.2%
Māori	43.9%	44.2%	38.2%	41.0%
Pacific	41.4%	43.3%	36.0%	41.4%

3.4. Cost Scenarios

For Māori, six items were identified as foods typically gathered or gifted rather than purchased. The modelled healthy diet reduces in cost more than the current diet when these foods are gifted, as all these foods were healthy. In rural areas, the healthy diet cost reduces by $28.34 per week and the current diet cost reduces by $15.00 while in urban areas these figures were $27.23 and $14.20 respectively. Both the healthy and current diets are cheaper in the urban area compared to the rural area, with the healthy diet costing 9.4% more and the current diet 7.6% more in rural areas.

4. Discussion

This study showed that in NZ, a diet modelled on dietary guidelines is not more expensive than the current, less healthy diet, however when the diets are equivalent in energy the healthy diet is more expensive than the current diet for all population groups. For the total population and Pacific, the cost of a healthy diet is slightly cheaper than the current, less healthy diet. The current diets are higher in energy than the healthy diets because household energy requirement is determined by the average current BMI for the current diet, which is higher than the BMI used for the healthy diet to maintain weight at a healthy BMI.

The input from the Māori and Pacific expert panels was invaluable to identify some popular foods and practices, the type of food to price, meal patterns, common type of retailers and the importance of gathered and gifted food.

An Australian pilot study using similar methodology found the modelled healthy diet cost approximately 12% less than the modelled current diet for a household of four [37]. The healthy diet had 9.6% less energy than the current diet. The energy requirement of the healthy diet was that required to maintain the current BMI and physical activity level of the population. In the New Zealand study, the energy requirement of the healthy diet was determined by a healthy BMI. In Australia, there is no GST on basic, healthy foods but 10% GST on discretionary foods, which contributed to the healthy diet being cheaper than the current diet.

The Otago Food Cost Survey [38] collects the price of a diet that meets the NZ Eating and Activity Guidelines and contains some less healthy snack foods but no alcohol or takeaways. The cost of three diets is calculated: basic (cheapest), moderate and liberal (most expensive, most variety). For a similar household of four, the costs of the healthy diets for Māori ($559) and Pacific ($527) in this study were between the cost of the basic ($482) and moderate ($628) diets in the Otago study, while the cost for the total population ($649) was slightly higher than the moderate diet.

There is no accepted benchmark for affordability of a healthy diet internationally, though other researchers consider a household is suffering from food stress if more than 25% of disposable income is spent on food [39]. Therefore, NZ households receiving the minimum wage or income support would be suffering from food stress with some households requiring half of their income to purchase a healthy diet. The percentage of household income required for other major costs such as housing and utilities also determines the income available for food. Affordability was similar for the healthy and current diets for Māori. The healthy diet was slightly more affordable for Pacific and the total population. However, for a household of four receiving income support or minimum wage, a considerable portion of household income is required to purchase either diet. Food insecurity is a concern with 7.3% of NZ households classified as having low food security in the 2008/09 national nutrition survey [2]. In NZ, all foods have 15% GST added [40]. If GST was removed from basic healthy foods, this would improve affordability more for the healthy diet than the current diet.

4.1. Strengths

Few reported studies have compared the cost of a hypothetical healthy diet and a current diet, particularly for different population groups. The current diet is based on the common foods reported by the population in a national nutrition survey. The healthy diet is developed to meet food-based dietary guidelines and Nutrient Reference Values. The energy requirement for the current diet reflected the actual BMI of the population rather than using the mean reported energy intake in the survey, which is always under-reported [41]. Takeaway foods and alcohol were included in the current diet as these are common. Overall, the healthy diet met more of the micronutrient recommendations than the current diet though the diet for the adult female (total population only) met the RDI for iron on the current diet but not the healthy diet. This study demonstrated that an expert panel is a useful method for gaining cultural input into the commonly consumed foods, dietary patterns and selection of retail outlets used by Māori and Pacific households. As the national nutrition surveys were not recent, the expert panels offered an up-to-date view on commonly consumed foods.

4.2. Limitations

Arbitrary decision points occur at all stages of the process from selecting common foods, selecting items to represent other foods, the amount of each food in the diets, the energy requirement, the definition of a healthy diet, sampling retail outlets and the price selected. The nutrient intake of the current diet was based on older nutrition surveys (2008/09, 2002/03) so may not reflect the nutrient intake of the current diet, however no other data were available.

There is a range of healthy menus that could fit the food-based dietary guidelines and recommended dietary intakes. Only one healthy and one current diet was developed for each population group, so this may not be representative of the average cost if a range of diets were priced. The healthy diet was modelled to be aspirational but when limited discretionary foods were added the cost was similar.

There are other inputs to the cost of producing a household meal, aside from food prices, which could underestimate diet cost, particularly for healthy diets, which may require more preparation. Inputs include time, cooking fuel, transport for groceries, storage, preparation, cooking utensils, cooking space and skills [10].

The cost of the diets was calculated using food prices collected at supermarkets, rather than actual household expenditure that may take into account brand loyalty or purchases from multiple stores. The prices for the different population groups were collected at different times and seasons: Pacific in September 2016, total population in November 2016, Māori in July 2017. The Food Price Index indicated that the price of foods increased by 3.0% from July 2016 to July 2017, particularly fruit and vegetables (8.2%) [42]. Therefore, the relative difference between the healthy and current diets of the different population groups was compared, not the absolute amount. The higher price of fruit and vegetables could be a factor in explaining why the Māori healthy and current diets were a similar price, rather than the healthy diet being slightly cheaper for the Pacific and total population diets. Seasons affect fruit and vegetable prices with fresh fruit and vegetables more expensive in July and September, and close to the average monthly price in November [42], therefore it is expected that the cost differences between the healthy and current diets would persist in seasons where prices are lower.

4.3. Implications

A diet modelled on dietary guidelines is not more expensive than the current diet when the reference household also shifts from the estimated current energy intake to the recommended energy intake. This is particularly important for those on low incomes because food costs are typically between a quarter and a half of household budgets indicating they are suffering from food stress. There is a perception that healthy diets are more expensive than those currently consumed [43,44]. However, this research and similar research in Australia [37] indicates it is possible to shift to a healthy diet (that does not exceed energy requirements) from the current, healthy diet without additional cost. Price is only one barrier to healthy eating. Other key influences are taste, traditions, convenience, knowledge and cooking skills [43]. Gathering and gifting food is important in reducing diet costs.

This paper describes the collection of the baseline data. After further price collections, it can be seen whether the healthy diet is increasing in cost at a different rate than the current diet. An analysis of foods in the NZ Food Price Index [45] over ten years indicates the price of healthy foods rose at a similar rate compared to unhealthy foods.

It is recommended that work be conducted with the expert panels on how to translate these findings into a practical health promotion tool for Pacific, Māori and low-income households. Monitoring the price and affordability of diets provides robust data and benchmarks to inform economic and fiscal policies [10]. As demonstrated in this study, having information on the prices of the current and healthy diets is invaluable to demonstrating the impact taxes and subsidies will have on diets.

5. Conclusions

Expert panels were invaluable in guiding development of the diets to be costed for specific population groups. In NZ, a lower-energy healthy diet is not necessarily more expensive than the current diet, but discretionary foods make up 36–41% of food costs in the current diet. Strategies to switch current spending on discretionary food and takeaways to healthy food need not cost more. However, overall food security is of concern as a considerable portion of income is required to purchase either a healthy or the current diet in NZ, especially for households receiving minimum wage or income support. In order to consume a healthy diet, policies are required to lower the cost of healthy food or ensure that households have sufficient income after fixed expenses to purchase nutritious, acceptable and safe food.

Supplementary Materials: The following are available online at http://www.mdpi.com/1660-4601/15/6/1255/s1. Table S1: Common foods added and removed from diets by Māori and Pacific expert panels, Table S2: Individual and household energy requirements for each population group, Table S3: Number of serves of each food group per week for each household member for healthy and current diets, Table S4: Nutrient intake of household members for healthy and current diets for each population group, Table S5: Edible amount of each common food in the current diet per fortnight for each population group, Table S6: Edible amount of each common food in the healthy diet per fortnight for each population group.

Author Contributions: S.M., A.L., S.V. and B.S. conceived and designed the study; S.M., T.B. and R.G. performed the study and analyzed the data; S.M. wrote the paper. E.K. and M.F.-T. provided expert advice and contributed to performing the study; All authors critically revised the manuscript.

Acknowledgments: This research was funded by a grant from the Health Research Council (3704724).

Conflicts of Interest: The authors declare no conflict of interest. The founding sponsors had no role in the design of the study; in the collection, analyses, or interpretation of data; in the writing of the manuscript, and in the decision to publish the results.

References

1. GBD 2016 Risk Factor Collaborators. Global, regional, and national comparative risk assessment of 79 behavioural, environmental and occupational, and metabolic risks or clusters or risks, 1990–2015: A systematic analysis for the Global Burden of Diseases Study 2015. *Lancet* **2016**, *388*, 1659–1724.
2. University of Otago and Ministry of Health. *A Focus on Nutrition: Key Findings of the 2008/09 New Zealand Adult Nutrition Survey*; Ministry of Health: Wellington, New Zealand, 2011.
3. Ministry of Health. New Zealand Health Survey 2016/17. Available online: https://www.health.govt. nz/nz-health-statistics/national-collections-and-surveys/surveys/current-recent-surveys/new-zealand-health-survey#published (accessed on 20 November 2017).
4. Swinburn, B.; Egger, G.; Raza, F. Dissecting obesogenic environments: The development and application of a framework for identifying and prioritizing environmental interventions for obesity. *Prev. Med.* **1999**, *29*, 563–570. [CrossRef] [PubMed]
5. Swinburn, B.; Sacks, G.; Vandevijvere, S.; Kumanyika, S.; Lobstein, T.; Neal, B.; Barquera, S.; Friel, S.; Hawkes, C.; Kelly, B.; et al. INFORMAS (International Network for Food and Obesity/non-communicable diseases Research, Monitoring and Action Support): Overview and key principles. *Obes. Rev.* **2013**, *14* (Suppl. 1), 1–12. [CrossRef] [PubMed]
6. Kumanyika, S.K. Environmental influences on childhood obesity: Ethnic and cultural influences in context. *Physiol. Behav.* **2008**, *94*, 61–70. [CrossRef] [PubMed]
7. Ministry of Health; Kahukura, T. *Māori Health Chart Book 2015*, 3rd ed.; Ministry of Health: Wellington, New Zealand, 2015.
8. Berghan, G.; Came, H.; Coupe, N.; Doole, C.; Fay, J.; McCreanor, T.; Simpson, T. Tiriti-Based Health Promotion Practice. STIR: Stop Institutional Racism. 2017. Available online: https://trc.org.nz/treaty-waitangi-based-practice-health-promotion (accessed on 7 February 2018).
9. Sorensen, D.; Jensen, S.; Rigamoto, M.; Pritchard, M. *Pacific People in New Zealand: How Are We doing?* Pasifika Futures Ltd.: Auckland, New Zealand, 2015.
10. Lee, A.; Ni Mhurchu, C.; Sacks, G.; Swinburn, B.; Snowdon, W.; Vandevijvere, S.; Hawkes, C.; L'Abbé, M.; Rayner, M.; Sanders, D.; et al. Monitoring the price and affordability of foods and diets globally. *Obes. Rev.* **2013**, *14* (Suppl. 1), 82–95. [CrossRef] [PubMed]
11. Ni Mhurchu, C.; Eyles, H.; Dixon, R.; Matoe, L.; Teevale, T.; Meagher-Lundberg, P. Economic incentives to promote healthier food purchases: Exploring acceptability and key factors for success. *Health Promot. Int.* **2012**, *27*, 331–341. [CrossRef] [PubMed]
12. Lloyd, S.; Lawton, J.; Caraher, M.; Singh, G.; Horsley, K.; Mussa, F. A tale of two localities: Healthy eating on a restricted income. *Health Educ. J.* **2011**, *70*, 48–56. [CrossRef]
13. Bowyer, S.; Caraher, M.; Eilbert, K.; Carr-Hill, R. Shopping for food: Lessons from a London borough. *Br. Food J.* **2009**, *111*, 452–474. [CrossRef]
14. Goedemé, T.; Storms, B.; Van den Bosch, K. *Pilot Project: Developing a Common Methodology on Reference Budgets in Europe*; European Commission: Brussels, Belgium, 2015.
15. Rao, M.; Afshin, A.; Singh, G.; Mozaffarian, D. Do healthier foods and diet patterns cost more than less healthy options? A systematic review and meta-analysis. *BMJ Open* **2013**, *3*, e004277. [CrossRef] [PubMed]
16. Kettings, C.; Sinclair, A.; Voevodin, M. A healthy diet consistent with Australian health recommendations is too expensive for welfare-dependent families. *Aust. N. Z. J. Public Health* **2009**, *33*, 566–572. [CrossRef] [PubMed]
17. Nathoo, T.; Shoveller, J. Do healthy food baskets assess food security? *Chronic Dis. Can.* **2003**, *24*, 65–69. [PubMed]
18. Statistics New Zealand. *Adult National Nutrition Survey 2008/09 Confidentialised unit Record Files*; Statistics New Zealand: Wellington, New Zealand, 2011.
19. National Institute of Diabetes and Digestive and Kidney Diseases. Body Weight Planner. Available online: https://www.niddk.nih.gov/health-information/weight-management/body-weight-planner (accessed on 6 April 2017).
20. Ministry of Health. Annual Update of Key Results 2013/14: New Zealand Health Survey. Available online: https://www.health.govt.nz/publication/annual-update-key-results-2013-14-new-zealand-health-survey (accessed on 20 November 2017).

21. FAO; WHO; UNU. *Report on Human Energy Requirements*; Food and Agricultural Organization; World Health Organization; United Nations University Expert Consultation: Rome, Italy, 2004.

22. CDC Growth Charts 2010. Available online: http://www.cdc.gov/growthcharts/index.htm (accessed on 11 January 2016).

23. Clinical Trials Research Unit and Synovate. *A National Survey of Children and Young People's Physical Activity and Dietary Behaviours in New Zealand: 2008/09: Key Findings*; Ministry of Health: Wellington, New Zealand, 2010.

24. Hall, K.; Butte, N.; Swinburn, B.; Chow, C. Dynamics of childhood growth and obesity: Development and validation of a quantitative mathematical model. *Lancet Diabetes Endocrinol.* **2013**, *10*, 97–105. [CrossRef]

25. Ministry of Health. *NZ Food NZ Children: Key Results of the 2002 National Children's Nutrition Survey*; Ministry of Health: Wellington, New Zealand, 2003.

26. Skeaff, S.; McLean, R.; Mann, J.; Williams, S. *The Impact of Mandatory Fortification of Bread with Iodine*; MPI Technical Paper No: 2013/025; Ministry of Primary Industries: Wellington, New Zealand, 2013.

27. Ministry of Health. Eating and Activity Guidelines for New Zealand Adults. 2015. Available online: https://www.health.govt.nz/publication/eating-and-activity-guidelines-new-zealand-adults (accessed on 20 November 2017).

28. NHMRC. *Nutrient Reference Values for Australia and New Zealand*; National Health and Medical Research Council: Canberra, Australia, 2006.

29. Xyris Software (Australia) Pty Ltd. *FoodWorks 7 Professional [computer program]*; Xyris Software (Australia) Pty Ltd.: Brisbane, Australia, 2012.

30. Dignan, C.; Burlingame, B.; Kumar, S.; Aalbersberg, W. *The Pacific Island Food Composition Tables*; Food and Agriculture Organization of the United Nations: Rome, Italy, 2004.

31. New Zealand Institute of Plant and Food Research. *FOODfiles 2013*; The New Zealand Institute of Plant and Food Research and the New Zealand Ministry of Health: Palmerston North, New Zealand, 2013.

32. Mackay, S.; Vandevijvere, S.; Xie, P.; Lee, A.; Swinburn, B. Paying for convenience: Comparing the cost of takeaway meals with their healthier home-cooked counterparts in New Zealand. *Public Health Nutr.* **2017**, *20*, 2269–2276. [CrossRef] [PubMed]

33. OECD Income Distribution and Poverty. 2016. Available online: http://stats.oecd.org/Index.aspx?DataSetCode=IDD (accessed on 30 May 2016).

34. Ministry of Social Development. Benefit Rates at 1 April 2016. Available online: http://www.workandincome.govt.nz/products/benefit-rates/benefit-rates-april-2016.html#null (accessed on 4 May 2016).

35. Inland Revenue. Estimate Your Working for Families Tax Credits 2016. Available online: http://www.ird.govt.nz/calculators/keyword/wff-tax-credits/calculator-wfftc-estimate-2016.html (accessed on 30 May 2016).

36. Employment New Zealand. The Minimum Wage. 1 April 2016. Available online: https://www.employment.govt.nz/hours-and-wages/pay/minimum-wage/ (accessed on 30 May 2016).

37. Lee, A.J.; Kane, S.; Ramsey, R.; Good, E.; Dick, M. Testing the price and affordability of healthy and current (unhealthy) diets and the potential impacts of policy change in Australia. *BMC Public Health* **2016**, *16*, 315. [CrossRef] [PubMed]

38. Department of Human Nutrition. *Information Package for Users of the New Zealand Estimated Food Costs 2016*; University of Otago: Dunedin, New Zealand, 2016.

39. Landrigan, T.; Kerr, D.; Dhaliwal, S.; Savage, V.; Pollard, C. Removing the Australian tax exemption on healthy food adds food stress to families vulnerable to poor nutrition. *Aust NZ J Public Health* **2017**. [CrossRef] [PubMed]

40. New Zealand Legislation. Goods and Services Tax Act 1985. Available online: http://www.legislation.govt.nz/act/public/1985/0141/latest/DLM81035.html (accessed on 30 August 2016).

41. Poslusna, K.; Ruprich, J.; de Vries, J.; Jakubikova, M.; van't Veer, P. Misreporting of energy and micronutrient intake estimated by food records and 24 h recalls, control and adjustment methods in practice. *Br. Nutr.* **2009**, *101* (Suppl. 2), S73–S85. [CrossRef] [PubMed]

42. Statistics New Zealand. Food Price Index: July 2017. Available online: http://www.stats.govt.nz/browse_for_stats/economic_indicators/prices_indexes/FoodPriceIndex_HOTPJul17.aspx (accessed on 10 October 2017).

43. Andajani-Sutjahjo, S.; Ball, K.; Warren, N.; Inglis, V.; Crawford, D. Perceived personal, social and environmental barriers to weight maintenance among young women: A community survey. *Int. J. Behav. Nutr. Phys. Act.* **2004**, *1*, 15. [CrossRef] [PubMed]

44. Funaki-Tahifote, M.; Fung, M.; Timaloa, Y.; Langi, T.; Lafuloa, S.; Manuopangai, V.; Johnston, O. *Better Quality and Reduced Quantity in Food/Drinks in Pacific Settings*; Health Promotion Agency: Wellington, New Zealand, 2016.

45. Statistics New Zealand. Food Price Index Selected Monthly Weighted Average Prices for New Zealand. 2017. Available online: http://www.stats.govt.nz/infoshare/SelectVariables.aspx?pxID=e3632d54-64c5-45c0-80f5-721bc77c2bca (accessed on 30 May 2017).

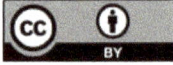

International Journal of
Environmental Research and Public Health

MDPI

Article

You Can't Find Healthy Food in the Bush: Poor Accessibility, Availability and Adequacy of Food in Rural Australia

Jill Whelan [1,*], Lynne Millar [2,3], Colin Bell [1], Cherie Russell [4], Felicity Grainger [4], Steven Allender [5] and Penelope Love [4,6]

1   School of Medicine, Global Obesity Centre, Deakin University, Geelong 3220, Australia;
    colin.bell@deakin.edu.au
2   Australian Health Policy Collaboration, Victoria University, Melbourne 3000, Australia;
    lynne.millar@vu.edu.au
3   Australian Institute for Musculoskeletal Science (AIMSS), The University of Melbourne and Western Health,
    St Albans 3021, Australia
4   School of Exercise and Nutrition Sciences, Deakin University, Geelong 3220, Australia;
    caru@deakin.edu.au (C.R.); fgrainge@deakin.edu.au (F.G.); penny.love@deakin.edu.au (P.L.)
5   School of Health and Social Development, Global Obesity Centre, Deakin University,
    Geelong 3220, Australia; steven.allender@deakin.edu.au
6   Institute for Physical Activity and Nutrition (IPAN), Deakin University, Geelong 3220, Australia
*   Correspondence: jill.whelan@deakin.edu.au; Tel.: +61-35-227-8039

Received: 12 September 2018; Accepted: 15 October 2018; Published: 21 October 2018

Abstract: In high-income countries, obesity disproportionately affects those from disadvantaged and rural areas. Poor diet is a modifiable risk factor for obesity and the food environment a primary driver of poor diet. In rural and disadvantaged communities, it is harder to access affordable and nutritious food, affecting both food insecurity and the health of rural residents. This paper aims to describe the food environment in a rural Australian community (approx. 7000 km² in size) to inform the development of community-relevant food supply interventions. We conducted a census audit of the food environment (ground truthing) of a local government area (LGA). We used the Nutrition Environment Measurement tools (NEMS-S and NEMS-R) to identify availability of a range of food and non-alcoholic beverages, the relative price of a healthy compared to a less healthy option of a similar food type (e.g., bread), the quality of fresh produce and any in-store nutrition promotion. Thirty-eight food retail outlets operated at the time of our study and all were included, 11 food stores (NEMS-S) and 27 food service outlets (NEMS-R). The mean NEMS-S score for all food stores was 21/54 points (39%) and mean NEMS-R score for all food service outlets was 3/23 points (13%); indicative of limited healthier options at relatively higher prices. It is difficult to buy healthy food beyond the supermarkets and one (of seven) cafés across the LGA. Residents demonstrate strong loyalty to local food outlets, providing scope to work with this existing infrastructure to positively impact poor diet and improve food security.

Keywords: rural; food supply; food security; obesity

1. Introduction

Globally, obesity is a leading cause of chronic disease and premature death [1]. In low and middle-income countries, it impacts the wealthy, shifting to the rural poor as the country's economy develops [1,2]. In high income countries, such as Australia, it impacts everyone but disproportionately affects those from more disadvantaged and rural areas [2]. Consequently, rural residents in Australia have higher rates of obesity and are more likely to die early from concomitant conditions including diabetes, heart disease and other chronic diseases [2,3].

Internationally and within Australia, poor diet has been identified as a leading modifiable risk factor contributing to the high burden of disease and obesity [3,4], and there is some evidence that the food environment is related to healthiness of diet among adults [5] and children [6]. These reviews highlight the lack of consistency in measurements of these associations which is to be expected in this emerging field but, nonetheless, some relationships are evident.

Some studies have identified that neighbourhoods without supermarkets have more diet-related health outcomes such as obesity and chronic disease [7]. In rural and/or disadvantaged communities, it is harder than in urban environments to access affordable and nutritious foods [8,9]. Availability varies as it is potentially constrained by the long distance required to travel to food stores [10], and limitations to fresh food supply delivery and increased prices occur with greater distance from the key metropolitan centres [11]. A consequence of these food supply constraints is that rural residents, and rural food retailers, in order to reduce the risk of waste, tend to purchase longer shelf-life foods [12], many of which may be less nutritious than the fresh options. Rural areas have a higher proportion of general stores to larger supermarkets compared to urban areas, providing fewer healthy options at higher prices and unpredictable quality [13,14]. These differences are most commonly attributed to limited transportation, storage and economies of scale for food distribution to rural areas [15].

Many rural areas experience diminishing population sizes, which reduces financial viability leading to the consolidation or closure of food stores [16,17]. With poor access to healthy food within close proximity, rural residents are reliant on transportation (public or private), incurring additional costs, and they frequently are forced to shop outside their local area, a phenomenon known as 'out-shopping' [17]. Out-shopping creates a vicious cycle for rural economies as revenue shifts to outside enterprises, and local businesses struggle to provide sufficient variety at low cost to attract and retain customers [17], adding further to rural economic decline. General stores, and 'take-away' food outlets, located in close proximity to residents, often with extended operating hours, may become the main source of food for rural communities [18], particularly those with limited mobility.

The food environment is defined as the "accessibility, availability and adequacy of food within a community or region" [19] and comprises three sub-environments: community, organizational and consumer. The community food environment (number, type, location and accessibility of retail food outlets); the organizational food environment (type and availability of healthy food within settings, such as workplaces, schools and at home); and the consumer food environment (price, promotion, placement, nutrition information, quality and availability of healthy food within retail food outlets) [19,20].

Importantly, food environment research should be considered alongside the concept of food insecurity, where people are unable to obtain a nutritious diet through socially acceptable means on a regular basis [21]. Within rural Australia, causes of food insecurity are discussed within five domains, these are: 1. access (economic and physical access to food), 2. inadequate supply (availability), 3. affordability, 4. inappropriate use of food (food safety, food preparation, nutritional status) and 5. trade policy [9]. Within this paper, we concentrate on three of these domains: access, supply/availability and affordability of food insecurity. The NEMS-S and NEMS-R tools are designed to collect data on food availability and access and do not aim to collect data on available food relief services, such as food pantries and community meals programs. The focus of this study is on the food and beverages stocked within retail food outlets in the area with a view to understanding access and availability of quality food produce at an affordable price. Whilst it might be expected that food insecurity would be linked with under-weight, research indicates that obesity is most prevalent amongst those at highest risk of food insecurity [22,23]. Other broad reaching health effects that have been identified in the literature include, disturbed sleep patterns, maternal depression, type 2 diabetes, anaemia poorer child health and higher rates of hospitalisation linked with poor infant feeding practices. Lifelong impacts include learning difficulties and adverse developmental outcomes [3].

These two major public health issues of obesity and food security should therefore be considered simultaneously, using local food environment data to inform positive environmental changes to enhance health.

Food environment interventions have the potential to improve population level diet quality in an equitable manner by ensuring an affordable, high quality food supply [24], and Glanz et al. argue that community and consumer food sub-environments should be given particular attention as they have the potential to promote and impact healthier choices at the point of purchase [20]. Measurement of community and consumer food environments is problematic, however, a recent review of retail food environment measures has provided some direction [25] by identifying the most common store types as supermarkets, grocery stores, convenience and corner stores. These store types are commonly categorized by number of registers [26,27] or sum of aisle length [28]. The review [25] also identified the two most frequently internationally used measures as the USDA's Thrifty Food Plan tool, developed to identify food and beverage purchases to meet minimum USA healthy diet requirements [29]; and the Nutrition Environment Measurement Survey for Stores (NEMS-S) which assesses the nutrition environment more broadly based on availability, price and quality [30]. NEMS-S is one of a suite of nutrition environment measurement tools that have been assessed for interrater reliability, test-re-test reliability and face and criterion validity; and adapted for use in several studies [30]. The NEMS-R tool comprises an observational checklist of 25 items [31] and is designed to assess the availability of healthier food and beverages on main and children's menus. In Australia, studies of food environments have focused on availability and access in urban settings and remote Indigenous communities, with most exploring food pricing [32].

Where nutrition environment measurement tools have been used in rural settings, either internationally or in Australia, they have presented with limitations to efficacy in these settings. For example, studies of food pricing commonly rely on a 'healthy food basket' conceptualization [33], where data include prices of a pre-defined list of 'healthy' foods in quantities representative of various household units, thereby enabling comparison across regions and over time [12]. However, exclusion of generic brands [34], exclusion of stores that contain fewer than 90% of the 44 items, and lack of quality assessment of fresh produce limit its usefulness and applicability in rural and remote areas.

While the definition of food environments is clear, and there is growing awareness of the need to intervene, less is known about the true disparity in the healthfulness of food environments in rural compared to urban areas. There is a paucity of evidence of the quality of rural food environments generally [15] and in Australian non-Indigenous communities specifically. The aim of this paper is to describe the food environment in a rural Australian community for use in future development of community-relevant food supply interventions.

2. Methods

2.1. Design

Census audit of rural food environment using the NEMS-S [30] and NEMS-R tools [31].

2.2. Context

This study took place in a rural, remote local government area (LGA) within Australia, as part of a broader community-wide obesity prevention study. Within the study, community stakeholders identified the local food supply as a determinant of unhealthy weight. Data published in 2014 show the LGA experienced a very poor chronic disease risk profile and above average adult prevalence of overweight and obesity at around 15% above the state average at that time. Concomitant health behaviours were of concern with high sugar sweetened beverage per capita consumption almost twice the state average and higher than average take-away meal consumption [35]. Located 350 km from the nearest capital city, the LGA has a total population of approximately 7000 people spread across approximately 7000 km^2 comprising farming land and several rural and remote towns with populations ranging from between 150 and 2302 people. The predominant crops include various grains and legumes which are be 'shipped out' for processing [36]. Within Australia there are four major chain supermarkets, and the smallest of these has a presence within this community.

2.3. Selection of Retail Food Outlets

We used the categories in Table 1 to define retail food outlets. These were adapted to the rural Australian context from Glanz et al. [20] and Innes-Hughes [26].

Table 1. Categorization of retail food stores and food service outlets.

Food Stores	Food Service
Supermarket—sells food products and other items, large scale, may open for extended hours on most days of the week. (Register numbers: 1 to 5)	Restaurants Sit-down—order and pay at table, table service, food eaten at outlet e.g.,: traditional restaurants
General—sells food products and other items, small scale, typically in a small town. General stores generally have reduced hours and usually are not open on weekends.	Fast-casual—order and pay at counter, may have table service, food eaten at outlet or taken away e.g.,: hotels (pubs) and cafés
Convenience stores (North American)—extended hours, stocking a limited range of household goods and groceries.	Fast-food—order, pay and served food at counter, quick service, food usually eaten away from outlet e.g.,: take-aways and bakeries

Thirty-nine retail food outlets were identified across the LGA using the community directory available on the LGA website. 'Ground truthing' (physically viewing and recording of outlets) identified that an additional four outlets had opened, and that three outlets had closed. Two petrol stations were excluded, as their food supply was extremely limited. All food outlets operating at the time of the study that met the definitions outlined in Table 1 were included (n = 38).

2.4. Selection of Food Environment Measurement Tools

We used the Nutrition Environment Measures Survey for Stores (NEMS-S) and Restaurants (NEMS-R) due to their validated status and peer-reviewed evidence of use in a variety of settings. NEMS-S scored high on reliability; percent agreement (92–100%), inter-rater reliability kappas (0.84–1.00) and test-retest (0.73–1.00) [30]. NEMS-R also scored generally high on inter-rater reliability, kappas mostly greater than 0.80 (0.27–0.97); percent agreement (77.6–99.5%), and test-retest: most kappa values greater than 0.80 (0.46–1.0) [31]. Scoring of the NEMS-S tool was based on the published scoring tool [30] and NEMS-R was scored using the revised scoring system provided in 2011 [37].

2.5. Nutrition Environment Measures Survey for Stores (NEMS-S)

The original, American-based, NEMS-S tool [30] includes 11 indicator food categories: milk, fruit, vegetables, ground/minced beef, hot dogs, frozen dinners, baked goods, beverages—diet soft drink and fruit juice, bread, chips, breakfast cereal. These food categories reflected the fat and calories of a typical diet and those most recommended for healthful eating at the time the tool was developed (2007) [30]. The following modifications were made to the NEMS-S tool for the Australian context. Measures were converted from imperial to metric, and chicken (skin on and skin off) was substituted for hotdogs (being a more commonly available and consumed food in Australia). Australian reference brands were used, and Australian seasonal fruit and vegetables were included. Common breakfast cereal and bakery options were also included. Due to the importance of calcium rich foods in the Australian Guide to Healthy Eating [38], data were collected on the availability and price comparisons of cheese and yoghurt, however, these were not included in the NEMS scoring protocol to allow comparison with previous studies.

The modified NEMS-S tool was piloted in three rural community retail food outlets to test for face validity. Our modified tool maintained the 11 categories as per the NEMS-S scoring tool with a maximum possible score of 54, (availability: maximum 30, pricing: maximum 18 and quality: maximum 6 (as fruit and vegetables only included)). Between one and three points were awarded for availability depending on product type and the number of varieties available. Affordability is assessed through comparative pricing. The price of food was scored comparatively with two points being awarded if the price of better nutrient profile food was cheaper than the regular varieties. Quality was scored as 'acceptable' or 'unacceptable' based on the appearance of the majority of a given type of fruits or vegetables; an unacceptable rating was applied if the produce was 'clearly bruised, old looking, over-ripe, or spotted' [30] (p. 284). As per the NEMS scoring protocol, a quality score of 1 was awarded if 25–49% of the produce met an acceptable standard, 2 points were awarded if between 50–74% of the produce was acceptable and 3 points awarded if 75% or more of the produce was 'acceptable'. An overall score combining all three dimensions was calculated. A higher score obtained in the NEMS-S tool equates to a healthier food environment.

2.6. Nutrition Environment Measures Survey for Restaurants (NEMS-R)

NEMS-R comprises a menu review and observational visit, (and if required, an interview with restaurant staff) to review the 25 items assessed for availability of healthier food and beverages on menus. Points are awarded for healthier options, for example: low fat dressings, whole grain breads, baked rather than fried foods, among others [31]. Factors that support or challenge healthy eating are measured and further points are awarded for signage/promotions, nutrition information and notations on menus. Points are deducted for unhealthy promotions such as super-sizing, all-you-can-eat offers, and unhealthy combo-meal deals [31]. Possible NEMS-R scores range from −5 to 23 (for establishments without a specific children's menu) and −8 to 32 (for establishments with a children's menu) [39].

Minor modifications to language were required to ensure NEMS-R was relevant to the Australian context. The term 'entree' in USA generally means main course and in Australia it means a smaller first course, therefore all references to entrée were removed and replaced with the Australian language of 'main course'. The size of the meal was captured through the retention of the question related to reduced-size portions offered on menu. NEMS-R collects data on 'low carb promotions' which was the 'diet fad' of choice at the time the tool was developed (2007). Instead we collected data on any 'diet fads' outside the Australian Guide to Healthy Eating (AGHE), such as raw foods or paleo diets that were popular at the time of data collection (2017). We also modified milk to include all lower fat milk options, typically 2% fat milk in Australia, (NEMS: 1% or non-fat). We administered the NEMS-R tool on all food service outlets in the study LGA. As there are no fast food chain outlets in the study LGA to enable a comparison between small family owned businesses and large chain store food outlets we administered the NEMS-R on a neighbouring large fast-food chain outlet. As per NEMS-S we pilot tested the modified NEMS-R for face validity. A higher score on NEMS-R also indicates a healthier food environment.

2.7. Data Collection

Prior to data collection, JW and PL undertook online NEMS training [40], then provided face-to-face training to CR and FG. Data were collected over four days from 19 to 22 June 2017. Retail food outlets were not informed of the assessment ahead of time, permission was obtained on entering the premises. Store owners were advised of the purpose of the study on entering the premises. Most of the data could be collected without interaction with the staff of the food premises. Where interaction was required, food retailers freely shared the required information.

All researchers conducted an initial NEMS-S and NEMS-R survey together and thereafter worked in pairs to ensure consistency between scoring. Test-retest reliability was performed on a 5% sample (n = 2/38) as per NEMS protocol. The results indicated a high level of test-retest reliability with NEMS-R kappa of 0.825 and NEMS-S kappa of 0.781. Surveys took between 20 and 60 min to complete dependent on the size of the outlet. Data were recorded using hard copy survey sheets and then entered into the relevant NEMS-S or NEMS-R Excel spreadsheet. A random sample of 25% of data entries was assessed for accuracy. No errors were found in this cross check. Ethical approval for this study was obtained through Deakin University [HEAG-H 80_2016].

2.8. Data Analysis

Data were prepared using NEMS Excel spreadsheets and the NEMS scoring system [30,37,39] and STATA release 15 [41]. Primary outcome measures were: availability, price and quality of healthy foods compared across store types (supermarkets and general stores), food service (restaurants, fast casual—hotels, fast casual—cafes, fast food), and geographic locations to identify if cost, availability, promotions, healthiness and quality of food varied across the LGA. Food was classified into the core food groups of the Australian Guide to Healthy Eating to determine if the foods recommended were available and if they were more or less expensive than unhealthier foods. Descriptive statistics on the availability of the Australian core food groups and discretionary foods were reported. For NEMS-S data, *t*-tests were used to compare the availability, price, quality of food between type of store (supermarket or general store) and separate linear regressions were used to compare the availability, price, quality between communities (north, central, south). For all statistics, *p*-values < 0.05 were deemed statistically significant.

Published studies appear to have applied different scoring protocols, therefore, we have converted our NEMS scores to percentage figures to enable comparison with other studies using these tools. In keeping with NEMS tools a higher percentage indicates a food environment more conducive to healthy eating.

3. Results

The exploration of the community food environment found a total of 38 outlets, all of which are included in the data analysis (100% RR), with 11 being food stores and 27 food service outlets (sit-down n = 13, fast-casual n = 7, fast food n = 7).

3.1. Food Stores

Of the 11 food stores, five were supermarkets and six were general stores. Table 2 shows the maximum possible score and mean scores for each of the three sub-categories of availability, price and quality for stores overall and by type of food store (the higher the score, the healthier the food environment). A total mean score of 21.0 (SD 4.6) out of a possible 54 points was obtained for the LGA as a whole. The overall NEM-S score was significantly higher for supermarkets (mean = 24.8, SD 2.6) than general stores (mean = 17.8 SD 3.2; t(2,9) = 3.9, *p* < 0.05) as was the availability of healthy foods score (supermarkets (mean = 21.4, SD 3.0); general stores (mean = 12.0, SD 3.0; t(2,9) = 5.2, *p* < 0.05).

Table 2. NEMS-S Food Stores Scores for all stores, grocery stores and general stores and *p* values resulting from *t*-tests between store type.

	Max	All Food Stores (n = 11)		Supermarkets (n = 5)		General Stores (n = 6)		*p*
		Mean	SD	Mean	SD	Mean	SD	
Availability	30	16.3	5.7	21.4	3.0	12.0	3.0	*p* < 0.05
Price	18	1.1	1.0	1.2	1.1	1.0	1.1	NS *
Quality	6	4.6	2.1	5.4	1.3	4.0	2.5	NS *
Total Score	54	21.0	4.6	24.8	2.6	17.8	3.2	*p* < 0.05

* NS—Non-significant at *p* ≥ 0.05.

Table 3 compares the mean NEMS-S scores for stores in the north (n = 3), central (n = 5) and south (n = 3) of the LGA. The mean NEMS-S score was highest in the central area at 24.8 (44%) where the two largest supermarkets were located. There were no statistically significant differences on any category between areas.

Table 3. NEMS-S score means from stores in the northern, central, and southern areas of the rural local government area.

Food Stores (n = 11)		North (n = 3)		Central (n = 5)		South (n = 3)	
	Max	Mean	SD	Mean	SD	Mean	SD
Availability	30	14.0	5.2	19.0	8.7	17.3	2.5
Price	18	1.2	1.1	1.3	1.2	0.7	1.2
Quality	6	4.8	1.6	6.0	0.0	3.0	3.0
Total Score	54	20.0	4.4	24.0	4.6	19.7	5.1

A breakdown of the availability of healthier choices and price differential across the Australian core food groups is shown in Appendix A. In most, but not all cases regardless of store types, healthier choices were more expensive and less available.

All supermarkets and general stores sold reduced fat milk. The price comparisons showed the price of reduced fat milk was more expensive than full fat milk in all stores. Low fat cheese and/or low fat yoghurt was only available in 27% of food stores and, where it was available' low fat options were more expensive than full fat. Wholegrain bread was available in all stores and more expensive than white bread in 27% of stores. Overall, healthier varieties of cereals (including rice, pasta, grains) were more expensive 60% of the time compared to their healthier counterparts. Low fat minced beef (ground beef) was available at two food stores across the Shire; at one of these it was more expensive than full fat minced beef and the other store stocked only low-fat minced beef so no price comparison was possible. The remaining nine stores stocked full fat varieties only. All five supermarkets and four of the six general stores stocked a wide variety of fruit and vegetables (10 or more). None of the food stores displayed any healthy eating promotions at the time of the surveys.

3.2. Food Service Outlets

Twenty-eight food service outlets were surveyed however, one café closed before collection of follow-up information and was excluded from the study (n = 27). All food service outlets were independent stores, with no fast food chain outlets in this rural community. Table 4 describes the type of food service establishment, number of outlets, explanation of the categorization, the mean and standard deviation NEMS-R score.

Table 4. Types and number of food service outlets across the Local Government Area and a comparison fast food chain outlet with their mean NEMS-R Scores and their scores as a percentage of the maximum NEMS-R Score (−5 to 23).

Food Service	Number of Outlets	NEMS-R SCORE		% of Max NEMS-R SCORE (−5 to 23)
	N	Mean	SD	%
Fast Casual: Hotels/pubs/restaurant	13	1.8	1.6	7.8
Fast Casual: Café	7	7.0	5.6	30.0
Fast Food: Take-aways	5	2.0	2.9	8.7
Fast Food: Bakeries	2	4.0	0.7	17.4
Total	27	3.0	4.0	13.0
Comparison	1	10.0	0.0	43.0

The mean NEMS-R score was low at 3 (SD 4.0) out of a possible 23, (excluding children's menu) [39] across the LGA. Nine of the 27 food service outlets offered a children's menu, eight of these scored two points, one scored five points (possible scoring range −3 to 9). One fast food outlet received a negative score indicating that the store sold almost exclusively unhealthy foods and encouraged over-consumption by promoting up-selling through 'meals deals' that comprise fried foods and sugar sweetened beverages at a price cheaper than purchasing items individually. Aside from one café in the central area scoring 17, no other food service outlet scored higher than eight. NEMS-R scoring of a comparison neighbouring fast food chain store, that predominately sold fried food, scored 10. Table 5 shows comparisons between different areas of the LGA, with the central area having a slightly better food environment as scored on NEMS-R.

Table 5. NEMS-R score means for the north, central and south of the Local Government Area.

	Score Range	NORTH			CENTRAL			SOUTH		
Number of outlets	27	9			13			5		
		MEAN	SD	% *	MEAN	SD	%	MEAN	SD	%
NEMS-R score	−8–32	2.0	1.0	6%	4.0	5.0	12%	3.0	3.0	9%

* percentage score calculated as a % mean of maximum possible score.

There was no statistically significant difference between these geographic boundaries or between types of outlets and the mean total. Table 6 reports NEMS-R according to food service outlet and compares means across the three measures of availability, facilitators and barriers to healthy eating. Means scores across hotels, cafes, fast food and bakeries were all low (maximum possible scores, means and standard deviations shown in the table). There were no statistically significant differences between these store types, though café's in general scored higher than hotels/pubs. Health promoting practices, as defined by NEMS-R, include signage/promotions, nutrition information/notations on menus, and reduced portion sizes.

Table 6. NEMS-R scores by type of food service outlet and health promoting practices.

Type of Outlet		Total		Hotels/Pubs/ Restaurant *		Cafes		Fast Food		Bakeries	
Outlets (n (%))		27 (100)		13 (48.1)		7 (25.9)		5 (18.5)		2 (7.4)	
NEMS-R items	Possible Score (A score closer to the maximum possible score indicates a healthier food environment.)	M	SD	M	SD	M	SD	M	SD	M	SD
Availability of healthy choices	0–15	2.8	2.5	1.4	1.4	5.3	3.1	2.6	1.5	3.5	0.7
Facilitators of healthy eating	0–8	0.4	1.4	0.2	0.4	1.1	2.6	−1.0	1.4	0.0	0.0
Barriers to healthy eating	−5–0	−0.3	0.8	0.0	0.0	−0.3	0.8	−1.0	1.4	0.0	0.0

* The scores of the one restaurant were combined with hotels/pubs to preserve anonymity.

The most frequent practice observed was the provision of diet soda (100% of food service outlets), and low fat milk (about two thirds of food service outlets) with two using it as the default option in hot and cold drinks. Across the area, 23% of food service outlets offered at least one main meal designated as 'healthy' according to NEMS-R standards. Fried, french fry-style potato chips were served at the majority (88%) of food service outlets. About a third (37%) offered a children's menu, from which one menu item met the NEMS-R definition of 'healthy' and two menu items included a healthy side as per published definition [31]. About a quarter (23%) offered unprocessed fruit for sale, 15% had non-fried vegetables identified on their menus. Across all food service outlets, just under half had wholemeal bread available, and just over half offered 100% fruit juice. Nutritional information and healthy menu items were identified in only one food service outlet. Bottled water was available for sale at all food service outlets, with some offering free tap water. Data on the collection of freely available tap water was not a component of the NEMS-R tool.

4. Discussion

The aim of this study was to describe the food environment in a rural Australian community in order to inform future community-relevant food supply interventions. We provide a comprehensive account of the community and consumer food environments in this LGA. The findings provide evidence that major changes to the food environment are needed for healthy foods to be available equitably to all community members. Food stores scored poorly on food availability and comparative pricing. Among food stores, healthier options were more expensive than their unhealthy alternative, and we observed variable quality of fresh fruit and vegetables. The availability of food service outlets (n = 27) was more predominant than food stores (n = 11), with the majority (n = 26) receiving low scores indicating healthy choices of prepared food were generally difficult to obtain across this LGA.

While NEMS tools have been used internationally across a variety of settings including rural environments [42,43], many have adapted the tool to local context thereby limiting direct comparability of these findings with our study. There are also no similar studies within Australia either measuring the food environment of a whole rural LGA or using the NEMS tools to undertake a comprehensive food environment audit.

4.1. Food Stores

Generally smaller store sizes have been correlated with lower NEMS-S scores and fewer healthy foods than larger supermarkets [44]. In our study, there was no statistically significant difference in the comparative pricing score between supermarkets and general stores, this may be due to a number of reasons. Firstly, both scores for comparative pricing (healthy vs. unhealthy price of a similar product), were very poor (1.2 and 1.0 respectively out of a possible 18 points); secondly, the small number of stores across the LGA limits statistical analysis, thirdly all supermarkets were small in size with the largest one having five registers, the smallest just one register, this limits the stock they can carry and may constrain their bargaining power in regards to food supply logistics to obtain healthy choices at a reasonable price. We consider the lack of variability in the quality score to be related to the quality scoring systems within the NEMS protocol where an 85% score translates to 100% on analysis. We consider some of our stores were over-scored on quality due to this protocol.

Our findings are consistent with studies that have identified rural areas typically have smaller and fewer supermarkets which equates to less variety, poorer quality and higher prices than in urban areas [7,43,45]. In Australia, four major supermarket chains exist, only the smallest of these was present in this community, all food stores in this LGA would be considered small in an urban context. In comparison with international studies, our food store environment score (39%) is lower than scores obtained in rural USA (around 60%) [7,42]. Our very low score indicates a food environment that is not conducive to healthy eating. However it also provides a baseline environment score and potential opportunity for food supply interventions to make a big impact on the availability of healthy choices.

Transport services to remote Indigenous communities are cited as barriers to a healthier food supply [46]. We contend that non-Indigenous rural and remote areas, locally and internationally, experience similar issues and all may benefit from food stores working together to negotiate lower freight costs [9], thereby, increasing supply and lowering prices. In the shorter term, interventions supported by food store owners show potential to improve healthier choices, these include: taste tests, free samples of healthier choices and communication interventions [47], also nutrition-style shelf labelling has been shown to be effective at nudging healthier choices [48].

Food store owners perceive that barriers to purchasing, stocking and promoting healthy food include consumer preferences for high fat, high sugar and low prices, along with lower wholesale availability of healthy food [47]. Within a small, low income, low profit-margin community, a useful strategy may be to provide financial incentives to healthy food procurement [8]. All interventions should not only focus on store proximity but availability of healthy choices [49]. Given that rural residents typically demonstrate strong loyalty to local food stores [50], these stores are well placed to positively impact dietary choices.

4.2. Food Service Outlets

Across the study area there are no major chain fast food outlets but 27 independent locally owned pubs, fast food outlets and cafes, with the majority of these providing inexpensive readily available high fat foods. Although the methodology differed, our findings are consistent with the Australian study by Innes-Hughes et al. (2012) [26] where take-away outlets in each town offered very few healthy foods, and high fat choices dominated menus.

Consistent with Pereira [43] we found the most widespread 'healthier practice' within food service outlets to be the availability of diet soda (100% in our study c.f. 80%). Healthy menu item availability was low with less than 30% of venues offering even one healthy choice (as defined by NEMS) [42,43]. The one food service outlet that scored well (74%) applies the State Government Healthy Choices Guidelines [51] supporting product promotion, placement and healthy meal deals. Other than this higher score, we observed that our comparison fast food chain outlet scored better than most of the food service outlets within the LGA, mainly due to the signage used rather than the health of the food on offer.

Our very low baseline restaurant score of 3 (SD 4.0) is indicative of an urgent need to intervene with multiple opportunities to improve the healthiness of food offerings within food service outlets [50]. Martinez-Donate (2015) [42] reported improved NEMS-R scores post introduction of a suite of strategies to promote healthier choices, including point-of-purchase labelling and promotions of healthier items. Children's menus could be improved through the introduction of healthy sides as default and reducing serving sizes [52]. Changing to healthier oils in takeaway outlets has been shown to reduce saturated fat intake in previous studies [53] and given the pervasiveness of deep fried food in the study area, a reduction in the use of unhealthy fats may be a useful first step in conjunction with the broader systemic changes required.

4.3. NEMS Tools for a Rural Australian Context

We identified limitations with the NEMS tools in the Australian rural context. With regards to NEMS-S, we considered the quality score protocol often created an over-statement of actual produce quality. Where we assigned a score of 75%, this was equated to 100% score in the overall score. In regards to NEMS-R we considered a smaller portion at a cheaper price should have been awarded a score. We also consider ready access to free tap water should receive additional points. We have some concerns about the importance placed on nutritional promotion given the example of our comparison store, which scored better than most stores, despite the mainly unhealthy food offerings.

4.4. Strengths

To our knowledge, this study is the first in Australia to apply the validated NEMS tools including all food stores across a single local government area, and is one of very few examining the food environment in a rural Australian context. Our study used ground-truthing to provide an accurate representation of the current food environment at a given point in time.

4.5. Limitations

By only collecting data within the LGA geographical borders, out-shopping to larger towns has not been accounted for. In this study there was no comparison group. The study was conducted at a single point in time so does not necessarily provide data on usual food availability, quality or pricing. One might expect seasonality would contribute to variation of produce, or variations in days of the week, which may be influenced by supplier drop off or residents' weekly shops. This study was limited to the rural, Australian context in which it was conducted, thus application of the results may not be appropriate for or applicable to other contexts. Also food environments can change rapidly, as evidenced in this and similar studies by businesses closing during the time of the audit [7].

5. Conclusions

Our findings showed that the healthfulness of the food environment for this remote local government area of rural Victoria is poor. Healthy options, nutrition information and nutrition promotion are not available at most food stores across the LGA.

Outside a supermarket it is very difficult to purchase healthy food in this rural community, made more challenging by the fact that supermarkets are often a significant distance from residents' homes. Given that food environments are a key determinant of obesity [54] and rural loyalty to local business [49], the current predominately unhealthy food environment provides scope to work with food retailers and consumers to ensure healthier options are more visible, available and affordable. This may enable consumers to make healthier choices and thereby impact positively on the health of this community.

Successful interventions have utilised multipronged strategies to improve both food supply and customer demand [8]. We consider it a priority to affect the food environment as a frontline intervention before embarking on, or alongside, any individual behaviour change strategies to ensure healthy food choices are available when consumers seek to choose these.

6. Recommendations

More research is required to explore the relationship between the food environment and food security in rural Australia and with health of those who reside there.

Author Contributions: Conceptualization, J.W., C.B. and P.L.; Data curation, J.W., C.R., F.G. and P.L.; Formal analysis, J.W., L.M., C.R., F.G. and P.L.; Funding acquisition, J.W.; Investigation, J.W. and P.L.; Methodology, J.W. and P.L.; Project administration, J.W. and P.L.; Resources, J.W. and P.L.; Supervision, J.W., L.M., C.B., S.A. and P.L.; Writing—original draft, J.W., L.M., C.B., C.R. and P.L.; Writing—review & editing, J.W., L.M., C.B., C.R., F.G., S.A. and P.L.

Funding: The first author (J.W.) received funding from the Royal Flying Doctors Service, Victoria.

Acknowledgments: Thanks to the local food stores for allowing us to collect this information.

Conflicts of Interest: The authors declare no conflict of interest. The funders had no role in the design of the study; in the collection, analyses, or interpretation of data; in the writing of the manuscript, or in the decision to publish the results.

Appendix A

Table A1. Availability of more healthful options, and pricing features for supermarkets and general stores, across the local government area, 2017.

Core Food Group (AGHE ref)	Total N = 11	Super-Markets N = 5	General Stores N = 6
Availability of healthier breakfast cereal > 2 varieties	9	5	4
n (%) cost healthy cereal < unhealthy	5	3	2
Whole grain bread availability	10	5	5
>2 varieties whole wheat bread	8	5	3
Price same for both	7	4	3
Price higher for whole wheat	3	1	2

Table A1. *Cont.*

Core Food Group (AGHE ref)	Total N = 11	Super-Markets N = 5	General Stores N = 6
DAIRY OR ALTERNATIVES			
Low-fat/skim **milk** available	11	5	6
Price Higher for low-fat/skim milk	11	5	6
Low-fat **cheese** available	3	3	0
Price Same for both	2	2	0
Price Higher for low-fat	1	1	
Low fat Yoghurt availability	3	3	0
Price Lower for lowest-fat	1	1	0
Price Same for both	1	1	0
Price Higher for low-fat	1	1	
FRESH FRUIT AVAILABILITY—NUMBER OF VARIETIES			
<5 varieties	1		1
5–9 varieties	3		3
10 varieties	7	5	2
FRESH VEGETABLES AVAILABILITY—NUMBER OF VARIETIES			
5–9 varieties	2	0	2
10 varieties	9	5	4
MEAT OR MEAT ALTERNATIVES			
Low-fat mince availability (beef or turkey)	2	2	0
Higher price for lean meat	1	1	
Chicken availability—skinless breast	5	4	1
Price Higher for skinless	3	3	
Legumes available (could also be classified as vegetables)	10	5	5
Eggs available	10	5	5
DISCRETIONARY FOODS			
Healthier snack alternatives to chips (e.g., Grain Waves) (Baked alternative to fried potato crisps)	4	4	0
Chips- Price- (Fried potato crisps)			
Price Lower for Grain Waves than Smiths Chips	0	0	0
Price Higher for Grain Waves than Smiths Chips	4	4	
Healthier dry biscuits available (e.g., water crackers)	11	5	6
Price Lower for water crackers than BBQ shapes (Savoury crackers)	10	5	5
Diet soft drinks available	10	5	5
Same price for both	10	5	5
100% Juice Availability-	9	5	4
Lower for 100% juice (2 L)	1	1	
Same for both	1		1
Higher for 100% juice (2 L)	4	2	2

References

1. Roberto, C.A.; Swinburn, B.; Hawkes, C.; Huang, T.T.K.; Costa, S.A.; Ashe, M.; Zwicker, L.; Cawley, J.H.; Brownell, K.D. Patchy progress on obesity prevention: Emerging examples, entrenched barriers, and new thinking. *Lancet* **2015**, *385*, 2400–2409. [CrossRef]

2. Australian Institute of Health and Welfare. *Australian Burden of Disease Study: Impact and Causes of Illness and Death in Australia 2011.S Bod 4*; AIHW, Ed.; Australian Institute of Health and Welfare: Canberra, Australia, 2016.

3. Swinburn, B.A.; Sacks, G.; Hall, K.D.; McPherson, K.; Finegood, D.T.; Moodie, M.L.; Gortmaker, S.L. The global obesity pandemic: Shaped by global drivers and local environments. *Lancet* **2011**, *378*, 804–814. [CrossRef]

4. Forouzanfar, M.H.; Alexander, L.; Anderson, H.R.; Bachman, V.F.; Biryukov, S.; Brauer, M.; Burnett, R.; Casey, D.; Coates, M.M.; Cohen, A.; et al. Global, regional, and national comparative risk assessment of 79 behavioural, environmental and occupational, and metabolic risks or clusters of risks in 188 countries, 1990–2013: A systematic analysis for the global burden of disease study 2013. *Lancet* **2015**, *386*, 2287–2323. [CrossRef]

5. Rahmanian, E.; Gasevic, D.; Vukmirovich, I.; Lear, S.A. The association between the built environment and dietary intake-a systematic review. *Asia Pac. J. Clin. Nutr.* **2014**, *23*, 183–196. [PubMed]

6. Engler-Stringer, R.; Le, H.; Gerrard, A.; Muhajarine, N. The community and consumer food environment and children's diet: A systematic review. *BMC Public Health* **2014**, *14*, 522. [CrossRef] [PubMed]

7. Vilaro, M.; Barnett, T. The rural food environment: A survey of food price, availability, and quality in a rural Florida community. *Food Public Health* **2013**, *3*, 111–118. [CrossRef]

8. Gittelsohn, J.; Rowan, M.; Gadhoke, P. Interventions in small food stores to change the food environment, improve diet, and reduce risk of chronic disease. *Prev. Chronic Dis.* **2012**, *9*. [CrossRef]

9. National Rural Health Alliance. *Food Security and Health in Rural and Remote Australia*; Australian Government: Rural Industries Research and Development Corporation: Canberra, Australia, 2016.

10. Health Canada. *Measuring the Food Environment in Canada*; Ministry of Health: Ottawa, ON, Canada, 2013.

11. Lebel, A.; Noreau, D.; Tremblay, L.; Oberlé, C.; Girard-Gadreau, M.; Duguay, M.; Block, J.P. Identifying rural food deserts: Methodological considerations for food environment interventions. *Can. J. Public Health* **2016**, *107*, 5353. [CrossRef] [PubMed]

12. Palermo, C.; McCartan, J.; Kleve, S.; Sinha, K.; Shiell, A. A longitudinal study of the cost of food in Victoria influenced by geography and nutritional quality. *Aust. N. Z. J. Public Health* **2016**, *40*, 270–273. [CrossRef] [PubMed]

13. Vilaro, M.; Barnett, T. The rural food environment: A survey of food price, availability, and quality in a rural florida community. *Food Public Health* **2013**, *3*, 10–5923.

14. Hardin-Fanning, F.; Rayens, M.K. Food cost disparities in rural communities. *Health Promot. Pract.* **2015**, *16*, 383–3911. [CrossRef] [PubMed]

15. Lenardson, J.D.; Hansen, A.Y.; Hartley, D. Rural and remote food environments and obesity. *Curr. Obes. Rep.* **2015**, *4*, 46–53. [CrossRef] [PubMed]

16. Byker Shanks, C.; Ahmed, S.; Smith, T.; Houghtaling, B.; Jenkins, M.; Margetts, M.; Schultz, D.; Stephens, L. Availability, price, and quality of fruits and vegetables in 12 rural Montana counties, 2014. *Prev. Chronic Dis.* **2015**, *12*, E128. [CrossRef] [PubMed]

17. Bardenhagen, C.J.; Pinard, C.A.; Pirog, R.; Yaroch, A.L. Characterizing rural food access in remote areas. *J. Commun. Health* **2017**, *42*, 1008–1019. [CrossRef] [PubMed]

18. Gantner, L.A.; Olson, C.M.; Frongillo, E.A.; Wells, N.M. Prevalence of nontraditional food stores and distance to healthy foods in a rural food environment. *J. Hunger Environ. Nutr.* **2011**, *6*, 279–293. [CrossRef]

19. Rideout, K.; Mah, C.; Minaker, L. *Food Environments: An Introduction for Public Health Practice*; National Collaborating Centre for Environmental Health British Columbia Centre for Disease Control: Vancouver, BC, Canada, 2015.

20. Glanz, K.; Sallis, J.F.; Saelens, B.E.; Frank, L.D. Healthy nutrition environments: Concepts and measures. *Am. J. Health Promot.* **2005**, *19*, 330–333. [CrossRef] [PubMed]

21. Rychetnik, L.; Webb, K.; Story, L.; Katz, T. *Food Security Options Paper: A Planning Framework and Menu of Options for Policy and Practice Intervention*; Nutrition Centre for Population Health: Sydney, Australia, 2003.

22. Burns, C. *A Review of the Literature Describing the Link between Poverty, Food Insecurity and Obesity with Specific Reference to Australia*; VicHealth: Melbourne, Australia, 2004.

23. Dhurandhar, E.J. The food-insecurity obesity paradox: A resource scarcity hypothesis. *Physiol. Behav.* **2016**, *162*, 88–92. [CrossRef] [PubMed]

24. Backholer, K.; Spencer, E.; Gearon, E.; Magliano, D.J.; McNaughton, S.A.; Shaw, J.E.; Peeters, A. The association between socio-economic position and diet quality in Australian adults. *Public Health Nutr.* **2016**, *19*, 477–485. [CrossRef] [PubMed]

25. Glanz, K.; Johnson, L.; Yaroch, A.L.; Phillips, M.; Ayala, G.X.; Davis, E.L. Measures of retail food store environments and sales: Review and implications for healthy eating initiatives. *J. Nutr. Educ. Behav.* **2016**, *48*, 280–288. [CrossRef] [PubMed]

26. Innes-Hughes, C.; Boylan, S.; King, L.A.; Lobb, E. Measuring the food environment in three rural towns in new south wales, Australia. *Health Promot. J. Aust.* **2012**, *23*, 129–133. [CrossRef]

27. Krukowski, R.A.; West, D.S.; Harvey-Berino, J.; Prewitt, T.E. Neighborhood impact on healthy food availability and pricing in food stores. *J. Commun. Health* **2010**, *35*, 315–320. [CrossRef] [PubMed]

28. Cameron, A.J. The shelf space and strategic placement of healthy and discretionary foods in urban, urban-fringe and rural/non-metropolitan Australian supermarkets. *Public Health Nutr.* **2018**, *21*, 593–600. [CrossRef] [PubMed]

29. United States Department of Agriculture. USDA Food Plans: Cost of Food. Available online: https://www.cnpp.usda.gov/USDAFoodPlansCostofFood (accessed on 22 July 2018).

30. Glanz, K.; Sallis, J.F.; Saelens, B.E.; Frank, L.D. Nutrition environment measures survey in stores (NEMS-S): Development and evaluation. *Am. J. Prev. Med.* **2007**, *32*, 273–281. [CrossRef] [PubMed]

31. Saelens, B.E.; Glanz, K.; Sallis, J.F.; Frank, L.D. Nutrition environment measures study in restaurants (NEMS-R): Development and evaluation. *Am. J. Prev. Med.* **2007**, *32*, 282–289. [CrossRef] [PubMed]

32. Hector, D.; Boylan, S.; Lee, A. *Healthy Food Environment Scoping Review*; PANORG: Sydney, Australia, 2016.

33. Palermo, C.; Wilson, A. Development of a healthy food basket for Victoria. *Aust. N. Z. J. Public Health* **2007**, *31*, 360–363. [CrossRef] [PubMed]

34. Chapman, K.; Innes-Hughes, C.; Goldsbury, D.; Kelly, B.; Bauman, A.; Allman-Farinelli, M. A comparison of the cost of generic and branded food products in Australian supermarkets. *Public Health Nutr.* **2013**, *16*, 894–900. [CrossRef] [PubMed]

35. Department of Health and Human Services. *Victorian Population Health Survey 2014: Modifiable Risk Factors Contributing to Chronic Disease*; Department of Health and Human Services, Ed.; State Government of Victoria: Melbourne, Australia, 2016.

36. Australian Bureau of Statistics. Data by Region. Available online: http://stat.abs.gov.au/itt/r.jsp?databyregion#/ (accessed on 25 July 2018).

37. Saelens, B.; Glanz, K.; Sallis, J.; Frank, L. NEMS-R Scoring Systems Dimensions. Available online: http://www.med.upenn.edu/nems/measures.shtml (accessed on 22 July 2018).

38. National Health and Medical Research Council. *Australian Guide to Healthy Eating*; NHMRC, Ed.; National Health and Medical Research Council: Canberra, Australia, 2013.

39. NEMS-R Scoring Systems Dimensions. Available online: https://www.med.upenn.edu/nems/measures.shtml (accessed on 20 July 2018).

40. University of Pennsylvania. NEMS Online Training. Available online: http://www.med.upenn.edu/nems/onlinetraining.shtml (accessed on 16 May 2018).

41. StataCorp. *Statacorp Stata Statistical Software: Release*, version 15; StataCorp: College Station, TX, USA, 2017.

42. Martínez-Donate, A.P.; Riggall, A.J.; Meinen, A.M.; Malecki, K.; Escaron, A.L.; Hall, B.; Menzies, A.; Garske, G.; Nieto, F.J.; Nitzke, S. Evaluation of a pilot healthy eating intervention in restaurants and food stores of a rural community: A randomized community trial. *BMC Public Health* **2015**, *15*, 136. [CrossRef] [PubMed]

43. Pereira, R.F.; Sidebottom, A.C.; Boucher, J.L.; Lindberg, R.; Werner, R. Assessing the food environment of a rural community: Baseline findings from the heart of new Ulm project, Minnesota, 2010–2011. *Prev. Chronic Dis.* **2014**, *11*. [CrossRef] [PubMed]

44. Cauchi, D.; Pliakas, T.; Knai, C. Food environments in Malta: Associations with store size and area-level deprivation. *Food Policy* **2017**, *71*, 39–47. [CrossRef]

45. Ghosh-Dastidar, M.; Hunter, G.; Collins, R.L.; Zenk, S.N.; Cummins, S.; Beckman, R.; Nugroho, A.K.; Sloan, J.C.; Dubowitz, T. Does opening a supermarket in a food desert change the food environment? *Health Place* **2017**, *46*, 249–256. [CrossRef] [PubMed]

46. National Rural Health Alliance. *Freight Improvement Toolkit—Getting Quality Healthy Food to Remote Indigenous Communities*; National Rural Health Alliance: Canberra, Australia, 2007.

47. Kim, M.; Budd, N.; Batorsky, B.; Krubiner, C.; Manchikanti, S.; Waldrop, G.; Trude, A.; Gittelsohn, J. Barriers to and facilitators of stocking healthy food options: Viewpoints of Baltimore city small storeowners. *Eco. Food Nutr.* **2017**, *56*, 17–30. [CrossRef] [PubMed]

48. Cameron, A.; Charlton, E.; Ngan, W.; Sacks, G. A systematic review of the effectiveness of supermarket-based interventions involving product, promotion, or place on the healthiness of consumer purchases. *Curr. Nutr. Rep.* **2016**, *5*, 129–138. [CrossRef]

49. Marshall, D.; Dawson, J.; Nisbet, L. Food access in remote rural places: Consumer accounts of food shopping. *Reg. Stud.* **2018**, *52*, 133–144. [CrossRef]

50. Cannuscio, C.C.; Tappe, K.; Hillier, A.; Buttenheim, A.; Karpyn, A.; Glanz, K. Urban food environments and residents' shopping behaviors. *Am. J. Prev. Med.* **2013**, *45*, 606–614. [CrossRef] [PubMed]

51. Healthy Eating Advisory Service. The Healthy Choices Framework. Available online: https://heas.health. vic.gov.au/sites/default/files/HEAS-healthy-choices-framework.pdf (accessed on 24 June 2018).

52. Ayala, G.X.; Castro, I.A.; Pickrel, J.L.; Williams, C.B.; Lin, S.-F.; Madanat, H.; Jun, H.-J.; Zive, M. A restaurant-based intervention to promote sales of healthy children's menu items: The kids' choice restaurant program cluster randomized trial. *BMC Public Health* **2016**, *16*, 250. [CrossRef] [PubMed]

53. Simmons, A.; Sanigorski, A.M.; Cuttler, R.; Brennan, M.; Kremer, P.; Mathews, L.; Swinburn, B. *Nutrition and Physical Activity in Children and Adolescents: Report 6: Lessons Learned from Colac's be Active Eat Well Project (2002-6)*; Department of Human Services Victoria, Melbourne, Vic.: Melbourne, Australia, 2009. Available online: http://dro.deakin.edu.au/view/DU:30021654 (accessed on 24 June 2018).

54. Butland, B.; Jebb, S.; Kopelman, P.; McPherson, K.; Thomas, S.; Mardell, J.; Parry, V. *Foresight: Tackling Obesities—Future Choices Project Report*; Government Office of Science: London, UK, 2007.

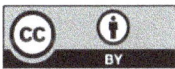

International Journal of
Environmental Research and Public Health

MDPI

Article

Undeserving, Disadvantaged, Disregarded: Three Viewpoints of Charity Food Aid Recipients in Finland

Anna Sofia Salonen [1,*], **Maria Ohisalo** [2] **and Tuomo Laihiala** [1]

[1]   Faculty of Social Sciences, University of Tampere, 33014 Tampere, Finland; tuomo.laihiala@uta.fi
[2]   Y-Foundation, 00531 Helsinki, Finland; maria.ohisalo@ysaatio.fi
*   Correspondence: anna.salonen@uta.fi

Received: 30 October 2018; Accepted: 13 December 2018; Published: 17 December 2018

Abstract: Since the economic recession of the 1990s, Finland has experienced the proliferation of charity food aid as a means of helping people who are afflicted by poverty. However, so far little research has been conducted regarding the food aid recipients. This article gives discursive, demographic, and experiential insights into charity food provision and reception in Finland. Drawing on quantitative survey data, online discussion data related to news published on Finnish newspapers' web pages, and observation and interviews with food aid recipients, this article sheds new light on Finnish food aid recipients from three perspectives. First, public perceptions about food aid often portray food recipients as dishonourable and responsible for their own poverty. Secondly, the survey data shows that the main reason for people resorting to charity food aid is deep economic disadvantage, and further, that there is an unequal accumulation of disadvantage among the food aid recipients, illustrating internal diversity. Third, observational and interview data show that from the food recipients' perspective, the food aid system has only a limited ability to answer even their immediate food needs, and for the recipients, food aid venues can become not only socially significant, but also socially demanding and emotionally burdening places.

Keywords: food aid; charity; Finland; welfare state; food aid recipient; deservingness; disadvantages; inequality

---

1. Introduction

Despite the almost thirty years of charitable food aid in Finland, so far little research has been conducted about the aid recipients. There have been a few studies examining the clientele of church diocese work and the food aid users at individual food banks [1–5]. This trend has changed only recently, as three studies have taken the initiative to explore Finnish charity food aid particularly from the users' perspectives [6–8]. In this article, we use the existing data from these three studies to give a comprehensive picture of what is known so far about people receiving food aid in Finland.

Recent decades have witnessed the growth of food aid across the affluent world [9,10]. The global expansion of this phenomenon raises serious questions concerning food insecurity, public policy, and the future of welfare states. Food aid has prompted a lot of research in different parts of the world. However, there is still a need for more research on the various societal contexts in which food aid proliferates and on the viewpoints of the aid users [11] in terms of both who they are and how they perceive the aid they receive. With the concept of charity food aid, we refer to the phenomenon where non-governmental organizations (NGOs) provide free food to people who are living in poor social and economic situations; in contrast to statutory welfare provision, the food aid is voluntarily organized by the NGOs.

The Nordic welfare state context makes the Finnish case peculiar in relation to the many other countries where food aid has proliferated. In principle in Finland, the state is assumed to provide universal social security against social risks, such as poverty, for all its citizens. However, since the recession of the 1990s, Finland has experienced the proliferation of charity-based food aid provision as a means of helping people who are afflicted by poverty, indicating that the welfare state does not feed everybody. In Finland, food aid was initially considered a short-term response to the consequences of the recession of the 1990s, but it has gradually grown into an unorganized field, with hundreds of actors sharing food throughout the country. Over a quarter of a century, breadlines have become one of the most visible and well-known portrayals of poverty in Finland [12,13].

In the first cross-national study of charity food aid in the 1990s, it was stated that food aid is characteristic of residual welfare states, whereas the universalist Nordic welfare states have been able to safeguard social rights, such as the human right to food [14]. However, the Finnish case has challenged this perception. In her recent study comparing food aid and its implications for the welfare state in Finland and Scotland, Mary Anne MacLeod found that the rise of food assistance in Finland is coupled with the dilemmas of welfare state identity. Food poverty and food aid are considered marginal to the welfare state; food aid questions the effectiveness of the welfare system, and it is associated with societal failure. According to MacLeod's study, in Finland, food is positioned as a public good, and thus charitable models of food aid provision are perceived as a threat to the social democratic welfare regime [15].

On the state level, it has been argued that the necessity for charity food aid contravenes the Finnish Constitution, which declares that everyone should have the right to a life of dignity guaranteed by the state. Section 19 in the Finnish constitution, 'the right to social security', explicitly lays the foundation for public social policy and social security, and points out the responsibility of the public authorities to safeguard social welfare and health. Finland has also signed the UN covenant on the Right to Food (RTF), which should guarantee freedom from hunger together with access to safe and nutritious food [9]. In other words, charity food aid raises particular disputes in the context of a Nordic welfare state that is presumed to guarantee basic social security for all its citizens.

Tellingly, food aid has even been called the 'open wound' of the welfare state [16] (p. 255). In public debates, it has been considered a deviant practice, since there should be no need for food aid in an affluent Finnish society with a comprehensive social security system. At the same time, the efforts of churches and NGOs to provide food aid have been applauded. The perception of food aid thus holds an ambivalent position in Finnish public discourse: charitable food assistance is not fitting for the Nordic welfare state, but it is an appropriate way for churches to help the needy [17]. Thus, Finland marks an interesting case where the strong constitutional responsibilities of the state meet widespread unofficial aid provided by a lively and diverse non-governmental sector.

Due to this particular discrepancy between the strong welfare state ideal and strong grassroots charity aid, the connection between professional social work and food aid is in principle absent in Finland. There is no referral system between charity food providers and social services, and it has even been considered unconstitutional for social workers to inform or guide their clients to charity food aid services [18,19]. In other words, there are no explicit connections between food aid and public social policy. Illustrative of this gap on the state level is the fact that the administration of the EU's food aid programme in Finland was first set up under the Ministry of Agriculture and Forestry—and later the Ministry of Employment and the Economy—instead of the Ministry of Social Affairs and Health ([13], p. 476). Interestingly, however, many of the non-governmental organizations providing food aid receive some public funding—from local municipalities, for example—to support their non-profit work. Nevertheless, this funding is not targeted at food aid per se, but to the infrastructures and general activities of the organizations. In practice, then, food aid is often publicly supported, though only partly and indirectly.

On the grassroots level, the characteristic features of Finnish charity food aid are a low-level of organization and a lack of eligibility control. Unlike in many other countries, there are hardly any intermediaries in Finland that could collect and store food and redeliver it to local charities. Instead, local actors most often collect, store, and redistribute the food independently and according to their own individual practices [20]. The methods of providing assistance vary across the individual food aid organizations, but very often food aid provision is based on the principles of low threshold and the absence of means tests. Some food aid providers might ask to see proof of the recipient's status as unemployed or a pensioner, for example, but a detailed income assessment is rarely conducted. The basic principle is that asking for food aid is in itself a sign that the recipient deserves the aid. Thus, in many assistance venues, technically anyone can ask for and receive charity food aid.

Due to a lack of coordination, shared practices, or comparable statistics, only rough approximations can be drawn about the volume of food aid in Finland. A 2013 survey estimated that food assistance was available in over 220 of the more than 300 municipalities throughout the country [20]. The food aid is distributed via various faith-based and other NGOs. The food comes from two main sources: the EU food aid programme and food companies and grocery stores donating their surplus food. In addition, public institutions such as schools have recently started to give out surplus meals to charities. Based on the assessment of food aid distributors, approximately 20,000 people received food aid rather regularly in 2013 [20]. However, a national-level survey asking whether respondents had used food aid at least once a year found that more than four times that number had received food aid [21]. The Evangelical-Lutheran Church in Finland gave food in the form of free or cheap meals or food packages to roughly 56,000 people in 2015 [22]. These are significant figures in a country with a population of approximately 5.5 million people. For comparison, in 2015, 634,000 people, or 11.7% of the Finnish population, were considered low-income—that is, they belonged to the population living on less than 60% of the equivalent median money income of all households [23].

Overall, the Finnish food aid system can be described as an unorganized yet widespread practice of unofficial, last-resort aid targeted at people living in difficult social and economic situations. Moreover, the system has no strict criteria for eligibility. This peculiar situation raises many questions. First of all, the lack of objective criteria for food eligibility provokes a normative debate concerning deservingness—that is, who should get what, and why [24,25]. Who should be granted the moral entitlement to use assistance that is in principle available to everyone, but which is at the same time contrary to the Finnish welfare ethos? Second, the situation raises a policy question concerning the populations involved in this widespread yet abnormal form of aid. In the absence of guidelines and practices shared between different food aid providers, it is very hard to estimate who the food assistance recipients are or to determine their reasons for using food aid. Third, such an unregulated and unofficial setting calls for an exploration of the experiences of the recipients. What are the repercussions of food aid use for these individuals? Without research addressing these questions, preconceptions flourish and colour the public and policy discussions on the issue.

In this article, we examine the Finnish charity food aid recipients from three distinct perspectives. First, we present findings from a study that analyses the online perceptions of food aid recipients to illustrate the discursive landscape in which Finnish charity food aid is rooted. Second, drawing on quantitative survey data collected among food aid recipients, we bring new light to the often-held assumptions about who the food aid recipients actually are. Third, we use observation and interview material from Finnish food banks to illustrate how the aid is experienced by the recipients. By bringing these findings together, we aim to provide a holistic picture of the food aid recipients in Finland. Together, the findings presented in this article provide discursive, demographic, and experiential insights into charity food provision and reception in the Finnish context, thus giving a novel account of charity food aid in an affluent, Nordic welfare state from the viewpoint of the people whom this aid concerns the most.

2. Materials and Methods

In this article, we present findings from recently conducted studies that utilize data from three sources. First, we present findings from online discussion data related to news published on Finnish newspapers' web pages to understand how the food aid recipients are perceived in public discourses. The data consist of 1294 comments collected from online discussions that were connected to news articles about food aid in nine prominent Finnish newspapers (*Aamulehti, Helsingin Sanomat, Iltalehti, Ilta-Sanomat, Länsiväylä, Metro, Satakunnan Kansa, Taloussanomat, Turun Sanomat*) in 2014 and 2015. The data were analysed with close reading, and a topic model was created with GUI Topic Modelling -programme to cover all the relevant themes. The themes that occurred in the data were interpreted in the light of Wim van Oorschot's criteria for deservingness, including need (the greater the level of need, the more deserving), control (poor people's control over their neediness, or their responsibility for it), identity (the identity of the poor, i.e., their proximity to the rich or their "pleasantness"), attitude (poor people's attitude towards support, or their docility or gratefulness), and reciprocity (the degree of reciprocation by the poor, or having earned support) [25]. The data collection and analysis is described in detail in [6].

Second, we present data from a quantitative survey that researched both the socio-economic status of food aid recipients and the accumulation of the recipients' disadvantages (see the Supplementary Materials for the English version of the survey form). This is the first and so far only study where the socio-economic position and disadvantages of the Finnish aid recipients has been studied with larger-scale survey data. The data were collected in a national food aid study (*N* = 3474) in 2012–2013 from 37 different charity food aid distributions in 11 Finnish municipalities. The food aid venues chosen for this study were known to be the largest in Finland in terms of the number of food aid recipients. As the number of people receiving food aid in Finland is unknown, the demographic sample does not necessarily represent all the food aid recipients in the country. However, the results from different municipalities are relatively uniform, indicating that the data sample captures a good overall picture of the food recipients. Surveys were distributed in three different languages—Finnish, Russian, and English—and the researchers who collected the surveys helped the respondents in translating them according to the situation. The study targeted the subjective well-being of the food aid recipients. The data were analysed with SPSS (IBM Corporation, Armonk, NY, USA) using multivariate methods, namely factor analysis, cluster analysis, and cross tabulations. The data collection and analysis is described in detail in [7].

Third, we present findings from a qualitative study that consist of observational notes from over seven months of participant observation in four food assistance organizations, written documents related to the operation of the organizations, and open-ended interviews with 25 food aid recipients. The data were collected from four food charity organizations in the city of Tampere, Finland, in 2012 and 2013. The selection of one of the large cities in Finland enabled the researchers to uncover possible variations in the different kinds of food aid venues and to reach a wider group of food recipients. The data were analysed with qualitative methods, such as qualitative inductive content analysis and grounded theory, where conceptions of different incidents, venues, people, and occasions were constructed and compared in order to develop a comprehensive understanding of the phenomenon. The data collection and analysis is described in detail in [8]. In this article, we discuss the findings that relate to the ability of food aid to meet the needs of the recipients.

In the subsequent sections, we first present the findings from these different data sets and then draw a synthesis of this recent body of knowledge on Finnish food aid recipients: we discuss how they are perceived by the public, who they actually are, and how they themselves see their own social position and the phenomenon they are engaged in (Figure 1). In the discussion section, we discuss these combined findings to show how they raise some significant issues regarding food aid recipients.

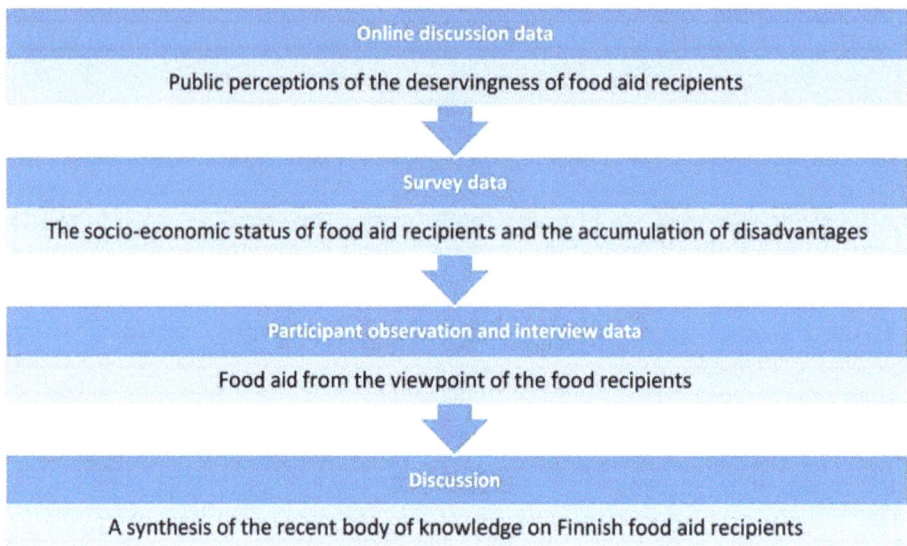

Figure 1. The outline of the study.

3. Results

3.1. Public Perceptions of Food Aid Recipients' Deservingness in Online Discussions

The online discussion data shows that Finnish food aid recipients are exposed to strong public criticism and blame. Of the themes covered in the discussions, the most prominent was the issue of need: the discussants questioned whether the food recipients were in need of food aid, for example, by suggesting that the recipients squander their money and then request assistance. The emphasis on need is surprising given that the needs-based arguments of deservingness do not fit well with the Finnish welfare state context.

The analysis of the online discussion data shows that the discussants differed based on how they related to the need of the food aid recipients and how they perceived the causes and reasons for the food aid use. The discussants who considered the food aid recipients to be in genuine need expressed their desire to help and give support and encouragement to the disadvantaged. Those who acknowledged the need but also blamed the recipients for their situation considered obtaining charity food aid acceptable only if the recipients were genuinely in need of help. However, the needs and motives of most of the recipients were questioned, and they were presumed to be caused by lifestyle choices. Furthermore, some of the online discussants maintained that food aid represents a systemic problem: in a good society, charity food aid should not be needed. The poor life situation of an individual is a matter for society and the welfare state rather than the fault of the individual. Finally, some of the discussants questioned the food recipients' need and pigeonholed them as undeserving scroungers.

Another central topic that surfaced in the discussions was the question of who is responsible for poverty. Unlike in previous quantitative research that found Finnish people tend to see poverty as a structural problem [26,27], a significant number of the online discussants considered the situation of the food aid recipients to be self-inflicted. The recipients' need was often questioned, and the recipients were considered a dishonourable group responsible for their own poverty. In its considerable resemblance to traditional aid for the poor, Finnish charity food aid enables this kind of discussion about deservingness, which fits poorly with an institutional welfare state.

Not all online discussants condemned the charity food aid recipients. Some defended the recipients' deservingness and considered them unfortunate, disadvantaged people who have to rely on charity food as a result of society's failures. Empathy, solidarity, and positive attitudes towards the recipients can be predicted by the discussant's personal or other close experiences with charity food aid and economic disadvantage in general. The analysis found that the discussants questioned the deservingness of the food aid recipients and emphasized their own responsibility particularly when the food aid recipients were not considered to belong to the same social group as them. The most conditional were the attitudes towards immigrant food recipients.

Unlike in studies that found gratitude and shame to be the prominent emotions expected of the food aid recipients [28], the Finnish online discussants rarely required the food recipients to perform emotional or attitude-related responses towards the aid or the aid providers. Instead, the food aid itself was seen by the discussants as humiliating, either for the food recipient or from the perspective of wider society.

3.2. The Socio-Economic Status of Food Aid Recipients and the Accumulation of the Recipients' Disadvantages

Perceptions of the extent of food aid in Finland, the position of aid recipients in the social security system, and their usage of services and benefits are often based on impressions rather than on systematic, empirical information. According to many food aid distributors, the picture of food aid recipients has diversified since the recession of the 1990s. Previously, it was often unemployed or homeless men queuing for food, but nowadays the charity food aid venues bring together people from a variety of backgrounds. The findings of the national food aid study presented here provide empirical evidence of the recipients' socio-economic position and disadvantages.

The socio-economic status of people receiving food aid was outlined with 11 questions. To begin with age, the biggest age group of food aid recipients was 46–65-year-olds. Young people tend not to be highly represented in Finnish food aid venues. There are several reasons for this; for example, students receive subsidized meals at the university level, and many of them complement their income by working part-time during their studies. Thus, the people receiving food aid seem to be older compared to the demographic structure of Finland in general (see Appendix A for the results compared to the general population of Finland).

Unlike in many other disadvantaged groups, the gender division among food aid recipients was nearly non-existent. There was only a small majority of women (51.7%, N = 1704) receiving food aid, even though men tend to be overrepresented in many disadvantaged groups. The majority of the people receiving food aid were native Finns (87.3%, N = 2817).

One stereotype about people receiving food aid in Finland is their assumed low educational background. However, the data partly challenge this supposition. In the food aid venues, there were more people with only a basic level of education (39.6%, N = 1270) and fewer people with a higher education background (20.4%, N = 656) compared to the general population in Finland. Nevertheless, the relative amount of the people with an upper secondary level education (40%, N = 1282) was nearly the same as it is among the wider Finnish population.

In terms of employment status, food aid recipients were characterized by a weak labour market position. Roughly four fifths of them were either pensioners (38.4%, N = 1260) or unemployed or laid off (38.4%, N = 1260). One in seven respondents were at home (7.3%, N = 240) or students (6.6%, N = 215). Many of the student respondents were working while studying, but their main occupation was recorded as 'student'. The phenomenon of the working poor is seen in food aid, as one in ten food aid recipients were people working part-time or on a fixed-term contract (5.6%, N = 185), or full-time (3.7%, N = 120).

In terms of housing, the majority of the respondents (78%, N = 2570) lived in a rented property, and only 16% (N = 527) owned their own home. On the national level in 2011, the percentages were nearly the reverse: 59% lived in owner-occupied dwellings, whereas only 29% of the people lived in rented dwellings. Homeless respondents (3.3%, N = 109) and people living in supported housing (2.8%, N = 92) were a small minority. However, these figures exceed the national levels, as roughly 8000 (0.15%) people in Finland were homeless at that time. The size of the household was measured by asking the number of adults and children living in the household. Of the respondents, over three fifths (60.5%, *N* = 2024) lived alone, whereas on the national level two fifths live in one-adult households [29].

In terms of the frequency of food aid use, nearly one third (*N* = 952) of the food aid recipients obtained charity food weekly. One quarter (25.9%, *N* = 816) received food aid approximately every two weeks, and one fifth (20.1%, *N* = 633) received food aid roughly once a month. Under a quarter (23.9%, *N* = 752) of the respondents received food aid only couple of times a year. A majority of the recipients of the food aid got the food for themselves (47.6%, *N* = 1544), but over two fifths (42.6 %, *N* = 1380) picked up food for themselves and their families. One in ten (9.8%, *N* = 317) got the food for themselves and other non-family members.

In terms of the money left over after each month's compulsory outgoings, the results show that nearly half of the respondents (44.5%, *N* = 1316) were left with 0–100 euros. One third (30.9%, *N* = 913) had 101–300 euros, and a quarter (24.7%, *N* = 730) had more than 301 euros per month.

It is known from Finnish national-level surveys that disadvantages tend to accumulate in three main dimensions: economic, social, and health [30]. When researching the disadvantages of the respondents, the findings show that the same dimensions found in studies representing the Finnish population were also found among the food aid recipients (Table 1). The results are statistically significant. One quarter of the respondents had not experienced severe economic disadvantage or accumulated disadvantages, although they were less well off when compared with the wider population. Typically, people belonging to this group were pensioners and the working poor living on social assistance or a guarantee pension and experiencing high levels of scarcity. Most of the people (three quarters) receiving food aid had deep economic problems, such as difficulties in making ends meet and paying debts. These were mainly young people, students, and people with families.

Notably, over two fifths of the people receiving charity food aid suffered from several simultaneous disadvantages. They not only had problems with their economic situation but also health disadvantages, such as poor mental and/or physical health and lower levels of life satisfaction. In addition, they experienced social disadvantages such as hunger, loneliness, and depression. In this group, the homeless, unemployed, substance abusers, and people with the least disposable income were overrepresented.

Overall, based on the data, people receiving food aid in Finland are a heterogeneous group. However, the group has a poorer employment status compared to the wider Finnish population, and is older, less educated, and on a lower income. People receiving food aid mostly suffer from economic deprivation. They are also more likely to live alone. Moreover, two fifths of the food aid recipients live with accumulated economic, social, and health disadvantages.

Table 1. Accumulation of disadvantages and people affected by economic, social, and health disadvantages.

How Do Disadvantages Accumulate?	Less well-off compared to the wider population, no accumulated disadvantage, 24.7% (N = 693)	Severe economic disadvantage (without other disadvantages), 33.7% (N = 945)	Strongly accumulated economic, social, and health disadvantage, 41.5% (N = 1163)
What does it mean?	Does not suffer from severe economic or accumulated disadvantage	Suffers from severe economic disadvantage, but not from social or health disadvantages; has difficulties in making ends meet and paying debts; is dissatisfied with the current standard of living and has experiences of insufficient support	Severe economic disadvantages; disadvantages in mental and physical health and lower levels of life satisfaction; social disadvantages such as hunger, loneliness, and depression
Who is affected?	Pensioners and the working poor living on social assistance or a guarantee pension and experiencing high levels of scarcity	Young people, students, and people with families	The homeless and people living in supported housing, the unemployed and laid-off, substance abusers, people considering themselves disadvantaged, people with the least money to spend freely, and people using last-resort social support

3.3. The Food Recipients' Viewpoint of Food Aid

The sections above illustrate that while the public perception of food aid recipients mostly presents these people as a homogeneous group, in reality food aid recipients come from various walks of life, and they experience disadvantages of various degrees and intensities. What, then, do these people themselves think about the assistance they receive? The qualitative data on the food aid recipients' perspectives of the assistance further complement the above findings. As in the survey data, the informants of the qualitative study were a heterogeneous group that came from various backgrounds. The common denominator for the informants was a low income and the concomitant need for material assistance. For these recipients, using food aid was a practical coping mechanism for dealing with a weak social and economic situation; it was relief that helped in managing everyday scarcity.

However, even though food aid alleviates the immediate food needs of the recipients, the study found out that there are limitations in the food aid system's ability to satisfy these needs. The finding is in line with previous research that suggests food aid does not address the root causes or structural problems behind food insecurity [31–33]. Furthermore, the study found that the food aid system has only a limited ability to meet the immediate food needs of the recipients. This was particularly the case due to the detachment of the food resources in the food assistance venues under study from the needs of the food recipients. Much of the food delivered to these venues was market surplus, and thus its quality and quantity was dependent on what happened to be left over from the primary food markets. Moreover, some of the venues also redistributed food from the EU's food programme, which did not completely align with the needs of the food recipients.

There were problems regarding both the amounts of food available and the quality of food: even though there was occasionally plenty of food available, the food recipients had difficulties in utilizing it. Thus, the occasional abundance of food highlights the inconsistency between the food needs and the food supply in the food aid venues. In terms of the material needs of the food recipients, food aid seems to be able to alleviate only the direct, immediate food needs of these people, and even those only insofar as the needs correspond with what happens to be available.

In addition to their food needs, many informants mentioned social reasons for coming to food aid venues, such as meeting other people, spending time, and enjoying the additional social and religious programmes that some of the food aid providers integrated in the food delivery events. This finding is in line with the quantitative survey study, which found that 53% of the respondents agreed with the statement that it is important for them to meet other people in the food aid venues [34].

Recently, the communal and social aspect of food assistance has gained prominence in Finnish public discussions about food assistance. There are efforts to remodel food aid to provide the participants with communal experiences. However, the findings of this study reveal that from the perspective of the food aid recipients, the communal and social aspect of food aid is not only a positive feature. Occasionally, the low threshold and lack of eligibility control that aimed at inclusiveness resulted in adverse outcomes, such as mutual surveillance among participants and both subtle and hash negotiations over who should receive food first. Thus, the study highlights that food banks are communities with various communal qualities, and not all of them are positive. For the recipients, food aid venues can be socially significant yet socially demanding and emotionally burdening places. From the perspective of the recipients, it is thus important to acknowledge that these venues are about 'more than bread'—both in the good, and in the bad.

In addition to the material and social challenges faced by the food aid recipients, the study found that the informants encountered restrictions on their ability to express their needs, expectations, and experiences related to the assistance. For example, the recipients could only subtly express criticism towards the quality or practical usability of the food items, even in matters regarding food safety. To give an example, one informant delicately noted when he realized that the expiry date of a food item had passed a while ago: 'I really don't dare to eat those meat products. I am not picky, but . . . ' In the context of food aid, the exercise of consumer choice was restricted and even resented. In everyday discussions, criticism was aimed at individuals who were considered choosy. One interviewee remarked aptly how, in the food aid context, '[y]ou have to be something like a piggy. You eat what comes. Yes. [. . .] If you choose, you starve!' The interviewee thus hints that in a food bank, exercising choice regarding food might lead to receiving nothing. As a further example, one recipient lamented how 'there are those finicky ones, who [do not eat particular food stuffs even though they] are not allergic, or anything. But if they can afford to...' Implicit in this statement is the idea that food aid recipients do not have the right to choose the content of the aid. As the latter part of the comment suggests, refusing certain food items indicates that one is not really in need of aid, which hints at the discussions of deservingness presented above.

The recipients' limited choices were also present in their limited ability to withdraw from food aid use. This became apparent in situations where the informants spoke about the social and emotional stress that food aid use caused for them. For example, one recipient stated, 'I feel that it would be easier not to come. But how do I cope then? Where do I get [food] then? I don't know where I would then get [food], and I don't know what I should do. But it is like, it is already quite depressing.' The restricted agency of the food recipients means that due to their harsh economic situations, they rarely have a chance to decide whether or not make use of the assistance food without tremendous disadvantages. However, they rarely have the ability to express their needs, outlooks, and feelings related to the assistance, either. In many ways, their needs and aspirations remain overlooked.

4. Discussion

The above findings shed new light on the recipients of Finnish food aid from various perspectives. First, public perceptions of food aid in the online discussions often portray the recipients as dishonourable and responsible for their own poverty. At the same time, the quantitative data reveal that the main reason for people resorting to charity food aid is deep economic disadvantage. Furthermore, the quantitative data show that there is an unequal accumulation of disadvantage, illustrating the internal diversity within food aid recipients. Finally, observational and interview data show that from the food recipients' perspective, food aid provision disregards the material and social needs of the food recipients. The assistance system has only a limited capacity to meet even the recipients' immediate food needs, and for the food assistance recipients, food aid venues can become not only socially significant, but also socially demanding and emotionally burdening places.

Together, these findings point out some significant issues regarding food aid recipients. First, the findings from the online discussions indicate that from perspective of outsiders, the food aid recipients are often seen as a homogeneous group, alien to the majority population. Paradoxically, the life situations of the food aid recipients are often evaluated by arguing that there should not be severe poverty in a Finnish welfare state. As a result, if and when one is afflicted by poverty, the need for help is questioned and the individual is blamed [35]. Hence, it is important to gather empirical data to understand who the food recipients really are and what their socio-economic status is. The survey data of the food aid recipients bring facts to the public discussion, where the stereotypical picture of a food aid recipient is an uneducated, poor, typically male substance abuser standing in a breadline. The data can reveal the inner diversity of this group and the fact that many of the recipients are living in weak social and economic positions when compared to the wider Finnish population.

Second, the quantitative data reveal that food aid recipients suffer from economic, social, and health disadvantages. In addition, qualitative data show that they suffer from disadvantages in the form of social exclusion from the consumer practices of the wider population. Further, the findings indicate the inner polarization among food aid recipients: the survey data show that there is an accumulation of disadvantages in certain groups, while the qualitative analysis of the experiences of the food recipients highlight experiences of social exclusion and being left without.

Finally, on the level of public perceptions, food aid recipients are judged based on their perceived deservingness. However, at the same time, from the perspective of the food recipients the question arises of whether the available food aid meets their needs in the first place. The study of the food aid from the perspective of the Finnish food assistance recipients highlights the ambivalent social position that the recipients hold. First of all, they are excluded from ways of acquiring food that are customary in contemporary society. At the same time, they are dependent on the consumer practices of the affluent population that secure the continuous flow of excess. Second, socialization into the food aid community might promote the institutionalization of food aid on the individual level and entrench the food aid recipients' social exclusion from wider society. Food aid serves as an instrument for polarization that distances the life worlds of the disadvantaged people and the well-off majority. As seen in the findings from the online discussions, the public perceptions of food aid recipients feed back into these experiences and aggravate the social divide.

5. Conclusions

There are certain limitations to this study that should be taken into account when interpreting the findings. First of all, the data used in this article were collected some years ago already, and thus they do not present the most recent situation. From a research perspective, it is unfortunate that there are no up-to-date data readily available. On the other hand, this situation well illustrates the ad hoc and unorganized field of food aid in Finland. There are no registers or any other reliable data available about food aid recipients in Finland. Charity food aid recipients comprise one of the so-called hard-to-survey populations [36]: people receiving food aid tend to be hard to find or contact, as they are not found via post or phone surveys; they are occasionally difficult to persuade to participate, as going to food aid is stigmatizing for many; and being anonymous is important for some [37]. Furthermore, they can be difficult to interview, as there is not always a common language, some might be illiterate, some might be intoxicated, and some might be generally reluctant to take part in research. These are only some of the difficulties faced in interviewing food aid recipients. We have relied on data from 2012–2013, because they represent the first and so far only consistent quantitative information about the Finnish food aid users.

Second, it is worth noting that the data from the online discussions about food aid is not representative when it comes to the general populations' perceptions and attitudes. About 80% of Finns follow online media sources. Still, relatively few readers use the opportunity to comment on and discuss the news online. Strong opinions and active debaters gain the most visibility online [38]. However, keeping this limitation in mind, the online discussions provide an interesting viewpoint to approach public perceptions about food aid, because they offer—albeit in aggravated form—an indication of the traits that represent the general public's attitudes. Furthermore, the mindsets expressed online have the potential to spread outside the online debates, and thus it is helpful to be aware of them.

Third, since this article uses existing sources of data that have been each collected for the particular purposes of the original studies, one should be cautious when discussing the combined findings. In this article, we have settled on discussing the connections between different data sets descriptively instead of conducting cross-data analyses about each domain of the results. The discussion of the findings shows that different data sources complement each other, and together they help to paint a more nuanced picture of the reality in which food aid takes place in Finland and where the food aid recipients make do. Further research is needed that more thoroughly integrates discursive, demographic, and experiential insights into charity food provision and reception.

Despite these limitations, the study offers valuable insights into Finnish food aid, as it brings together the current body of knowledge about Finnish food aid recipients. In doing so, it shows that unlike in other Nordic countries such as Norway and Sweden, where the food aid clientele often represents the very margins of society [39,40], the recipients in Finland make up a relatively wide and diverse group. The food aid recipients are more typically of an older age, lower education, and lower income compared to the wider Finnish population. They are also more likely to have a weaker employment status and live in a one-person household. At the same time as the public debates about their deservingness, the food recipients themselves suffer from (often accumulated) economic, social, and health disadvantages. For them, the aid is important—if not necessary—to cope in their everyday life, even though they simultaneously struggle to make use of the aid, which does not always fall in line with their wants and needs.

Despite the general image of Finland as an affluent welfare state, there are tens of thousands of people who need to resort to charitable food aid in order to cope in their everyday lives. In February 2018, the annual fundraising campaign of the Finnish Lutheran Church, called the 'Common Responsibility Campaign' (*Yhteisvastuukeräys*), launched its annual campaign with the theme of hunger and poverty. With the domestic part of the proceeds, the campaign aims to provide one-off subsidies and food aid for low-income households in Finland. With its poignant hashtag #foodtrends, the campaign underlies the ambiguity of today's Finnish society where some people feast while others fast or starve [41]. This example illustrates that the issue of food aid is far from diminishing in Finnish society. Rather, it is becoming institutionalized, and it is gaining public recognition. One distinguishing feature of Finnish food aid has been the relative absence of a charitable culture attached to the aid; this is in contrast to the United States and Canada, for example, where private individuals and corporations are invited and encouraged to donate food for charitable purposes through prominent popular campaigns [42,43]. In the future, the proliferation of visible 'hunger campaigns' in Finland might influence who receives food aid, how the aid is experienced, and how its recipients are perceived by the public. More research is needed about food aid recipients in this changing landscape.

With charity food aid, the issues of poverty and food insecurity have been shifted to the margins and the purview of NGOs and third-sector voluntary aid. However, it is ideally a public responsibility to take care of people who experience poverty. Leaving the responsibility for the care of this vulnerable group to voluntary and religious actors indicates a neglect of the constitutional and basic rights of these people, especially the right to food [10,13].

Poor relief is always stigmatizing. People who receive last-resort charitable aid are exposed to public judgement, which is likely to weaken their well-being. Charity food aid also provokes discourses of deservingness that are alien to the universalist welfare model [24]. In the light of the findings, there is a legitimate need for assistance. However, this need cannot be met solely by giving people food as charity. Rather than deservingness, the focus of public concern ought to be on how the official social security system could be developed so that it can respond to the life situations of those who are afflicted by poverty. Mapping the actual needs and reasons for food aid use requires more research knowledge on the life worlds of the people who live in vulnerable social and economic positions.

Finally, charitable food aid venues are often one of the only places where the most deprived members of society can be found. This fact could be used as an asset when planning more effective ways to tackle poverty and food insecurity. Information and research knowledge about food aid in general, and food aid recipients' wellbeing and experiences in particular, should be systematically gathered and made available in order to alleviate poverty and food insecurity more effectively.

Supplementary Materials: The following are available online at http://www.mdpi.com/1660-4601/15/12/2896/s1, S1: research on food aid 2012.

Author Contributions: Conceptualization, A.S.S.; Methodology, A.S.S., M.O. and T.L.; Formal Analysis, M.O. and T.L.; Investigation, A.S.S., M.O. and T.L.; Writing-Original Draft Preparation, A.S.S. and M.O; Writing-Review & Editing, A.S.S., M.O. and T.L.; Project Administration, A.S.S.

Funding: The APC and proofreading were funded by the Academy of Finland under the project (Im)moderation in everyday food consumption (decision number 316141) at the University of Tampere.

Conflicts of Interest: The authors declare no conflict of interest.

Appendix A

Table A1. Socio-economic background of food aid recipients compared to the general population in Finland (2012–2013).

	Food Aid Recipients		General Population of Finland
	N	%	%
Age (in full years)			
16–25	199	6	12.2
26–35	356	10.7	12.6
36–45	512	15.4	12.1
46–55	789	23.7	13.7
56–65	893	26.9	14.2
Over 65	574	17.3	18.8
Gender			
Male	1592	48.3	49.1
Female	1704	51.7	50.9
Nationality			
Finnish	2817	87.3	96.4
Other	410	12.7	3.6
Education			
Comprehensive school	1270	39.6	32
Upper secondary school/Vocational school	1282	40	40
University	656	20.4	28
Employment status			
At home	240	7.3	
Pensioner	1260	38.4	
Unemployed or laid off	1260	38.4	
Student	215	6.6	
Working fixed term or part-time	185	5.6	
Working under permanent contract	120	3.7	
Housing			
Home owner	527	16	59
Rental accommodation	2162	65.6	29.1
Council accommodation	408	12.4	
Supported living	408	2.8	
Homeless	109	3.3	0.15
Recipient of food aid during the last year			
A few times a year	752	23.9	-
Approximately once a month	633	20.1	-
Approximately every other week	816	25.9	-
Every week	952	30.2	-
Getting food			
Only for myself	1544	47.6	-
For myself and my family	1380	42.6	-
For myself and others	317	9.8	-
Number of adults in a household			
1	2024	60.5	41
2 or more	1324	39.5	59
Number of children in a household			
0	2403	71.6	
1	412	12.3	
2 or more	543	16.2	
Money (€) left after each month's compulsory outgoings			
0	607	20.5	
1–100	709	24	
101–300	913	30.9	
301–500	429	14.5	
Over 500	301	10.2	

References

1. Iivari, J.; Karjalainen, J. *Diakonian Köyhät. Epävirallinen Apu Perusturvan Paikkaajana*; Stakes: Helsinki, Finland, 1999.
2. Jokela, U. *Diakonian Paikka Ihmisten Arjessa*; Diak: Helsinki, Finland, 2011.

3. Juntunen, E.; Grönlund, H.; Hiilamo, H. *Viimeisellä Luukulla. Tutkimus Viimesijaisen Sosiaaliturvan Aukoista ja Diakoniatyön Kohdentumisesta*; Kirkkohallitus: Helsinki, Finland, 2006.

4. Kettunen, P. *Leipää vai Läsnäoloa? Asiakkaan Tarve ja Diakoniatyöntekijän Työnäky Laman Puristuksessa*; Kirkon Tutkimuskeskus: Tampere, Finland, 2001.

5. Siiki, A. Myllypuron ruokajono—Esimerkki hyvinvointiköyhyydestä. In *Toisten Pankki. Ruoka-Apu Hyvinvointivaltiossa*; Hänninen, S., Karjalainen, J., Lehtelä, K., Silvasti, T., Eds.; Stakes: Helsinki, Finland, 2008; pp. 127–161.

6. Laihiala, T. Kokemuksia ja Käsityksiä Leipäjonoista: Huono-Osaisuus, Häpeä ja Ansaitsevuus. Ph.D. Thesis, University of Eastern Finland, Kuopio, Finland, February 2018.

7. Ohisalo, M. Murusia Hyvinvointivaltion Pohjalla: Leipäjonot, Koettu Hyvinvointi ja Huono-Osaisuus. Ph.D. Thesis, University of Eastern Finland, Kuopio, Finland, June 2017.

8. Salonen, A.S. Food for the Soul or the Soul for Food: Users' Perspectives on Religiously Affiliated Food Charity in a Finnish City. Ph.D. Thesis, University of Helsinki, Helsinki, Finland, October 2016.

9. Riches, G.; Silvasti, T. (Eds.) *First World Hunger Revisited. Food Charity or The Right to Food*, 2nd ed.; Palgrave Macmillan: Basingstoke, UK, 2014.

10. Riches, G. *Food Bank Nations. Poverty, Corporate Charity and the Right to Food*; Routledge: London, UK; New York, NY, USA, 2018.

11. Caraher, M.; Cavicchi, A. Old crises on new plates or old plates for new crises? Food banks and food insecurity. *Br. Food J.* **2014**, *116*. [CrossRef]

12. Hiilamo, H. Rethinking the role of church in a socio-democratic welfare state. *Int. J. Sociol. Soc. Policy* **2012**, *32*, 401–414. [CrossRef]

13. Silvasti, T. Food aid—Normalising the abnormal in Finland. *Soc. Policy Soc.* **2015**, *14*, 471–482. [CrossRef]

14. Riches, G. Hunger, food security and welfare policies: Issues and debates in first world societies. *Proc. Nutr. Soc.* **1997**, *56*, 63–74. [CrossRef] [PubMed]

15. MacLeod, M. Understanding the Rise of Food Aid and Its Implications for the Welfare State: A study of Scotland and Finland. Ph.D. Thesis, University of Glasgow, Glasgow, UK, June 2018.

16. Silvasti, T. Elintarvikejärjestelmä globalisoituu—Ruokaturvasta yksityinen liikesuhde? In *Toisten Pankki. Ruoka-apu Hyvinvointivaltiossa*; Hänninen, S., Karjalainen, J., Lehtelä, K., Silvasti, T., Eds.; Stakes: Helsinki, Finland, 2008; pp. 241–262.

17. Silvasti, T.; Karjalainen, J. Hunger in a Nordic welfare state: Finland. In *First World Hunger Revisited. Food Charity or the Right to Food?* 2nd ed.; Riches, G., Silvasti, T., Eds.; Palgrave Macmillan: Basingstoke, UK, 2014; pp. 72–86.

18. Demokraatti.fi. Available online: https://demokraatti.fi/polemiikki-vantaan-sosiaalitoimi-ohjaa-leipajonoihin-arajarvi-loukkaavaa/ (accessed on 10 October 2018).

19. Kaks.fi. Available online: https://kaks.fi/uutiset/polemiikki-uutiset-professori-pentti-arajarvi-vantaan-leipajonotapauksesta-kyse-vakavasta-oireesta/ (accessed on 10 October 2018).

20. Ohisalo, M.; Eskelinen, N.; Laine, J.; Kainulainen, S.; Saari, J. *Avun Tilkkutäkki. Suomalaisen Ruoka-Apukentän Monimuotoisuus*; RAY: Helsinki, Finland, 2014.

21. Lehtelä, K.-M.; Kestilä, L. Kaksi vuosikymmentä ruoka-apua. In *Suomalaisten Hyvinvointi 2014*; Vaarama, M., Karvonen, S., Kestilä, L., Moisio, P., Muuri, A., Eds.; Terveyden ja Hyvinvoinnin Laitos: Helsinki, Finland, 2014; pp. 270–281.

22. Kirkkohallitus. *Kirkon Diakoniarahaston Avustustoiminta v. 2015. Kirkon Diakoniarahasto*; Kirkkohallitus: Helsinki, Finland, 2016; Available online: Http://sakasti.evl.fi/sakasti.nsf/0/E3537B3D390324C5C22578E10047CB71/$FILE/KDR%202015.pdf (accessed on 14 January 2017).

23. Tilastokeskus. Available online: https://www.stat.fi/til/tjt/2015/01/tjt_2015_01_2017-03-03_kat_001_fi.html (accessed on 26 November 2018).

24. Larsen, C.A. The Institutional Logic of Welfare Attitudes: How Welfare Regimes Influence Public Support. *Comp. Political Stud.* **2008**, *41*, 145–168. [CrossRef]

25. Van Oorschot, W. Who should get what and why? On deservingness criteria and the conditionality of solidarity among the public. *Policy Politics* **2000**, *28*, 33–48. [CrossRef]

26. Niemelä, M. Perceptions of the causes of poverty in Finland. *Acta Sociol.* **2008**, *51*, 23–40. [CrossRef]

27. Kallio, J.; Niemelä, M. Kuka ansaitsee tulla autetuksi? Kansalaisten asennoituminen toimeentulotuen saajiin Suomessa vuonna 2015. *Janus* **2017**, *25*, 144–159.

28. Van der Horst, H.; Pascucci, S.; Bol, W. The 'dark side' of food banks? Exploring emotional responses of food bank receivers in the Netherlands. *Br. Food J.* **2014**, *116*, 1506–1520. [CrossRef]

29. Findikaattori: Asuntokuntien Koko. Available online: https://findikaattori.fi/fi/93 (accessed on 10 October 2018).

30. Vaarama, M.; Karvonen, S.; Kestilä, L.; Moisio, P.; Muuri, A. *Suomalaisten Hyvinvointi 2014*; Terveyden ja Hyvinvoinnin Laitos: Helsinki, Finland, 2014.

31. Poppendieck, J. *Sweet Charity? Emergency Food and the End of Entitlement*; Penguin Books: New York, NY, USA, 1999.

32. Tarasuk, V.; Eakin, J.M. Charitable food assistance as symbolic gesture: An ethnographic study of food banks in Ontario. *Soc. Sci. Med.* **2003**, *56*, 1505–1515. [CrossRef]

33. Tarasuk, V.; Eakin, J.M. Food assistance through 'surplus' food: Insights from an ethnographic study of food bank work. *Agric. Hum. Values* **2005**, *22*, 177–186. [CrossRef]

34. Kainulainen, S. Ruoka-avun hakijoiden hyvinvointi. In *Kuka Seisoo Leipäjonossa?* Ohisalo, M., Saari, J., Eds.; KAKS—Kunnallisalan Kehittämissäätiö: Helsinki, Finland, 2014; pp. 59–69.

35. Goffman, E. *Stigma. Notes on the Management of Spoiled Identity*; Penguin Books: London, UK, 1963.

36. Tourangeau, R.; Edwards, B.; Johnson, T.; Wolter, K.; Bates, N. *Hard-to-Survey Populations*; Cambridge University Press: Cambridge, UK, 2014.

37. Laihiala, T.; Kallio, J.; Ohisalo, M. Personal and social shame among the recipients of charity food aid in Finland. *Res. Finn. Soc.* **2017**, *10*, 73–85.

38. Pöyhtäri, R.; Haara, P.; Raittila, P. *Vihapuhe Sananvapautta Kaventamassa*; Tampere University Press: Tampere, Finland, 2013.

39. Farnes, S.B.H. Fattigdom og Frivillig Velferd i Norge En Kvalitativ Studie av Brukere ved Robin Hood Huset i Bergen. Master's Thesis, Sosiologisk Institutt, Universitetet i Bergen, Bergen, Norway, 2014.

40. Engebrigtsen, A.I.; Haug, A.V. *Evaluering av Tilskuddsordningen for Humanitære Tiltak til Tilreisende EØS-Borgere som Tigger*; NOVA Notat 2/2018; Norsk Institutt for Forskning om Oppvekst, Velferd og Aldring: Oslo, Norway, 2018.

41. DeLind, L.B. Celebrating hunger in Michigan: A critique of an emergency food program and an alternative for the future. *Agric. Hum. Values* **1994**, *11*, 58–68. [CrossRef]

42. Salonen, A.S. Religion, poverty and abundance. *Palgrave Commun.* **2018**, *4*, 1–5. [CrossRef]

43. Caplan, P. *Feasts, Fasts, Famine: Food for Thought*; Berg Occasional Papers in Anthropology, No. 2; Berg Publishers: Oxford, UK, 1994.

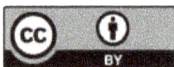

International Journal of
Environmental Research and Public Health

MDPI

Article

Charitable Food Systems' Capacity to Address Food Insecurity: An Australian Capital City Audit

Christina M. Pollard [1],* , Bruce Mackintosh [2] , Cathy Campbell [1], Deborah Kerr [1] ,
Andrea Begley [1] , Jonine Jancey [1], Martin Caraher [3] , Joel Berg [4] and Sue Booth [5]

[1]   Faculty of Health Science, School of Public Health, Curtin University, GPO Box U1987, Perth 6845, Australia;
      Cathy.Campbell555@gmail.com (C.C.); D.Kerr@curtin.edu.au (D.K.); A.Begley@curtin.edu.au (A.B.);
      J.Jancey@curtin.edu.au (J.J.)
[2]   School of Agriculture and Environment, The University of Western Australia, 35 Stirling Highway, Crawley,
      Perth 6009, Australia; bruce.mackintosh@uwa.edu.au
[3]   Centre for Food Policy, City University of London, Northampton Square, London EC1V 0HB, UK;
      m.caraher@city.ac.uk
[4]   Hunger Free America, 50 Broad Street, Suite 1103, New York 10004, NY, USA; JBerg@hungerfreeamerica.org
[5]   College of Medicine & Public Health, Flinders University, GPO Box 2100, Adelaide 5000, Australia;
      sue.booth@flinders.edu.au
*   Correspondence: C.Pollard@curtin.edu.au; Tel.: +61-8-9224-1016

Received: 18 April 2018; Accepted: 31 May 2018; Published: 12 June 2018

Abstract: Australian efforts to address food insecurity are delivered by a charitable food system (CFS) which fails to meet demand. The scope and nature of the CFS is unknown. This study audits the organisational capacity of the CFS within the 10.9 square kilometres of inner-city Perth, Western Australia. A desktop analysis of services and 12 face-to-face interviews with representatives from CFS organisations was conducted. All CFS organisations were not-for–profit and guided by humanitarian or faith-based values. The CFS comprised three indirect services (IS) sourcing, banking and/or distributing food to 15 direct services (DS) providing food to recipients. DS offered 30 different food services at 34 locations feeding over 5670 people/week via 16 models including mobile and seated meals, food parcels, supermarket vouchers, and food pantries. Volunteer to paid staff ratios were 33:1 (DS) and 19:1 (IS). System-wide, food was mainly donated and most funding was philanthropic. Only three organisations received government funds. No organisation had a nutrition policy. The organisational capacity of the CFS was precarious due to unreliable, insufficient and inappropriate financial, human and food resources and structures. System-wide reforms are needed to ensure adequate and appropriate food relief for Australians experiencing food insecurity.

Keywords: food insecurity; charitable food services; food charity; food system; nutrition; voluntary failure

1. Introduction

The health consequences of socio-economic disadvantage, including homelessness, are increasingly seen in high income countries, including Australia [1–4]. Food insufficiency is closely associated with poor mental and physical health [5–8] and is common among people who are homeless [5,9,10].

Cities attract vulnerable populations experiencing food insecurity as they provide concentrated food and support services. The types of people accessing inner-city charitable food services (CFS) are highly variable and include people who are homeless or domiciled and in financial difficulty due to a range of circumstances, those living in hostel and shelters, backpackers, and women fleeing from domestic violence. The inner-city precinct of Perth, the capital city of Western Australia, covers

10.9 square kilometres with a population of about 32,000 people. The Perth Homeless Registry showed that the number of street-present people increased from 192 to 319 between 2012 and 2016 [11]. Over 80% had been homeless for six months or more and 52% had complex comorbidities of existing medical conditions, mental illness and substance use disorders [11].

Concerns have been raised regarding the ongoing capacity of food relief systems in both Australia and the United States (U.S.) to meet the increasing demand [12,13]. There is also evidence of sub-optimal nutritional quality in the food provided [14,15]. Australia's response to food insecurity is at a critical point given the increasing need, the absence of government-funded food assistance such as in the U.S. [15] and the diminishing welfare safety net [16]. Australian Government welfare policies designed to reduce poverty—for example, the Australian Age Pension [17], Family Tax Benefit and the Child Care Subsidy [18] and Newstart Allowance [19]—provide assistance to low income earners and may assist in improving food security; however, the evidence for the increasing demand for food relief suggests they are inadequate.

Food charity, the delivery of donated, unsaleable, or waste food by the voluntary (non-profit) sector, is the dominant response to food insecurity in Australia [12]. This charitable food system (CFS), originally designed to provide immediate short-term food relief, is struggling as food insecurity and the demand for food assistance is chronic and increasing [12,20]. In 2015, there were 3000 to 4000 food relief services nationally [12]. The demand for food relief services increased in 2016, up 8% from 2015 [21].

Although short-term need is assumed in Australia [22], there is evidence of long-term reliance on the CFS [23,24]. The Australian response to food insecurity has been described as ad hoc with numerous small voluntary organisations providing food assistance [25]. Internationally, researchers have questioned whether the expansion and reliance on food charity and food banking is the appropriate response to food insecurity in developed countries, based on users' negative experiences of shame and being stigmatised and poor quality or limited food choices [26]. The CFS consists of both "in-direct" services (IS) (food banking and rescue organisations who collect, bank and/or distribute unsaleable food) and 'direct' services (DS) who provide the food to those in need.

The non-profit (NP) sector's ability to effectively address problems such as food insecurity has also been questioned in the academic literature, which has been critical of food banks based on users' experiences such as shame, stigma and eligibility criteria in high-income countries [20,27]. Salamon's theory of voluntary failure was developed in 1987 to explain the effectiveness of the voluntary response to issues such as food insecurity [28]. His theory described market failure, voluntary failure, and third-party government failure in delivering effective welfare-government relationships in the United States. The CFS NP voluntary response in Australia has arisen as a result of both a market and a third-party government failure in delivering the "collective good" of providing a welfare safety net to prevent food insecurity. The Commonwealth Department of Social Services acknowledges the existence of Emergency Relief as "services delivered by community organisations".

Salamon's four types of voluntary failure include (i) philanthropic insufficiency, the "inability to generate resources on a scale that is both adequate enough and reliable enough to cope with the human-service problems" [28] (p. 39); (ii) philanthropic particularism, which occurs when "some subgroups of the community may not be adequately represented in the structure of voluntary organizations" [28] (p. 40) where the focus is on treating "the more 'deserving' of the poor" leaving serious service gaps or duplicating services and wasting resources; (iii) philanthropic paternalism, which refers to the notion that "those with the greatest resources have influence over the definition of community need" [28] (p. 41); and (iv) philanthropic amateurism, described as "amateur approaches to coping with human problems" [28] (p. 42). A current assessment of CFS in Perth shows evidence of one type of voluntary failure, namely philanthropic insufficiency [24].

There has been limited exploration of the scope and organisational capacity of the Australian CFS [12,29] and none in Western Australia. In 2014, due to increasing demand, food relief organisations expressed a need to understand the current and future capacity of the CFS in inner-city Perth to meet their clients' needs [25]. Understanding the practical organisational issues facing the CFS is important when considering options for change to improve end-user services [30]. The aim of this paper is to document the scope, nature and organisational capacity of the CFS located in or serving inner-city Perth.

2. Methods

Between July and September 2015, an organisational capacity audit was undertaken of the CFS located in or serving inner-city Perth. The audit identified and mapped component organisations, their values, human and financial resources, their networks, nutrition policies, and food service operations.

A research advisory group comprising the research team and five representatives from key organisations working with homelessness, social disadvantage and relief services identified the CFS organisations located in or serving inner-city Perth. They provided initial contact details which were confirmed via telephone or web search. A nomenclature for the types of food service models and their inter-relationships was agreed, for example IS and DS.

Two semi-structured interview schedules were developed for the IS and DS. The assessment of organisational capacity was guided by the approach used to improve nutrition for vulnerable groups, children in childcare in Australia [31] and food bank users in the United States [15]. The instrument was adapted from the Research Tools for Use in Studying Nutrition Policies and Practices in the Emergency Food Bank Network [15] and Food Service Planning in Child Care in Western Australia [32] surveys, which assessed organisational capacity for a safe, nutritious and appropriate food service. Table 1 provides an overview of the interview schedule.

Table 1. Semi-structured interview schedule.

Topics Covered	Indirect Services	Direct Services
Organisational values, length of operation, funding sources	Asked	Asked
Food service models/types, location, timing, description of recipients	Asked	Asked
Workforce profile including volunteers and training	Asked	Asked
Food storage capacity	Asked	Asked
Nutrition and food safety training, policy and practices	Asked	Asked
Sources of foods	Asked	Asked
Food transport (for food received and distributed)	Asked	Asked
Perception of donors influence on charitable food services (CFS)	Asked	Asked
Impact of government actions on CFS	Asked	Asked
Preferences for specific foods	Asked	Asked
Challenges and opportunities to increasing nutritious food	Asked	Asked
Agencies receiving food, quantities and recipients	Asked	Not asked

The surveys were trialed with senior managers from two CFS organisations, with changes made to the order and phrasing of questions post-pilot to ensure clarity. Background information was obtained from organisational websites, and interviewees were asked to provide written documentation such as annual reports or service brochures.

Two researchers (Bruce Mackintosh and Cathy Campbell) with extensive experience in food relief and public health nutrition conducted the interviews. Thirty DS and five IS were telephoned to screen for interview suitability. If the organisation played a role in food service delivery in inner-city Perth, the chief executive officer, director or manager, or a nominated proxy was invited for face-to-face interview. Twelve face-to-face interviews were conducted (nine DS and three IS). Eight telephone interviews were conducted with DS offering limited food relief; for example, only supermarket vouchers or one-off cash payments to their clients. Both researchers attended each interview, filled in the written questionnaire and took additional notes. The three lots of data—the audit of the websites, interviewee responses to the survey instrument and interviewer notes—were collated, reported in tables where appropriate, and general findings were summarised by the interviewers. The study was conducted according to guidelines in the Declaration of Helsinki and all procedures involving human subjects were approved by the Curtin University Human Research Ethics Committee (HR183/2015). Written informed consent was obtained from all subjects.

3. Results

This study is the first to describe the organisational capacity of the CFS located in or servicing a capital city in Australia. The inner-city Perth CFS comprised three indirect services (IS) who sourced, banked and/or distributed food to 15 direct services (DS), who in turn provided food to recipients. DS offered 30 different food services at 34 locations feeding over 5670 people/week via 16 models including mobile and seated meals, food parcels, supermarket vouchers, and food pantries: see Table 1.

The CFS organisational capacity is described in terms of purpose; years of operation; funding sources and workforce structure; food supply and food service models offered; commitment to and structures to support the provision of nutritious food; the influence/impact of government regulation or legislation. The organisational overview of the CFS serving inner-City Perth is shown in Figure 1, and the audit results described for IS and then for DS followed by the barriers to improvement and interviewee recommendations.

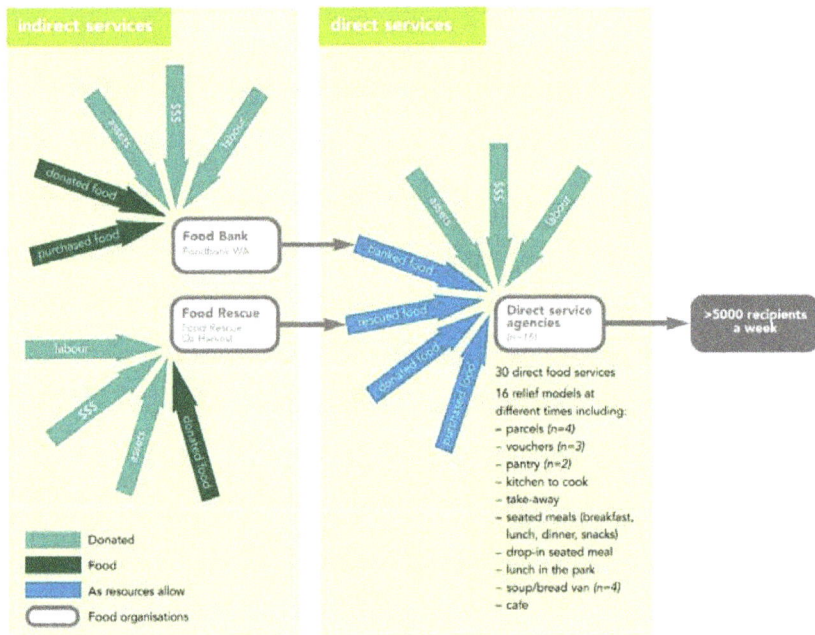

Figure 1. Model of the charitable food sector in inner-city Perth.

3.1. Indirect Services

Three IS were either located in or serviced inner-city Perth at the time of the research who procured food and either banked, sorted or directly distributed it to DS; Supplementary Table S1 shows the characteristics of the IS.

3.1.1. Organisational Intent, Funding and Workforce

Foodbank WA (Perth Western Australia), had operated for 21 years in, compared to 2 and 5 years for OzHarvest and Food Rescue WA, respectively. All three IS aimed to rescue surplus food and reduce food waste to provide for people in need, either via DS or directly. Foodbank WA and Food Rescue WA included reducing hunger with nutritious food and Foodbank WA and OzHarvest mentioned quality food. Food Rescue WA merged with Uniting Care West, a community services agency of the Uniting Church in Australia Synod of WA in 2013.

IS managers said their funding was ad hoc, unreliable, and from different sources including corporate and private donations, sponsorships and government grants. Foodbank WA also charged DS a per-kilogram handling fee to cover operating costs which generated AUD$3.78 million in 2017 [33]. OzHarvest and Food Rescue WA relied entirely on donations.

The workforce varied with organisational size: the number of paid full-time equivalent (FTE) staff ranged from two to 50 (Food Rescue WA and Foodbank WA respectively). Foodbank and OzHarvest employed nutritionists/dietitians (10 FTE and 1 casual respectively), one chef (1 FTE and 1 casual respectively) and hosted student placements. All three IS relied heavily on volunteers: Food Rescue WA had 2 paid staff and 100 volunteers (1:50), Foodbank WA has 1:45 and OzHarvest 1:25.

3.1.2. Food Types, Sources, Collection and Distribution

All IS sourced donated food through partnerships with the local food and grocery industry or retailers. Foodbank WA estimated that it receives over 80% of all donated food in WA and the larger DS in inner-city Perth sourced food from them. The type of food collected varied: 74% of Foodbank WA food was packaged non-perishable; 99% of Food Rescue WA and OzHarvest's food is perishable (e.g., fruit and vegetables, frozen meals, sushi, prepared sandwiches and quiches), collected in refrigerated vans from cafes, restaurants, supermarkets, caterers and bakeries. Overall, food donations did not meet demand and, despite an interest in discouraging unhealthy food donations, IS all accepted them.

Foodbank WA established their 'key staples program' (KSP) to meet the demand for healthy food. KSP is an alliance with suppliers who donate or subsidize the cost of ingredients, packaging and delivery of nine products (flour, pasta sauce, oats, spaghetti, and canned baked beans, tomatoes, fruit, vegetables and soup). Foodbank WA's expenditure on KSP represented 8.95% of their total expenditure in 2017 [33].

3.1.3. Facilities, Size and Function

IS varied in facilities, size and function. Foodbank WA's, the largest, has premises located 27 kilometres from CBD. They operate as a food storage depot and 510 DS collect food from them, paying a small handing fee. There is substantial warehouse storage with refrigeration and freezers and a commercial kitchen. A fleet of trucks collects food from major supermarkets and they prepare 2000 meals each week onsite and freeze them to sell to DS. A small number of people, referred by DS, can purchase food from directly as well.

Food Rescue WA has premises 10 km from the CBD with refrigerated and freezer storage space where they sort and repack the food they collect in two refrigerated trucks from supermarkets, then deliver to DS. They also use 'cargo carts' to collect and redistribute sandwiches and wraps from cafes in the CBD each day. OzHarvest distributes the food to DS immediately.

In 2016, Foodbank WA rescued 2.8 million kg of food, OzHarvest rescued 348,627 kg and distributed it to 84 DS [34] and Food Rescue WA distributed 478,000 kg of food [33]. Most (75%) of OzHarvest's food is rescued from supermarkets.

Overall, despite rescuing and redistributing significant quantities of food, the IS said they were unable to meet the demand and provide a sustainable, consistent supply of nutritious food to DS agencies who consequently had to make daily modifications to their services.

3.1.4. Nutrition Policy and Capacity

No IS had a formal nutrition policy to specify the types of foods procured. The Foodbank WA interviewee said that the presence of the nutrition staff encouraged a preference for nutritionally preferable KSP and the amount of sugar-sweetened beverages and potato crisps they distributed had declined. Food Rescue WA mainly focused their effort on the procurement of fresh fruit and vegetables.

All paid food preparation staff at Foodbank WA were food safety trained and premises were regularly inspected by local government officers. The two food rescue organisations said they did not accept unsafe food so did not train staff in food safety. OzHarvest offered two sessions of their Nutrition Education Sustenance Training (NEST) nutrition education program for staff, volunteers and service recipients.

3.1.5. Organisational Relationships

Some DS were not aware of the extent and nature of Foodbank WA's services and capacity to supply, at no or a very small cost, many of the items they were purchasing at full price from supermarkets. Some of those who were aware did not use Foodbank WA because they lacked regular transport and the distance from the CBD was a barrier. Others who accessed Foodbank WA purchased energy dense-nutrient poor foods such as potato crisps because they were cheaper by weight than heavier nutritious foods.

3.2. Direct Services

3.2.1. Organisational Intent, Funding and Workforce

The DS had provided food charity in inner-city Perth for many years: for example, the Salvation Army has provided food relief for 125 years while others have done so for 35 to 60 years. Ten of the 15 organisations had faith-based origins. Humanitarian values with a commitment to human dignity and a finding pathway out of food security guided most, typified by one interviewee's comment: "We believe that by nourishing the homeless and the vulnerable in a non-judgmental and compassionate way, we give hope, raise awareness about poverty and provide better outcomes for the wider community".

Funding sources were described as diverse and difficult to quantify. Three of the 15 DS received government funding (e.g., grants from State Government (Departments of Health or Child Protection and Family Support) or the Commonwealth Department of Social Services via their Emergency Relief Fund). Faith-based DS relied on parent organisations such as their church as well as corporate or public donations. Non-faith-based DS relied on philanthropic donations, fundraising activities, and community grants from funders such as Lotterywest, the official State lottery for WA. Specific information on corporate donors was not provided for confidentiality reasons.

The DS workforce structure is summarized in Table 2. The reliance on volunteers was high at a paid staff to volunteer ratio of 1:37. Although many interviewees said that they would value input from a nutritionist or dietitian, only two DS had access to formally trained nutrition personnel. One had employed a full-time dietitian but terminated the position in December 2015 due to lack of funds and the other dietitian was only employed on a casual basis to plan menus.

Table 2. Snapshot of the types and extent of direct food service in inner-city Perth, January 2015.

Funding	Food Source	Food Model	Days of Operation							Serve	Staff	
			M	T	W	T	F	S	Su	/wk	Paid	Vol
G (CP)	D	S, S/W (MS)	✓	✓	✓	✓	✓	✓	✓	500	4	565
CH	D	Parcels		✓		✓				-		
CH	D	BBQ Monthly								-		
G (CP, H)	P	Kitchen	✓	✓	✓	✓	✓	✓	✓	-		
D	D (f&P), B, R	TA noon	✓	✓	✓	✓	✓	✓		1250	5	200
CH	D (f&P)	BF (SM)	✓	✓	✓					30–45		
CH	D (f&P)	Lunch (SM)	✓	✓	✓			✓		30–45		
CH	D (f&P)	D (SM)				✓	✓	✓		120		
D, CH	D (f&P), B, R	BF (SM)	✓	✓	✓	✓				150	6	
D, CH	D (f&P), B, R	Food Any	✓	✓	✓	✓		✓		-		
D, CH	D (f&P), B, R	Lunch						✓		-		
D, CH	D (f&P), B, R	Parcel	✓	✓	✓	✓	✓			-		
D, CH	D (f&$), B, R	Voucher	✓	✓	✓	✓	✓			-		
Lottery	D	Parcel	✓	✓	✓	✓	✓			5		
Lottery	D	Voucher	✓	✓	✓	✓	✓			-		
G (CP)	D, R	MT	✓	✓	✓	✓	✓			650	4	40
CH	D (f&$)	S Kitchen						✓		20–50		
G (CP, H)	B, R	All meals	✓	✓	✓	✓	✓	✓	✓	144	4	6
Lottery	D	S/W	✓	✓	✓	✓	✓			5		
CH	D	Pantry	✓	✓	✓	✓	✓			75		
CH	D (f&P), B, R	Café	✓	✓	✓	✓	✓			-	2	153
CH	D (f&P), B, R	Parcel/Pantry	✓	✓	✓	✓	✓			250		
CH	D (f&P), B, R	Voucher $20	✓	✓	✓	✓	✓			150		
CH	D (f&P), B, R	S, S/W (Van)	✓	✓	✓	✓		✓	✓	350		
CH	D (f&P), B, R	S, S/W (Van)						✓	✓	150		
CH	D (f&P), B, R	All meals	✓	✓	✓	✓	✓	✓	✓	600	4	20
CH, G CP	D (f&P), B, R	Drop-in (SM)	✓	✓	✓	✓	✓			500	1	1
Total										5029	30	985

✓: yes; &: and; G: government; CP: Department of Child Protection; CH: church; H: Department of Health; TA: take-away, P: purchased; D: donated; f: food; $: money; B: bank; R: rescue; SM: seated meal; UCW: Uniting Care West; BF: breakfast; MT: morning tea; L: lunch; D: dinner; S: soup; S/W: sandwich; M: Monday; T: Tuesday; W: Wednesday; T: Thursday; F: Friday; S: Saturday; Su: Sunday; wk: week; Fed: Federal; Vol: volunteers.

3.2.2. Food Service Models, Number and Facilities

Table 2 outlines the types of food service models and number of facilities (4 mobile services, 7 with premises, 2 shelters and 4 for specific client groups, e.g., people at risk of HIV/AIDS). There were 16 food service models offered at different locations on various days in the week: mobile and seated meals food parcels and pantries, and vouchers. Most DS recipients were homeless men, with a high proportion of Aboriginal and/or Torres Strait Islander people. Weekend coverage was limited. Four vans distributed prepared food in parks: one offered a three-course lunchtime meal 5-days/week, one offered soup, pies, sandwiches, tea and coffee each morning, another soup and bread each evening, and the fourth offered sandwiches to young people on the street 5 days/week.

Seven DS with premises had food preparation and serving areas and offered seated meals, usually on weekdays in one large room. Based on an eligibility assessment of need, five provided food parcels and pantry (a small storeroom with mostly non-perishable food items arranged on shelves) visits. A staff member accompanied eligible recipients to the pantry where they choose a set number of free food items or a food parcel, deemed sufficient for 1–2 days to enable a single person or a family to "get back on their feet". Pantry visits are restricted to once or twice a year.

Two DS only provided vouchers or "gift cards" to purchase food from supermarkets with eligibility based on DS-assessed need. Vouchers can be redeemed for food and/or any supermarket items other than cigarettes and alcohol. Recipients often purchase non-food items: for example, toiletries or dog food. Several DS provided school breakfasts or delivered frozen meals to other agencies.

3.2.3. Food Sources

Figure 1 shows DS food sources. Most DS use more than one source of food (either from IS or from direct food donations or purchased directly from supermarkets using donated money) and quantities varied from week to week. Some went to Foodbank WA for free food but chose lighter food by weight due to the handling fee while others relied on food rescue delivered daily. Church groups and philanthropic supporters intermittently offered food to DS. Most of the DS food supply was non-perishable and shelf-stable such as pasta or canned tuna, with the exception of daily rescued food. Interviewees said they needed more donations of perishable whole foods, particularly fruit and vegetables, meat, fish and dairy products.

3.2.4. Nutrition Policy and Capacity

Interviewees said that DS were generally wanting to improve nutrition standards but none had a formal nutrition policy and only one listed nutrition and food safety as program priorities. Interviewees did not believe that their reliance on donated food would influence nutrition policy actions they might choose to implement, but also said that they were unwilling to refuse donations of poor nutrition quality. The increasing and unmet demand for food, uncertain and unreliable food supply, and the salience of nutrition messages among volunteers and recipients were listed as barriers to improving the healthfulness of the food DS provided. The interviewers noted the poor nutrition knowledge of interviewees.

Interviewees were aware of the importance of nutrition and the relationship between the food provided and recipients' health. They said that some recipients had special dietary needs due to diabetes, heart disease, poor oral health, excessive body weight, or drug or alcohol dependency.

Food handling and safety training was rare for staff and not available for volunteers. The exception was DS with premises, such as the aged care nursing home, whose license required that all staff be trained to meet Australian food safety standards. Although no DS received government funding to deliver nutrition education, four had nutrition programs adapted from the FOODCents© budgeting, purchasing, and cooking skills development program [35,36] and several expressed interest in nutrition and budgeting training.

3.2.5. Influence of Government Policies or Legislation

DS interviewees said that state or federal government food-related policies were limited and had little or no day to day influence on the operations of DS. However, local government parking and public nuisance by-laws negatively impacted mobile services by limiting the locations where they could operate. DS referred to "Good Samaritan" legislation that protected them from liability for any unintended consequences of their activity and they were aware that food safety regulations did not currently apply to them as they did not sell food.

When asked about what was needed to improve DS, they wanted more meat, fish and dairy, fresh fruit and vegetables, sliced bread, facilities and equipment (larger kitchen, more vans, refrigerators, commercial bread slicers), the capacity to extend their weekend outreach services, including a bus with more refrigeration and a barbecue onboard, and the resources and capacity to serve a three-course seated meal.

3.2.6. Overall Barriers to CFS Meeting Demand for Nutritious Food

There is no overarching system or policies directing the CFS in inner-city Perth. Many interviewees did not know or communicate with other services. Even though IS said they preferred to supply nutritious foods to DS, they all received and passed-on donated food (for example, cakes, pastries, soft drinks and other unhealthy foods and drinks, particularly those from bakeries and supermarkets). IS said that their reliance on donated food was the main influence on the food they supplied to DS; they cannot predict their food inventory and are often not able to meet DS needs. Foodbank WA and Food

Rescue WA had more consistent donations, but OzHarvest said that donations were unreliable in the type and quantity of food and that they never know what they will get from donors and remarked on the challenges this presents. The IS recommended that food donors be educated regarding the importance of healthy food.

While one DS said they preferred to provide fruit juice and not carbonated sugar-sweetened beverages, another said that "food is food" and they did not hesitate to provide any food. Mobile services purchased and distributed meat pies because they were convenient, easy to prepare and recipients preferred them. One DS interviewee said it was important to give people the occasional "treat" food.

4. Discussion

The findings of this study need to be considered in the context of neo-liberal market economies, where a decline in social welfare creates conditions for individual insecurity and stress [37]. Efforts to reduce pressure on government spending has seen a rise in third sector or voluntary organisations involved in efforts to address complex human problems such as food insecurity [38,39]. The study findings show the CFS in inner-city Perth is complex, with disparate organisations working in an uncoordinated way in difficult conditions. A significant number of operational challenges face both IS and DS, limiting their ability to deliver nutritious or appropriate food relief to recipients. These include the increasing demand and long-term nature of food insecurity (with some models consisting of 1–2 days of emergency relief); their human resource capacity being heavily reliant on volunteers; declining and/or unreliable financial support; an unreliable and inconsistent food supply based primarily on donated or rescued waste food; no food safety or nutrition policy or regulatory framework; and limited nutrition capacity and expertise. No organisation has a standalone ratified nutrition policy supporting the regular acquisition of a nutrition-focused food supply. Disconnected and incoherent policy making is a key challenge in global food systems [40] but equally applies to charitable food systems. In CFS, the policy disconnect and incoherence occurs because decisions are being made in different spaces by diverse policy actors, e.g., government departments, IS, DS, food donors and referring social welfare agencies, which serve diverse interests. Good policy requires a clear understanding of what we want to achieve; so, in this example, is it reducing food waste or reducing food poverty?

DS have offered food relief for up to 125 years demonstrating both the long-term nature of food insecurity and their commitment to providing food to people in need. IS, a more recent addition to the CFS, bring a sophisticated business proposition to food rescue, particularly Foodbank WA based on its organisational capacity. The intent of DS was that they were aspiring to achieve what Hamm and Bellows (2003) call community food security, "a situation in which all community residents obtain a safe, culturally acceptable, nutritionally adequate diet through a sustainable food system that maximizes community self-reliance, social justice, and democratic decision-making" (p. 37) [41,42], whereas IS focused on redistributing food waste without the emphasis on empowering people out of food security.

The inner-city Perth CFS exhibit all three failures (market, government and voluntary) of welfarism described 30 years ago by Lester Salamon [28]. The inability of some citizens to be able to afford to purchase sufficient food in a wealthy country such as Australia is evidence of market failure. The size, scope, expansion and longevity of the food relief sector is a marker of both Government social policy failure in terms of living and income standards and dignified food access [20]. It is also a government failure in terms of the Nation states obligation with respect to the right to food for all citizens—namely to respect, protect and fulfill. Evidence of the four voluntary failures of the non-profit sector includes the following.

4.1. Philanthropic Insufficiency

The increasing demand for food relief and the failure of the CFS to meet that demand is evidence of philanthropic insufficiency. The unreliable and inadequate funding, workforce, food and limited facilities undermine the capacity to support the provision of appropriate food relief. The length of CFS organisations' operation supports the findings of a 2012 review of the WA Emergency Relief sector, which concluded that it will always exist as a safety net, arguing that government should make it a program within a legitimate framework with a funding process [25]. The current findings suggest insufficient government policy, in particular, to assist the CFS to provide safe, reliable and nutritious food to recipients who represent a population sub-group vulnerable to poor health.

CFS relied heavily on corporate, philanthropic and individual donors in inner-city Perth and Victoria due to the limited and unreliable government funding [20]. Charities contribute a significant proportion of their income to CFS; for example, food accounted for 62% of the assistance provided by St Vincent de Paul Inc. in WA in 2017, an expenditure of AUD$1.15 million [43]. During the same period, the Victorian arm provided AUD$14.9 million in material aid, of which 71% was food-related (47% as food vouchers or gift cards) [44]. Getting food to recipients is the focus of effort, leaving little if any time for evaluation of activities for effectiveness or efficiencies. There is some concern that charitable donations have been declining in WA; for example, in 2014–2015 the Salvation Army's income was AUD$700,000 short of its donation target [45].

Interestingly the sentiment expressed by interviewees in this study was that there was enough food, but that it was not able to be distributed effectively, and that resources were wasted. As far back as the 1890s, there was a recommendation that charities in a local area should coordinate to achieve their common purpose and there is limited evidence of co-ordination in our study [28].

4.2. Philanthropic Particularism

DS who focused their donations towards particular subgroups—for example, only providing sandwiches for homeless young people on the street or food for people with HIV—were evident. Particularism also extended to local government, who prefer "pop-up" commercial food trucks catering for transient community events. As a consequence of this example, DS mobile vans and their recipients were regularly asked to move on.

4.3. Philanthropic Paternalism

There was a discord between DS organisations' intent to relieve hunger and promote pathways out of food insecurity and the current practice. The unreliable food supply and lack of nutrition policy meant DS were unlikely to refuse food or beverages of poor nutritional value. The lack of a nutrition policy in Australia is well known [12,26]. Yet, interviewees did not feel that complying with a nutrition policy would limit their food acquisition, consistent with previous research that has found no detriment to services with the establishment of nutrition policy that increases nutritious food acquisition and provision [13,14,46]. A more formal and professional approach is needed to ensure recipients of food relief needs are met.

4.4. Philanthropic Amateurism

Philanthropic amateurism was demonstrated by a lack of food service and/or nutrition training, in part due to the reliance on a "well-meaning but largely untrained workforce to deliver the service". As in other Australian cities, volunteers underpin the CFS workforce in inner-city Perth, suggesting a need for specific volunteer and staff training [20]. Volunteers were mainly retired older people, students, or from large corporate organisations who gift their workforce's time for community service. Although there are acknowledged benefits of reciprocity, there are also challenges relating to the health, financial resources and the preferred contribution of the workforce [47,48]. Complying with Australian standards for volunteering (matching roles to skills, supporting and developing the workforce, protecting their safety and wellbeing, recognizing contribution and continuously improving) [24] is difficult.

The lack of supportive government policy and legislation contributed to the CFS voluntary failure. Mobile food services were vulnerable to local government regulations who can withdraw permission to operate at their discretion. Interviewees described numerous examples of services being moved on due to construction, festivals, parking restrictions, or conflict. Locating DS indoors would alleviate these problems and provide dignified seated meal services and socialisation, critical for people who are socially isolated [24]. This would also facilitate contact with additional services (e.g., health, accommodation, or supports for employment readiness). The FreshPlace model is an example of this type of integrated service which provides both food and assists pathways out of food insecurity [49].

Maintaining food safety along the logistics supply chain is likely to be difficult in the current CFS given the reliance on rescuing perishable waste food that may be past or close to expiry, and untrained volunteers handling food. Ensuring food handling and safety practices could protect this high-risk population sub-group against foodborne illness. Food safety legislation was designed to reduce the public health risk to the individual, yet the Western Australian Civil Liabilities Act 2002 Volunteers and Food and other Donors Act "protects persons who donate food or grocery products from incurring civil liability for personal injury resulting from the consumption of that food or the use of those grocery products, and for related purposes." [50] (p. 1).

CFS-focussed hospitality training would build the confidence and efficiency of the workforce in food service management, food procurement, menu planning, food preparation, occupational health and safety, food safety, and nutrition.

4.5. Equity, Effectiveness and Efficiency

This current study also provides evidence of inadequacy and the corresponding need for action to address all three areas of the 'iron triangle of hunger relief' described by Sengul Orgut et al. (2017) [51]. The three areas are equity (serving the needs of the recipient fairly in regard to both the quantity and quality or type of food received), effectiveness (the ability to meet the needs of the food insecure recipient), and efficiency (cost of resources needed to collect, manage, store and distribute donated food). Each dimension is in turn affected by supply (uncertain monetary supply, donations, and perishability), distribution (uncertain demand) and capacity factors (physical storage, transportation, workforce, and budget). Inefficient food redistribution is exacerbated by a lack of communication between CFS organisations and concerns were raised about overlapping or even competing services, and apparent lack of coordination.

4.6. Strategic Partnerships—The Way Forward

Based on the findings of this organisational audit, there are seven recommendations to guide action to improve the capacity of the CFS to provide a food service that meet the needs of its recipients. The recommendations are ranked in order of priority and given the similarities of the CFS in other Australian States and Territories, we believe they have national applicability.

1. Government-led framework with strategic coordinated partnerships with policy, licensing and funding supports

Streamlining the coordination and collaboration to reduce duplication and provide a better-quality service is recommended. The voluntary sector's weaknesses correspond to government strengths, and vice versa. In the case of the CFS, all levels of government (national, state and local) could partner with the DS and IS. Each level of government has a different imperative; for example, local area health plans are required to address significant health needs of the community, statewide departments act as system managers to set policy priority and conduct monitoring and surveillance activities, and the Federal government sets national standards, develops quality improvement schemes and is responsible for emergency response and social welfare decision making. Funding opportunities and decisions could then occur across all three levels of government and with all partners. Special care would need to be taken to ensure this is achieved without the loss of autonomy or flexibility for the CFS to meet recipient's needs.

2. Refocus, resource and prioritise the requirements for a nutrition-focussed CFS.

Planned menus are integral to the provision of a safe, nutritious and appropriate food service, and a reliable food supply is essential. The scope and nature of the IS suggest that the timing is right for them to focus on nutritious food acquisition with a formalized policy, such as that achieved with nutrition-focussed food banking [13]. Government can support the policy development and implementation through appropriate licensing and/or regulation to address any food safety or nutrition risk and sustain the change with additional resources.

3. Establish CFS principles and standards for appropriate food service needs.

The duty of care is described and controls (policy, licensing, legislation, accreditation and/or training) are implemented in other areas where foodservices are offered to vulnerable population sub-groups; for example, for children (in childcare centers, schools, or day care [31,32]) or people in custodial facilities, aged care facilities, or hospitals where recipients are reliant of the food provided to meet their welfare needs. At a local government level, compliance with food safety regulations for events such as festivals, music concerts are tightly controlled but do not apply for CFS.

Local government is currently considering licensing mobile CFS, including standards that translate nutrition needs across the continuum of care into the types and amounts of foods that should be acquired and supplied to meet CFS recipients' needs in a timely, cost-effective way to improve CFS. Work needs to be undertaken to determine both the content and 'format' (how the food is distributed, utilised and mechanisms for social inclusion) as was undertaken in Belgium [52]. A realistic individual assessment of the length of time the DS is needed should be included in the assessment.

Food safety training should be a mandatory requirement for all CFS workers handling food. As with retail food business, measures should be taken to ensure food safety. The large and changeable volunteer workforce and limited funding may hamper training opportunities; however, given the types of perishable foods distributed, particularly eggs, meat, prepared meals, sushi, there is likely an increased risk of food poisoning in a system without a food safety and handling framework.

4. Explore options to increase the sufficiency and efficiency of the food supply

Efficiencies are needed in both the distribution of food from IS to DS to recipients and its transformation into appropriate forms suitable for different food service models. With coordination, many options are available to improve food supply logistics and efficiencies. Technology-based online inventories of donated food used to improve food distribution efficiencies in other developed countries [53–55] are not used in Perth. These systems could improve efficiencies by signposting food availability earlier based on "use-by" or "best-by" dates; increasing donations of perishable items; assisting small CFS with limited food storage and with disaster relief emergency responses for food at short notice and in large quantities.

For a sustainable CFS system, government and the commercial and voluntary sector should consider the following: what are the cost benefits of redistributing food waste from the retail sector? Who pays, and what are the costs at each stage of the supply chain, including the food service end? Are there other preferred options? Improving efficiencies may also lead to resources being freed up to re-direct to other priorities; for example, providing meal services on weekends and during holiday periods where they are currently not provided.

5. Training and development of the CFS workforce is needed

Develop and provide CFS workforce training to enable delivery of services to meet their organisational intent and recipient's needs, framed as providing community food security. Cost-effective options should be investigated such as using the massive open online course (MOOC) platform, which enables flexible participation and uses a contemporary educational design to show case studies and provide opportunities for interactive learning and has been shown to be effective [56,57]. The "Developing Food Bank Nutrition Policy to Procure Healthful Foods" (Canvas.net) MOOC for food banks provides a precedent [58]. Local government, peak volunteering bodies, or hospitality training colleges or universities could consider offering gratis training for CFS staff and volunteers.

6.   Develop a CFS measurement system monitoring demand, distribution, impact and economic benefit

The CFS works to provide community food security, yet currently measures their impact in terms of kilograms of food rescued or meals provided. Consistent system-wide measures would enable all players in the CFS to articulate its value in terms of achieving community food security. Specific cross-discipline higher degree research should be a university research and government funding priority.

7.   Reorient the CFS to create pathways to build sustained food insecurity for recipients

The values of DS organisations suggest that the aim of the CFS approach should be to ensure "community food security" which focusses on local sustainable solutions to ensure ongoing food security rather than just providing short-term food relief. Inherent in any CFS response is the need for higher degrees of citizen empowerment and food democracy, not evident in Perth CFS recipient views [24]. Reducing food insecurity is also an internationally acknowledged government public health priority. Placing people's lived experiences at the centre of decision delivers better integrated policy solutions and effective pathways out of food insecurity [40]. The lack of uptake of innovative social enterprises as a response to food insecurity in Australia has been attributed to the resistance from dominant commercial players and restrictive government legislation [20]. There is a need to work with these actors to support the development and trialing of alternative models to address the market, government and voluntary failures that exist in the current CFS.

4.7. Strengths, Limitations and Further Research

This study is the first comprehensive examination of the scope and operational capacity of the charitable food sector in inner-city Perth and provides a detailed picture of the workings of the sector in an Australian capital city. Specific information on corporate donors and funding was not provided due to confidentiality; however, additional information was sought from financial reports. Service delivery achievements and shortfalls were inconsistently expressed across organisations; for example, millions of meals served versus tonnes of food waste diverted from landfill and numbers of people provided meals. Turn away rates due to short falls in food supply were not available but would assist in the assessment of the effectiveness of the CFS. The findings of this study are limited to the CFS provided in inner-city Perth and provide only a snapshot at a point in time; however, they are likely to be relevant to other the inner-city precincts of Australian and international capital cities with a welfare safety net.

Further research is needed to quantify the types, amount and form of food supplied and the environment in which it is delivered. This will help to determine the suitability and capacity of CFS to meet of the needs of their recipients in terms of food security, nutrition status, and social inclusion. Current decision-making is divorced from lived experience. Decision makers are crafting solutions devoid of an understanding of those who are affected by the problem. Further research validating people lived experience of food insecurity and trialing new responses which offer pathways out is a priority.

Further research recommendations include an economic cost-benefit analysis of the efficiencies of the CFS; further exploration of the government (federal, state and local) and private sector roles in the CFS; and the development and piloting of other models of food relief with an emphasis on social inclusion and pathways out of food insecurity.

5. Conclusions

This research is a timely contribution that shines a light on the NP sector as it struggles to cope with the chronicity of embedded food insecurity, the ad hoc nature of donated food, declining funding and resource constraints. The lack of formalised nutrition policy and training is likely to hinder the acquisition and provision of nutritious and appropriate food relief for people vulnerable to food insecurity. Coordination, reliable funding and food acquisition, food handling and nutrition policy and training and volunteer support is needed to build the capacity of the sector. The findings suggest a CFS at breaking point and highlight the urgent need for debate and investigation of other models to better address food insecurity.

Supplementary Materials: The following are available online at http://www.mdpi.com/1660-4601/15/6/1249/s1, Table S1: Characteristics of Charitable Food System Indirect Service organisations servicing or located in the inner-city Perth.

Author Contributions: C.M.P., S.B., A.B., D.K., J.B., B.M., M.C. and J.J. conceived the study design and research objectives, all authors and the research advisory team developed the research questions and interview guide; B.M. and C.C. conducted the interviews; B.M., C.C., C.M.P., and S.B. analyzed the data; B.M., C.C., C.M.P., and S.B. wrote the paper; all authors reviewed and edited the manuscript.

Acknowledgments: This work was funded by Healthway, the Western Australian Health Promotion Foundation, who funded Curtin University to undertake this Special Research Initiative entitled "Charitable Food Services and the Needs of Homeless and Disadvantaged People" (Grant number 24266). Healthway had no role in the design, analysis or writing of this article. We wish to acknowledge the partner organisations (The Salvation Army, United Care West, Noongar Patrol Services, Australian Red Cross, Foodbank, Western Australian Council of Social Services WACOSS—Emergency Relief Forum, Vincentcare, Perth City Council) who formed the research advisory group. We would like to thank members of the research team who have contributed to the work of the project particularly Lieutenant Kris Halliday from The Salvation Army's Doorways Community Programs and Bernie Fisher from WACOSS, Rex Milligan from Foodbank WA as well as the interviewees who willingly gave their time and shared their insights and experience with the ambition of creating a better CFS.

Conflicts of Interest: The authors declare no conflicts of interest. B.M. is a long-term volunteer for the CFS, Cathy Campbell. is a former and Christina M Pollard a current Foodbank WA board member, J.B. is the C.E.O. of Hunger Free America. The founding sponsors had no role in the design of the study; in the collection, analyses, or interpretation of data; in the writing of the manuscript, and in the decision to publish the results.

References

1. Seligman, H.K.; Laraia, B.A.; Kushel, M.B. Food insecurity is associated with chronic disease among low-income NHANES participants. *J. Nutr.* **2010**, *140*, 304–310. [CrossRef] [PubMed]
2. Marmot, M. Inclusion health: Addressing the causes of the causes. *Lancet* **2017**, *10117*, 186–188. [CrossRef]
3. McKee, M.; Reeves, A.; Clair, A.; Stuckler, D. Living on the edge: Precariousness and why it matters for health. *Arch. Public Health* **2017**, *75*, 13. [CrossRef] [PubMed]
4. Fazel, S.; Geddes, J.R.; Kushel, M. The health of homeless people in high-income countries: Descriptive epidemiology, health consequences, and clinical and policy recommendations. *Lancet* **2014**, *384*, 1529–1540. [CrossRef]
5. Baggett, T.P.; Singer, D.E.; Rao, S.R.; O'Connell, J.J.; Bharel, M.; Rigotti, N.A. Food insufficiency and health services utilization in a national sample of homeless adults. *J. Gen. Intern. Med.* **2011**, *26*, 627–634. [CrossRef] [PubMed]
6. Cook, J.T.; Black, M.; Chilton, M.; Cutts, D.; Ettinger de Cuba, S.; Heeren, T.C.; Rose-Jacobs, R.; Sandel, M.; Casey, P.H.; Coleman, S. Are food insecurity's health impacts underestimated in the U.S. population? Marginal food security also predicts adverse health outcomes in young us children and mothers. *Adv. Nutr.* **2013**, *4*, 51–61. [CrossRef] [PubMed]
7. Hamelin, A.-M.; Hamel, D. Food insufficiency in currently or formerly homeless persons is associated with poorer health. *Can. J. Urban Res.* **2009**, *18*, 1.
8. Quine, S.; Kendig, H.; Russell, C.; Touchard, D. Health promotion for socially disadvantaged groups: The case of homeless older men in Australia. *Health Promot. Int.* **2004**, *19*, 157–165. [CrossRef] [PubMed]
9. Lee, B.A.; Greif, M.J. Homelessness and hunger. *J. Health Soc. Behav.* **2008**, *49*, 3–19. [CrossRef] [PubMed]

10. Crawford, B.; Yamazaki, R.; Franke, E.; Amanatidis, S.; Ravulo, J.; Steinbeck, K.; Ritchie, J.; Torvaldsen, S. Sustaining dignity? Food insecurity in homeless young people in urban Australia. *Health Promot. J. Austr.* **2014**, *25*, 71–78. [CrossRef] [PubMed]

11. Ruah. *Ruah Community Service*; Registry Week 2016 Report; Ruah: Perth, Australia, 2016.

12. Lindberg, R.; Whelan, J.; Lawrence, M.; Gold, L.; Friel, S. Still serving hot soup? Two hundred years of a charitable food sector in Australia: A narrative review. *Aust. N. Z. J. Public Health* **2015**, *39*, 358–365. [CrossRef] [PubMed]

13. Simmet, A.; Depa, J.; Tinnemann, P.; Stroebele-Benschop, N. The nutritional quality of food provided from food pantries: A systematic review of existing literature. *J. Acad. Nutr. Diet.* **2017**, *117*, 577–588. [CrossRef] [PubMed]

14. Campbell, E.; Webb, K.; Michelle, R.; Crawford, P.; Hudson, H.; Hecht, K. *Nutrition-Focused Food Banking*; Institute of Medicine: Washington, DC, USA, 2015.

15. Campbell, E.C.; Ross, M.; Webb, K.L. Improving the nutritional quality of emergency food: A study of food bank organizational culture, capacity, and practices. *J. Hunger Environ. Nutr.* **2013**, *8*, 261–280. [CrossRef]

16. Pollard, C.; Begley, A.; Landrigan, T. The rise of food inequality in Australia. In *Food Poverty and Insecurity: International Food Inequalities*; Caraher, M., Coveney, J., Eds.; Springer International Publishing Switzerland: Basel, Switzerland, 2016; pp. 89–103.

17. Australian Government Department of Human Services. Age Pension. Available online: https://www.humanservices.gov.au/individuals/services/centrelink/age-pension (accessed on 18 April 2018).

18. Australian Government Department of Human Services. Families. Available online: https://www.humanservices.gov.au/individuals/families (accessed on 18 April 2018).

19. Australian Government Department of Human Services. Newstart Allowance. Available online: https://www.humanservices.gov.au/individuals/services/centrelink/newstart-allowance (accessed on 18 April 2018).

20. Wills, B. Eating at the limits: Barriers to the emergence of social enterprise initiatives in the australian emergency food relief sector. *Food Policy* **2017**, *70*, 62–70. [CrossRef]

21. Foodbank Hunger Report 2016. Available online: https://www.foodbank.org.au/wp-content/uploads/2016/05/Foodbank-Hunger-Report-2016.pdf (accessed on 1 December 2017).

22. Wingrove, K.; Barbour, L.; Palermo, C. Exploring nutrition capacity in australia's charitable food sector. *Nutr. Diet.* **2016**, *74*, 495–501. [CrossRef] [PubMed]

23. Wicks, R.; Trevena, L.J.; Quine, S. Experiences of food insecurity among urban soup kitchen consumers: Insights for improving nutrition and well-being. *J. Acad. Nutr. Diet.* **2006**, *106*, 921–924. [CrossRef] [PubMed]

24. Booth, S.; Begely, A.; Mackntosh, K.A.; Jancy, J.; Caraher, M.; Whelan, J.; Pollard, C.M. Gratitude, resignation, and the desire for dignity: Lived experience of food charity recipients and their recommendations for improvement, Perth, Western Australia. *Public Health Nutr.* **2018**. accepted for publication.

25. Western Australian Council of Social Service. *Giving Shape to the Emergency Relief Sector*; Western Australian Council of Social Service: West Perth, Australia, 2012.

26. Middleton, G.; Mehta, K.; McNaughton, D.; Booth, S. The experiences and perceptions of food banks amongst users in high-income countries: An international scoping review. *Appetite* **2018**, *120*, 698–708. [CrossRef] [PubMed]

27. Booth, S.; Whelan, J. Hungry for change: The food banking industry in Australia. *Br. Food J.* **2014**, *116*, 1392–1404. [CrossRef]

28. Salamon, L.M. Of market failure, voluntary failure, and third-party government: Toward a theory of government-nonprofit relations in the modern welfare state. *Nonprofit Volunt. Sect. Q.* **1987**, *16*, 29–49. [CrossRef]

29. McKay, F.H.; McKenzie, H. Food aid provision in metropolitan Melbourne: A mixed methods study. *J. Hunger Environ. Nutr.* **2017**, *12*, 11–25. [CrossRef]

30. Harris, E.; Wise, M.; Hawe, P.; Finlay, P.; Nutbeam, D. *Working Together: Intersectoral Action for Health*; Australian Government Publishing Service: Canberra, Australia, 1995.

31. Pollard, C.; Lewis, J.; Miller, M. Start right–eat right award scheme: Implementing food and nutrition policy in child care centers. *Health Educ. Behav.* **2001**, *28*, 320–330. [CrossRef] [PubMed]

32. Pollard, C.M.; Lewis, J.M.; Miller, M.R. Food service in long day care centres—An opportunity for public health intervention. *Aust. N. Z. J. Public Health* **1999**, *23*, 606–610. [CrossRef] [PubMed]

33. Foodbank Western Australia Annual Report 2017. Available online: https://www.foodbankwa.org.au/wp-content/blogs.dir/5/files/2017/10/FB-AR-17_online.pdf (accessed on 12 April 2018).
34. The Ozharvest Effect 2016. Available online: https://www.ozharvest.org/wp-content/uploads/2014/04/OZHF0034F_OzHarvest_AnnualReport_Book2_FA3_LR41.pdf (accessed on 12 April 2018).
35. Foley, R.M.; Pollard, C.M. Food cent $—Implementing and evaluating a nutrition education project focusing on value for money. *Aust. N. Z. J. Public Health* **1998**, *22*, 494–501. [CrossRef] [PubMed]
36. Pettigrew, S.; Moore, S.; Pratt, I.S.; Jongenelis, M. Evaluation outcomes of a long-running adult nutrition education programme. *Public Health Nutr.* **2016**, *19*, 743–752. [CrossRef] [PubMed]
37. Offer, A.; Pechey, R.; Ulijaszek, S. Obesity under affluence varies by welfare regimes: The effect of fast food, insecurity, and inequality. *Econ. Hum. Biol.* **2010**, *8*, 297–308. [CrossRef] [PubMed]
38. Enjolras, B.; Salamon, L.M.; Sivesind, K.H.; Zimmer, A. *The Third Sector as a Renewable Resource for Europe: Concepts, Impacts, Challenges and Opportunities*; Springer: Berlin/Hamburg, Germany, 2018.
39. Casey, J. *The Nonprofit World: Civil Society and the Rise of the Nonprofit Sector*; Kumarian Press: Sterling, VA, USA, 2016.
40. Hawkes, C. The role of law, regulation, and policy in meeting 21st century challenges to the food supply. In *Food Governance Conference*; Sydney University: Sydney, Australia, 2016.
41. Bellows, A.C.; Hamm, M.W. U.S.-based community food security: Influences, practice, debate. *J. Study Food Soc.* **2002**, *6*, 31–44. [CrossRef]
42. Hamm, M.W.; Bellows, A.C. Community food security and nutrition educators. *J. Nutr. Educ. Behav.* **2003**, *35*, 37–43. [CrossRef]
43. St Vincent de Paul Society (WA) Inc. Annual Review 2017: Restoring Hope. Available online: https://www.vinnies.org.au/icms_docs/276248_Vinnies_WA_2017_Annual_Report.pdf (accessed on 12 April 2018).
44. St Vincent de Paul Society (Victoria) Inc. 2016–2017 Annual Review Face to Face Side by Side Walking together. Available online: https://www.vinnies.org.au/icms_docs/276542_2016-2017_Annual_Report.pdf (accessed on 12 April 2018).
45. Claire, D. *Salvation Army May Cut Services in WA as Donations Decline for Third Year in a Row*; ABC New 2015; Australian Broadcasting Commission: Perth, Australia, 2015.
46. Simmet, A.; Depa, J.; Tinnemann, P.; Stroebele-Benschop, N. The dietary quality of food pantry users: A systematic review of existing literature. *J. Acad. Nutr. Diet.* **2017**, *117*, 563–576. [CrossRef] [PubMed]
47. Stephens, C.; Breheny, M.; Mansvelt, J. Volunteering as reciprocity: Beneficial and harmful effects of social policies to encourage contribution in older age. *J. Aging Stud.* **2015**, *33*, 22–27. [CrossRef] [PubMed]
48. Wheeler, J.A.; Gorey, K.M.; Greenblatt, B. The beneficial effects of volunteering for older volunteers and the people they serve: A meta-analysis. *Int. J. Aging Hum. Dev.* **1998**, *47*, 69–79. [CrossRef] [PubMed]
49. Martin, K.S.; Colantonio, A.G.; Picho, K.; Boyle, K.E. Self-efficacy is associated with increased food security in novel food pantry program. *SSM-Popul. Health* **2016**, *2*, 62–67. [CrossRef] [PubMed]
50. Government of Western Australia; Department of Communitities. *Volunteers and Food and Other Donors (Protection from Liability) Act 2002*; Government of Western Australia; Department of Communitities: Perth Western, Australia, 2016; Volume 32.
51. Orgut, I.S.; Brock, L.G., III; Davis, L.B.; Ivy, J.S.; Jiang, S.; Morgan, S.D.; Uzsoy, R.; Hale, C.; Middleton, E. Achieving equity, effectiveness, and efficiency in food bank operations: Strategies for feeding America with implications for global hunger relief. In *Advances in Managing Humanitarian Operations*; Springer: Berlin/Hamburg, Germany, 2016; pp. 229–256.
52. Stepman, E.; Uyttendaele, M.; De Boeck, E.; Jacxsens, L. Needs of beneficiaries related to the format and content of food parcels in Ghent, Belgium. *Br. Food J.* **2018**, *120*, 578–587. [CrossRef]
53. Bazerghi, C.; McKay, F.H.; Dunn, M. The role of food banks in addressing food insecurity: A systematic review. *J. Community Health* **2016**, *41*, 732–740. [CrossRef] [PubMed]
54. Chow Match. *Food Sharing Database*; Chow Match: San Francisco, CA, USA, 2015.
55. Corbo, C.; Fraticelli, F. The use of web-based technology as an emerging option for food waste reduction. In *Envisioning a Future Without Food Waste and Food Poverty: Societal Challenges*; San-Epifanio, L.E., Scheifler, M.D.R., Eds.; Wageningen Academic Publishers: Wageningen, The Netherlands, 2015; pp. 1–2.
56. Bozkurt, A.; Akgun-Ozbek, E.; Yilmazel, S.; Erdogdu, E.; Ucar, H.; Guler, E.; Sezgin, S.; Karadeniz, A.; Sen-Ersoy, N.; Goksel-Canbek, N. Trends in distance education research: A content analysis of journals 2009–2013. *Int. Rev. Res. Open Distrib. Learn.* **2015**. [CrossRef]

57. Adam, M.; Young-Wolff, K.C.; Konar, E.; Winkleby, M. Massive open online nutrition and cooking course for improved eating behaviors and meal composition. *Int. J. Behav. Nutr. Phys. Act.* **2015**, *12*, 143. [CrossRef] [PubMed]

58. Webb, K.; Campbell, E.M.R. Developing Food Bank Nutrition Policy to Procure Healthful Foods (Canvas.Net). Available online: https://www.canvas.net/browse/cwh/courses/food-bank-nutrition-policy (accessed on 12 April 2018).

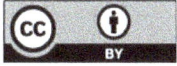

International Journal of
Environmental Research and Public Health

MDPI

Article

'Sustainable' Rather Than 'Subsistence' Food Assistance Solutions to Food Insecurity: South Australian Recipients' Perspectives on Traditional and Social Enterprise Models

Sue Booth [1,*], Christina Pollard [2], John Coveney [3] and Ian Goodwin-Smith [4]

1   College of Medicine and Public Health, Flinders University, Adelaide 5000, Australia
2   Faculty of Health Sciences, School of Public Health, Curtin University, Perth 6102, Australia;
    C.Pollard@curtin.edu.au
3   College of Nursing & Health Sciences, Flinders University, Adelaide 5000, Australia;
    john.coveney@flinders.edu.au
4   College of Business, Government and Law, Flinders University, Adelaide 5000, Australia;
    ian.goodwinsmith@flinder.edu.au
*   Correspondence: sue.booth@flinders.edu.au; Tel.: +61-8-7221-8464

Received: 14 August 2018; Accepted: 19 September 2018; Published: 21 September 2018

Abstract: South Australian (SA) food charity recipients' perspectives were sought on existing services and ideas for improvement of food assistance models to address food insecurity. Seven focus groups were conducted between October and November 2017 with 54 adults. Thematically analysed data revealed five themes: (1) Emotional cost and consequences of seeking food relief; (2) Dissatisfaction with inaccessible services and inappropriate food; (3) Returning the favour—a desire for reciprocity; (4) Desiring help beyond food; and, (5) "It's a social thing", the desire for social interaction and connection. Findings revealed that some aspects of the SA food assistance services were disempowering for recipients. Recipients desired more empowering forms of food assistance that humanise their experience and shift the locus of control and place power back into their hands. Some traditional models, such as provision of supermarket vouchers, empower individuals by fostering autonomy and enabling food choice in socially acceptable ways. Improvement in the quality of existing food assistance models, should focus on recipient informed models which re-dress existing power relations. Services which are more strongly aligned with typical features of social enterprise models were generally favoured over traditional models. Services which are recipient-centred, strive to empower recipients and provide opportunities for active involvement, social connection and broader support were preferred.

Keywords: food assistance; food insecurity; food charity; food service; social enterprise models

1. Introduction

Despite comprehensive social welfare provisions in Australia, such as unemployment benefits and universal health care, increasing neoliberalism and economic pressures have resulted in insufficient and inadequate levels of income support for vulnerable groups [1]. The United Nations Committee on the Rights of the Child recommended that Australia improve its social services (for education, health, income support, disability services and employment to strengthen their responsiveness for those at risk) [1]. Liberal state welfare models increase reliance on markets, individual responsibility and charitable responses rather than the state acting to universally respect, protect and fulfil the needs of vulnerable citizens [2]. As a consequence of the liberal model of welfare capitalism [3], more Australians are experiencing poverty, leading to food inequality [4] and a reliance on food assistance. In countries without robust, adequate welfare safety nets, people rely on food relief provided by charitable organisations such as foodbanks, faith-based groups and non-government organisations [5,6].

South Australia has experienced an economic downturn due in part to key industries relocating, resulting in unemployment and population subgroups at increasing risk of food insecurity [7,8]. In 2015, approximately 75,000 South Australians (4.2% of the population) were classified as food insecure, with higher prevalence among: women (4.9% compared to 4.1% of men); the unemployed (12.3% compared to 2.2% of full-time employed); households with an income of less than AUD$20,000 (12.1% compared to 1.2% of income over AUD$80,000); and Aboriginal and Torres Strait Islander people (16% compared to 4.4% non-Indigenous) [9]. The demand for food relief has increased, with recipients described as socially isolated, homeless, unemployed, financially struggling and marginalised [10]. Complex client needs, intergenerational poverty, limited education and employment opportunities contribute to the demand [11]. There is also evidence of food insecurity and reliance on food charity among middle-income Australian families [12]. The growing number of 'working poor' may reflect the unaffordability of household utility costs [13].

Australian food relief is predominantly provided by charitable food services [6,14]. In 2015, the Federal government provided ~AUD$64 million to support the provision of emergency relief, which was estimated to provide food assistance for up to eight percent of the population [14]. State governments assist in managing the distribution of funds and may allocate additional grant funding for targeted programs, for example, school breakfast programs. Between 3000 and 4000 emergency relief services provided short-term, immediate food assistance to eligible recipients in 2015 [14]. Seventy percent of emergency relief agencies reported increasing demand for food assistance in 2016, up by eight percent since 2015 [15].

The effectiveness and appropriateness of the traditional charitable food assistance model, has been questioned by government and academics, in light of the increasing demand for food assistance and an emerging interest in social enterprise models [16]. The South Australian Government's former Department of Communities and Social Inclusion (DCSI) (now Human Services) and SA Health commissioned research to explore recipients' experience of charitable food services and their recommendations for service improvements.

Traditional food assistance models are delivered via partnerships between the non-profit sector and supermarket chains—often with some government funding—with the aim of redistributing food waste to those living below the poverty line [17]. Food services are diverse and include mobile soup vans, food parcels, supermarket vouchers, pantries, seated meal services, food hubs and food banks [6,14]. The food provided is usually donated by supermarkets to food banks, where it is collected by direct services or "rescued" and delivered by food rescue organisations and faith-based groups, or purchased directly from supermarkets. Food is usually provided to recipients free or at a minimal cost. There is limited information on the types of foods provided in Australia; however, internationally, the types of food provided by these types of services have been found likely to exacerbate recipients' diet-related chronic disease conditions [6,18,19].

There are consistent reports from other jurisdictions of the recipients of traditional charitable food assistance being dissatisfied with the quality and quantity of food provided [20–22]. In addition to negative experiences due to limited food choice and poor food quality, recipients report feelings of shame, and describe the stigma and embarrassment associated with using food banks [23–25]. In Australia similar results are reported particularly concerning gratitude and shame: dissatisfaction with the variety, quality and types of food offered [26–28].

Social enterprise food assistance models, such as community or social supermarkets, social cafes, buying groups, and co-operatives, are uncommon in Australia, but are emerging as alternatives to the traditional charitable model [16]. Social enterprise broadly means 'trading for a social purpose', that is to say not for profit and for public benefit. However, there is little uniformity on what they are or do [29,30]. In other words, social enterprises are diverse, heterogeneous types of organisations using multiple activities to address the social needs of different client groups [31,32]. They vary in approach, but include: nonprofits' income earning strategies; voluntary organisations contracted to deliver public services; democratically controlled organisations primarily aiming to benefit the community with limited profits for external investors; commercial businesses operating in public welfare fields or with a social conscience; and, locally driven community enterprises combatting a shared problem [29,30].

Market, government and voluntary sector failures have been identified as the reason for the lack of uptake of social enterprise models in Australia, even though social enterprise models have the potential to address all three failures [16]. When reviewing these models in Australia, Wills (2017) found that resistance to them may be a consequence of commercial stakeholders fearing devaluation of their product range, lack of government legislative support, and/or current legislation undermining practices that social entrepreneurs wish to take [16].

There is no research on Australian food assistance recipients' perspectives on the likely benefits and limitations of social enterprise models to address food insecurity. Yet, the views of current food assistance recipients bring the lived experience perspective on receiving food assistance as well as helping to identify the elements of service delivery that are important to better meet needs. This study aimed to investigate recipients' views on both of these approaches (traditional and social enterprise), compare food relief models and their perspectives on each model's potential to meet the needs of food insecure people.

2. Materials and Methods

This study used a qualitative focus group methodology. Ethical approval was granted by the Flinders University Social and Behavioural Research Ethics Committee (Project No. 7770).

2.1. Recruitment and Data Collection

The DCSI provided researchers with an email contact list of South Australian emergency food relief services which they fund. Purposive sampling was used to capture inner metropolitan, outer metropolitan and country areas, as well as a diversity of service types. This enabled researchers to capture multiple and different perspectives. An email was sent to the CEO or similar explaining the study. Of the twelve organisations invited, seven (2 inner city, 3 outer metropolitan and 2 country) were agreeable and provided the name and contact details of their service manager to assist with focus group recruitment. The researchers were in regular contact with service managers regarding the most convenient day, and time to run the focus group. During times of food relief operations, the service manager and researchers would randomly approach recipients, advise them of the study and invite them to participate. All service managers were invited to attend the focus groups which were run in conjunction with a scheduled food relief session. Three experienced researchers (SB, JC and I G-S) conducted the focus groups in pairs. Service staff approached food relief participants and invited them to participate using a standard verbal script outlining the time and location of the focus group. The focus groups were held on site in a private room approximately an hour later. Invitees were provided with a study information sheet and consent form and a verbal explanation was given and written consent was obtained before the focus group commenced.

Each group was digitally recorded, field notes were written up afterwards and a commercial service transcribed each group. Participants were given a AUD$30 supermarket gift card as a token of appreciation for their time and contribution.

2.2. Focus Group Guide

A semi-structured guide was developed by the research team to direct the discussion while allowing for diversions reflective of participants' statements. Participants were asked to describe the type of charitable services they had used in the last year and the appropriateness and effectiveness of these services. A set of visual prompts were then used to assist participants to consider the pros and cons of traditional charitable and emerging social enterprise food relief service models. Finally, the group was asked to describe their ideal service for food relief provision.

2.3. Visual Prompts and Ranking of Preferences

A set of eight pictorial flash-cards was developed by the researchers. Each card had a short description of the type of service on the back to assist participants in considering the pros and cons of a variety of different food assistance models. The cards were used to stimulate focus group discussion and for an assessment of overall preference for services (Figure 1). The cards were divided into 2 groups based on availability. The first five cards showed and described traditional charitable food relief options commonly available in South Australia: (i) Food parcels, (ii) Food pantries, (iii) Gift cards/vouchers, (iv) Seated meal services, and (v) and Foodbank Food hubs. The remaining three cards showed social enterprise models of food relief which were not available in South Australia, but examples existing interstate or internationally. These were (vi) Social café program, (vii) Food co-operatives, and (viii) Social supermarkets. Each Group was asked to place the cards in rank order, starting with the service type they would be least likely to use. In each focus group, discussion continued until consensus was reached on the preferential ranking of cards. The discussions during the group ranking exercise highlighted some of the potential positive and negative attributions of services.

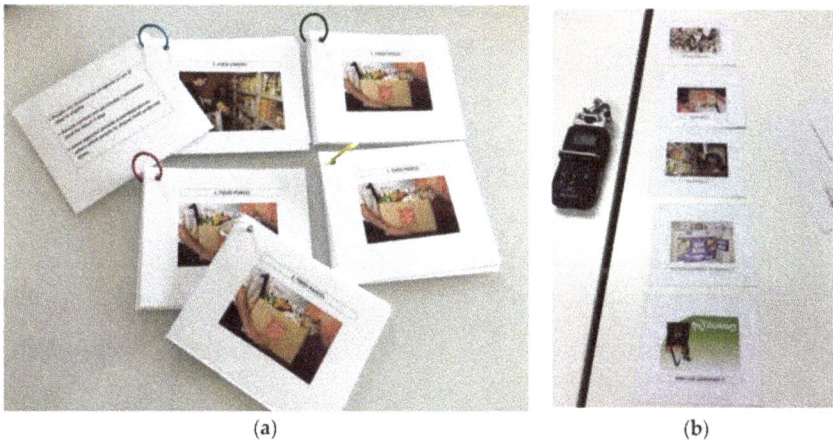

Figure 1. (a) The visual flash cards; (b) Visual flash cards in ranked order of preference during a focus group.

2.4. Data Analysis

Focus group recordings and notes were transcribed and de-identified. CMP and SB read and re-read all the transcripts and a sub-sample were read by the remaining researchers. The data was then analysed using the qualitative software program QSR NVivo (version 11.4.3, QSR International, Doncaster, Victoria, Australia). Deductive codes were initially developed from the focus group schedule as well as from the researchers' knowledge of the literature on experiences of charitable food service users. Inductive codes were developed from the focus group participant responses and discussed with the team to ensure rigour [33]. A thematic analysis was conducted by CMP with the codes and emergent themes cross-checked with the other members of the team until consensus was reached. SB double-coded three of the seven focus group transcript and any disagreements with the coding structure were discussed and the codes subsequently revised. Throughout the analysis, the data was further tested with the literature and subsequent focus groups in an iterative process. Data on the preferential ranking of service models across all focus group was tabulated. Verbal comments on the reasons for the ranking, pros, cons and recommendations to improve models were included in the thematic analysis.

3. Results

Fifty-four adults, 34 males and 20 females, who were recipients of food relief, participated in seven focus groups. Table 1 provides details of focus group location, service types from which participants were recruited and their gender.

Table 1. Location of focus group services, brief description, date and number of participants.

Group	Location	Service Description	Participants (*n*) Gender Split
1	Inner city	Seated breakfast program and emergency food relief appointments (Voucher)	(10) 7 men, 3 women
2	Inner city	Emergency food relief appointments (Food pantry access), free bread service	(7) 6 men, 1 woman
3	Country	Emergency food relief appointments (Food hub)	(7) 5 men, 2 women
4	Country	Emergency food relief appointments (Food parcels)	(4) 2 men, 2 women
5	Outer metropolitan	Volunteer run food hub—free food plus access to some items at reduced prices	(9) 2 men, 7 women
6	Outer metropolitan	Emergency food relief appointments (Food pantry access)	(7) 5 men, 2 women
7	Outer metropolitan	Food pantry, free bread, fruit and vegetables	(10) 3 men and 7 women

Overall, participants had used nine different food relief models, often accessing multiple services to overcome service food restrictions on frequency and amount. Several vulnerabilities led participants to use charitable food services, these included: homelessness; precarious employment; low income due to insufficient welfare payments; relationship breakdown; gambling addiction; and rises in the cost of living. The long-term nature of the need for food relief was evident, for example the chronicity recorded in the field note of SB,

> *"A woman on the far side of the table from me is of medium-thick build with shoulder-length strawberry blonde hair. She has broad facial features and makes intermittent eye contact. She tells the group she has been on the streets since she was 11 and she's now about 41. She looks much older. She has diabetes and food allergies. After the focus group she says I look familiar to her. We work out that I interviewed her for my PhD on homeless youth and food insecurity in 2000. She is terribly excited by this and tells everyone in the vicinity . . . She shouts she can't believe it and tells the people she is sitting with the story."* Field note extract, SB Focus Group 1.

Participants' views on the pros, cons, and recommendations for improvement for the five traditional and three social enterprise food service models were varied and to some extent dependent on their current circumstances, as shown in Table 2.

Table 2. Participants' perspectives on the pros and cons of food service models and their recommendations to improve them.

Model	Pros	Cons	Recommendation
Food Parcel	• Commonly available • Grateful for parcels when have nothing	• 'Harsh' eligibility criteria • Inappropriate amount of food for family, types of food for special diets • Inadequate nutritious foods • No choice • Short term (1–3 day) solution • Food expires if you get more • Incomplete meals—no meat • Homeless people cannot carry	• Respectful and dignifying eligibility processes • Appropriate amounts and type of food to suit nutrition needs (e.g., meat, recipes, full meals, nutritious foods, length of time to cover) • Ability to choose items
Food Pantry	• Allows choice • Other items available (toiletries, washing powder etc.) • Fresh produce • Suitable if have access to cooking facilities	• Limits to number of items • Close to expired food • Limited types of foods, e.g., meat • Can only use twice a year • Must prove need • Difficulty securing an assessment appointment • Insufficient daily appointments • Have to waiting for appointment despite immediate need • Not suitable if no cooking facilities	• Respectful and dignifying eligibility processes • Reduce appointments waiting time, e.g., free calls or 1800 number • Appropriate amounts and type of food to suit nutritional needs (meat, recipes, full meals, nutritious foods) • Align food quantity with need • Increase access during holidays and weekends
Supermarket gift card	• Allows choice • Can buy other essential items • Easy to carry • Dignifying and 'normal' way to acquire food	• 'Harsh' eligibility criteria • Amount ($20) is inadequate • Only allowed to spend at major supermarket chains where food is expensive	• Increase supermarket voucher card value • Relax eligibility criteria • Cash for purchases from alternative food businesses
Seated meal services	• Best for people without dwelling, social isolated or cooking facilities • Able to combine with other services (e.g., shower, phone charging) • Social engagement with volunteers	• Families with young children too noisy • Sometimes unpleasant environment/people • Do not want children to experience the stigma • Cost to recipient • Can miss out on food because there is not enough and waiting time is too long • No-one sits down to and talks to you • Agency referral needed	• Combine with other services • Maintain pleasant, quiet, dignified atmosphere • Tailor food service to client needs • Universal eligibility • Socially connect with recipients
Foodbank Food Hubs	• Membership-based • Reward/incentive program • Discounts towards end of year, pre-saving for Christmas hampers • Free bread, fruit and vegetables	• Agency-issued vouchers require assessment appointments. Viewed as judgemental, embarrassing and undignified • Food that is unsaleable or approaching its use by date or expired.	• Universal eligibility or respectful and dignifying eligibility processes • Membership includes rewards scheme for every dollar spent • Food is purchased using own money • Blended model—free food and some discounted for purchase • Increase access during holidays and weekends

Table 2. *Cont.*

Model	Pros	Cons	Recommendation
Co-operative	• Dignifying • Dietitian assessed low-cost food packs with recipes for preparing at home • Offer toiletries, toys etc. • Best with other services including seated meals	• Membership fee • Having to pay for food if no income	• Include other services, e.g., seated meals or cafes • Make it more accessible to people e.g., transport • Increase access—Open during school holidays, weekends and major holidays
Social cafe	• Allows access to mainstream café—normalising experience • Helps isolated individuals • An outing for a special occasion	• Agency eligibility and assessment • Meal subsidy is time limited • Does not allow for family members and children • Dependent on participating café in local area	• Universal eligibility or respectful and dignifying eligibility processes • Incorporate access for children and family members • Free community barbecues to reduce social isolation and provide a treat/family outing
Social supermarket	• Opportunity for capacity building and volunteerism • Associated café providing cheap meals • Membership and discounted food • Supermarket style format, can exercise individual food choice • Other services can be accessed via the social supermarket—the idea of linked service valued • One-stop shop • Opportunity for socialisation, community connection	• Stocked with food that may be expired or close to use by date. Purchased food may have a shorter life span?	• Increased access—Open during school holidays, weekends and major holidays

Consensus on the preferential ranking of the five existing food service models varied across focus groups, depending on participants' social circumstances. Preference also varied for the three new models presented; however, social supermarkets were ranked highest by half of the groups, see Table 3.

Table 3. Focus group consensus ranking scores for participants' preference for five traditional models and three social enterprise food service models.

Ranking *	Traditional Models					Social Enterprise Models		
Focus group	Hub	Voucher	Pantry	Seated Meal	Parcel	Social Supermarket	Co-op	Social Café
1	5	2	3	1	4	2	3	1
2	5	4	3	2	1	2	1	3
3	1	2	3	5	4	1	3	2
4	2	1	3	5	4	1	3	2
5	1	4	3	2	5	1	2	3
6	2	1	3	5	5	2	1	3
7	1	3	2	5	4	1	2	3
Total	17	17	20	25	27	10	15	17

* Traditional models ranked from 1 most preferred to 5 least preferred (total possible 35) and social enterprise models from 1 most preferred to 3 the least preferred (total possible = 21).

When participants ranked the traditional food assistance service models, the hub, supermarket voucher and pantry were the most preferred. Discussions of the pros and cons revealed that these models enabled choice and allowed recipients to behave as mainstream consumers, that is, to engage in socially acceptable methods of food procurement. These types of food service models were the most likely to create a sense of empowerment for those who used them. Participants' recommendations to improve the traditional models generally focussed on universal eligibility or, if not possible, timely, dignified and respectful eligibility assessment processes. Traditional food assistance services also need to be re-engineered to provide the appropriate types and amounts of food to meet recipient's physical needs, specifically for: family composition, nutrition requirements, duration of food insecurity; and availability of food preparation facilities. They believed that services should also be re-engineered to provide opportunities reduce social isolation and foster social connection over a meal, for example, to incorporate seated meal services including cafes.

When participants ranked the three social enterprise food assistance service models, the social supermarket was first, co-operatives second and social cafe third. Again, the preference was to engage in socially acceptable models of food procurement. When informed about these models, participants viewed them favourability, particularly the normalising of food procurement processes, and the opportunity for neighbourhood and community connection. Social supermarkets and co-operatives were viewed as offering a dignified eligibility process, as a member rather than a recipient, and the opportunity to access additional services to assist recipients out of food insecurity. The opportunity to visit a café was viewed as highly desirable but out of reach for most participants. The main barriers to the social café model were the short-term nature, agency eligibility assessment, and the fact that recipients could not bring along their family members.

Five key themes emerged from all of the focus group and model ranking discussions (Figure 2). These were: (1) Emotional cost and consequences of seeking food relief; (2) Dissatisfaction with inaccessible services and inappropriate food; (3) Returning the favour—a desire for reciprocity; (4) Desiring help beyond food; and (5) "It's a social thing", the desire for social interaction and connection.

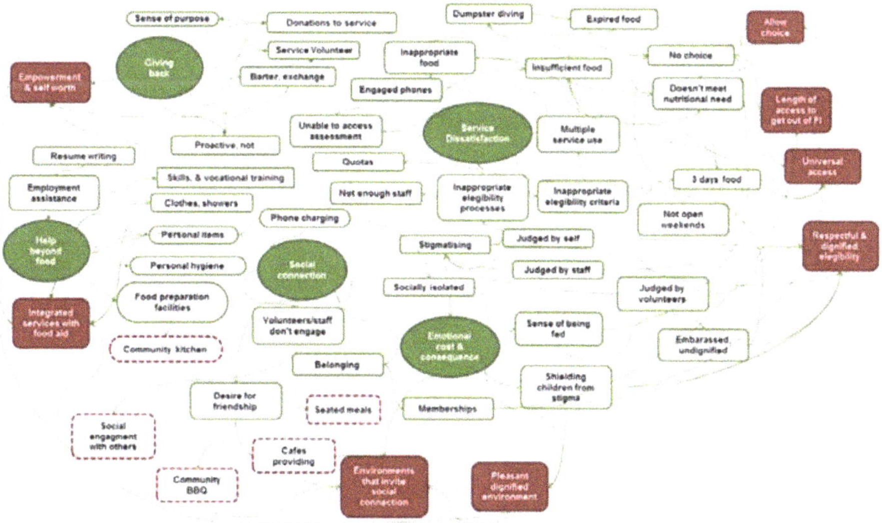

Figure 2. The thematic of food charity recipient perspectives on existing services and ideas for improvement—major themes (solid green), sub-themes (green outline), recipient recommendations (red outline), and final recommendations (solid red).

Each theme is described below.

3.1. Theme One: Emotional Cost and Consequences of Seeking Food Relief

Feelings of stigma, embarrassment, being judged or patronised as a result of many of the food service procedures or eligibility requirements. As one male said, *"I think the stigma should be the highlight I think and you shouldn't be made to feel embarrassed because, you know, you're sort of in need".*

Negative comments regarding strict eligibility criteria for food relief were made in most groups and the notion of being referred by an agency to a particular service was seen as degrading and embarrassing,

"Yeah, if you have more than two visits you've got to take all these documents and you asked all the questions 'what do you do with the money, with the pension?' They say 'I get the same. How come I can do it and you can't do it?" Male, Focus Group 1.

"See, the problem with most of those is that, like you said, you have to go to an agency where they make you feel so degraded. They're like 'how much do you earn? What do you do with that money? Why don't you have any money to buy food?' and it is embarrassing whereas here you don't have to explain yourself and the food co-op you don't have to explain yourself, you go in, buy what you want or get what you want and you walk out the door. They're not looking at you like 'oh my God what.'" Female, Focus Group 2.

Operational inefficiencies had an emotional impact on recipients, contributing to their frustration and despair, for example, constantly engaged telephone lines that limited the opportunity for appointments to assess food assistance eligibility (Focus Group 6). One female participant showed the group her mobile telephone record of 39 calls logged trying to get an assessment appointment the morning of the interview. Delays in food eligibility assessments meant no food, and participants sometimes waited without food for up to three days for an appointment.

The impact of experiencing humiliation, judgment, embarrassment, or indignity during the food assistance process had some recipients stating they would not return to specific services, *"They make me feel this small. I never went there again."* Male, Focus Group 1.

Participants wanted services that were accepting and non-judgmental, *"If I could go somewhere that did not make me feel degraded to ask for help, that'd be awesome."* Female, Focus Group 5.

Some types of food relief models were seen as less stigmatising, for example, supermarket gift cards,

"Well, the card system is okay because there's no sort of stigma, is not it? Some people feel sort of embarrassed or ashamed in entering places like these and if you go in a place like this and, you know, if a card is given to you, I mean you're free to go and buy without no sort of stigma attached because nobody knows." Male, Focus Group 2.

3.2. Theme Two: Inaccessible Services with Inappropriate Food

Food services were appreciated, but this was tempered by dissatisfaction due to problems related to food services, including: access, food types, the amount, and quality. Several participants mentioned that services were only available Monday to Friday and this made their life difficult, especially for those experiencing acute food shortages and needing emergency help.

"Yeah I think just even general –like in general, not just food or whatever, for the homeless, for the shutting down on the weekend, you know, people have crises on weekends, people have crises—you know, it is a real business structure and does not conform to business hours." Female, Focus Group 2.

Supermarket vouchers and gift cards usually had a AUD$20 value. The amount was considered meagre and, although possibly suitable to pay for an individual's food for one day, the amount was viewed as insufficient for a family,

"They [cards] are very useful but realistically what can you get out of them, $20? I have a family of eight." Female, Focus Group 4.

Some participants said that the food offered was generally poor or may have exacerbated their existing health conditions, for example, diabetes, eating disorders, irritable bowel, allergies or mental health issues.

"I'm allergic to tomatoes and things like that so literally for myself, like trying to find—something like macaroni and cheese for me would be all right but I'm not supposed to eat too much pasta because of my diabetes so I'd have to actually find a way of being able to split that into two because two nights of—that whole meal would put me in hospital because of how much gluten's in it so I'm probably queen of the fuss but I'd just still rather be healthy by what I'm eating as well." Female, Focus Group 1.

"Pies are bad for diabetics because of the pastry. Pastry is really bad." Female, Focus Group 1.

Ready-made emergency food parcels also caused concern for people with existing health conditions because participants said they may contain food they were unable to eat. Negotiating to change the parcel contents or asking for a supermarket voucher instead caused some participant to experience guilt,

" . . . if I was to say 'look, I've got food issues and the food parcel that you've just given me, I really can't eat anything out of that' I would feel really—I feel guilty getting a [supermarket voucher/ gift] card." Female, Focus Group 2.

Supermarket vouchers and food pantries were preferred over ready-made food parcels because they afforded the opportunity for individuals to choose their own food items, with the statements below being typical:

"if you've got the card (supermarket gift card), you feel free to pick up what you want . . . " Male, Focus Group 2.

I like the . . . *"Food pantry because then you get to choose it."*Female, Focus Group 1.

Some service aspects and management strategies seemed to work better for recipients,

" . . . we paid $2. You get a little card. For every dollar you spend it gets accumulated up and at a Christmas time that amount would come off a Christmas hamper that they'd do, which I thought was absolutely fantastic. Go in there if you've made anything. If you've grown veggies or fruit you could take it in there and they give back to you. Like you give them that, you can get a couple of meals." Female, Focus Group 4.

To enable individuals to better manage their food insecurity, rather than seek help from food relief agencies, one Focus Group suggested a person's entire welfare payment should be directly deposited into supermarkets. They said this would avoid the money for food not being available if individually managed,

"You give it to—whatever shopping centre you use, you give it to them, the whole cheque, and so, okay, you can spend this much every week or every fortnight. You can't spend the whole lot in one hit. That will allow people to go there when they need something for tea or breakfast or whatever. They can grab the specific items and then go home 'oh well, I can make a meal and everything now' and then tomorrow comes 'well, I need this. I need onions and I need carrots and stuff'. Go in and buy them because if you gave someone a cheque they'd just go in and blow the whole lot." Male, Focus Group 1.

3.3. Theme Three: Returning the Favour—Reciprocity

Some participants engaged with services as both volunteers and recipients of food relief. Others desired to volunteer at services; however, the degree to which both men and women wanted to reciprocate at a 'pop up' service was sometimes unable to be accommodated. One comment indicated that children had also offered to volunteer at this same service. The quotes below are illustrative,

"We have on average maybe seven requests to volunteer every week. Well we don't [take more volunteers on]—I mean we're not ungrateful but we don't need them . . . " Female, Focus Group 6.

"I volunteer and then sort of just pick some bits and pieces during my shift to take home to help out the family. I also am on a single parent pension so coming here for food relief by the volunteering . . . " Female, Focus Group 7.

For some, the volunteering at a food relief service was driven by a desire to reciprocate for the assistance they had received.

"(I was) one of the people that lined up every week and then I started volunteering and I actually like returned the favour, giving back to the community." Female, Focus, Group 5.

Duties included staffing the café, preparing and/or re-packaging food items for distribution, or chatting to people lining up. Volunteers empathised with the circumstances and feelings of those seeking food relief variously commenting,

"We're not judging them", and *"we don't hold ourselves higher than what they are. We're one of them."* Female, Focus group 5.

Potential volunteer duties at food relief services were variable with garden maintenance on the premises suggested. Others suggested donating fresh home grown produce to food relief services as an acknowledgement of previous help or using produce to barter for pre-prepared meals or other food items,

" . . . people could be working on an idea of providing food for—and people could contribute to that facility, if you know what I mean, and providing food for people on a regular basis, so people would be going there for meals and working in the garden and socialising . . . " Male, Focus Group 2.

"'oh the lemon tree is nearly ready for picking' and then they go 'oh we'll bring lemons'. You know, big boxes like this that they've walked down the street with in wheelbarrow . . . things or oranges, mandarins. If people have got trees they bring in the stuff to share back, like to say thank you to us." Female, Focus Group 5.

"Go in there if you've made anything. If you've grown veggies or fruit you could take it in there and they give back to you. Like you give them that, you can get a couple of meals." Female, Focus Group 4.

3.4. Theme Four: Help Beyond Food

Many participants described a need for help with other parts of their lives. For example, there was a need for items like nappies and toiletries, homeless people needed access to showers, laundry facilities and phone charging, domiciled people needed white goods (fridges, washing machines). Phone charging was important to keep people connected and the removal of free power points in the city mall was noted. Alternative charging stations were used including at McDonald's restaurants, suburban train carriages, some street locations, and libraries. Existing shower services were sometimes described as "hopeless" and the lack of showers in places like parklands were noted, prompting suggestions for alternative showers.

"Most people will pay . . . $20 and go to the bus terminal, give $20 over because it is a $20 deposit for the key and get the key and you can have a shower as long as you like. Then you go hand your key back and get your $20 back. That is how a lot of people get their showers . . . . And sometimes they let you put your phone [in] and go in the shower." Male, Focus Group 1.

"Can I just say something about the showers? I was talking to Orange Sky* not long ago because Orange Sky showers are going to be hopefully starting in January." Male, Focus Group 1 (Orange Sky is free of charge mobile laundry service).

Some participants wanted financial assistance and management, others were interested in support to increase the likelihood of employment such as resume development or assistance from a social worker.

" . . . you go to Centrelink and they go 'oh, it is nice if you start looking for work'—like before I had the babies—and it is like well, how do you put a resume together?" Female, Focus Group 4.

" . . . there needs to be like a social worker or someone that can be there to listen . . . " Female, Focus Group 4.

There were positive comments on the social supermarket model, centred around learning and training opportunities, which offered pathways out of poverty and a reliance on food relief.

"I really like the fact that with that one you're actually doing something as well. I just think that anything where people can learn to become better . . . . I would see it as a building and a stepping stone even more so because you get training . . . . They're the sort of things and for me that gives a person hope. That builds hope that I can get out of this position and get a bit better in life. You know, that I love." Female, Focus Group 7.

These suggestions, along with giving back, indicate a desire to gain skills and resources to seek financial independence or employment and get out of poverty.

3.5. Theme Five: "It's a Social Thing"—Desire for Social Interaction and Connection

In seeking food assistance, participants simultaneously sought meaningful social interaction and connection in a friendly atmosphere. They described how they wanted opportunities to engage with other regulars and volunteers, laugh, converse over coffee, or a meal or engage in fun activities.

"I'd rather the person that is handing the meal out, when you've finished handing the meals out sit down and talk to us, spend time with us. Don't just hand the meal out and go 'zoom' and take off and go somewhere else." Male, Focus Group 4.

"I'd rather go to [Service] because they sit down and talk and laugh and have fun and everything like that." Male, Focus Group 5.

Participants who had used food relief and who now volunteered their time registered the importance of providing social support for recipients,

"We get a lot of people that don't come here for the food; they come here because they know they can have a chat. Sometimes we're the only people in the whole entire week that they've spoken to . . . " Female, Focus group 5.

An outcome of social connection at food relief services included the development of friendships, and in one case marriage and cohabitation,

"Those people that are getting married, be it that they're elderly but they were facing nursing homes because they had no-one to look after them. They were living on their own and they met here. They've now moved in together. They don't have to move into nursing homes." Female, Focus Group 8.

4. Discussion

The aim of this study was to investigate food assistance recipients' views on both existing services in South Australia and on examples of social enterprise models. We also sought to understand how food assistance might be improved more broadly to better meet the needs of food insecure people. Five themes emerged from the discussions: (i) considerable emotional costs and consequences in receiving food assistance, (ii) dissatisfaction with inaccessible services and inappropriate food, (iii) desire to reciprocate for food assistance by volunteering at services, (iv) the need for help goes beyond food, and (v) a strong desire for social connection.

Participants desired food assistance models that afforded some of the features characteristic of social enterprise models, particularly the opportunity to exercise food choice, meet their desire for social connection and commensality, and provide access to other services such as training or skills development. Social supermarkets offer an innovative model of food assistance which could address some of these points, but are unavailable in Australia [34]. Internationally, there are a variety of novel food assistance practices that have the potential to transform incrementally and interact with other food systems to deliver pathways out of food poverty [35]. Our work suggests that recipients support the re-making of traditional food relief models as a way to support individual empowerment and pathways out of food insecurity.

The findings highlighted the power imbalances inherent in the provision of food assistance and suggests that they are deeply embedded at an operational level in existing South Australian services. The intrinsic design and delivery of charitable food assistance can be either disempowering or empowering. Forms of assistance which are empowering help vulnerable people climb out of their neediness and offers real pathways out of food insecurity. In contrast, disempowering assistance traps clients in a continuous, chronic food assistance cycle.

This study found evidence of disempowerment within traditional South Australian food charity models such as stigma or embarrassment, having to prove their eligibility, need or worthiness for assistance. Empowering options aligned more strongly with social enterprise models.

4.1. Disempowering Food Assistance

Although recipients were grateful for food assistance, there were several aspects of the system that were experienced as disempowering, which contributed to the emotional costs and consequences in receiving food relief including loss of power, similar to those described by van der Horst et al. (2014) [36]. Aspects of traditional food assistance models inadvertently impact the emotional wellbeing of recipients by fostering negative feelings such as judgment, embarrassment and stigma. The emotional consequences of having to ask for food assistance in the first place speaks to an admission of failure that one cannot provide food for oneself. This can be so overwhelming for some people that they would rather avoid seeking food assistance [36]. These findings are consistent with evidence from other wealthy industrial countries for recipients of food bank users and other types of food charities [25].

The power imbalance is also evidenced by the dissatisfaction with inaccessible and inappropriate food services, particularly recipient's inability to enforce their right to food, their freedom to choose food the food they want in socially acceptable ways, or eat in dignified settings. Riches (2018) asserts that it is "the universal right of vulnerable individuals and families to be able to feed themselves with choice and human dignity" (p. 3) [37]. Recipients were frustrated with the lack of choice in the current system and desired the dignity of being able to choose their own food, recommending models that were considered empowering and less stigmatising, such as supermarket gift cards. These finding were consistent with those of recipients in Perth, Western Australia [27].

4.2. Empowering Food Assistance

Study participants expressed a desire to receive flexible, recipient-oriented services that were empowering, encouraged independence and autonomy. They had a strong desire for giving back—that is, wanting to 'return the favour'—for example, by volunteering at services when their circumstances allowed them to. Applying Mauss's 1925 framework of gift exchange, food [charity] is this context is essentially a gift which cannot be reciprocated and may render the recipient powerless [38]. Inherent in Mauss's theory of gift giving is the obligation to reciprocate. This may explain the strong desire of participants to 'return the favour', namely, to regain a modicum of situational power by donating fruit or volunteer labour.

Recipients described the need for 'Help beyond food'. Their desire for empowerment went beyond food. Participants spoke positively of food assistance models that extended to the social purpose of tackling food insecurity and offered a viable pathway out of chronic reliance on food assistance. The current findings align with the UK's All-Party Parliamentary Group (AAPG) recommendations on the Hunger and Food Poverty inquiry into foodbanks in the UK [39]. The AAPG called for models to end food poverty which were 'sustainable' rather than offering 'subsistence' and recommended a 'food bank plus model', as described by Paget et al. (2015) [40]. The nature of the 'food plus model' included multiple services, all of which should be considered when reviewing funding to food assistance services in South Australia.

In Australia, charitable food assistance services rely on foodbanks and food rescue organisations to redistribute retail food waste. The participants in this current study, although grateful, were dissatisfied with the food provided by services, describing issues with the appropriateness and quality of food and the reliance on charity, and ultimately their inability to attain a varied and healthy diet in an autonomous way. The conversations rang true to the sentiment of 'Left over food for left over people' previously described by Dowler [41]. Participants wanted to 'fit in' and to shop at supermarkets and eat at cafes like 'normal people', and they did not want their children to know they were struggling. The findings suggest the retail sector reconsider their moral and social obligation in light of the right to food for the most vulnerable citizens residing in countries where they operate. For example, as part of their retail practice they could directly provide dignified access to appropriate food by assisting people during times of economic hardship to access their goods in socially acceptable ways.

The current study findings also highlight the acceptability of some of the aspects of social enterprise models to address food insecurity among recipients. A well-developed example of a social enterprise model to food insecurity are social supermarkets (SSMs). SSMs are a retail formula where the outlet receives free surplus food and consumer goods from partner companies and sells them at symbolic prices to people who are at risk of, or living in poverty (Holweg and Lienbaucher 2010) [34]. They may also operate as retail training grounds to assist people who are long term unemployed or disabled re-integrate into society. In doing so, SSMs provide opportunities for work and immediate positive fulfilment and feedback; they provide a wage rather than government handouts and subsidies, and they build individual confidence and resilience [42]. SSMs are widespread in continental Europe, with more than 1000 in operation in 2013 [43], but few, if any, examples exist in Australia. Despite being widespread, however, there is no available literature evaluating the effectiveness of social supermarkets.

Successful programs for food assistance and other support pathways are likely to be ones that are co-produced with recipients [39] and the current findings highlight the value in obtaining recipient reviews on current and future service options. Co-production has become synonymous with innovative approaches to service delivery and been defined as "A meeting of minds coming together to find a shared solution. It involves people who use services being consulted, included and working together from the start to the end of any project that affects them" (p.7) [44].

4.3. The Desire for Social Interaction and Connection

Participants desired meaningful social interaction and connection, recognition and acknowledgement, and friendship networks. The sense of isolation and loneliness experienced by homeless people or those living in poverty is well documented and may constitute a risk to survival [45]. Loneliness is adversely associated with physical and mental health and lifestyle factors [46]. The experience of social pain, defined as the unpleasantness that is associated with actual or potential damage to one's sense of social connection or social value (owing to social rejection, exclusion, negative social evaluation or loss) may involve an overlap of the neural circuitry underpinning physical pain (defined as the unpleasant experience that is associated with actual or potential tissue damage) [47].

High levels of concern about the consequences of loneliness experienced by all ages has prompted calls for it to be considered a public health issue [48]. The strong preference for seated shared meal services, commensality and connection with others in the current study suggest that social enterprise models integrated with cafes and restaurant dining are an option [49,50].

The study has several strengths and limitations. A strength of this study is that the 54 participants were recipients of food assistance from different geographic locations (metropolitan, regional and country areas) in South Australia. They provided a real-life perspective on the issues and potential solutions. The presentation of three novel social enterprise options to provide food assistance enabled participants to think beyond the current system; however, as there are few social enterprise options in Australia [16], they did not have an experience of using these types of services. Only three social enterprise models were presented, with very little description (one image and three to four descriptive sentences), further research is needed to identify and pilot the effectiveness of social enterprise models for food assistance in Australia.

A limitation of the current research is that it was not designed to explore options to address food insecurity other than food assistance. There are numerous social and economic policy actions that should be explored as to their effectiveness in addressing food insecurity, for example, increasing the minimum welfare payments, employment schemes or other economic options that are under the auspice of government. There was a noticeable absence of government policy and/or accountability in the food assistance system in South Australia, and indeed in Australia. Further research is needed to describe options for an integrated food assistance system that includes government, commercial sector and voluntary organisations.

The findings suggest that the retail sector may have an important role to play in addressing food insecurity, outside the current food waste redistribution paradigm. Recipient dissatisfaction with the food currently available suggests that food acquisition and distribution models need to be critically analysed for their ability to address food insecurity. Exploration of effective Corporate Social Responsibility commitments to address food insecurity that are not reliant on redistributing waste food is warranted.

5. Conclusions

Food systems, including charitable food systems, need to work for everyone, especially those who are vulnerable. This study has revealed aspects of the existing South Australian food assistance system that can be disempowering to recipients. Disempowering forms of food assistance can trap recipients in a cycle of food charity. Participants desired empowering forms of assistance that humanise the charitable food system, shift the locus of control and place power back into the hands of users. Improvement in the quality of existing food relief models, should focus on recipient-informed models (co-production) which re-dress existing power differentials. Services which are more strongly recipient-centred, strive to empower clients and provide opportunities for active involvement, social connection and broader support are needed.

Author Contributions: Conceptualisation, S.B., J.C., C.P. and I.G.-S.; Methodology, S.B., J.C., C.P. and I.G.-S.; Focus group facilitation, S.B., I.G.-S., and J.C.; Focus Group Themed Analysis, C.P.; Secondary analysis S.B., Resources, S.B., C.P.; Writing-Original Draft Preparation, S.B. and C.P.; Writing-Review & Editing, S.B., J.C., C.P. and I.G.-S.; Project Administration, I.G.-S.; Funding Acquisition, I.G.-S.

Funding: This research was funded by the South Australian Government's former Department of Communities and Social Inclusion (DCSI) (now Human services) and SA Health.

Acknowledgments: The authors would like to acknowledge the service managers, volunteers and recipients of food assistance who participated in the study.

Conflicts of Interest: The authors declare no conflict of interest. C.P. is a Board Member of Foodbank Western Australia. The other authors have no conflict of interest to declare. The funders had no role in the design of the study; in the collection, analyses, or interpretation of data; in the writing of the manuscript, and in the decision to publish the results.

References

1. United Nations. Committee on the Rights of the Child Sixtieth Session 29 May–15 June 2012. Available online: http://docstore.ohchr.org/SelfServices/FilesHandler.ashx?enc=6QkG1d%2fPPRiCAqhKb7yhsk5X2w65LgiRF%2fS3dwPS4NXPtJlvMuCI3J9Hn06KCDkN8AgEce%2bNlwRMULqb84PSl9FicZROAZolAudnAZ3CxmRZ%2fzxW2Yn8qOrVcMCd9xFL (accessed on 21 September 2018).
2. Claeys, P. The right to food: Many developments, more challenges. *Can. Food Stud.* **2015**, *2*, 60–67. [CrossRef]
3. Esping-Andersen, C. *The Three Worlds of Welfare Capitalism*; Polity Press: Cambridge, UK, 1990.
4. Pollard, C.; Begley, A.; Landrigan, T. The rise of food inequality in Australia. In *Food Poverty and Insecurity: International Food Inequalities*; Springer International: Cham, Switzerland, 2016; pp. 89–103.
5. McKee, M.; Reeves, A.; Clair, A.; Stuckler, D. Living on the edge: Precariousness and why it matters for health. *Arch. Public Health* **2017**, *75*, 13. [CrossRef] [PubMed]
6. Pollard, C.M.; Mackintosh, B.; Campbell, C.; Kerr, D.; Begley, A.; Jancey, J.; Caraher, M.; Berg, J.; Booth, S. Charitable food systems' capacity to address food insecurity: An Australian capital city audit. *Int. J. Environ. Res. Public Health* **2018**, *15*, 1249. [CrossRef] [PubMed]
7. Jericho, G. Why South Australians Are Older, Poorer and on Their Way Interstate. *The Guardian Newspaper.* 14 March 2018. Available online: https://www.theguardian.com/business/grogonomics/2018/mar/15/south-australia-dragged-down-by-demographics (accessed on 18 March 2018).
8. BankSA, Manufacturing South Australia's Future. Trends—November 2017—A Bulletin on Economic Development in South Australia. 2017. Available online: https://www.banksa.com.au/content/dam/bsa/downloads/bsa-media-trends-nov-2017.pdf (accessed on 18 September 2018).
9. Anglicare. *Improving Individual and Household Outcomes in South Australia—Discussion Paper*; Anglicare SA: Adelaide, Australia, 2017. Available online: https://dhs.sa.gov.au/__data/assets/pdf_file/0007/59812/Anglicare-SA-Response-to-Food-Security-Discussion-Paper.pdf (accessed on 18 September 2018).
10. Wingrove, K.; Barbour, L.; Palermo, C. Exploring nutrition capacity in Australia's charitable food sector. *Nutr. Diet.* **2017**, *74*, 495–501. [CrossRef] [PubMed]
11. McKay, F.; McKenzie, H. Food aid provision in metropolitan Melbourne: A mixed methods study. *J. Hunger. Environ. Nutr.* **2017**, *12*, 11–25. [CrossRef]
12. Kleve, S.; Davidson, Z.; Gearon, E.; Booth, S.; Palermo, C. Are low to middle income households experiencing food insecurity in Victoria, Australia? An examination of the Victorian Population Health Survey 2006–2009. *Aust. J. Prim. Health* **2017**, *23*, 249–256. [CrossRef] [PubMed]
13. Ramsay, R.; Giskes, K.; Turrell, G.; Gallegos, D. Food insecurity amongst adults residing in disadvantaged urban areas: Potential health and dietary consequences. *Public Health Nutr.* **2012**, *15*, 227–237. [CrossRef] [PubMed]
14. Lindberg, R. Still serving hot soup? Two hundred years of a charitable food sector in Australia: A narrative review. *Aust. N. Z. J. Public Health* **2015**, *39*, 358–365. [CrossRef] [PubMed]
15. Foodbank, W.A. Foodbank WA Annual Report 2015. Available online: https://www.foodbankwa.org.au/wp-content/blogs.dir/5/files/2015/10/Annual-Report-Final-2015_web.pdf (accessed on 14 September 2018).

16. Wills, B. Eating at the limits: Barriers to the emergence of social enterprise initiatives in the Australian emergency food relief sector. *Food Policy* **2017**, *20*, 62–70. [CrossRef]

17. Richards, C.; Kjaernes, U.; Vik, J. Food security in welfare capitalism: Comparing social entitlements to food in Australia and Norway. *J. Rural Stud.* **2016**, *43*, 61–70. [CrossRef]

18. Seligman, H.; Lyles, C.; Marshall, M.; Prendergast, K.; Smith, M.; Headings, A.; Bradshaw, G.; Rosenmoss, S.; Waxman, E. A pilot food bank intervention featuring diabetes appropriate food improved glycemic control among clients in three states. *Health Aff.* **2015**, *34*, 1956–1963. [CrossRef] [PubMed]

19. Miewald, C.; Ibanez-Carrasco, F.; Turner, S. Negotiating the local food environment: The lived experience of food access for low-income people living with HIV/AIDS. *J. Hunger. Environ. Nutr.* **2010**, *5*, 510–525. [CrossRef]

20. Hamelin, A.; Beaudry, M.; Habicht, J. Characterization of household food insecurity in Quebec: Food and feelings. *Soc. Sci. Med.* **2002**, *54*, 119–132. [CrossRef]

21. McNeill, K. Talking with Their Mouths Half Full: Food Insecurity in the Hamilton Community. Ph.D. Thesis, The University of Waikato, Hamilton, New Zealand, 2011.

22. Loopstra, R.; Tarasuk, V. The relationship between food banks and household food insecurity among low-income Toronto families. *Can. J. Public Health* **2012**, *38*, 497–514. [CrossRef]

23. Garthwaite, K. Stigma, shame and 'people like us': An ethnographic study of foodbank use in the UK. *J. Poverty Soc. Justice* **2016**, *24*, 277–289. [CrossRef]

24. Purdam, K.; Garrett, E.A.; Esmail, A. Hungry? Food insecurity, social stigma and embarrassment in the UK. *Sociology* **2016**, *50*, 1072–1088. [CrossRef]

25. Middleton, G.; Mehta, K.; McNaughton, D.; Booth, S. The experiences and perceptions of foodbank amongst users in high income countries: An international scoping review. *Appetite* **2018**, *120*, 698–708. [CrossRef] [PubMed]

26. Booth, S. Eating Rough—Food Insecurity Amongst Homeless Young People in Adelaide. Ph.D. Thesis, Flinders University, Adelaide, Australia, 2003.

27. Booth, S.; Begley, A.; Mackintosh, B.; Kerr, D.A.; Jancey, J.; Caraher, M.; Whelan, J.; Pollard, C.M. Gratitude, resignation and the desire for dignity: Lived experience of food charity recipients and their recommendations for improvement, Perth, Western Australia. *Public Health Nutr.* **2018**, *21*, 2831–2841. [CrossRef] [PubMed]

28. Middleton, G. Evaluation of a Community Food Banking Model in South Australia. Honours Thesis, Flinders University, Adelaide, Australia, 2015.

29. Teasdale, S. What's in a name? Making sense of social enterprise discourse. *Public Policy Adm.* **2011**, *27*, 99–119. [CrossRef]

30. Teasdale, S. How can social enterprise address disadvantage? Evidence from an inner city community. *J. Non-Profit Public Sect. Mark.* **2010**, *22*, 89–107. [CrossRef]

31. Shaw, E.; Carter, S. Social entrepreneurship: Theoretical antecedents and empiricle analysis of entrepreneurial processes and outcomes. *J. Small Bus. Enterp. Dev.* **2007**, *14*, 418–434. [CrossRef]

32. Sharir, M.; Lerner, M.; Yitshaki, R. Long term survivability of social ventures: Qualitative analysis of external and internal explainations. In *International Perspectives of Social Entrepreneurship*; Robinson, J., Mair, J., Hockerts, K., Eds.; Palgrave Macmillan: Basingstoke, UK, 2009.

33. Henninck, M.; Hutter, I.; Bailey, A. *Qualitative Reseach Methods*; Sage Publications: Thousand Oaks, CA, USA, 2011.

34. Holweg, C.; Lienbacher, E.; Zinn, W. Social supermarkets-a new challenge in supply chain management and sustainability. *Supply Chain Forum* **2010**, *11*, 50–58. [CrossRef]

35. Hebinck, A.; Galli, F.; Arcuri, S.; Carroll, B.; O'connor, D.; Oostindie, H. Capturing change in european food assistance practices: A transformative social innovation perspective. *Local Environ.* **2018**, *23*, 398–413. [CrossRef]

36. van der Horst, H.; Pascucci, S.; Bol, W. The "dark side" of food banks? Exploring emotional responses of food bank receivers in the netherlands. *Br. Food J.* **2014**, *116*, 1506–1520. [CrossRef]

37. Riches, G. *Food Bank Nations. Poverty, Corporate Charity and the Right to Food*; Routledge: New York, NY, USA, 2018.

38. Mauss, M.T. *The Gift: The Form and Reason for Exchange in Archaic Societies*; Routledge Classics: London, UK, 1990.

39. All-Party Parliamentary Group on Hunger and Food Poverty. *Feeding Britain: A Strategy for Zero Hunger in England, Wales, Scotland and Northern Ireland, the Report of the All-Party Parliamentary Inquiry into Hunger in the United Kingdom*; Children's Society: London, UK, 2014.

40. Paget, A. *Community Supermarkets Could Offer a Sustainable Solution to Food Poverty*; Demos: London, UK, 2015.

41. Caraher, M.; Furey, S. *The Economics of Emergency Food Aid Provision: A Financial, Social and Cultural Perspective*; Springer International: Cham, Switzerland, 2018.

42. Schneider, F. The evolution of food donation with respect to waste prevention. *Waste Manag.* **2013**, *33*, 755–763. [CrossRef] [PubMed]

43. Cocozza, P. 'If I Shop Here I've Got Money for Gas': Inside the UK's First Social Supermarket. Available online: http://www.theguardian.com/society/2013/dec/09/inside-britains-first-social-supermarket-goldthorpe-yorkshire (accessed on 5 August 2018).

44. Council of the Ageing. The Voice of Consumers in Home Care: A Practical Guide. 2014. Available online: https://www.cota.org.au/publication/the-voice-consumers-in-home-care-guide/ (accessed on 14 September 2018).

45. Pantell, M.; Rehkopf, D.; Jutte, D.; Syme, S.L.; Balmes, J.; Adler, N. Social isolation: A predictor of mortality comparable to traditional clinical risk factors. *Am. J. Public Health* **2013**, *103*, 2056–2062. [CrossRef] [PubMed]

46. Richards, A.; Rohrmann, S.; Vandeleur, C.L.; Schmid, M.; Barth, J.; Eichholzer, M. Loneliness is adversely associated with physical and mental health and lifestyle factors: Results from a Swiss national survey. *PLoS ONE* **2017**, *12*, e0181442. [CrossRef] [PubMed]

47. Eisenberger, N. The pain of social disconnection: Examing the shared neural underpinnings of physical and social pain. *Nat. Rev. Neurosci.* **2012**, *13*, 421–434. [CrossRef] [PubMed]

48. Matthews, T.; Danese, A.; Caspi, A.; Fisher, H.L.; Goldman-Mellor, S.; Kepa, A.; Moffitt, T.E.; Odgers, C.L.; Arseneault, L. Lonely young adults in modern Britain: Findings from an epidemiological cohort study. *Psychol. Med.* **2018**, *1*. [CrossRef] [PubMed]

49. Lambie-Mumford, H.; Dowler, E. Hunger, food charity and social policy–challenges faced by the emerging evidence base. *Soc. Policy Soc.* **2015**, *14*, 497–506. [CrossRef]

50. Linares, E. Food services for the homeless in Spain: Caritas programme for the homeless. *Public Health Nutr.* **2001**, *4*, 1367–1369. [PubMed]

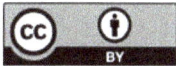

International Journal of
Environmental Research and Public Health

MDPI

Article

Healthy Choice Rewards: A Feasibility Trial of Incentives to Influence Consumer Food Choices in a Remote Australian Aboriginal Community

Clare Brown [1,*], Cara Laws [1], Dympna Leonard [2], Sandy Campbell [3], Lea Merone [1], Melinda Hammond [1], Kani Thompson [1], Karla Canuto [1,4] and Julie Brimblecombe [5]

[1] Apunipima Cape York Health Council, 4870 Cairns, Australia; cara.laws@apunipima.org.au (C.L.); lea.merone@apunipima.org.au (L.M.); melinda.hammond@apunipima.org.au (M.H.); kani.thompson@apunipima.org.au (K.T.); karla.canuto@jcu.edu.au (K.C.)
[2] Australian Institute of Tropical Health and Medicine, College of Public Health Medical and Veterinary Sciences, James Cook University, 4870 Cairns, Australia; dympna.leonard@jcu.edu.au
[3] Centre for Indigenous Health Equity Research, Central Queensland University, 4870 Cairns, Australia; s.campbell@cqu.edu.au
[4] Wardliparingga Aboriginal Health, South Australian Health and Medical Research Institute, 5001 Adelaide, Australia
[5] Department of Nutrition, Dietetics and Food, Monash University, 3168 Melbourne, Australia; julie.brimblecombe@monash.edu
* Correspondence: clare.brown@apunipima.org.au; Tel.: +7-4037-7483

Received: 16 November 2018; Accepted: 28 December 2018; Published: 3 January 2019

Abstract: Poor diet including inadequate fruit and vegetable consumption is a major contributor to the global burden of disease. Aboriginal and Torres Strait Islander Australians experience a disproportionate level of preventable chronic disease and successful strategies to support Aboriginal and Torres Strait Islander people living in remote areas to consume more fruit and vegetables can help address health disadvantage. Healthy Choice Rewards was a mixed methods study to investigate the feasibility of a monetary incentive: store vouchers, to promote fruit and vegetable purchasing in a remote Australian Aboriginal community. Multiple challenges were identified in implementation, including limited nutrition workforce. Challenges related to the community store included frequent store closures and amended trading times, staffing issues and poor infrastructure to support fruit and vegetable promotion. No statistically significant increases in fruit or vegetable purchases were observed in the short time frame of this study. Despite this, community members reported high acceptability of the program, especially for women with children. Optimal implementation including, sufficient time and funding resources, with consideration of the most vulnerable could go some way to addressing inequities in food affordability for remote community residents.

Keywords: Aboriginal and Torres Strait Islander; remote; community store; fruit and vegetables; incentive; subsidy; food security; nutrition; diet

1. Introduction

Food security is a major global issue [1]. Strategies to achieve physical and economic access to sufficient, safe and nutritious food are important for all and this is especially important for Indigenous Peoples who often experience the most severe economic and health disparities [2]. Australia is a wealthy country but high levels of food insecurity have been documented for Aboriginal and Torres Strait Islander people compared to other Australians (22% versus. 3.7%) [3]. In Australia, food insecurity is highest among Aboriginal and Torres Strait Islander people living in remote locations (31%) compared to non-remote (20%) [3].

The life expectancy gap of 10–11 years between Aboriginal and Torres Strait Islander people and non-Indigenous Australians is well known [4]. Recent national survey reports indicate that Aboriginal and Torres Strait Islander people consume a diet that is relatively poor compared to other Australians, with lower intakes of fruit and vegetables and higher intakes of sugar sweetened beverages and nutritionally poor foods [3]. Chronic diseases, much of which are diet-related were responsible for 70% of the gap in health between Aboriginal and Torres Strait Islanders and non-Indigenous Australians in 2011 [5]. Contributing to this are the higher rates of overweight and obesity, cardiovascular disease, chronic kidney disease and type two diabetes [4].

Many factors influence the nutritional status of Aboriginal and Torres Strait islander people, including socioeconomic disadvantage and other historical, social, environmental and geographical factors [6–8]. Healthy foods in remote Aboriginal and Torres Strait Islander communities cost more than urban areas [9–11]. The 2016 Census shows the median household weekly income in the remote region of interest is AUD $987 for a mean household size of 3.8 people [12]. This is 70% of the median state of Queensland household income of AUD $1402 per week with a lower average household size of 2.6 people [12]. On this lower income, remote area residents in Queensland pay 41% more for fruit and 12% more for vegetables compared with Queenslanders living in urban areas [9]. Research has shown that when food choices are made under budget constraints, consumer purchasing behaviour is driven by maximising energy value for money (dollars per megajoule), resulting in the purchase of fewer nutrient rich foods such as fruit and vegetables and more nutrient poor, energy dense foods [13,14].

There is a well-established link between increased fruit and vegetable consumption and improved health outcomes [15]; consequently, increasing consumption of fruit and vegetables has been identified as an important measure to achieve health gains nationally [16]. In addition to improved health, it has been estimated that if vegetable consumption in Australia was 10% higher, government expenditure on health care could be reduced by AUD $100 million annually [17]. If all Australians met the recommended daily intake of vegetables this saving would increase nine fold [17]. The potential savings are likely to be more pronounced for Aboriginal and Torres Strait Islander people living in remote areas due to the higher burden of disease experienced and the high costs of delivering remote health services.

In the context of increasing health care costs and government budget cuts threatening progress in the prevention of chronic disease [18], it is important to investigate cost effective measures to address health disadvantage for Aboriginal and Torres Strait Islander people living in remote communities and provide clear recommendations for policy makers. There is a growing body of research demonstrating the potential for food price changes to influence diet quality and drive positive population health gains [19–24]. Government policy options in pricing strategies include unhealthy food taxation, healthy food subsidies and price discount schemes to promote healthy food environments [25,26]. In Australia, two large supermarket price discount randomised controlled trials have recently been completed, both showing the effectiveness of price discounts on fruit and vegetable purchasing [22,23]. One of these projects, the Stores Healthy Options at Remote Indigenous Communities (SHOP@RIC) was implemented in 20 remote communities in Northern Territory and achieved a 12.7% increase in purchases of fruit and vegetables [22].

Strategies to make fruit and vegetables more accessible to Aboriginal and Torres Strait Islander families living in remote communities have the potential to reduce health inequality and subsequent health care costs. Here we report on a feasibility trial of a monetary incentive to promote fruit and vegetable purchasing in one remote community. To our knowledge, the effectiveness of immediately rewarding healthy purchasing behaviours has not yet been explored in a remote Aboriginal and Torres Strait Islander community context.

2. Materials and Methods

2.1. Setting

Apunipima Cape York Health Council (Apunipima) community nutrition project staff conducted a study in 2015 to assess the feasibility of implementing a fruit and vegetable incentive in a very remote Australian community store in far north Queensland, located around 2500 km from the nearest major city. This remote community has approximately 1400 residents with most (90.4%) identifying as Aboriginal and/or Torres Strait Islander [27]. The community experiences low levels of formal education, low income, reliance on social security payments and high dependency ratios [27]. While the people of this community value traditional foods and traditional food systems, the community store is the main source of food for residents for their daily needs. The next nearest grocery store is 200 km away; a three hour drive by dirt road.

2.2. Design

A mixed methods approach was used and included collection of qualitative data using semi-structured interviews, participant observation, a weekly electronic survey on store and wider community contextual information and a quantitative assessment of store sales data. Feasibility of the intervention was assessed in terms of acceptability, voucher uptake, implementation issues and impact on fruit and vegetable sales. All customers of the store were eligible to participate. Study implementation was led by Apunipima community nutrition staff.

2.3. Healthy Choice Rewards Program

The Healthy Choice Rewards (HCR) program offered community store customers an incentive of a fruit and vegetable voucher to the value of AUD $10 each time a set minimum amount was spent on fruit and vegetables. Store staff participated in semi-structured interviews prior to the study to inform the reward system design and determine what supports would need to be in place for implementation. Two phases of the minimal amount spent were trialed: phase one required a AUD $20 spend on fresh fruit and vegetables to receive a AUD $10 HCR voucher to be redeemed on the date of purchase; phase two required a AUD $15 spend on fresh fruit and vegetables to receive a AUD $10 HCR voucher to be redeemed within three days. Frozen, tinned and dried fruit and vegetables were not included as part of the minimum spend as they could not be easily distinguished in the store's electronic grocery management system. The vouchers were redeemable for fresh, frozen, tinned or dried fruit and vegetables and excluded tinned fruit in syrup and frozen potato chips and wedges. Vegetable packs valued at AUD $10 were available for sale. The store was reimbursed for the value of any vouchers used.

The incentive was available for 32 weeks; phase one ran for 15 weeks, followed immediately by phase two for 17 weeks. The HCR vouchers appeared as black and white plain text print outs at the end of customer store dockets. The reward offer was promoted in English and local language using posters, flyers, radio advertisements and electronic register screen displays at the store.

Project staff visited the community monthly during the intervention period to promote HCR. During the visits they delivered healthy cooking demonstrations, distributed healthy recipe flyers, spoke with community members on how to utilise the offer and assisted store staff in merchandising the fruit and vegetable display. Between visits the project team provided weekly phone and email support to the store manager to maintain program promotion and assist with processing the vouchers.

2.4. Data Collection

To determine the feasibility of the HCR program the primary outcome measures included: acceptability of the voucher incentive to customers and store staff, voucher uptake and redemption and identification of the opportunities and challenges of implementation. A secondary measure included per capita total fruit and vegetable intake derived from store sales purchasing data.

2.4.1. Acceptability

Following completion of both phases of the intervention, we invited store staff and store customers (community members) to provide feedback through semi-structured face-to-face interviews (customer or staff satisfaction interviews). Demographics on age, gender, Aboriginal and Torres Strait Islander status, and employment were collected. Project staff (one of whom is a Torres Strait Islander woman) with training and experience interviewing Aboriginal and Torres Strait Islander community members conducted the interviews. To promote the feedback opportunities to the community, the team engaged in local activities including performing a healthy cooking demonstration and organising a group fishing trip with a healthy lunch. All customer and store staff interviewees ($n = 34$) received a fruit and vegetable voucher to the value of AUD $10 to acknowledge their time contributed. In addition to the customer satisfaction interviews conducted at the completion of the program, four customer interviews were conducted during phase one to inform intervention changes for phase two.

2.4.2. Voucher Uptake

Weekly HCR voucher redemption data were collected using the stores' electronic point of sale system.

2.4.3. Implementation

Interview data was also used to assess implementation issues. Project staff also routinely recorded observational data with hand written notes on their regular community visits.

2.4.4. Fruit and Vegetable Sales

Electronic point-of sale data including product description, unit weight, number of units sold, and dollar value were collected weekly for all food and drink sales for the duration of the project period and the same time-period in the previous year. A purpose built weekly electronic survey used in the SHOP@RIC trial [22] collected descriptive data from the store manager on potential factors influencing usual food and drink purchasing such as population movements, community events and activities, frequency of food delivery to the store and retail management practices. This data collection aimed to contextualise store sales data and account for community-level factors that may have influenced purchasing behaviours during the intervention.

2.5. Data Analysis

2.5.1. Acceptability and Implementation

Interview data and project observations were collated in Excel. Two project staff members independently coded interview responses and grouped these into emerging themes. Apunipima staff members who had research experience reviewed the coding results and resolved inconsistencies by consensus.

2.5.2. Voucher Uptake

To evaluate HCR voucher uptake, we compared the number of vouchers issued and number of vouchers redeemed across both program phases.

2.5.3. Fruit and Vegetable Sales

A pre-post point-of-sale analysis of purchasing was completed by Menzies School of Health Research in January 2016. Weekly point-of-sale data were uploaded to a purpose-built Microsoft Access database and coded into relevant food groups. Aggregated weekly point-of-sale data for the 32 week study period were compared to the same time-period in the previous year, to account for seasonal variation. Per capita daily fruit and vegetable consumption for the community was estimated by dividing the average sales for the study period by 32 weeks $\times$ 7 days and the usual population estimates obtained from 2011 Australian Bureau of Statistics national census data. The average per capita daily amounts of fruit and vegetables purchased were converted from weights measured in grams to average number of serves using Australian Dietary Guideline definitions for standard fruit and vegetable weights (i.e., 150 g per serve for fruit and 75 g per serve for vegetables) [16]. Statistical analysis was performed using the paired t-test technique to compare sales in phase 1 and phase 2 with the baseline time-periods in the previous year. p Values of less than 0.05 were considered statistically significant. Contextual factors were uploaded into an Access Database and frequency of occurrence was graphed on a weekly timescale and considered against the results reported from the purchase data to identify potential variables impacting store sales and to assist interpretation of the impact of the incentive on the outcome measures.

2.6. Ethical Approval

James Cook University Human Research Ethics Committee (HREC H5938) and the combined Northern Territory Department of Health and Menzies School of Health research Human Research Ethics Committee (HREC 2014-2313) granted ethical approval for the study.

3. Results

3.1. Acceptability

A total of 28 post program customer satisfaction interviews were completed. The majority of customers interviewed identified as Aboriginal and/or Torres Strait Islander people (82.1%) and were women (71.4%). Additionally, 68% of responders reported being employed at the time of the interview. Of those interviewed, more women that were employed than not employed reported using the HCR voucher. All respondents reported they would like the offer to continue and 61% of respondents indicated that HCR encouraged their family to consume more fruit and vegetables. All store staff interviewed following the completion of the project ($n = 6$) reported they wanted the offer to occur again. Community members identified that healthy eating was important for health but there were many challenges and competing priorities to eat a healthy and nutritious diet. They also provided suggestions for improving the program.

3.1.1. Community Perceptions of Healthy Eating

Healthy eating was viewed as important for participants and HCR was seen as a valuable program as it promoted healthy food choices, as one grandmother said, "It's important, it is very important. Kids need to eat healthy. We don't want to see our kids wither away, we want them to have a healthy choice"

The HCR program was also seen as a good reminder to consume fruit and vegetables, "Like you remind kids, 'don't do that', it's good to remind us Aboriginal people to eat more fruits and vegetables because sometimes we forget" [Female Elder].

Healthy eating was seen as especially important for women with children or young families, as one female participant responded, "Being healthy is especially important for kids to grow strong, good clean blood for [to prevent] anaemia . . . [it is] good for people with plenty of children, good for their health".

3.1.2. Challenges and Competing Priorities to Consume a Healthy Diet

Community members described facing many challenges to healthy eating including high food costs and limited available money to spend on healthy food, as one participant described, "It's expensive here, there is hardly enough money to buy food".

Although the HCR program was valued and seen to encourage fruit and vegetable consumption, it was not enough to alleviate the high cost of food as one respondent indicated, "It was really good. It encourages people to get more fruit and vegetables. AUD $10 doesn't get you much, but it's good".

While another participant reported, "AUD $10 only gets you two or three fruit and vegetables because of costings of the shop".

Other reported challenges to consuming healthy eating included limited access to health hardware such as no fridge to store food at home, limited availability of fresh produce and concerns over quality of this produce by the time it arrives in the community. It was also noted that community members have increasing dependency on takeaway foods rather than preparing homemade meals. Another concern was that children are now preferring the taste of sweet discretionary foods from the store rather than traditional bush foods.

Some responders also reported that healthy eating was not a priority for everyone, for example there may be other competing priorities based on social factors that are viewed as more important or there may be basic challenges such as the inability to shop for groceries. This was particularly thought to be the case for people with little money, those who did not live at one fixed address (living between multiple houses), those relying on meals provided by family (such as the frail elderly) and even people who struggled with addictions such as alcohol, drugs or gambling.

3.1.3. Suggestions for Improving the HCR Program

Feedback from the customer interviews suggested that future incentives may be more effective if the reward system was tailored specifically for women with children and used electronic store loyalty cards instead of paper-based vouchers. Other recommendations from the interviews included: increased flexibility of redemption parameters, more support from store staff (such as explaining the voucher and helping determine AUD $10 worth of fruit and vegetables so it is more convenient for the customer), offering higher incentives and strengthening promotion through increased community involvement. Store staff observed an increase in customer interest in HCR following promotion by the visiting nutrition team and noted that customers reported that uptake of the incentive could have been be improved with greater promotion.

3.2. Voucher Uptake

Voucher redemption rates averaged 28.6% (95% CI: 26, 31) for the duration of the study. A total of 2150 vouchers were issued and 632 redeemed. Redemption rates were higher during phase two of the study compared to phase one, averaging 30% (95% CI: 30, 31) and 27% (95% CI: 21, 32) respectively. The highest redemption rate (44%) was recorded on a week when project staff were at the store performing cooking demonstrations raising awareness about the project and assisting with merchandising of fresh produce.

3.3. Implementation

Four of the six staff interviewed reported having issues with the reward offer and required more support to run the offer. Issues identified by store staff included: being unsure of how to process the voucher in the store electronic grocery management system; having too many customers at once to help other customers claim their voucher; limited time to prepare the AUD $10 fruit and vegetable packs for customers to redeem; customers complaining of losing their receipts and customers refusing the voucher as it meant they needed to queue up a second time to redeem their reward.

Several challenges that impacted on project implementation at the store level were observed by project staff including store infrastructure issues; support for store staff to run the offer; and support for store managers to promote fresh produce. Fresh produce displays were impacted by transport issues; infrastructure issues, such as limited equipment to display produce; the hot climate affecting the temperature control of open display refrigeration units; and store air-conditioning and refrigeration units often breaking down. Supporting store staff proved challenging due to a shortage of trained and experienced staff; high turnover and low attendance among store staff; variable expertise among store management in merchandising of fresh produce and limited capacity of Community and Store Nutritionists to provide sufficient support to store staff. In addition, due to issues impacting the community during the study period such as community unrest, forced store closures and amended trading hours were reported on 23 out of 32 weeks.

Implementation of the project was strengthened by the existing rapport of project staff with community and regular presence in the community; strong partnerships with industry and the research sector; and support from community, local Council and the Store Group to implement the project.

3.4. Fruit and Vegetable Sales

The voucher incentive was not successful in increasing fruit and vegetable store sales during the study period compared to sales for the same time period in the previous year. In fact, despite including voucher purchases, a 7% reduction in total fruit sales was observed between the two periods, decreasing from 41 to 38 g/person/day (0.27 to 0.25 serves/person/per day), $p = 0.01$. Non-significant reductions in sales of vegetables and overall food and drink sales were also observed.

4. Discussion

This feasibility study describes a monetary incentive strategy to promote fruit and vegetable consumption in a remote Aboriginal community in Australia. While we were unsuccessful in increasing fruit and vegetable purchases during the intervention period, qualitative data indicates that there was a high level of acceptability of the program by community members. This study also highlights the many challenges to be considered in implementing food subsidy strategies to improve nutritional health in the remote community context.

The HCR project was completed in 2015 as part of implementing a key objective of the Cape York Food and Nutrition Strategy—to ensure equitable food affordability, availability and access comparable to urban Australia [28]. This project therefore works towards addressing the high costs of nutritious foods in remote Aboriginal and Torres Strait Islander communities; a known barrier to healthy eating.

Although the project staff made frequent trips to the community, store staff and management identified the need for more support. Furthermore, interview data suggested that voucher uptake could have been improved with strengthened promotion. These findings are consistent with other studies demonstrating that consumers need to be made aware of promotional offers [29]. Limited funding for this project and limited community nutrition workforce on the ground restricted promotion efforts. Sufficient resource allocation for promotion and nutrition workforce should be prioritised in future programs. Additionally, interview data indicated that the paper-based voucher system was not always well understood by customers and was reported to be a barrier to participation and could have therefore influenced voucher uptake. An electronic store loyalty card system was recommended by stakeholders as a preferred alternative. This option was explored in the early phases of study, however, the cost of implementing the system with such limited funding was prohibitive but should be considered in any future interventions.

Women who were employed were most likely to report using the HCR in customer satisfaction interviews. Qualitative data indicated that healthy eating was considered by community members to be more of a priority for women with children or young families. Given that improving access to nutritious food for at-risk mothers, infants and children is a key priority of the 2013–2023 National Aboriginal and Torres Strait Islander Health Plan [30], these findings warrant further investigation. If a reward incentive or subsidy were to be targeted towards smaller population subgroups such as women with children, an individual or household level measure of food and drink purchasing would be needed rather than store population level purchasing data.

This study provided information of fruit and vegetable consumption data for this community which differ from other information sources. Average fruit and vegetables sales were estimated to be equivalent to 0.25 serves/person/day for fruit and 0.92 serves/person/day for vegetables during the study period. These results are lower than self-reported data from the 2012–2013 National Aboriginal and Torres Strait Islander Nutrition and Physical Activity Survey (NATSINPAS) which reported

Aboriginal and Torres Strait Islander people living in remote areas across Australia consume on average 0.9 serves of fruit and 1.7 serves of vegetables per day [31]. The NATSINPAS combines results from remote and very remote areas and includes fruit and vegetable components from mixed food sources (such as lasagna), which will likely result in a higher reported intake [31]. While observed differences may also be the result of the different methodology used, a recent comparison of dietary estimates from the very remote sample of the NATSINPAS to food and beverage purchase data from 20 remote Northern Territory community stores suggests over-reporting of fruit and vegetable consumption with self-reporting data [32]. A strength of using sales data is that in a very remote community where there is only one food retail store it provides an objective proxy of population diet [32,33]. For this study, the closest alternative food retail store is 200 km away from the community. Our results are more consistent with a Northern Territory study which reported an average of 0.3–0.7 serves of fruit and 1.1–2.1 serves of vegetables sold per person per day across three remote Aboriginal communities [34].

The limitations of this study are that it was conducted in one remote community only and for a short time period, with limited staffing. These factors reflect the currently limited resources available for nutrition promotion in this setting, compared to previous investments [35]. With additional resources, more support could be provided to the store for implementation, and other factors contributing to the low uptake of the vouchers and reductions on sales of fruit and vegetables could be clarified and addressed. It is likely however that the issues impacting the community at the time which resulted in a high number of forced store closures and amended trading hours influenced voucher uptake and purchases of fruit and vegetables. A strength of HCR was that the voucher incentive was well received by community members and the majority of participants in the evaluation indicated that it helped their family to consume more fruit and vegetables. It was particularly seen as important for mothers with children who needed fruit and vegetables for a healthy start in life.

Another strength of this project was the strong partnerships and relationships formed by the project team with the community, particularly with the local community store as HCR was supported by store managers, staff and at management levels of the store group. Store Managers play an important role in food supply in remote Aboriginal and Torres Strait Islander communities and are therefore essential partners in helping to improve dietary intake [36]. This project illustrates how the store managers can be effectively supported by nutritionists to actively promote the incentive, resulting in increased uptake.

Remote community stores have an important influence on community health through their ability to control the availability and accessibility of both healthy and unhealthy foods [36]. Significant store implementation challenges were observed in this study. This highlighted the difficulties remote retailers face in maintaining normal store operations, in addition to the ability to adequately support health promotion efforts. Investing in assistance for remote retailers to provide healthy foods to communities is critical to the success of any efforts to improve fruit and vegetable purchase and consumption in remote Aboriginal and Torres Strait Islander communities.

5. Conclusions

This mixed methods feasibility study showed high levels of acceptability of the program by community. It also resulted in the identification of several challenges to be considered when implementing a food subsidy strategy or incentive in remote Australia. Investing in remote retailers to overcome the challenges in providing healthy foods is critical to the success of any efforts to improve fruit and vegetable consumption in remote Aboriginal and Torres Strait Islander communities. Additionally, increased investment in a nutrition prevention workforce to implement healthy remote store practices and support retailers to promote nutrition is required.

Feedback from customer interviews suggested that future incentives may be more effective if the reward program was tailored specifically for women with children. A larger scale controlled study targeting women and children may provide greater insight into the use and appropriateness of a fruit and vegetable subsidy in the remote community context.

Consumer food subsidy schemes can help overcome financial barriers and increase affordability of healthy food and drink in remote areas. The high rates of food insecurity in remote Aboriginal and Torres Strait Islander communities are largely a consequence of high rates of unemployment and low incomes compounded by high food costs. Government commitment is needed to reduce the underlying social inequality and to address the affordability of healthy food choices to help close the gap in Aboriginal and Torres Strait Islander health.

Author Contributions: Conceptualization, M.H., C.L., D.L., J.B. and C.B.; Methodology, J.B., C.L., M.H, K.T. and C.B.; Formal Analysis, J.B.; Project administration, C.L.; Supervision, J.B.; Writing-Original Draft Preparation, C.B. and C.L., Writing-Review & Editing, C.B., L.M., C.L., M.H., S.C., J.B., K.C., K.T. and D.L.

Funding: This research received no external funding.

Acknowledgments: The authors sincerely thank the store staff and store group, Aboriginal Shire Council members, and community members involved in this study. The authors also thank Susan Jacups and Yvonne Cadet-James who contributed to the development of the paper and Jemma McCutcheon for reviewing the final draft.

Conflicts of Interest: The authors declare no conflict of interest.

References

1. FAO; IFAD; UNICEF; WFP; WHO. The State of Food Security and Nutrition in the World 2018. Building Climate Resilience for Food Security and Nutrition. Available online: http://www.who.int/nutrition/publications/foodsecurity/state-food-security-nutrition-2018-en.pdf?ua=1 (accessed on 20 October 2018).

2. Kuhnlein, H.; Erasmus, B.; Spigelski, D.; Burlingame, B. Indigenous People's Food Systems and Wellbeing: Interventions and Policies for Healthy Communities Food and Agriculture Organization of the United Nations. Available online: http://www.fao.org/docrep/018/i3144e/i3144e.pdf (accessed on 20 October 2018).

3. Australian Bureau of Statistics. Australian Aboriginal and Torres Strait Islander Health Survey: Nutrition Results- Food and Nutrients, 2012-13 Cat No. 4727.0.55.005. Available online: http://www.ausstats.abs.gov.au/ausstats/subscriber.nsf/0/5D4F0DFD2DC65D9ECA257E0D000ED78F/$File/4727.0.55.005%20australian%20aboriginal%20and%20torres%20strait%20islander%20health%20survey,%20nutrition%20results%20%20-%20food%20and%20nutrients%20.pdf (accessed on 20 October 2018).

4. Australian Institute of Health and Welfare. Australia's Health 2018 Cat No. AUS 221. Available online: https://www.aihw.gov.au/getmedia/7c42913d-295f-4bc9-9c24-4e44eff4a04a/aihw-aus-221.pdf.aspx?inline=true (accessed on 20 October 2018).

5. Australian Institute of Health and Welfare. *Australian Burden of Disease Study: Impact and Causes of Illness and Death in Aboriginal and Torres Strait Islander People 2011*; AIHW: Canberra, Australia, 2016.

6. Lee, A.; Ride, K. *Review of Nutrition among Aboriginal and Torres Strait Islander People*; Australian Indigenous HealthInfoNet: Perth, Australia, 2018.

7. Brimblecombe, J.; Maypilama, E.; Colles, S.; Scarlett, M.; Dhurrkay, J.G.; Ritchie, J.; O'Dea, K. Factors Influencing Food Choice in an Australian Aboriginal Community. *Qual. Health Res.* **2014**, *24*, 387–400. [CrossRef] [PubMed]

8. Lee, A.J. The Transition of Australian Aboriginal Diet and Nutritional Health. *World Rev. Nutr. Diet.* **1996**, *79*, 1–52. [PubMed]

9. Queensland Health. Healthy Food Access Basket. Available online: https://www.health.qld.gov.au/research-reports/reports/public-health/food-nutrition/access (accessed on 15 October 2018).

10. Department of Health. *Northern Territory Market Basket Survey 2016*; Northern Territory Government of Australia: Darwin, Australia, 2017.

11. Pollard, C.; Savage, V.; Landrigan, T.; Hanbury, A.; Kerr, D. *Food Access and Cost Survey 2013 Report*; Department of Health: Perth, Australia, 2015.

12. Australia Bureau of Statistics. 2016 Census QuickStats. Available online: http://quickstats.censusdata.abs.gov.au/census_services/getproduct/census/2016/quickstat/IREG303 (accessed on 1 November 2018).

13. Brimblecombe, J.; O'Dea, K. The role of energy cost in food choices for an Aboriginal population in northern Australia. *Med. J. Aust.* **2009**, *190*, 549–551. [PubMed]

14. Drewnowski, A.; Darmon, N. Food choices and diet costs: An economic analysis. *J. Nutr.* **2005**, *135*, 900–904. [CrossRef] [PubMed]

15. World Health Organization. Increasing Fruit and Vegetable Consumption to Reduce the Risk of Noncommunicable Diseases. Available online: https://www.who.int/elena/titles/fruit_vegetables_ncds/en/ (accessed on 1 November 2018).

16. National Health and Medical Research Council. *Australian Dietary Guidelines*; National Health and Medical Research Council: Canberra, Australia, 2013.

17. Deloitte Access Economics. *The Impact of Increasing Vegetable Consumption on Health Expenditure*; Deloitte Access Economics: Canberra, Australia, 2016.

18. Wilson, A. Budget cuts risk halting Australia's progress in preventing chronic disease: Investing in prevention is essential to our nation's long term productivity. *Med. J. Aust.* **2014**, *200*, 558–589. [CrossRef] [PubMed]

19. Thow, A.M.; Jan, S.; Leeder, S.; Swinburn, B. The effect of fiscal policy on diet, obesity and chronic disease: A systematic review. *Bull. World Health Organ.* **2010**, *88*, 609–614. [CrossRef] [PubMed]

20. Thow, A.M.; Downs, S.; Jan, S. A systematic review of the effectiveness of food taxes and subsidies to improve diets: Understanding the recent evidence. *Nutr. Rev.* **2014**, *72*, 551–565. [CrossRef] [PubMed]

21. An, R. Effectiveness of subsidies in promoting healthy food purchases and consumption: A review of field experiments. *Public Health Nutr.* **2013**, *16*, 1215–1228. [CrossRef] [PubMed]

22. Brimblecombe, J.; Ferguson, M.; Chatfield, M.D.; Liberato, S.C.; Gunther, A.; Ball, K.; Moodie, M.; Miles, E.; Magnus, A.; Mhurchu, C.N.; et al. Effect of a price discount and consumer education strategy on food and beverage purchases in remote Indigenous Australia: A stepped-wedge randomised controlled trial. *Lancet Public Health* **2017**, *2*, e82–e95. [CrossRef]

23. Ball, K.; McNaughton, S.A.; Le, H.N.; Gold, L.; Ni Mhurchu, C.; Abbott, G.; Pollard, C.; Crawford, D. Influence of price discounts and skill-building strategies on purchase and consumption of healthy food and beverages: Outcomes of the Supermarket Healthy Eating for Life randomized controlled trial. *Am. J. Clin. Nutr.* **2015**, *101*, 1055–1064. [CrossRef] [PubMed]

24. Black, A.P.; Vally, H.; Morris, P.S.; Daniel, M.; Esterman, A.J.; Smith, F.E.; O'Dea, K. Health outcomes of a subsidised fruit and vegetable program for Aboriginal children in northern New South Wales. *Med. J. Aust.* **2013**, *199*, 46–50. [CrossRef] [PubMed]

25. Thow, A.M.; Downs, S.M.; Mayes, C.; Trevena, H.; Waqanivalu, T.; Cawley, J. Fiscal policy to improve diets and prevent noncommunicable diseases: From recommendations to action. *Bull. World Health Organ.* **2018**, *96*, 201–210. [CrossRef] [PubMed]

26. World Health Organization. *Fiscal Policies for Diet and Prevention on Noncommunicable Diseases Technical Meeting Report, 5–6 May 2015*; World Health Organization: Geneva, Switzerland, 2016.

27. Queensland Government Statistician's Office. Queensland Regional Profiles. Available online: https://statistics.qgso.qld.gov.au/qld-regional-profiles (accessed on 22 October 2018).

28. Steering Committee for the Cape York Food and Nutrition Strategy 2012–2017. *Cape York Food and Nutrition Strategy 2012–2017*; Queensland Health: Brisbane, Australia, 2012.

29. Ferguson, M.; O'Dea, K.; Holden, S.; Miles, E.; Brimblecombe, J. Food and beverage price discounts to improve health in remote Aboriginal communities: Mixed method evaluation of a natural experiment. *Aust. N. Z. J. Public Health* **2017**, *41*, 32–37. [CrossRef] [PubMed]

30. Commonwealth of Australia. National Aboriginal and Torres Strait Islander Health Plan 2013–2023. Available online: http://www.health.gov.au/internet/main/publishing.nsf/content/B92E980680486C3BCA257BF0001BAF01/5File/health-plan.pdf (accessed on 22 October 2018).

31. Australian Bureau of Statistics. Australian Aboriginal and Torres Strait Islander Health Survey: Consumption of Food Groups from the Australian Dietary Guidelines, 2012–13. Available online: http://www.abs.gov.au/AUSSTATS/abs@.nsf/Lookup/4727.0.55.008Main+Features12012-13?OpenDocument (accessed on 29 October 2018).

32. McMahon, E.; Wycherley, T.; O'Dea, K.; Brimblecombe, J. A comparison of dietary estimates from the National Aboriginal and Torres Strait Islander Health Survey to food and beverage purchase data. *Aust. N. Z. J. Public Health* **2017**, *41*, 598–603. [CrossRef] [PubMed]

33. Brimblecombe, J.; Liddle, R.; O'Dea, K. Use of point-of-sale data to assess food and nutrient quality in remote stores. *Public Health Nutr.* **2013**, *16*, 1159–1167. [CrossRef] [PubMed]

34. Brimblecombe, J.; Ferguson, M.; Liberato, S.; O'Dea, K. Characteristics of the community-level diet of Aboriginal people in remote northern Australia. *Med. J. Aust.* **2013**, *198*, 380–384. [CrossRef] [PubMed]
35. Vidgen, H.; Adam, M.; Gallegos, D. Who does nutrition prevention work in Queensland? *Nutr. Diet.* **2015**, *74*, 88–94. [CrossRef] [PubMed]
36. Lee, A.J.; Bonson, A.P.; Powers, J.R. The effect of retail store managers on Aboriginal diet in remote communities. *Aust. N. Z. J. Public Health* **1996**, *20*, 212–214. [CrossRef] [PubMed]

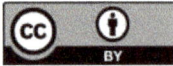

International Journal of
Environmental Research and Public Health

MDPI

Article

Health-Promoting Food Pricing Policies and Decision-Making in Very Remote Aboriginal and Torres Strait Islander Community Stores in Australia

**Megan Ferguson [1,2,]*, Kerin O'Dea [3], Jon Altman [4], Marjory Moodie [5]
and Julie Brimblecombe [2,6]**

[1] School of Public Health, The University of Queensland, Brisbane 4072, Australia
[2] Wellbeing and Preventable Chronic Diseases, Menzies School of Health Research, Darwin 0811, Australia;
   julie.brimblecombe@monash.edu
[3] Division of Health Sciences, University of South Australia, Adelaide 5001, Australia;
   Kerin.O'Dea@unisa.edu.au
[4] Alfred Deakin Institute for Citizenship and Globalisation, Deakin University, Burwood 3125, Australia;
   jon.altman@anu.edu.au
[5] Deakin Health Economics, Centre for Population Health Research, Deakin University, Geelong 3220, Australia;
   marj.moodie@deakin.edu.au
[6] Faculty of Medicine, Nursing and Health Sciences, Monash University, Melbourne 3168, Australia
* Correspondence: megan.ferguson@uq.edu.au; Tel.: +61-7-3365-5546

Received: 8 November 2018; Accepted: 14 December 2018; Published: 19 December 2018

Abstract: Aboriginal and Torres Strait Islander people living in remote communities in Australia experience a disproportionate burden of diet-related chronic disease. This occurs in an environment where the cost of store-purchased food is high and cash incomes are low, factors that affect both food insecurity and health outcomes. Aboriginal and Torres Strait Islander storeowners and the retailers who work with them implement local policies with the aim of improving food affordability and health outcomes. This paper describes health-promoting food pricing policies, their alignment with evidence, and the decision-making processes entailed in their development in community stores across very remote Australia. Semi-structured interviews were conducted with a purposive sample of retailers and health professionals identified through the snowball method, September 2015 to October 2016. Data were complemented through review of documents describing food pricing policies. A content analysis of the types and design of policies was undertaken, while the decision-making process was considered through a deductive, thematic analysis. Fifteen retailers and 32 health professionals providing services to stores participated. Subsidies and subsidy/price increase combinations dominated. Magnitude of price changes ranged from 5% to 25% on fruit, vegetables, bottled water, artificially sweetened and sugar sweetened carbonated beverages, and broadly used 'healthy/essential' and 'unhealthy' food classifications. Feasibility and sustainability were considered during policy development. Greater consideration of acceptability, importance, effectiveness and unintended consequences of policies guided by evidence were deemed important, as were increased involvement of Aboriginal and Torres Strait Islander storeowners and nutritionists in policy development. A range of locally developed health-promoting food pricing policies exist and partially align with research-evidence. The decision-making processes identified offer an opportunity to incorporate evidence, based on consideration of the local context.

Keywords: food security; diet-related chronic disease; policy; food pricing

1. Introduction

Aboriginal and Torres Strait Islander people living in remote areas generally experience the poorest health outcomes and hold the worst economic position in Australia [1,2]. Aboriginal and Torres Strait Islander people experience unemployment at 4.2 times, and have an average disposable income 70% of, non-Indigenous Australians [3]. Poverty is greatest for Aboriginal and Torres Strait Islander people living in very remote areas and is growing [2]. The life expectancy of Aboriginal and Torres Strait Islander people is approximately 10 years less than non-Indigenous Australians. The majority of this gap is due to chronic disease, especially cardiovascular disease and cancer, and injury for the 35–74 years age group [4]. The gap is largest in remote areas where Aboriginal and Torres Strait Islander people experience a burden 2.4 times that of non-Indigenous people [5]. Dietary intake is a key risk factor contributing to this gap [4,5].

Nutrient-rich traditional, non-market food continues to contribute to dietary intake [6], though the rapid nutrition transition resulting from colonization has led to a population diet high in sugar, salt and fat and low intakes of vegetables, fruit and other nutrient-rich foods [7]. In remote Aboriginal and Torres Strait Islander communities, Western foods are predominantly purchased from the single retail food outlet, referred to as the store, operating in a challenging, remote environment, which contributes to the high cost of food. Many stores are community-owned, providing a unique opportunity for local policy development [8].

The remote store landscape has undergone considerable change in the last decade, particularly in policy and services. In 2008, a Close the Gap statement of intent was agreed to by a number of Aboriginal and Torres Strait Islander people and organizations and the Australian Government [9]. In the same year, the Council of Australian Governments released the Closing the Gap Strategy that aimed to achieve health equity within 25 years [10] and in 2009 developed the National Strategy for Food Security in Remote Indigenous Communities which linked food security (i.e., the ability to acquire appropriate and nutritious food in a regular and socially acceptable manner) and nutrition with the national Closing the Gap targets [11]. Two years prior to this in the Northern Territory (NT) of Australia, the Northern Territory Emergency Response was implemented and included a number of measures indirectly related to food 'security'. One of these was for the compulsory income management of welfare recipients [12] (i.e., restriction of available cash and purchase of specific products), which has since been extended beyond the NT [13]. A second measure was the introduction of a regulatory framework for the operation of remote stores, including minimum standards relating to food security; this remains effective today [14]. The Australian National Audit Office reports however, that government policies have made minimal contribution to addressing food insecurity in remote communities [15]. Reports on the Closing the Gap targets show mixed outcomes, though importantly that the target to close the life expectancy gap is not on track [10] and that outcomes are worse in remote than non-remote areas [2]. The Productivity Commission highlights the importance of developing an evaluation culture in Aboriginal and Torres Strait Islander policy where policy evaluation informs future policy [16].

During this time of policy change there has also been a growth in organizations that provide retail management services to remote community storeowners, alongside an increasing recognition of the role that the stores play in the health of the communities [17–21]. The historical tension between economic and health outcomes may be giving way as organizations publicly demonstrate valuing health outcomes as an objective of sustainable business [19,21–25]. In remote Aboriginal and Torres Strait Islander community stores, there are examples of local policies (i.e., the rules of operation determined by the governing body [26]), which aim to promote health outcomes within a sustainable business model [24,25,27]. There is significant opportunity in this dynamic remote retail context to work with storeowners and the systems they operate within to influence local store food policy to create health-promoting environments.

Food pricing is considered one of the more effective practices to influence consumer purchasing patterns [28]. Health-promoting food pricing policies exist in remote stores, but there is little understanding of the decision-making process informing their design development including the magnitude of the price increase or decrease and promotion of the policy [29]. Policy analysis can help understand the process of design development and thereby identify opportunities to strengthen design and improve health outcomes through the store [30,31]. Policy development models have evolved to consider trade-offs between multiple and often conflicting objectives [32]; they may have utility in understanding efforts in the remote retail context where governing bodies deal with the dual and potentially conflicting objectives of consumer health outcomes alongside commercial viability of stores. Decision-making which incorporates evidence will hopefully lead to consideration of a greater range of policy options and result in more effective outcomes [33].

This paper describes health-promoting food pricing policies including their alignment with evidence, and the decision-making processes in their development in very remote Aboriginal and Torres Strait Islander community stores in Australia. We specifically refer to 'food policy' as the local-level food policy implemented in stores aimed at modifying the price of food/beverages in order to promote health.

2. Methods

2.1. Context

Approximately 175 stores supply food in some of the 1187 discrete Indigenous communities in remote locations across Australia [8,34]. A total of 92,960 Aboriginal and Torres Strait Islander people and a small number of non-Indigenous people reside in these communities. Seventeen communities have a population greater than 1000 and almost 75% are located in very remote locations [34]. Our study included very remote communities only [35]. These are located largely in the NT, Queensland (Qld), South Australia (SA) and Western Australia (WA). Some stores are owned by the government or are privately owned, though the most common model is of incorporated community ownership where Aboriginal and Torres Strait Islander residents comprise the membership. These stores function as either not-for-profit or business enterprises and are often responsive to community priorities. The owners of community-owned stores employ a store manager/s or engage the services of a retail organization to manage the store's operation, with the latter model accounting for approximately 55% of stores in remote Aboriginal and Torres Strait Islander communities in Australia [17–21]. In addition to operating an effective retail operation, a number of stores and retail organizations aim to employ local Aboriginal and Torres Strait Islander people and promote positive nutrition outcomes and healthy lifestyles [8].

2.2. Design

A qualitative study was conducted that applied a methodology informed by Thow's framework used in the Pacific Region. This framework was informed by policy theories related to lesson drawing to understand the form of food policies and how to engage with policy-makers [30]. It was successfully used to describe the common elements of policy processes across the diversity of policy processes identified in different countries in the Pacific Region. Our methodology was informed by this framework as we similarly anticipated a diversity of policy processes across different remote communities, states and territories and governance models. We first focused on determining the range of pricing policies in place in remote stores and secondly on an understanding the stages of the process [32], the people involved [30,33], identification of objectives [32], consideration of assessment criteria applied [32] including a list of pre-determined criteria previously used in food policy assessment (i.e., feasibility, sustainability, acceptability, importance, effectiveness, unintended consequences [36–39]), and the evidence considered.

2.3. Data

Purposive sampling was employed, informed by the snowball method, to maximize coverage of the types of policies implemented. Participants were: (i) retailers, who were the store managers employed by the owners of a community store or store managers and retail management staff employed by a retail organization, and (ii) health professionals, including public health nutritionists (hereafter, nutritionists) and others working in roles with stores employed by a retail organization, government or non-government organization. Participants were required to identify that they had knowledge of health-promoting food pricing policy in remote Aboriginal and Torres Strait Islander community stores. At least one retailer and where applicable, the nutritionist from each of five retail organizations representing the majority of these entities, and all nutritionists in service provision and food supply policy known to Megan Ferguson and Julie Brimblecombe operating in remote NT, Qld, SA and WA, were invited to participate. Participants were invited by email from the lead researcher or by a potential participant in the study. This study did not seek to quantify policy implementation by store, store governance model or state/territory.

A semi-structured interview guide was used in all interviews. It focused on two sets of data. The first was the health-promoting food pricing policies in stores. We included price increases and subsidies in the form of price discounts, rewards, vouchers and free product give-away. We excluded takeaway food outlets as a setting and government policy instruments that might impact on food purchases such as income management. The second set of data focused on the decision-making process for one of the policies reported. Interviews lasted on average 50 min, and were conducted by Megan Ferguson, a nutritionist who has worked in both the remote health and retail sectors. This background was important in terms of understanding the context and relating to participants' experiences. Interviews were conducted in English, in person or by phone. In one case, responses to the interview questions were e-mailed by a participant. Participants provided consent and all interviews were audio-recorded, transcribed verbatim and returned to participants for checking. Documents describing food pricing policies were sourced or provided by participants and used to complement interview data. Data were uploaded and managed in NVivo (QSR International Pty Ltd. Version 11, Melbourne, Victoria, Australia, 2012). Ethical approval for this study was provided by Human Research Ethics Committees in the NT (HREC NTDHMSHR 2012–1711; CAHREC HREC-12-13; CDU HREC H12096), Qld (FNQ HREC HREC/16/QCH/35-1041) and WA (WACHS HREC 2016/13; WAAHEC 715; KAHPF 2016-006). Informed consent was obtained from all participants.

2.4. Analysis

The dataset was reviewed independently by two researchers, Megan Ferguson and Julie Brimblecombe, who have extensive research, policy and practice experience in the remote retail and health sectors. This strengthened the analysis by ensuring research quality and relevance. The authors discussed and agreed on the coding framework. The data were coded by Megan Ferguson and the findings reviewed with Julie Brimblecombe.

Firstly, a data content analysis relating to the types and design of food pricing policies was conducted, with allowance for additional codes. The coding framework included the following: Under the three pre-determined codes, *subsidy, price increase, subsidy/price increase combination*; the sub-codes relating to each code of *targeted food or beverage, magnitude of price change, duration, administration, complementary strategies, other design elements*; and, a fourth emergent code, *business fundamentals*. Secondly, a deductive, thematic analysis of the decision-making process was conducted to identify why, how and who was involved.

3. Results

3.1. Participants

Between September 2015 and October 2016, 47 interviews were conducted with 15 retailers, 28 nutritionists and four health professionals servicing communities in NT, Qld, WA and SA. Forty-two more people were invited to participate by Megan Ferguson; two delegated the interview invitation to staff under their supervision, 21 did not respond to the email invitation and 19 declined, with the most common response being that they did not have sufficient knowledge relevant to the study objectives.

3.2. Health-Promoting Food Pricing Policies

The most commonly implemented food pricing policies across very remote Australia were subsidies and subsidy/price increase combinations as shown in Table 1. These policies mostly targeted fruit, vegetables, bottled water, artificially sweetened and sugar sweetened carbonated beverages, in addition to groups of foods broadly referred to as 'healthy/essential' foods and 'unhealthy' foods. Magnitude of price changes ranged from 5% to 25%. The policies were largely ongoing. A number of these, predominantly those targeting fruit, vegetables and 'healthy/essential' and 'unhealthy' foods, had been in place for many years including in some locations for over 35 years, where the beverage policies were first introduced in 2010. Short-term discounts were applied more recently and were usually up to two weeks duration. Stores generally funded the long-term policies, such as fruit and vegetables discounts, while more recently implemented policies were partly funded by the suppliers and manufacturers. Pricing policies were at times supported by one or more merchandising strategies involving product availability (e.g., specific brand, quality), placement (e.g., shelf space allocation, planograms) and promotion (e.g., in-store announcements, use of local celebrities), though implementation of these strategies seemed more ad hoc than planned. Promotion of the ongoing pricing policies did not occur and was identified as a missed opportunity in communicating the policy to customers.

> *"I reckon that it is not visible to the average person in terms of what pricing policies stores have ... and therefore not as effective. ... I don't think that translates to the customer that they're getting a good deal on whatever they're getting a good deal on."* (Interviewee 47, Health professional)

Finally, retailers and health professionals stressed the requirement of efficient and effective retail operations as the key condition for the development of health-promoting pricing policies.

3.3. Decision-Making

3.3.1. Process of Decision-Making

The process of decision-making reported included some level of deliberation and procedure, though this was generally described as flexible. The processes described by those in retail organizations were more structured with specific stages of development, than those described for stores operating independently. However, there were often more people involved in the decision-making processes of retail organizations than in individual community stores.

Table 1. Health-promoting food pricing policies in very remote Aboriginal and Torres Strait Islander community stores in Australia.

Food/Beverage Targeted	Impact on Selling Price	Duration	Administration
Subsidy—Price discount			
Fruit and vegetables—all fresh	**Approximately 20% to 25% discount or equal to, to ≤30% of urban retail prices**	**Ongoing**	**Store**
Fruit and vegetables—all fresh, frozen, canned and dried	**Approximately 20% discount**	**Ongoing**	**Store**
Water—bottled	**Various, example $0.53, $1.00 and $2.00 for 600 mL**	**Ongoing**	**Store and manufacturer**
Fruit and vegetables—a small range of fresh items	5% to 10% discount or comparable to urban retail prices	Short-term, rotating	Store and supplier
Dairy products—fresh milk, yoghurt and cheese	Approximately 20% discount	Ongoing	Store
Dairy products—low-fat fresh milks	Low-fat milk retailed for the price of full cream milk	Ongoing	Store; Store and manufacturer
Bread—multigrain and wholemeal bread	$1.00 less than white bread	Ongoing	Store
Healthy foods [1]	n/a	Ongoing and short-term	Store; Store and supplier
Beverages—bottled water and artificially sweetened soft-drink	Various, example bulk packs of bottled water retailing for less than the equivalent volume achieved in single units	Short-term, rotating	Store and manufacturer
Subsidy—Reward			
Fruit and vegetables—fresh; fresh, frozen, canned and dried	Various, example a $10 fruit and vegetable gift following a $20 fruit and vegetable purchase	Short-term, including feasibility assessment	Store; Health organization [2]
Fruit, vegetables, meat [3] and bottled water	$25 voucher for health assessment participation	Ongoing	Health organization
Subsidy—Free			
Water—chilled via a bubbler outside the store	Free	Ongoing	Store
Price increase			
Sugar sweetened carbonated beverages	19% increase	Ongoing	Store
Sugar sweetened carbonated beverages	$0.30 increase per 375 mL can and $1.00 per 1.25 L bottle	Ongoing	Store
Subsidy/price increase combination			
Reduction on healthy foods and increase on unhealthy foods [1]	**n/a**	**Ongoing**	**Store**
Reduction on artificially sweetened carbonated beverages and increase on sugar sweetened carbonated beverages	**Various ranging from 6% to 22%, and in places a widening gap [4]**	**Ongoing**	**Store; Stores and manufacturer**

Note: The policies most commonly reported are in bold (i.e., subsidy on fruit and vegetables—all fresh; fruit and vegetables—all fresh, frozen, canned and dried; water—bottled and subsidy/price increase combination on healthy and unhealthy foods and artificially sweetened carbonated and sugar sweetened carbonated beverages). All values are in AUD (AUD1.00 = USD0.77 in 2016). [1] Healthy and unhealthy foods were not specified though healthy foods often reported to include commodity groups which were largely though not solely considered to be healthy/core foods such as fruit, vegetables, bread, milk, meat, eggs and infant foods, or items deemed to be essential food items such as tea, sugar and margarine and unhealthy foods often reported to include foods commonly considered to be discretionary foods such as crisps, confectionery, chocolate, biscuits, bakery lines and sugar sweetened beverages. [2] Health organization is a local or regional Aboriginal health organization. [3] Meat included lean and non-lean cuts of meat. [4] It was unclear if this price gap always included a price increase to sugar sweetened carbonated beverages.

3.3.2. Decision-Makers

Three groups of people were identified as being involved in policy development, namely retailers, nutritionists employed by retail organizations, and Aboriginal and Torres Strait Islander and non-Indigenous store committee/board members. There were a few cases where nutritionists or health professionals employed by the health sector contributed directly to the process. Retailers and/or nutritionists employed by retail organizations reported that they primarily identified the need for, and designed policies, though the need for a policy was said to be identified sometimes by Aboriginal and Torres Strait Islander storeowners.

> *"...we are working with (X) communities at the moment to reduce the sale of full sugar soft drink. And I must note the communities or the storeowners approached us about it. So we talk about the health stats every quarter. But now that there's more education around you know, the impacts of diet and poor health and those things. Now storeowners are saying, 'What can we do to improve these outcomes?'"* (Interviewee 40, Retailer)

Policies were reported to be approved by the store committee/board, and at times, by retailers. Examples were provided where store committees/boards were reported to actively direct and monitor policy, whereas others provided support or opposition to policy proposals initiated by retailers.

3.3.3. Policy Objectives

Price manipulation was seen by most participants as a means to increase purchases of healthy foods and to reduce purchases of unhealthy foods and hence improve the quality of dietary intake, with participants acknowledging the high rates of overweight and obesity, diet-related chronic diseases and lower life expectancy of Aboriginal and Torres Strait Islander people. A second policy objective described, although to a lesser extent, was one of addressing equity and providing access to healthy food at prices comparable to that of all Australians.

These two objectives were not considered in isolation, with operating costs and commercial viability raised largely, though not solely, by retailers as significant pertinent factors. The cost of food to the store was seen as a significant barrier in implementing health-promoting pricing policies. Participants described the balance required between pricing and profit. Examples were described where storeowners chose to invest their profits in reduced food prices. It was proposed that there is an opportunity to reframe the discourse around profit, by engaging new terms such as 'retailing for health.'

3.3.4. Decision-Making Criteria

Participants were first asked about the use of six predetermined criteria in policy-making in their context. They were then asked which criteria they considered most important to the process and to identify any gaps in the criteria used. These predetermined criteria were feasibility, sustainability, effectiveness, importance, acceptability and unintended consequences. In describing which criteria were applied, participants described the meaning these criteria had in their context.

Feasibility and sustainability were reported by both retailers and health professionals to be considered in the policy-making processes. A feasible policy was described as one which is achievable in both economic and practical terms, including being a good fit with the existing system, aligning with the available human resource skill set and capacity and the supply of product and infrastructure required to deliver the policy. A sustainable policy was considered to be one which could be continued or scaled-up. A small number of health professionals viewed sustainability as the need for a policy to have appeal to, or be aligned with government policy.

The potential effectiveness of a policy was considered by both retailers and health professionals in policy-making though often with a caveat, such as they 'assumed', 'hoped', or 'thought' a policy might be effective, rather than describing having confidence in a policy's potential effectiveness. Participants referred to policy as being influenced by the poor population-level health status of Aboriginal and

Torres Strait Islander people and current and recommended dietary intake. Rarely however, was research-informed evidence of effectiveness reported to inform policy development.

Participants reported less consideration of the criteria of importance and acceptability. Importance included an assessment of how worthwhile a policy was considered, which was almost solely related to health outcomes. Acceptability related to a policy's appropriateness to the recipients (i.e., customers) and implementers (i.e., store managers). Both retailers and health professionals reported that it was important to have community buy-in, or that policies be community-driven or at least community-partnered and support capacity enhancement of Aboriginal and Torres Strait Islander storeowners.

Unintended consequences were rarely reported as being considered, though where they were, this was by both retailers and health professionals.

> *"Unintended consequences—I don't think we really considered at all. It's definitely not, if we do, if we drop the price of milk, what will happen next? I don't think we considered that at all. We, our presumption is always that they (i.e., customers) will continue to spend more money in the store."* (Interviewee 9, Retailer)

Unintended consequences were perceived as factors that may positively or negatively impact on a health or business outcome. Organization or store brand image and positive or negative publicity were highlighted as emerging unintended consequences that were perceived to impact on business outcomes and recently informed policy development. In relation to health outcomes, one retailer referred to the group of Aboriginal and Torres Strait Islander storeowners he worked with, considering equity across the population in policy development.

Participants were asked to nominate criteria that they considered most important to decision-making and any gaps. All six pre-determined criteria were considered important to decision-making, with the exception that approximately half of the retailers considered assessment of unintended consequences as unnecessary. The order of importance placed on these criteria was generally considered to be context- and policy-specific. No new criteria were identified.

3.3.5. Evidence Informing Decision-Making

There was limited use of research-informed evidence in the processes reported. The three key forms of information used largely originated from the retail sector. Firstly, health professionals, more so than retailers, noted the 'diffusion of ideas' or benchmarking as a method which commonly informed local policy. Policy was also informed by food price survey reports and urban store pricing. Secondly, retailers and health professionals referred to the use of store sales in a variety of ways: to conduct retail modelling to inform policy design, to measure retail performance and sales of a targeted product when a pricing policy is implemented, and to provide ongoing monitoring to staff and storeowners in relation to top sellers or targeted products. A reliable point-of-sale system was seen as a requirement for implementing pricing policies, as was the importance of understanding data and disseminating user-friendly reports.

> *"So a Board that's not getting nutritional reports back to them, from the store is really not being told enough of the key information. ... So that it's always in their mind and they can see what the store's doing and then they start to think about their own, well, what if we did this, why can't we do that, you know. 'Cause management (i.e., retailers) doesn't have all the answers."* (Interviewee 23, Retailer)

The third key information source described was retail, and especially remote retail, industry knowledge. Retailers often described their thinking as influenced by employing the strategies known to work in the retail industry to promote or disincentivize targeted products to shape a health-promoting environment.

3.4. Strengthening the Decision-Making Process

3.4.1. Supporting Roles of Decision-Makers

The Aboriginal and Torres Strait Islander and non-Indigenous store committee/board members, retailers and nutritionists, and the relationships between these decision-makers were considered crucial to the process. Opportunities to enhance the current process were proposed: (i) to further support/engage Aboriginal and Torres Strait Islander storeowners, staff and customers in the identification and design of policies, and (ii) to support greater participation of nutritionists, by addressing barriers which included nutritionists either not having the opportunity or not recognizing a role for themselves or their capacity to contribute to policy-making.

Suppliers, whilst not considered to be central to the decision-making process, appeared to have an increasing support role as shown in Table 1. Some suppliers were reported to be supportive having shared values; others, however, were seen as having a poor understanding of the context and promoted unhealthy products even as retailers tried to secure deals on healthy products.

3.4.2. Accessing and Strengthening the Evidence Base

Retailers and health professionals identified three forms of evidence as being potentially useful to the process. The first was accessing research-informed evidence through user-friendly dissemination methods.

"...all the journal articles and big reports and what not are nice, but even people within our (health) organization wanted like almost sound bites, like stories and we needed options in the community and say, 'This is what's been done before, here's the stories and you can choose from these options.'" (Interviewee 11, Health professional)

The second was further development of locally-informed evidence through improved evaluation and timely feedback to communities. Time and resources were identified as the limiting factor in conducting quality evaluation, not the lack of data. Notably, retailers and health professionals referred to reduced capacity to support activities such as evaluation owing to government funding cuts, resulting in the loss of nutritionist positions in retail and non-government organizations dedicated to working with stores. The third was a better understanding of the factors that drive purchasing decisions, including income and cost of living data and the impact of price on the purchasing of targeted products. Participants sensed that price elasticity of demand varied for different products, that price impacted differently across population groups and that customer response to price is changing. There was also a sense that customers generally may not have all the necessary information available to them in a useable form to make an informed purchasing decision in relation to price.

4. Discussion

Health-promoting food pricing policies implemented in very remote Aboriginal and Torres Strait Islander community stores in Australia were dominated by subsidies and subsidy/price increase combinations. These had a small to moderate impact on food prices of fruit, vegetables, bottled water, artificially sweetened and sugar sweetened carbonated beverages, and broadly used 'healthy/essential' and 'unhealthy' food classifications. Decision-making was a deliberative process, which evaluated policy feasibility and sustainability, though generally lacked incorporation of research-informed evidence.

4.1. Designing Health-Promoting Food Pricing Policy

The dominance of subsidies and subsidy/price increases reported in this study is in line with recommendations to support healthier choices in low socioeconomic populations with the subsidy/price increase combination possibly mitigating concerns about the potential regressive nature of taxes [40,41]. The range of products targeted only partially align with the current evidence. The lack of criteria applied to the 'healthy' category for example, results in a misalignment with guidelines for good health and a lost opportunity to promote a healthy diet. Targeting artificially sweetened carbonated beverages may not support positive health outcomes as reducing the price of these is unlikely to decrease the consumption of sugar sweetened carbonated beverages [42–45]. Additionally, there are calls for a greater focus on policy targeting discretionary foods [43,46]. Magnitude of price changes were at best in line with recommendations for modifying purchasing [47]. Equity was the objective of decision-making in some cases, and the magnitude of the price changes went some way to achieving this [48]. The ongoing nature of most policies which are not routinely advertised to customers prevented the use of price as a signal to customers; this was described by participants and supported by others as a significant missed opportunity [49].

Food pricing policies in this context which aim to improve health would be more aligned with research evidence if there was: (i) further targeting of products (e.g., specify healthy foods, foods likely to have a greater response to price changes [43]); (ii) increased magnitude of price change [47,50]; (iii) use of price and price promotion to send a signal to customers, such as through a price increase alone or dynamic, rotating subsidies and promoting the change in price to customers [29,47,49,51]. Policies need to be assessed within the local context and may require new avenues for funding, such as by manufacturers, suppliers and wholesalers, by government or through evaluation of current food pricing policy or funds dispersal.

4.2. Enhancing Policy Development Processes

This analysis indicates that the process of decision-making was deliberative [32]. Improved health, and to a lesser extent equity, were key objectives in the decision-making process. These objectives of health and equity inform policy development differently, including the sources of evidence required. Whilst assessment of effectiveness was considered a priority, participant response and the design of current policies, indicates limited use of research-informed evidence. Although consideration of unintended consequences was not universally viewed as important to the process, research-informed evidence would go some way to inform the assessment of this criterion whether it was explicitly included or not. Acceptability and importance were not well-considered criteria, although they were regarded a priority and likely to be best addressed through further engagement with Aboriginal and Torres Strait Islander storeowners and others they elect to involve. Given articulating and communicating problems is a crucial stage in decision-making [32], the processes reported in this context are likely to be improved with further assessment of the criteria, acceptability, importance, effectiveness and unintended consequences of potential policies. The processes were generally focused on a single policy rather than evaluation of a suite of options. They were based on analysis of retail data, informed by an assessment of cost in terms of retail impact though not cost-effectiveness, nor health impact, and limited in terms of robust monitoring and evaluation. Greater incorporation of research-informed evidence into the design of food pricing policies which have an objective of dietary or health improvement, is likely to result in more effective policy, and was called for by study participants [33].

Complex policy with multiple and potentially conflicting objectives, is likely to create tension [32]. There appears to be a shift in the well-documented tension between commercial profit and health outcomes in remote stores [22,23]. Opportunities exist for well-designed health-promoting food pricing policies to be considered within the suite of business practices by storeowners, and precedent has been set for this as described in our study. Currently, retailers are front and center of the decision-making process in remote stores, hence the reliance on retail-focused evidence and criteria in the decision-making process. Current processes offer opportunities to further progress health-promoting policy, such as using the role of benchmarking against other stores and organizations as a potential mechanism for dissemination of good practice. Mechanisms to support decision-makers to access research-informed evidence and to assess acceptability, importance and unintended consequences of policies for the local context could lead to more effective health-promoting policies.

This might involve a greater role for Aboriginal and Torres Strait Islander storeowners and nutritionists in decision-making.

4.3. Strengths and Limitations

This study has captured the views and experiences of retailers and health professionals across remote Aboriginal and Torres Strait Islander communities in Australia. Effort was made to ensure retailers operating in independent stores were included, though without a census of all stores, this is a more challenging cohort to identify and locate. The resources for this study did not allow for the conduct of interviews in remote communities with Aboriginal and Torres Strait Islander store committee/board members. Interviewing those persons known to work closely with storeowners provided insight into the roles and processes which could be further explored. Participants were invited to contribute where health-promoting food pricing policies were implemented and as such, this is likely to represent the best-case scenario rather than the situation in all remote Aboriginal and Torres Strait Islander community stores. The case considered was food pricing policies, and the process of policy development may be different to that of other health-promoting food policies in stores.

5. Conclusions

Remote Aboriginal and Torres Strait Islander community stores provide a crucial setting if health outcomes of their customers are to improve. While owners and operators face major challenges, community ownership provides an opportunity to make a difference to the foods purchased from community stores. The urgency of the situation for Aboriginal and Torres Strait Islander storeowners and those who work to support them is not unlike that of low- and middle-income countries currently leading the way in implementing food-related policies [31,52]. This study identifies opportunities that exist to further shape the store food environment through incorporation of research-informed evidence. In doing so, it offers lessons on how locally-developed and -implemented policies can be formulated to shape other food retail environments for health outcomes. However, addressing equity and positively shaping healthy retail environments should not be a task for storeowners and retailers alone. There is a role for government, manufacturers and wholesalers to work with Aboriginal and Torres Strait Islander storeowners and those who support their efforts, to implement evidence-informed policy to support healthy environments.

Author Contributions: Conceptualization, M.F.; data curation, M.F.; formal analysis, M.F., J.B.; validation, J.B., K.O., J.A. and M.M.; investigation, M.F.; resources, M.F.; writing—original draft preparation, M.F.; writing—review and editing, K.O., J.A., M.M, J.B.; supervision, J.B., K.O., J.A. and M.M.; project administration, M.F.; funding acquisition, M.F.

Funding: M.F. received funding through a National Health and Medical Research Council (NHMRC) Postgraduate Scholarship (#1039074). J.B. received funding through a National Heart Foundation Fellowship (#100085). M.M. is supported by a NHMRC funded Centre for Research Excellence in Obesity Policy and Food Systems (#1041020). The contents of the published material are solely the responsibility of the individual authors and do not reflect the views of the NHMRC.

Acknowledgments: The authors are grateful to the study participants for providing such valuable insights into food policy decision-making in stores across very remote Australia. We are grateful to Anthony Gunther for his review of the manuscript.

Conflicts of Interest: M.F., K.O. and M.M. declare no conflict of interest. J.B. is a Non-Executive Director on the Board of Outback Stores. J.A. is a Director of Jimmy Little Thumbs Up Limited a charity looking to provide health and nutrition education to remote Indigenous communities. The funders had no role in the design of the study; in the collection, analyses, or interpretation of data; in the writing of the manuscript, or in the decision to publish the results.

References

1. Vos, T.; Barker, B.; Begg, S.; Stanley, L.; Lopez, A.D. Burden of disease and injury in Aboriginal and Torres Strait Islander Peoples: The Indigenous health gap. *Int. J. Epidemiol.* **2009**, *38*, 470–477. [CrossRef]
2. Markham, F.; Biddle, N. *Income, Poverty and Inequality, CAEPR 2016 Census Paper No. 2*; Centre for Aboriginal Economic Policy Research; The Australian National University: Canberra, Australia, 2018.
3. Australian Institute of Health and Welfare. *The Health and Welfare of Australia's Aboriginal and Torres Strait Islander Peoples 2015*; Cat. No. IHW 147; AIHW: Canberra, Australia, 2015.
4. Australian Institute of Health and Welfare. *Australia's Health 2016*; Australia's Health Series No. 15. Cat. No. AUS 199; AIHW: Canberra, Australia, 2016.
5. Australian Institute of Health and Welfare. *Australian Burden of Disease Study: Impact and Causes of Illness and Death in Aboriginal and Torres Strait Islander People 2011*; AIHW: Canberra, Australia, 2016.
6. Ferguson, M.; Brown, C.; Georga, C.; Miles, E.; Wilson, A.; Brimblecombe, J. Traditional food availability and consumption in remote Aboriginal communities in the Northern Territory, Australia. *Aust. N. Z. J. Public Health* **2017**, *41*, 294–298. [CrossRef]
7. Brimblecombe, J.; Ferguson, M.; Liberato, S.; O'Dea, K. Characteristics of the community-level diet of Aboriginal people in remote northern Australia. *Med. J. Aust.* **2013**, *198*, 380–384. [CrossRef]
8. House of Representatives Aboriginal and Torres Strait Islander Affairs Committee. *Everybody's Business Remote Aboriginal and Torres Strait Community Stores*; Commonwealth of Australia: Canberra, Australia, 2009.
9. Australian Human Rights Commission. Close the Gap: Indigenous Health Equality Summit—Statement of Intent. Available online: https://www.humanrights.gov.au/publications/close-gap-indigenous-health-equality-summit-statement-intent (accessed on 18 September 2017).
10. Commonwealth of Australia, Department of the Prime Minister and Cabinet. *Closing the Gap Prime Minister's Report 2017*; Commonwealth of Australia: Canberra, Australia, 2017.
11. Council of Australian Governments. National Strategy for Food Security in Remote Indigenous Communities. Available online: http://webarchive.nla.gov.au/gov/20130329094202/http://www.coag.gov.au/node/92 (accessed on 18 September 2017).
12. Altman, J.; Klein, E. Lessons from a basic income programme for Indigenous Australians. *Oxf. Dev. Stud.* **2017**, *46*, 132–146. [CrossRef]
13. Parliament of Australia. Social Services Legislation Amendment (Cashless Debit Card) Bill 2017. Available online: http://www.aph.gov.au/Parliamentary_Business/Committees/Senate/Community_Affairs/CashlessDebitCard (accessed on 18 September 2017).
14. Australian Government. *Stronger Futures in the Northern Territory: A Ten Year Commitment to Aboriginal People in the Northern Territory July 2012*; Commonwealth of Australia: Canberra, Australia, 2012.
15. Australian National Audit Office. *Food Security in Remote Indigenous Communities*; Commonwealth of Australia; Commonwealth of Australia: Canberra, Australia, 2014.
16. Productivity Commission. *National Indigenous Reform Agreement, Performance Assessment 2013-4*; Commonwealth of Australia: Canberra, Australia, 2015.
17. Regional Merchandising Solutions. Homepage. Available online: http://regionalmerchandising.com.au/ (accessed on 19 December 2016).
18. Outback Stores. Map of Stores. Available online: http://outbackstores.com.au/map-of-stores/ (accessed on 19 December 2016).
19. Community Enterprise Queensland. Store Locations. Available online: http://www.ceqld.org.au/store-locations/ (accessed on 17 July 2017).
20. The Arnhem Land Progress Aboriginal Corporation. Where We Operate. Available online: http://www.alpa.asn.au/pages/Where-we-operate.html (accessed on 19 December 2016).
21. Mai Wiru. Mai Wiru Stores. Available online: http://www.maiwiru.org.au/stores (accessed on 19 December 2016).
22. Department of Health. *FoodNorth: Food for Health in North Australia*; Government of Western Australia: Perth, Australia, 2003.
23. Brimblecombe, J. *Enough for Rations and a Little Bit Extra: Challenges of Nutrition Improvement in an Aboriginal Community in North-East Arnhem Land*; Charles Darwin University: Darwin, Australia, 2007.
24. The Arnhem Land Progress Aboriginal Corporation. Nutrition Policy. Available online: http://www.alpa.asn.au/pages/Nutrition-Policy.html (accessed on 9 February 2014).

25. Outback Stores. Nutrition Strategy. Available online: http://outbackstores.com.au/wp-content/uploads/2013/09/Nutrition-Strategy.pdf (accessed on 11 February 2014).

26. Guba, E.G. The effect of definitions of policy on the nature and outcomes of policy anlaysis. *Educ. Leadersh.* **1984**, *42*, 63–70.

27. Nganampa Health Council and Ngaanyatjarra Pitjantjatjara Yankunytjatjara Women's Council. *Mai Wiru—Process. and Policy Regional Stores Policy and Associated Regulations for the Anangu Pitjantjatjara Lands*; Nganampa Health Council and Ngaanyatjarra Pitjantjatjara Yankunytjatjara Women's Council: Alice Springs, Australia, 2002.

28. Chandon, P.; Wansink, B. Does food marketing need to make us fat? A review and solutions. *Nutr. Rev.* **2012**, *70*, 571–593. [CrossRef]

29. Ferguson, M.; O'Dea, K.; Holden, S.; Miles, E.; Brimblecombe, J. Food and beverage price discounts to improve health in remote Aboriginal communities: Mixed method evaluation of a natural experiment. *Aust. N. Z. J. Public Health* **2016**, *41*, 32–37. [CrossRef]

30. Thow, A.M.; Swinburn, B.; Colagiuri, S.; Diligolevu, M.; Quested, C.; Vivili, P.; Leeder, S. Trade and food policy: Case studies from three Pacific Island countries. *Food Policy* **2010**, *35*, 556–564. [CrossRef]

31. Thow, A.; Quested, C.; Juventin, L.; Kun, R.; Khan, A.; Swinburn, B. Taxing soft drinks in the Pacific: Implementation lessons for improving health. *Health Promot. Int.* **2011**, *26*, 55–64. [CrossRef]

32. Walker, W.E. Policy analysis: A systematic approach to supporting policymaking in the public sector. *J. Multi-Crit. Decis. Anal.* **2000**, *9*, 11–27. [CrossRef]

33. Hanney, S.; Gonzalez-Block, M.; Buxton, M.; Kogan, M. The utilisation of health research in policy-making: Concepts, examples and methods of assessment. *Health Res. Policy Syst.* **2003**, *1*, 2. [CrossRef] [PubMed]

34. Australian Bureau of Statistics. *Housing and Infrastructure in Aboriginal and Torres Strait Islander Communities*; Cat. No. 4710.0; ABS: Canberra, Australia, 2007.

35. Australian Bureau of Statistics. 1270.0.55.005—Australian Statistical Geography Standard (ASGS): Volume 5—Remoteness Structure, July 2016. Available online: http://www.abs.gov.au/AUSSTATS/abs@.nsf/Lookup/1270.0.55.005Main+Features1July%202016?OpenDocument (accessed on 7 December 2018).

36. Braun, K.L.; Nigg, C.R.; Fialkowski, M.K.; Butel, J.; Hollyer, J.R.; Barber, L.R.; Bersamin, A.; Coleman, P.; Teo-Martin, U.; Vargo, A.M.; et al. Using the ANGELO Model to Develop the Children's Healthy Living Program Multilevel Intervention to Promote Obesity Preventing Behaviors for Young Children in the US-Affiliated Pacific Region. *Child. Obes.* **2014**, *10*, 474–481. [CrossRef] [PubMed]

37. Snowdon, W.; Lawrence, M.; Schultz, J.; Vivili, P.; Swinburn, B. Evidence-informed process to identify policies that will promote a healthy food environment in the Pacific Islands. *Public Health Nutr.* **2010**, *13*, 886–892. [CrossRef] [PubMed]

38. Snowdon, W.; Potter, J.; Swinburn, B.; Schultz, J.; Lawrence, M. Prioritizing policy interventions to improve diets? Will it work, can it happen, will it do harm? *Health Promot. Int.* **2010**, *25*, 123–133. [CrossRef] [PubMed]

39. Swinburn, B.; Gill, T.; Kumanyika, S. Obesity prevention: A proposed framework for translating evidence into action. *Obes. Rev.* **2005**, *6*, 23–33. [CrossRef]

40. Thow, A.; Jan, S.; Leeder, S.; Swinburn, B. The effect of fiscal policy on diet, obesity and chronic disease: A systematic review. *Bull. World Health Organ.* **2010**, *88*, 609–614. [CrossRef] [PubMed]

41. Purnell, J.Q.; Gernes, R.; Stein, R.; Sherraden, M.S.; Knoblock-Hahn, A. A systematic review of financial incentives for dietary behavior change. *J. Acad. Nutr. Diet.* **2014**, *114*, 1023–1035. [CrossRef]

42. Ball, K.; McNaughton, S.A.; Le, H.N.; Gold, L.; Mhurchu, C.N.; Abbott, G. Influence of price discounts and skill-building strategies on purchase and consumption of healthy food and beverages: Outcomes of the Supermarket Healthy Eating for Life randomized controlled trial. *Am. J. Clin. Nutr.* **2015**, *101*, 1055–1064. [CrossRef]

43. Brimblecombe, J.; Ferguson, M.; Chatfield, M.D.; Gunther, A.; Liberato, S.; Ball, K.; Moodie, M.; Miles, E.; Magnus, A.; Ni Mhurchu, C.; et al. Effect of a price discount and consumer education strategy on food and beverage purchases in remote Indigenous Australia: A stepped-wedge randomised controlled trial. *Lancet Public Health* **2017**, *2*, e82–e95. [CrossRef]

44. Popkin, B.M.; Hawkes, C. Sweetening of the global diet, particularly beverages: Patterns, trends, and policy responses. *Lancet Diabetes Endocrinol.* **2015**, *4*, 174–186. [CrossRef]

45. Imamura, F.; O'Connor, L.; Ye, Z.; Mursu, J.; Hayashino, Y.; Bhupathiraju, S.N.; Forouhi, N.G. Consumption of sugar sweetened beverages, artificially sweetened beverages, and fruit juice and incidence of type 2 diabetes: Systematic review, meta-analysis, and estimation of population attributable fraction. *Br. Med. J.* **2015**, *351*, h3576. [CrossRef] [PubMed]

46. Capewell, S.; Lloyd-Williams, F. Promotion of healthy food and beverage purchases: Are subsidies and consumer education sufficient? *Lancet Public Health* **2017**, *2*, e59–e60. [CrossRef]

47. World Health Organization. Fiscal Policies for Diet and Prevention of Noncommunicable Diseases. In *Proceedings of the Technical Meeting Report, 5–6 May 2015, Geneva, Switzerland*; World Health Organization: Geneva, Switzerland, 2016.

48. Ferguson, M.; O'Dea, K.; Chatfield, M.; Moodie, M.; Altman, J.; Brimblecombe, J. The comparative cost of food and beverages at remote Indigenous communities, Northern Territory, Australia. *Aust. N. Z. J. Public Health* **2016**, *40*, S21–S26. [CrossRef]

49. Hawkes, C. Sales promotion and food consumption. *Nutr. Rev.* **2009**, *67*, 333–342. [CrossRef] [PubMed]

50. Waterlander, W.; de Boer, M.; Schuit, A.; Seidell, J.; Steenhuis, I. Price discounts significantly enhance fruit and vegetable purchases when combined with nutrition education: A randomized controlled supermarket trial. *Am. J. Clin. Nutr.* **2013**, *97*, 886–895. [CrossRef] [PubMed]

51. Waterlander, W.E.; Ni Mhurchu, C.; Steenhuis, I. Effects of a price increase on purchases of sugar sweetened beverages. Results from a randomized controlled trial. *Appetite* **2014**, *78*, 32–39. [CrossRef] [PubMed]

52. Colchero, M.A.; Popkin, B.M.; Rivera, J.A.; Ng, S.W. Beverage purchases from stores in Mexico under the excise tax on sugar sweetened beverages: Observational study. *Br. Med. J.* **2016**, *352*, h6704. [CrossRef]

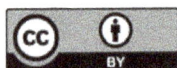

International Journal of
*Environmental Research
and Public Health*

MDPI

Commentary

Re-Evaluating Expertise: Principles for Food and Nutrition Security Research, Advocacy and Solutions in High-Income Countries

Danielle Gallegos [1,2,*] and Mariana M. Chilton [3]

1   School of Exercise and Nutrition Sciences, Queensland University of Technology; Brisbane 4059, Australia
2   Center for Children's Health Research, Institute of Health and Biomedical Innovation, Queensland
     University of Technology, Brisbane 4101, Australia
3   Department of Health Management and Policy, Dornsife School of Public Health, Drexel University,
     Philadelphia, PA 19104, USA; mmc33@drexel.edu
*   Correspondence: danielle.gallegos@qut.edu.au; Tel.: +61-7-3138-5799

Received: 7 December 2018; Accepted: 13 February 2019; Published: 15 February 2019

Abstract: Drawing on examples from Australia and the United States, we outline the benefits of sharing expertise to identify new approaches to food and nutrition security. While there are many challenges to sharing expertise such as discrimination, academic expectations, siloed thinking, and cultural differences, we identify principles and values that can help food insecurity researchers to improve solutions. These principles are critical consciousness, undoing white privilege, adopting a rights framework, and engaging in co-creation processes. These changes demand a commitment to the following values: acceptance of multiple knowledges, caring relationships, humility, empathy, reciprocity, trust, transparency, accountability, and courage.

Keywords: food and nutrition security; research; values; co-creation; trauma-informed

1. Introduction

Food insecurity is a symptom of our social, economic, political, and ecological systems in crisis. Hunger is not due to a lack of food production or availability but rather to the unequal and unjust distribution of people's entitlements to social and economic support [1]. The economically, politically, and socially powerful also control access to food and conditions under which food is available, effectively limiting the capabilities of others. These crises have at their root the continued legacy of colonization and the overarching neoliberal principles of the market economy and personal responsibility. These conditions perpetuate the structural and social institutions that undermine individual and collective agency. The result for people who are low-income is limited access to healthy food and other basic needs such as safe and affordable housing, utilities, gainful employment, and opportunities for political and civic participation.

Rising obesity rates across all social strata, overall low breastfeeding rates, and continued disparities in food insecurity point to systems failures and to inadequate approaches to improve nutrition and food security. Included in these failures is the lack of engagement with appropriate experts with lived experience. Experts from dominant classes have become adept at aligning with powerful authorities in order to interpret and translate complex issues into "health-speak" while viewing people who lack income as passive recipients of expert nutrition and financial knowledge. In high-income countries a primary response to food and nutrition insecurity has been the growth of the charitable food sector, while government and public support for adequate wages and entitlements to basic needs, adequate means for earning money, and a publicly funded safety net have been receding or are under threat [2–4]. The lack of success in addressing food and nutrition insecurity indicates that there is a serious gap between supposed knowledge sitting with the "experts" from academia, law, non-governmental organizations (NGOs), corporations, and other arenas of social and political power, and the realities of people who struggle with food insecurity. This gap is an indication that experts with financial resources and power do not truly understand the causes and experiences of food insecurity, and thereby promote solutions that are misplaced or inadequate.

While there are many examples of people with lived experiences with poverty and food insecurity that are active in academia in a way that informs their work and strengthens their approaches, the academic research community overall has failed to effectively work with and learn from people who have lived experience in a manner that can promote lasting change [5,6]. Though there are several inspiring exceptions such as The Food Action Research Centre (FoodArc) in Nova Scotia, Canada and the Poverty and the Social Exclusion Program in the United Kingdom, the tendency in the academic study of food insecurity is to drown out, exclude, or marginalize the experiences of people with lived experience [7–9]. Additionally, those with lived experience with food insecurity within academia can help to lead the way for researchers and others, yet due to potential stigma and structural barriers, they may not be willing to do so [10]. As there are growing numbers of people who have experienced poverty and also report food insecurity during college years [11,12], engaging with people with lived experiencing in food insecurity in all arenas will strengthen and inform solutions that have otherwise been lacking.

We encourage researchers, policy makers and non-profit organizations to ensure that the lived experience and wisdom of those who experience food and nutrition insecurity, including those in academia and other professional occupations, are central in the conceptualization of food and nutrition security challenges and solutions. We identify some challenges for doing so. Focusing our efforts on governments, social services agencies, NGO's, and civil society (rather than on public private partnerships that engage the corporate sector) we characterize ways in which experts of all kinds can work together to identify the local, regional and national solutions that lead to effective nutrition and food security.

This paper emerges from research undertaken by the authors working in different paradigms (nutrition and anthropology) with individuals and communities that are economically oppressed which include but are not limited to; indigenous peoples, migrants and refugees, and those experiencing hunger, poverty, and trauma. We acknowledge that we are both white and privileged; and that we are products of and operate within the colonialist structures of education, health and welfare. Our context likely limits our viewpoints and clouds our own understanding of what we have learned so far about solutions to food insecurity. We outline here what we hope can be the beginning of a dialogue about our own limitations and the limitations of the research community. We start with our experiences in addressing poverty and food insecurity through our lenses as people who have had the privilege to work with families and communities that have experienced food and nutrition insecurity. Gallegos has worked as a public health nutritionist among Torres Strait and Pacific Islander communities, migrant and refugee communities, and marginalized youth in Australia. Chilton has worked with the Southern Cheyenne and Arapaho tribes in the United States and with caregivers of young children participating in public assistance in the United States who are primarily African American and Latinx.

First, we identify the significance of working in partnership with experts with lived experience of food insecurity, we then address the challenges to collaboration and co-creation, and finally we describe the necessary principles and values that can help to drive potential solutions.

2. Examples and Insights on Benefits of Shared Expertise

We are aware that there are many types of programs that have partnered with people who know food insecurity and hunger first-hand with indigenous groups, farmers and community activists [13,14]. However, in the interest of utilizing our own experiences as grounding for our conviction that partnership is key, we focus on specific examples from Australia and the United States. The Australian example provides insight into how co-creation of solutions can be developed in programs already prescribed by health and political structures. It could be argued that the solutions developed in this program were expedient and immediate, framed by the structures in which the program was embedded. The U.S. example demonstrates the additional step around developing capacity for political action that go to root causes of food insecurity such as violence and discrimination, and the systems that perpetuate these dynamics.

2.1. Australia

Good Food for New Arrivals (GFNA) was a nutrition intervention program funded by the Commonwealth Department of Health through the national child nutrition program and the Department of Family and Community Services from 2001 to 2008 [15,16]. The original aim of GFNA was not to address food and nutrition security but rather to develop nutrition resources to "educate" newly arrived refugee families about nutrition within the western context. Originally the program set out to change what were unhealthy food choices as determined by nutrition and health promotion professionals. Rather than rely on this second-hand knowledge, the program undertook a community participatory approach that engaged members of identified communities (South Sudanese, Hazara Afghani, African 'Grand Lacs' (Democratic Republic of Congo, Rwanda, Burundi), Iraqi and Iranian [17]. Community members identified iron deficiency, poor appetite in children, food safety and foods appropriate for school as key issues. GFNA was also the first program to identify that food and nutrition insecurity was an issue for refugees settling in Australia with 70% of households running out of money for food [18]. Over the program's duration GFNA developed a set of resources that addressed multiple issues identified by both communities and health professionals. However, an evaluability assessment of the program identified that the underlying funding premise was that refugees were "doing something wrong". After engagement with communities GFNA identified that the deficits lay within the infrastructural constraints of the system and with health professionals [19]. This realization led to the identification of a broader range of activities including the development of nutrition champions from within communities and influencing system changes such as the speed at which welfare payments were processed on arrival. The examples of the reasons for running out of food clearly demonstrated a link to trauma and adverse childhood events and included: high medical costs associated with amputation due to a landmine, having family back in the country of origin and feeling guilty about eating, and also moving from having no food to having some food [18].

2.2. United States

Witnesses to Hunger (Witnesses) is an ongoing participatory action program that works with women who know hunger first-hand to increase their meaningful participation in the national dialogue on poverty. Witnesses began in Philadelphia in 2008 with 42 mothers of young children that then expanded to multiple cities to reach over 100 participants. Most members of Witnesses were eager to share their experiences of poverty, their ideas on ways to overcome it, and to inform key decision-makers about the importance of improving labor laws, neighborhood zoning codes, education, tax and labor policies, and to recognize the true value of each person, of motherhood, childhood, and family struggle. Utilizing a human rights approach where the rights-holders participate in shaping the problem, challenges, and solutions, members of Witnesses to Hunger have not only contributed to ethnographic and qualitative research, but also mounted over 30 exhibits of their photographs in locations such as the US Senate, the US House of Representatives, city halls and state houses for audiences that include elected officials, federal, city and state agency administrators, community leaders, the press and the lay public [20,21]. Exhibits also include public forums, hearings and formal testimonies with elected officials. In addition to exhibits, policy briefs, individual and group visits to elected officials, members of Witnesses launched their own blog series and developed a social media presence. They speak at conferences and have co-authored scholarly publications and newspaper opinion essays that demand focus on root causes of food insecurity such as violence (institutional racism, community violence, interpersonal violence, and policy violence), discrimination, and inadequate health and welfare systems.

2.3. Benefits and Insights

From these two case studies of co-creation and mutual engagement, there emerged four significant insights: (1) solutions should recognize personal and collective agency and seek to promote freedom and opportunity; (2) complex issues are dependent on policy change across interlocking systems, and solutions therefore need to be broadly conceptualized across and not within systems (e.g., political, health, economic, welfare); (3) root causes as identified by experts with lived experience should inform the solutions; (4) and co-creation efforts require building trust and transparency.

First, the immediate solutions usually generated by researchers and advocates alike are those that are "top-down" that view the food insecure person, family or community as passive recipients of assistance. For example, many researchers suggest that if we improve public nutrition assistance programming, or seek to improve other aspects of the safety net such as improving access to housing vouchers or healthcare, people's lives will improve [22–24]. This was the case for GFNA, although there was an intent to build capacity in developing "nutrition champions", the onus was on improving access to the elements of the current "broken" system. This system was filled with delays in getting access to income and food resulting in an increased reliance on individuals and organizations to fill the gap. The engagement with Witnesses identified that policy solutions needed to go beyond simply "improving the safety net." Members of Witnesses viewed the safety net as an untrustworthy system that remains broken, inadequate, and undesirable. Members of Witnesses did not want to receive more government assistance; rather, they had a strong desire for freedom and opportunity in developing more entrepreneurship, improving access to education for themselves and their children, and to safe neighborhoods which included ridding their neighborhoods of drug dealers and users, and greater investment in public services such as improved playgrounds, blight alleviation, garbage pickup, and other opportunities for neighborhood improvements.

Secondly, GFNA and Witnesses identified that food and nutrition security was not just the remit of a single system but involved policy change across systems. Food and nutrition security are not simply about lack of food but are an indication of a failure of income, housing and health systems to deliver. Members of Witnesses were eager to learn about how to shape policy. Yet, as training was provided to those who were interested in advocating for solutions, the members quickly discovered that available policy solutions were too siloed. They preferred approaches to be more holistic. For instance, they saw a direct relationship between the trade-offs of paying for food and housing, and therefore, they wanted to advocate for programs that incentivized higher paying jobs and entrepreneurship, so people could pay for their own food and market rate rents. Their frustration with the official policy process was tangible, and they have mostly abandoned standard policy-related solutions and turned their attention to more home-grown solutions that involve neighborhood clean-ups, clothing exchanges, and improved access to local housing.

Thirdly, members of Witnesses have insisted that food insecurity was *not* their most significant issue; whereas, exposure to violence and lack of safety were the central problems that tied all other problems together [21,25]. This was also evident for GFNA. But despite the program being sponsored by a torture and trauma agency, food and nutrition was effectively compartmentalized away from these issues. For Witnesses however, the insistence on the importance of safety led the research team into a new area of research and policy focus on exposure to violence and trauma [26,27]. With this new knowledge about the centrality of trauma and adversity, and the need for individual and collective resilience and, holistic, group-oriented approaches to social services, the research team developed a new intervention effort called the Building Wealth and Health Network (The Network). The Network works with caregivers of young children through a trauma-informed peer support approach (to address exposure to violence), financial empowerment education and new savings accounts, where people's savings are doubled (to address economic insecurity) [28,29]. The Network has reduced the odds of economic insecurity and improved mental health and income. Without that intentional and long-term engagement and magnanimous expertise of members of Witnesses, they would never have been able to develop effective solutions.

Finally, while GFNA undertook a participatory approach and there was recognition of individual and collective agency, the capabilities of community members were not fully realized. On reflection, part of this was a failure of those in power to fully trust experts with lived experience and their conceptualization of the issues and the solutions. This lack of trust often masqueraded as lack of time to develop partnerships, difficulty in engaging individuals and communities, as well as empathy regarding the overwhelming number of issues community members faced. The project officers undertook a wide range of activities and advocacy on behalf of the community members [15,16]. On the flip-side, GFNA was one of the first projects to employ members of the community as project consultants in order to provide cultural and experiential expertise (previously community members were expected to volunteer their services). In Witnesses to Hunger, the long-standing nature of the relationship between members of Witnesses (primarily Black and Latinx women) and the research team (racially diverse, with majority white leadership in terms of funding and decision-making) engendered some feelings of mutual trust and accountability, especially as all engagement by members of Witnesses was treated as professional work for which members were paid market-rate wages and honoraria. However, partnering across racial barriers and the spoken memory of generations of mistrust, misunderstanding, and oppression among black women by white women has generated ongoing challenges that bring to light questions about racism, leadership, and misaligned priorities, mission and goals.

Throughout both of these examples of partnered research it is clear that the best solutions are not simply based in science and standard empirical evidence, but also in what Maria Miess asserts is the wisdom that comes from experience and struggle [30].

3. Challenges of Sharing Expertise and Co-Creation of Solutions

There are many challenges to sharing expertise among traditional, highly educated and well-resourced experts (this includes those with lived experience that adopt a traditional scientific approach) and experts who have lived experience and who do not share the tools, resources and power of academia. These include the refusal to look at food insecurity as related to social factors such as (1) historical and contemporary racism and discrimination, (2) the culture of academia, (3) siloed thinking, and (4) marginalization and cultural differences in meaning.

3.1. Historical and Contemporary Racism and Discrimination

Our first challenge to overcome is our lack of willingness to identify the discriminatory social structures that cause poverty, deprivation, and trauma. As a single example among so many for African Americans, in 1898 with the publication of the Philadelphia Negro, sociologist William Edward Burghardt Du Bois identified how the struggles within the black community—poor health, unemployment and deplorable living conditions—are due to racial segregation. These directly stem from a socially constructed racial hierarchy that isolates, segregates and disenfranchises black people. He asserted that segregation and discrimination results in devastating poverty. The 1968 Kerner Commission Report described that the single most important issue for the struggles of African American people in terms of housing, poor nutrition, poor health, and low educational attainment in the United States is that whites systematically discriminate against and marginalize people of color [31], for example in its municipal, city, state and regional housing policies, in media coverage, and in general American society. Yet nutrition and food security researchers in the United States continuously ignore the dynamics of racism and discrimination that underlie poverty. Against this backdrop, it is only in the past few years that researchers in nutrition are beginning to call out discrimination and lack of equity as significant to the experience of food insecurity, obesity, and other nutrition-related conditions. The multiple forms of discrimination and oppression (systemic, interpersonal, structural, historical, etc.) are difficult to measure, and often do not fit in a simple model, yet researchers have begun to identify how lifetime, historical and systemic exposure to racism as associated with food and nutrition insecurity [32–34].

Australia has also demonstrated repeated failure to significantly address the blatant harms caused by discrimination. The same year as the Kerner Commission, William Edward Hanley Stanner delivered the nationally acclaimed Boyer Lecture "The Great Australian Silence" which argued that the history of invasion and the theft of lands and the genocide of Aboriginal and Torres Strait Islanders has been ignored [35]. Since this time, the Australian state has generally continued to ignore harms committed against Indigenous peoples [36]. In 2008 the Closing the Gap initiative was launched following a Social Justice report identifying serious inequity in health and life expectancy between Indigenous and white people. For instance, there are much higher mortality rates among Indigenous infants, and Indigenous men are dying more than 10 years earlier than their white counterparts [37]. Clearly, Australian health professionals failed to address the underlying structural power imbalances, intergenerational trauma and racism contributing to poor health [38,39]. Over time, nutrition researchers have all highlighted the inequalities related to food and nutrition for Aboriginal and Torres Strait Islander peoples and have identified the role of colonialism on the quantity and quality of food for Indigenous communities [40–43]. However, most are still describing the problem rather than identifying the root causes, that is, institutionalized racism, discrimination, poverty and marginalization.

3.2. Culture of Academia

The culture of academia and the legacy of western European influences in scientific investigation creates blind spots that allow for scientists to ignore or obfuscate how discrimination shapes economic insecurity, illness and health. The definition of food insecurity itself—the lack of access to enough food for an active and healthy life due to economic circumstances [44]—lacks connection to social and political circumstances such as lack of access to living wages, lack of political power of people who are low-income, and to discrimination and exclusion. An improved definition would draw attention to context behind "economic circumstances" to include concepts of "economic exploitation" and "marginalization" that demonstrate how food insecurity is a concept that is in relationship to societal dynamics. Despite Krieger's 1994 call to action for epidemiologists to move beyond biomedical individualism to acknowledge how health and disease have their roots in history, social relationships and political structures [45], food insecurity research published in English language research journals has been mired in the risk-exposure binary that still dominates health research. As Zuberi and Bonilla-Silva assert, researchers continue to ignore the large societal conditions that drive poor health and poor nutrition, and ignore their own place in perpetuating those conditions [46].

Most research and funding for research emanates from universities, well-resourced public policy centers, and from government sources, where a majority of people who are carrying out the research, making funding decisions, and generating research questions and methods are people without lived experience, and who do not see how the systems in which they are involved (i.e., education and government) are perpetuating poverty. While it is common knowledge in research circles that among food insecurity and poverty researchers there are people who have lived experiences with poverty, it is unclear how many there are, as this has not been previously studied or counted, and it is possible that such researchers would not readily describe these experiences due to real and perceived stigma as mentioned above. The culture of academia could also improve to be more accepting and inclusive of research scientists with lived experiences to help deepen understanding of the experiences and emphasize the importance of innovative approaches grounded in experience. Class, race and gender inequities are not solely among individual researchers, but are also built into institutional practices. As an example, universities and health systems have a long history of causing gentrification that further isolates people of color and people who are poor from mainstream resources [47]. Additionally, scientific methods demand strict definition of measurable problems, and center around testing of hypotheses of limited measures of covariates and outcomes. The pressures of producing peer reviewed research to establish academic credibility, and incentives for promotion in academia that utilize metrics unrelated to impact or how much engagement and authentic collaboration there is with research participants both work to devalue, isolate or discourage participatory research. Additionally, there is little to no incentive or recognition of the intensive time and trust building processes necessary for effective participatory research [48]. Overall the glorification of mainstream science and the pressures of academia to publish scientific research prioritize only one way of knowing about social problems such as food insecurity. This has led to a lack of appreciation for lived experience and wisdom from the streets, the farm, the reservation, and the neighborhood.

Qualitative researchers may view themselves as less engaged in research that ignores broader contexts of discrimination and inequality. However, we argue that most qualitative research still relies on a one-way process that extracts stories and experience from people who have lived experience, that generally enhances the investigator's career through publishing books and articles, while those studied remain unseen, without political power, economic security, and legal recourse. We suggest that research move beyond the relatively simple process of gathering insight and stories from individuals and groups, and move into the co-creation of understanding and move to mutual problem solving in partnership. There are strong traditions from which to draw, such as action research by Sol Tax, applied anthropology, critical participatory action research [49–51], and indigenous methodologies where knowing and knowledge is built through relationality via yarning circles (Australian) [52], *talanoa* (Pacific/Maori) [53]. These methodologies are conversational techniques that involve the sharing of stories. They have at their core equal respectful engagement and the co-creation of knowledge [54].

3.3. Siloed Thinking

Reducing health inequalities and addressing social determinants of health requires greater integration across government and civil society. Sir Michael Marmot and colleagues have identified that action however is limited by organizational boundaries and "siloes" [55] (p. 86). Additionally, in most neoliberal high-income countries, funding streams are aligned with discrete government agencies that are based on outdated systems. In the US, it is well known that funding streams cannot be easily merged or braided together without acts of Congress. Even when federal agencies seek to work together, there becomes a territoriality of concern regarding programs where agency leaders are afraid of losing funding if they share some of their funding with other programs [22,56]. In Australia and the UK there is strong rhetoric about "whole-of-government" approaches for persistent social and environmental challenges. However, the three primary barriers for horizontal governance or "joined-up" government are identified as: a deeply entrenched program focus based on funding streams that remain siloed, centralized decision-making that undermine devolved decision-making, and the reliance on co-locating services rather than adjusting the underlying operating systems [57,58]. Overall, this siloed thinking is what Rebecca Costa refers to as a "super meme"—a way of thinking that is simply accepted despite the fact that it is irrational—that stymies innovative action to solve society's most intractable problems such as hunger [59].

3.4. Marginalization and Cultural Differences in Meaning

The poor are marginalized or excluded by multiple systems such as zoning laws, school funding laws (as in the US), higher education discrimination, housing discrimination, as well as the systems of academic inquiry. An example of this is how from the perspective of academic researchers, sex workers, people who are homeless, or people who are "disconnected" from public welfare programs are considered "hard to reach" because of recruitment methods that have limited timeframes during the day, extensive costs to the individuals, and inadequate community engagement [60]. Additionally, food insecurity researchers tend to look at food insecurity over a short period of time, usually in cross-sectional studies, or in a one-two year time frame, with a few exceptions. Yet some groups have a very different view. Indigenous peoples may view their experiences with hunger and ill-health as stemming from times of genocide of their peoples and through ongoing injustices of broken treaty rights (where treaties exist) or failure to recognize sovereignty through constitutional reform [61,62]. Additionally, they may consider hunger to be an issue consistent with the violation of their sovereignty and the rights of nature [63].

4. New Principles for Food and Nutrition Security Research

While the challenges mentioned above are serious, they can be overcome through new ways of thinking about our work, and through adopting core principles and values. Developing solutions for food and nutrition insecurity, particularly when the issue involves marginalized groups in high-income countries. New approaches require a change in mindset and in our ways of working. We argue here for a set of core principles and values that should underpin and inform our actions in research and in devising evidence-based solutions. These principles draw from a variety of traditions such as civic agriculture and civic dietetics, trauma-theory, emancipatory education, and indigenous worldviews. Learning from these frameworks we propose four core principles that should guide our work in alleviating household food insecurity: (1) a critical consciousness that requires individuals to constantly question their own and others' positions; (2) working to deconstruct white supremacy; (3) a rights-based approach that ensures engagement with people with lived experience, and (4) actively engaging in co-creation processes where power is shared and all expertise is regarded as meaningful.

4.1. Use Critical Consciousness and Emancipatory Processes That Transgress Boundaries

Critical consciousness lies at the heart of working "inside out" to question perceptions of ourselves, of privilege and of the social and structural institutions that seek to maintain divisions in society. Critical consciousness highlights the need for a reflexive approach (that is not just thinking but also acting) to understand and change inequities in power and privilege. It requires reorientation to a commitment to love for humanity and social justice [64,65]. This raising of consciousness leads to what Freire described as engaged discourse, collaborative problem-solving and a re-humanization of our social relationships. Critical consciousness is required to understand that marginalization is not inherent within an individual but is rather a result of the structural and social forces that create that lived experience [66]. For example, just focusing on the food insecure individual or household locates the marginalized person as "the problem," whereas the problem is located within the social and political context.

While Freire's original conceptualization was focused on those who were experiencing oppression and or marginalization, increasingly it is being applied to all types of participants in social programs including the researcher or those involved in developing and delivering programs [67]. Critical consciousness therefore has three essential elements: critical reflection—an analysis and rejection of the social inequities that limit agency and contribute to poor health and wellbeing; political efficacy—the perceived capacity to effect social and political change individually or collectively; and critical action—the actions taken to change aspects of society that are unjust [68]. Integrating feminist and intersectional approaches is also important to integrate attention to multiple, intersecting identities such as race, gender and sexuality, that consider a whole person approach, and that puts the authority of lived experiences at the center of inquiry. This approach helps all experts involved to transgress boundaries of race, gender, age, class, sexuality and beyond to resist and subvert patriarchal oppression and white supremacy [69]. These practices can be put into action in ongoing nutrition education efforts, participatory action endeavors, and other types of qualitative research efforts. In Witnesses to Hunger, these principles were utilized in every group meeting, where members were invited to explore from their own experiences how policies fell short, and worked together to identify their ideas for solutions that were then crafted into the exhibits, information booklets, and postcards for bringing along to meetings with legislators. This community self-empowerment education approach is also utilized by the Poverty Truth Commissions that were first established in Scotland and spread to other cities in the UK, currently hosted and promoted by Church Action on Poverty [70,71].

4.2. Utilize an Anti-Oppression Framework and a Trauma-Informed Lens

An anti-oppression framework is one that seeks to undo the effects of oppression, oppose the roots of all forms of oppression, and to adopt an emancipatory approach to social change. Anti-oppressive practice has penetrated a variety of fields, and became most highly developed in social work practice and psychology, where attention to breaking down status quo definitions of identity, eliminating boundaries of social division based on gender, race, ethnicity, age, and other identities can help to improve the therapeutic relationship as well as bring about societal change. The approach also seeks to call attention to power differentials in our relationships. An anti-oppressive approach demands not only the practice of actively seeking to ensure we do not oppress others, but also to continuously recognize our own roles in perpetuating our privilege and power that can lead to oppression. This means actively taking a decolonization stance, employing approaches and methodologies that disrupt and reverse the ongoing exploitation and subjugation of people who have been marginalized, excluded and oppressed [9,53].

The intergenerational and interpersonal trauma associated with colonialism and imperialism and the vast arrays of "isms" and phobias such as racism, sexism, ableism, classism, homophobia, and xenophobia, can be acknowledged and addressed in our everyday actions and in our policy proposals. Trauma informed practice realizes the widespread impact of trauma, and pathways to recovery, recognizes symptoms of trauma in clients, participants, families, staff, systems, and in ourselves, responds to fully integrate trauma-knowledge to improve and inform policies procedures and practices, and actively resists re-traumatization [72]. Given decades of evidence that exposure to violence such as intimate partner violence, child abuse, neglect and other adverse childhood experiences, suicide attempts and ideation, and post-traumatic stress disorder are strongly associated with household food insecurity [26], taking a trauma-informed lens to co-creating solutions is fundamentally important.

A trauma-informed approach to self-organization was essential in the methods of Witnesses to Hunger [21], and later created the foundation of The Building Wealth and Health Network [73], which significantly reduced food insecurity. Other trauma-informed approaches are being integrated throughout many school districts across the United States [74,75], and there are more calls for trauma-informed policy-making [76,77].

4.3. Utilize a Human Rights Approach

The right to food and to be free from hunger are fundamental human rights in the Universal Declaration of Human Rights and in the International Covenant on Economic, Social and Cultural Rights (ICESCR). It incorporates being able to have access to culturally appropriate and healthy food in order to live a healthy and fulfilling life without fear. Viewing food security as a human rights issue means that good nutrition should not be left to benevolence or charity, relegated to the remit of the charitable food sector. Instead food security should be respected, protected, and fulfilled by governments and NGOs to promote the health, security, and wellbeing of all people [78,79]. In order to advance the right to food, it is necessary to ensure that there is a national plan to respect, protect, and fulfil the right to food, and a comprehensive approach to ensure participation of many stakeholders (especially those who are most affected by food insecurity), in the development of solutions, as well as for redress and repair when the right to food is violated. Having a national measurement mechanism for monitoring and accountability is essential. The governments of Australia, UK and New Zealand (among others) fail to regularly monitor food insecurity and issues related to access and provision of food. This keeps comprehensive solutions to food and nutrition insecurity unknown or ad hoc. While national monitoring is not the only way to get started with a human rights approach, it can help to provide information and empirical evidence for monitoring and evaluation of interventions.

Adopting a rights framework is a key tenet of the recommended approach to ensure:

- Solutions ensure equitable access to nutritious food regardless of one's circumstances;

- Solutions move beyond charitable approaches to those that address capabilities and enhance individual freedoms to achieve health and wellbeing;
- Trauma and stigma are not inflicted or exacerbated and healing opportunities that build resilience are integrated into food-related programming;
- Food sovereignty is respected and promoted;
- Policy development does not exacerbate inequalities or contravene other human rights in recognition that all human rights are universal, inalienable, indivisible, interdependent and interconnected;
- Rights holders have a central role in bringing about solutions.

Advancing human rights, and the right to food is very challenging. This is especially true in high income countries such as Australia and the United States, where there are major cultural assumptions by a powerful elite that trivialize and downplay the importance of economic and social rights [3,78,80]. Additionally, the focus on food, rather than on the social, economic and political conditions that cause food insecurity limit the understanding and adoption of the rights framework. The emphasis on charitable food provision, the slow dismantling of an already inadequate social security safety net, and reliance on "trickle-down" economics to alleviate poverty are serious obstacles to helping civil society adopt a rights framework and to demand right to food [78,81,82]. Despite these challenges, if the research and advocacy communities in high income countries could begin to adopt a broader justice framework, and promote such solutions among advocates, the press, and policy-makers, it can help support the current efforts of civil society to ensure people can be empowered to demand their right to food, and to health and wellbeing. Efforts such as the Participation and the Practice of Rights (PPR) in Northern Ireland, Detroit Black Community Food Security Network and the Southern Rural Black Women's Initiative for Economic and Social Justice (SRBWI) and other organizations of the US Human Rights Network, the international campaign La Via Campesina which advocates for food sovereignty, and the Right to Food Coalition in Australia, are just a few of many examples where economic social and cultural rights are being advanced by civil society despite the above-listed challenges. The research community has much to learn from these ongoing efforts.

4.4. Seek Co-Creation of Problems and Solutions

There is growing recognition in research circles that there needs to be a different paradigm of knowledge production [83] and a fundamental shift from privileging experimental expertise to experiential expertise [84]. Characterizing problems from the perspective of the scientific "expert" is using knowledge as a form of "discursive power in ways that privilege some definitions of health and social problems and marginalize others" [85]. If change is to occur, those in positions of knowledge "expert" status need to reorient their inquiries from describing the problem to research that seeks to understand the effectiveness of interventions [85].

In undertaking collective processes of inquiry, empowerment and action, the experimental and experiential experts need to work to remove power differentials and utilize their respective strengths to co-create a mutual understanding of: the life-world, the dispositions and aspirations of those who live in that life-world, the problem as socially-constructed and the solutions that will be best fit in that context [86]. In taking this approach we agree with other scholars that it is no longer possible or ethical to separate the "research" from the ensuing policy discussion. In the case of food and nutrition security the understanding of the problem and the solutions requires both experimental and experiential experts to lend their voices to ongoing policy discussions [49,85]. Indeed as Fine indicates, "it is the obligation of the scholar to not only expose social injustice but to transform unjust conditions" [49] (p. 116). Examples of such co-creation are efforts by Witnesses to Hunger, and the Poverty and the Social Exclusion in the United Kingdom research project funded by the Economic and Social Research Council consisting of collaboration between the University of Bristol (lead), Heriot-Watt

University, The Open University, Queen's University Belfast, University of Glasgow and the University of York [8,87].

5. Values for Sharing Expertise and Co-Creation

Underpinning the principles are a set of underlying values informing approaches to researching and programming for food security. Table 1 characterizes the values that inform this process and help to create an ethos of action that questions the status quo, empowers partnership development and makes use of different forms of expertise. These qualities require self and political awareness.

Table 1. Underlying Values for Sharing Expertise.

Value	Description
Knowledges	Recognize that knowledge comes in a variety of forms and is not limited to book learning and the scientific method. Different forms of knowledge extend to different forms of expertise. Each participant brings a unique set of expertise to problem identification and solution creation that can be brought together to construct new knowledge.
Relationships	Build relationships that are genuine and long-lasting. These relationships need to be built on trust, reciprocity and an understanding of and explicit attention to differences that create power inequities.
Humility	For those with the power, education and privilege it is essential that we express an understanding of how our unearned privilege and societal rank limits our skill sets, and that these skills are not necessarily better than those of others. Coming to the work with humility and a beginner's mind helps to undo power differentials based on education, gender, sexual orientation, economic resources, race, class, cultural background and spiritual beliefs.
Empathy	Build a powerful imagination in order to understand the life situations of others in order to be able to respond to social inequities. Empathy requires an understanding of the differences between self and other and an ability to understand and relate to another's perspective, emotion and experience.
Reciprocity	Exchange material resources, ideas, social obligations and power for mutual benefit. Reciprocity is fundamentally steeped in conceptualizing balance and an interconnectedness across time and space. Reciprocity requires giving and receiving.
Trust	Trust is premised on respect, transparency, accountability and reciprocity. There needs to be mutual trust in the process and outcomes of the co-creation of knowledge and solutions.
Transparency and accountability	Recognize that there are mutual accountabilities for individuals and organizations. There may be accountabilities to education institutions, funders and donors, political ideologies, families, communities, and cultural traditions. There will be tensions between these accountabilities but in order for trust to develop transactions and encounters need to be transparent. In this way the primary accountability is to social change and to the disruption of institutional and social structures that maintain inequity.
Courage	Understand that to work in a different way, to be politically active and to challenge the status quo takes self-knowledge, fearlessness and a willingness to be vulnerable and uncomfortable.

These values transcend any one field of study and action and can provide some grounding to to continue to address the challenges of racism and discrimination, the limited culture of academia, siloed thinking, and marginalization and cultural differences in meaning and time horizons.

6. Conclusions

Co-creation of solutions and sharing expertise across boundaries of race, class, education level, gender and age are beneficial and necessary for devising meaningful, effective and lasting changes in food and nutrition insecurity. The co-creation of solutions on food and nutrition insecurity will however not come easily. The challenges of racism and discrimination, the culture of academia, our siloed thinking, and cultural differences will consistently be in the backdrop of our efforts, and may actively get in the way of creating and then implementing solutions. We propose here some organizing principles and values to help overcome these challenges. Without actively engaging with these, researchers may be perpetuating inequality and injustices that drive poor nutrition and health. Embracing multiple forms of knowledge, humility and courage, among many other values, may be difficult and unrewarded currently in our own spheres. Yet we suggest that the rewards of improving food and nutrition insecurity for millions far outweighs the discomfort many of us might have with shaking up and altering our ways of doing. We invite the rest of the food insecurity research community, especially those with lived experience, to weigh in on these principles and values, and we hope they will join us in establishing a shared international consensus for co-creating solutions that promote the right to food, and promote health and wellbeing for all.

Author Contributions: D.G. and M.M.C. contributed equally to this manuscript.

Funding: This research received no external funding.

Conflicts of Interest: The authors declare no conflict of interest.

References

1. Sen, A. Ingredients of famine analysis: Availability and entitlements. *Q. J. Econ.* **1981**, *96*, 433–464. [CrossRef] [PubMed]
2. Fisher, A. *Big Hunger: The Unholy Alliance Between Corporate America and Anti-Hunger Groups*; MIT Press: Cambridge, MA, USA, 2017.
3. Riches, G. *Food Bank Nations: Poverty, Corporate Charity and the Right to Food*; Routledge: London, UK, 2018.
4. Caraher, M.; Furey, S. Growth of food banks in the UK (and Europe): Leftover food for leftover people. In *The Economics of Emergency Food Aid Provision: A Financial, Social and Cultural Perspective*; Palgrave Pivot: London, UK, 2018; pp. 25–48.
5. Cale, G. Confessions Of A Poverty-Class Academic-In-Training. Available online: https://conditionallyaccepted.com/2015/09/01/workingclass-pt1/ (accessed on 15 January 2019).
6. Sarcozona, Poverty in the Ivory Tower, in Tenure, She Wrote. Available online: https://tenureshewrote.wordpress.com/2014/01/16/succeeding-in-graduate-school-despite-poverty/ (accessed on 15 January 2019).
7. Food Action Resource Center. Food ARC: Research Inspiring Change. Available online: https://foodarc.ca/ (accessed on 17 January 2019).
8. Poverty and Social Exclusion. PSE: Poverty and Social Exclusion, Reporting Research, Examining Policy, Stimulating Debate. Available online: http://www.poverty.ac.uk/ (accessed on 15 January 2019).
9. Smith, L.T. *Decolonizing Methodologies: Research and Indigenous Peoples*; Zed Books Ltd.: New York, NY, USA, 2013.
10. Heller, J.L. The enduring problem of social class stigma experienced by upwardly mobile white academics. *McGill Sociol. Rev.* **2011**, *2*, 19–38.
11. Goldrick-Rab, S.; Richardson, J.; Schneider, J.; Hernandez, A.; Cady, C. *Still Hungry and Homeless in College*; Wisconsin Hope Lab, 2018. Available online: https://hope4college.com/wp-content/uploads/2018/09/Wisconsin-HOPE-Lab-Still-Hungry-and-Homeless.pdf (accessed on 14 February 2019).
12. Gallegos, D.; Ramsey, R.; Ong, K.W. Food insecurity: Is it an issue among tertiary students? *High. Educ.* **2014**, *67*, 497–510. [CrossRef]
13. Activating Change Together for Community Food Security: Knowledge Mobilization Working Group. Knowledge Mobilization in Participatory Action Research: A Synthesis of the Literature. 2014. Available online: https://foodarc.ca/wp-content/uploads/2014/09/ACT-for-CFS-Knowledge-Mobilization-in-PAR-Jan-2014.pdf (accessed on 5 December 2018).
14. White, M. Environmental reviews & case studies: D-town farm: African American resistance to food insecurity and the transformation of Detroit. *Environ. Pract.* **2011**, *13*. [CrossRef]
15. Ellies, P.; Gallegos, D. *Good Food for New Arrivals: Final Report*; Association for Services to Torture and Trauma Survivors and East Metropolitan Population Health Unit: Perth, Australia, 2004.

16. Vicca, N.; Straton, R.; Gallegos, D. *Good Food for New Arrivals: Final Evaluation Report*; Association for Services to Torture and Trauma Survivors and Centre for Social and Community Research, Murdoch University: Perth, Australia, 2009.

17. Gallegos, D.; Ellies, P. Good Food for New Arrivals: A case study of inclusive health practice. In *Settling in Australia: The Social Inclusion of Refugees*; Colic-Peisker, V., Tilbury, F., Eds.; Centre for Social and Community Research, Murdoch University: Perth, Australia, 2007; pp. 97–107.

18. Gallegos, D.; Ellies, P.; Wright, J. Still there's no food! Food in a refugee population in Perth, Western Australia. *Nutr. Diet.* **2008**, *65*, 78–83. [CrossRef]

19. Durham, J.; Gillieatt, S.; Ellies, P. An evaluability assessment of a nutrition promotion project for newly arrived refugees. *Health Promot. J. Aust.* **2007**, *18*, 43–49. [CrossRef]

20. Chilton, M.; Rabinowich, J.; Council, C.; Breaux, J. Witnesses to Hunger: Participation through photovoice to ensure the right to food. *Health Human Rights* **2009**, *11*, 73–86. [CrossRef] [PubMed]

21. Knowles, M.; Rabinowich, J.; Gaines-Turner, T.; Chilton, M. *Witnesses to Hunger: Methods for Photovoice and Participatory Action Research in Public Health*; Human Organization: Oklahoma City, OK, USA, 2015; Volume 74.

22. Bartfeld, J.; Gundersen, C.; Smeeding, T.; Ziliak, J.P. (Eds.) *SNAP Matters: How Food Stamps Affect Health and Well-Being*; Stanford University Press: Stanford, CA, USA, 2015.

23. Sandel, M.C.D.; Meyers, A.; Ettinger de Cuba, S.; Coleman, S.; Black, M.; Casey, P.; Chilton, M.; Cook, J.; Shortell, A.; Heeren, T.; et al. Co-enrollment for child health: How receipt and loss of food and housing subsidies relate to housing security and statutes for streamlined, multi-subsidy application. *J. Appl. Res. Child. Informing Policy Child. Risk* **2014**, *5*, 2.

24. Seligman, H.K.; Berkowitz, S.A. Aligning programs and policies to support food security and public health goals in the United States. *Annu. Rev. Public Health* **2019**, *40*, 2.1–2.19. [CrossRef] [PubMed]

25. Chilton, M.M.; Rabinowich, J.R.; Woolf, N.H. Very low food security in the USA is linked with exposure to violence. *Public Health Nutr.* **2014**, *17*, 73–82. [CrossRef] [PubMed]

26. Sun, J.; Knowles, M.; Patel, F.; Frank, D.A.; Heeren, T.C.; Chilton, M. Childhood adversity and adult reports of food insecurity among households with children. *Am. J. Prevent. Med.* **2016**, *50*, 561–572. [CrossRef] [PubMed]

27. Chilton, M.; Knowles, M.; Bloom, S.L. The intergenerational circumstances of household food insecurity and adversity. *J. Hunger Environ. Nutr.* **2017**, *12*, 269–297. [CrossRef] [PubMed]

28. Booshehri, L.; Dugan, J.; Patel, F.; Bloom, S.; Chilton, M.M. Trauma-informed Temporary Assistance for Needy Families (TANF): A Randomized Controlled Trial with a Two-Generation Impact. *J. Child Family Stud.* **2018**, *27*, 1594–1604. [CrossRef] [PubMed]

29. Sun, J.; Patel, F.; Kirzner, R.; Newton-Famous, N.; Owens, C.; Welles, S.L.; Chilton, M. The Building Wealth and Health Network: Methods and baseline characteristics from a randomized controlled trial for families with young children participating in temporary assistance for needy families (TANF). *BMC Public Health* **2016**, *16*, 583. [CrossRef] [PubMed]

30. Mies, M.; Shiva, V. *Ecofeminism*; Zed Books: London, UK, 2014; 328p.

31. Gillon, S.M. *Separate and Unequal: The Kerner Commission and the Unraveling of American Liberalism*, 1st ed.; Basic Books: New York, NY, USA, 2018; 374p.

32. Kumanyika, S. *Getting to Equity in Obesity Prevention: A New Framework*; National Academy of Medicine: Washington, DC, USA, 2017.

33. Odoms-Young, A.; Bruce, M.A. Examining the impact of structural racism on food insecurity: Implications for addressing racial/ethnic disparities. *Family Community Health* **2018**, *41* (Suppl. 2), S3–S6. [CrossRef] [PubMed]

34. Burke, M.P.; Jones, S.J.; Frongillo, E.A.; Fram, M.S.; Blake, C.E.; Freedman, D.A. Severity of household food insecurity and lifetime racial discrimination among African-American households in South Carolina. *Ethn. Health* **2018**, *23*, 276–292. [CrossRef] [PubMed]

35. Collins, J.; Thompson, W.K. Reconciliation in Australia? Dreaming beyond the cult of forgetfulness. In *Reconciliation in Conflict-Affected Communities: Practices and Insights from the Asia-Pacific*; Jenkins, B., Subedi, D.B., Jenkins, K., Eds.; Springer: Singapore, 2018; pp. 185–206.

36. McMillan, M.; Rigney, S. Race, reconciliation, and justice in Australia: From denial to acknowledgment. *Ethn. Racial Stud.* **2018**, *41*, 759–777. [CrossRef]

37. Deravin, L.; Francis, K.; Anderson, J. Closing the gap in Indigenous health inequity—Is it making a difference? *Int. Nurs. Rev.* **2018**, *4*, 477–483. [CrossRef]

38. Pholi, K. Is' Close the Gap'a useful approach to improving the health and wellbeing of Indigenous Australians? *Aust. Rev. Public Aff.* **2009**, *9*, 1–13.

39. Gannon, M. Indigenous health: Closing the gap-10 year review. *Aust. Med.* **2018**, *30*, 25.

40. Gracey, M. Historical, cultural, political, and social influences on dietary patterns and nutrition in Australian Aboriginal children. *Am. J. Clin. Nutr.* **2000**, *72*, 1361S–1367S. [CrossRef] [PubMed]

41. McDermott, R.; O'Dea, K.; Rowley, K.; Knight, S.; Burgess, P. Beneficial impact of the Homelands Movement on health outcomes in Central Australian Aborigines. *Aust. N. Z. J. Public Health* **1998**, *22*, 653–658. [CrossRef] [PubMed]

42. Brimblecombe, J.; Maypilama, E.; Colles, S.; Scarlett, M.; Dhurrkay, J.G.; Ritchie, J.; O'Dea, K. Factors influencing food choice in an Australian Aboriginal community. *Qual. Health Res.* **2014**, *24*, 387–400. [CrossRef] [PubMed]

43. Lee, A.J.; Leonard, D.; Moloney, A.A.; Minniecon, D.L. Improving Aboriginal and Torres strait islander nutrition and health. *Med. J. Aust.* **2009**, *190*, 547–548. [PubMed]

44. Bickel, G.; Nord, M.; Price, C.; Hamilton, W.; Cook, J. *Measuring Food Security in the United States: Guide to Measuring Household Food Security*; US Department of Agriculture, Food and Nutrition Service, Office of Analysis and Evaluation: Alexandria, VA, USA, 2000.

45. Krieger, N. Epidemiology and the web of causation: Has anyone seen the spider? *Soc. Sci. Med.* **1994**, *39*, 887–903. [CrossRef]

46. Zuberi, T.; Bonilla-Silva, E. *White Logic, White Methods: Racism and Methodology*; Rowman & Littlefield Publishers: Lanham, ML, USA, 2008; 416p.

47. Gomez, M.B. *Race, Class, Power, and Organizing in East Baltimore: Rebuilding Abandoned Communities in America*; Lexington Books: Lanham, ML, USA, 2013; 271p.

48. Minkler, M.; Wallerstein, N. *Community-Based Participatory Research for Health: From Process to Outcomes*, 2nd ed.; Jossey-Bass: San Francisco, CA, USA, 2008; 508p.

49. Fine, M. *Just Research in Contentious Times: Widening the Methodological Imagination*; Teachers College Press: New York, NY, USA, 2017.

50. Daubenmier, J.M. *The Meskwaki and Anthropologists: Action Anthropology Reconsidered*; Critical Studies in the History of Anthropology; University of Nebraska Press: Lincoln, RI, USA, 2008; 416p.

51. Bennett, L.A.; Whiteford, L.M.; National Association for the Practice of Anthropology (U.S.). *Anthropology and the Engaged University: New Vision for the Discipline Within Higher Education*; Annals of Anthropological Practice; Wiley Subscription Services, Inc.: Hoboken, NJ, USA, 2013; 204p.

52. Martin, B. Methodology is content: Indigenous approaches to research and knowledge. *Educ. Philos. Theory* **2017**, *49*, 1392–1400. [CrossRef]

53. Suaalii-Sauni, T.; Fulu-Aiolupotea, S.M. Decolonising Pacific research, building Pacific research communities and developing Pacific research tools: The case of the talanoa and the faafaletui in Samoa. *Asia Pac. Viewpoint* **2014**, *55*, 331–344. [CrossRef]

54. Walker, M.; Fredericks, B.; Mills, K.; Anderson, D. "Yarning" as a method for community-based health research with Indigenous women: The Indigenous Women's Wellness Research Program. *Health Care Women Int.* **2014**, *35*, 1216–1226. [CrossRef]

55. Marmot, M. Social determinants of health inequalities. *Lancet* **2005**, *365*, 1099–1104. [CrossRef]

56. Dean, S. Testimony of Stacy Dean, Vice President for Food Assistance Policy Before the House Committee on Agriculture's Subcommittee on Department Operations, Oversight, and Nutrition, O. House Committee on Agriculture's Subcommittee on Department Operations, and Nutrition, Editor. 2014. Available online: https://www.cbpp.org/testimony-of-stacy-dean-vice-president-for-food-assistance-policy-before-the-house-committee-on-0 (accessed on 14 February 2019).

57. O'Flynn, J.; Buick, F.; Blackman, D.; Halligan, J. You win some, you lose some: Experiments with joined-up government. *Int. J. Public Adm.* **2011**, *34*, 244–254. [CrossRef]

58. Carey, G.; Crammond, B.; Keast, R. Creating change in government to address the social determinants of health: How can efforts be improved? *BMC Public Health* **2014**, *14*, 1087. [CrossRef] [PubMed]

59. Costa, R.D. *The Watchman's Rattle: Thinking Our Way Out of Extinction*; Vanguard Press: Philadelphia, PA, USA, 2010; 346p.

60. Bonevski, B.; Randell, M.; Paul, C.; Chapman, K.; Twyman, L.; Bryant, J.; Brozek, I.; Hughes, C. Reaching the hard-to-reach: A systematic review of strategies for improving health and medical research with socially disadvantaged groups. *BMC Med. Res. Methodol.* **2014**, *14*, 42. [CrossRef] [PubMed]

61. Pickering, K.; McShane-Jewell, B.; Brydge, M.; Gilbert, M.; Black Elk, L. *National Commission on Hunger: Invited Written Testimony on Food Insecurity, Plains Indian Tribes, Pine Ridge and Rosebud Indian Reservations, U;* National Commission on Hunger: Washington, DC, USA, 2015. Available online: https://cybercemetery.unt.edu/archive/hungercommission/20151217003520/https://hungercommission.rti.org/Portals/0/SiteHtml/Activities/WrittenTestimony/InvitedWritten/NCH_Invited_Written_Testimony_Kathleen_Pickering.pdf (accessed on 10 November 2018).

62. Jalata, A. The impacts of English colonial terrorism and genocide on Indigenous/black Australians. *SAGE Open* **2013**, *3*, 2158244013499143. [CrossRef]

63. Wittman, H. Food sovereignty: A new rights framework for food and nature? *Environ. Soc. Adv. Res.* **2011**, *2*, 87–105.

64. Freire, P. *Pedagogy of the Oppressed;* Continuum: New York, NY, USA, 2007.

65. Freire, P. *Education for Critical Consciousness;* Bloomsbury Publishing: London, UK; New York, NY, USA, 1974.

66. Godfrey, E.B.; Burson, E. Interrogating the intersections: How intersectional perspectives can inform developmental scholarship on critical consciousness. In *Envisioning the Integration of an Intersectional Lens in Developmental Science. New Directions for Child and Adolescent Development;* Santos, C.E., Toomey, R.B., Eds.; Jossey-Bass: San Francisco, CA, USA, 2018; pp. 17–38.

67. Kumagai, A.K.; Lypson, M.L. Beyond cultural competence: Critical consciousness, social justice, and multicultural education. *Acad. Med.* **2009**, *84*, 782–787. [CrossRef] [PubMed]

68. Watts, R.J.; Diemer, M.A.; Voight, A.M. Critical consciousness: Current status and future directions. *New Dir. Child Adolesc. Dev.* **2011**, *134*, 43–57. [CrossRef] [PubMed]

69. Hooks, B. *Teaching to Transgress: Education as the Practice of Freedom;* Routledge: New York, NY, USA, 1994; 216p.

70. Church Action on Poverty. Poverty Truth Commissions. Available online: http://www.church-poverty.org.uk/povertytruth (accessed on 15 January 2019).

71. Faith in Community Scotland. Poverty Truth Commission. 2019. Available online: https://www.faithincommunityscotland.org/ (accessed on 15 January 2019).

72. Substance Abuse and Mental Health Services Administration. *SAMHSA's Concept of Trauma and Guidance for a Trauma-Informed Approach;* In HHS Publication No. (SMA) 14-4884; Office of Policy, Planning and Innovation, Substance Abuse and Mental Health Services Administration, HHS.: Rockville, MD, USA, 2014.

73. Booshehri, L.G.; Dugan, J.; Patel, F.; Bloom, S.; Chilton, M. Trauma-informed Temporary Assistance for Needy Families (TANF): A randomized controlled trial with a two-generation impact. *J. Child Family Stud.* **2018**, *27*, 1594–1604. [CrossRef] [PubMed]

74. Walkley, M.; Cox, T.L. Building trauma-informed schools and communities. *Child. Schools* **2013**, *35*, 123–126. [CrossRef]

75. Substance Abuse and Mental Health Services Administration. Trauma-Informed Care in Behavioral Health Services. In *Treatment Improvement Protocol (TIP) Series;* Health and Human Services, Ed.; Substance Abuse and Mental Health Services Administration: Rockville, MD, USA, 2014.

76. Hecht, A.A.; Biehl, E.; Buzogany, S.; Neff, R.A. Using a trauma-informed policy approach to create a resilient urban food system. *Public Health Nutr.* **2018**, 1–10. [CrossRef] [PubMed]

77. Prewitt, E. State, Federal Lawmakers Take Action on Trauma-Informed Policies, Programs. 2014. Available online: http://acestoohigh.com/2014/04/30/state-federal-lawmakers-take-action/ (accessed on 21 September 2014).

78. Chilton, M.; Rose, D. A rights-based approach to food insecurity in the United States. *Am. J. Public Health* **2009**, *99*, 1203–1211. [CrossRef] [PubMed]

79. Gallegos, D.; Booth, S.; Kleve, S.; McKechnie, R.; Lindberg, R. Food insecurity in Australian households: From charity to entitlement. In *A Sociology of Food and Nutrition: The Social Appetite;* Germov, J., Williams, L., Eds.; Oxford University Press: Oxford, UK, 2017; pp. 55–74.

80. Booth, S. Food. In *First World Hunger Revisited;* Riches, G., Silvasti, T., Eds.; Palgrave Macmillan: London, UK, 2014.

81. Dowler, E.A.; O'Connor, D. Rights-based approaches to addressing food poverty and food insecurity in Ireland and UK. *Soc. Sci. Med.* **2012**, *74*, 44–51. [CrossRef] [PubMed]

82. Poppendieck, J. *Sweet Charity? Emergency Food and the End of Entitlement*; Viking Press: New York, NY, USA, 1998.

83. Popay, J. What will it take to get the evidential value of lay knowledge recognised? *Int. J. Public Health* **2018**, *63*, 1013–1014. [CrossRef] [PubMed]

84. El Ansari, W.; Phillips, C.J.; Zwi, A.B. Narrowing the gap between academic professional wisdom and community lay knowledge: Perceptions from partnerships. *Public Health* **2002**, *116*, 151–159. [CrossRef] [PubMed]

85. Murphy, K.; Fafard, P. Knowledge translation and social epidemiology: Taking power, politics and values seriously. In *Rethinking Social Epidemiology: Towards a Science of Change*; O'Campo, P., Dunn, J.R., Eds.; Springer: Dordrecht, The Netherlands, 2012; pp. 267–283.

86. Popay, J.; Williams, G.; Thomas, C.; Gatrell, T. Theorising inequalities in health: The place of lay knowledge. *Sociol. Health Ill.* **1998**, *20*, 619–644. [CrossRef]

87. Kent, G. Community Engagement in Challenging Times, Poverty and Social Exclusion in the UK, in Working Paper—Methods Series No. 25. 2013. Available online: http://www.poverty.ac.uk/editorial/community-engagement-challenging-times (accessed on 14 February 2019).

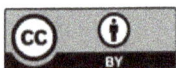

MDPI

St. Alban-Anlage 66

4052 Basel

Switzerland

Tel. +41 61 683 77 34

Fax +41 61 302 89 18

www.mdpi.com

International Journal of Environmental Research and Public Health Editorial Office

E-mail: ijerph@mdpi.com

www.mdpi.com/journal/ijerph